Chiropractic Management of Spine Related Disorders

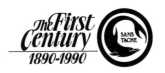

Chiropractic Management of Spine Related Disorders

MERIDEL I. GATTERMAN, D.C.

Director, Division of Chiropractic Sciences
Canadian Memorial Chiropractic College
Toronto, Ontario, Canada

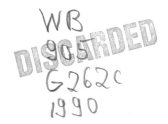

WILLIAMS & WILKINS

Baltimore • Hong Kong • London • Sydney

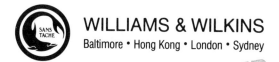

Editor: Jonathan W. Pine, Jr.
Associate Editor: Linda Napora
Copy Editor: Anne K. Schwartz
Designer: Norman Och
Illustration Planner: Lorraine Wrzosck
Production Coordinator: Adèle Boyd-Lanham

Printed in the United States of America

ISBN 0-683-03438-3

This book is dedicated to

My teachers that their knowledge may thus be shared

All students of chiropractic who will use this knowledge

for the benefit of chiropractic patients

and

Chiropractic patients who will have the advantage of

chiropractic management of spine-related disorders.

PREFACE

This book is designed to provide a practical guide for the evaluation and management of spine-related disorders that are commonly treated by doctors of chiropractic. An attempt has been made to provide not only information but also a philosophy supported by scientific data that relate the observed results from chiropractic care to generally accepted principles of anatomy, physiology, kinesiology, and pathology.

Neuromusculoskeletal disorders are emphasized because they comprise the major component of the typical chiropractic practice. Considerable space has been allocated to the biomechanical dysfunction of the vertebral motion segments from a chiropractic perspective. This perspective appreciates the interdependence of the nervous system with all body parts and a holistic approach to health care. Because biomechanical lesions rarely occur in the absence of surrounding tissue pathology, both pathomechanics and histological changes must receive attention in the formulation of the diagnosis and management of the patient.

The primary therapeutic tool used by doctors of chiropractic is spinal manipulation. While not unique to the chiropractic profession, the art of manipulation has been developed and refined to a greater degree by chiropractors than by those in other professions. In addition to specific spinal manipulation, chiropractors have traditionally utilized mobilization techniques, trigger point therapy, soft tissue massage, and adjunctive physiological procedures. Finally, of equal importance is the consideration of the contraindications to manipulation.

The purpose of this book is to provide the practicing chiropractor with the most scientifically supported rationale for treatment. Though mainly written for chiropractic physicians, this book has also been created to foster better understanding of the principles and practices of chiropractic for all those involved in treating patients with spine-related disorders.

CONTRIBUTORS

Scot G. Fechtel, B.S., D.C.

Portland, Oregon

Meridel I. Gatterman, D.C.

Director, Division of Chiropractic Sciences
Canadian Memorial Chiropractic College
Toronto, Ontario, Canada

Donald R. Goe, Ph.D., D.C.

Dayton, Washington

Bonnie L. McDowell, R.P.T., D.C.

Postgraduate Faculty
Fellow International Academy of Clinical Acupuncture
Western States Chiropractic College
Portland, Oregon

David M. Panzer, D.C.

Assistant Professor
Department of Chiropractic Science
Western States Chiropractic College
Portland, Oregon

Cynthia Peterson, R.N., D.C., D.A.C.B.R.

Assistant Professor
Chairperson Department of Radiology
Postgraduate Faculty
Western States Chiropractic College
Portland, Oregon

Tyrone Wei, B.S., D.C., D.A.C.B.R.

Resident
Radiology Department
Assistant Professor of Radiology
National College of Naturopathic Medicine
Postgraduate Faculty
Western States Chiropractic College
Portland, Oregon

Michael R. Wiles, B.S., M.Ed., D.C., F.C.C.S.(C)

Associate Professor
Formerly Director, Division of Chiropractic Science
Postgraduate Faculty
Canadian Memorial Chiropractic College
Toronto, Ontario, Canada

ACKNOWLEDGMENTS

Writing a textbook of this nature is too great a task for a single individual and I am most grateful to the many who have contributed their time and expertise to see this project through to completion.

Above all I extend a special thanks to the contributing authors Dr. Scot Fechtel, Dr. Don Goe, Dr. Bonnie McDowell, Dr. David Panzer, Dr. Cindy Peterson, Dr. Tyrone Wei, and Dr. Michael Wiles for adding diversity and expertise. I am grateful for the special effort put forth by Dr. Christina Peterson and Dr. Art Walker in completing the tables on the differential diagnosis of headaches and the effectiveness of manipulation.

I especially appreciate the many hours Dr. Bill Dold, Dr. Don Goe, and Dr. Norman Singer spent reviewing and editing rough manuscript.

Appreciation is also expressed to Dr. Alan Adams, Dr. Len Faye, Dr. Frank Ferraro, Dr. Scott Haldeman, Dr. Dan Hansen, Dr. Joseph Howe, Dr. Paul Jaskoviak, Dr. Reed Phillips, Dr. Raymond Sandoz, Dr. Dick Stonebrink, Dr. Phil Soliceto, and Dr. Herb Vear for their expert review of selected material and their many helpful suggestions.

I am indebted to Ellen Shapiro and Lydia Kibial for their original drawings and to Dr. Terry Yochum and Dr. Lindsay Rowe for permission to reproduce the figures taken from their textbook *Essentials of Skeletal Radiology*.

The patience and generous assistance of my friend Dick Meissner is duly appreciated for the many hours spent taking the photographs, and a special thanks to the two models Marina Carr and Melissa Jamison.

I am extremely grateful to Leanne Harmon, Heidi Purnell, and Susan Hawkins for the long, tedious hours spent typing the manuscript.

The assistance in obtaining essential reference material provided by Dr. Geffery Anderson and Dr. Blaine Auerkamp, and Kay Irvine and Lynn Attwood at the Western States Chiropractic College library is also much appreciated.

Special gratitude is expressed to the staff of Williams & Wilkins for bringing the manuscript to publication. I offer special thanks to my patient editor Jonathan Pine, to the ever-helpful Adèle Boyd, and to Terry Minton for the initial inspiration.

To my numerous friends who have provided the encouragement necessary to complete this lengthy project, I am deeply grateful.

I am especially appreciative of my friendship with the late Earl Homewood and the many delightful hours spent with him discussing chiropractic principles. While we sometimes disagreed, his legacy is inherent in this textbook.

Finally, my love and appreciation go to my husband, Mike, for his support, understanding, and gracious acceptance of the many hours I've spent completing this book.

CONTENTS

INTRODUCTION

Chiropractic is a branch of the healing arts specializing in the correction by spinal manual therapy of what chiropractors identify as biomechanical disorders of the spinal column. They carry out spinal diagnosis and therapy at a sophisticated and refined level (1).

NATURE AND SCOPE OF CHIROPRACTIC PRACTICE

The primary therapeutic tool utilized by doctors of chiropractic is spinal manipulation (2). Spinal manipulative therapy (the chiropractic adjustment) has been traditionally utilized to restore normal joint function, reversing pathological processes. Chiropractic manipulation is characterized by the implementation of specific short-lever, high-velocity forceful thrusts of controlled amplitude directed as specific articulations (3). There has been a gradual shift within the chiropractic profession from a preoccupation with the correction of static mechanisms (spinal misalignment) to a focus on the reversal of dynamic aberrations of function (joint fixation).

Although the precise nature of biomechanical dysfunction of spinal joints has not been demonstrated scientifically, the theories presented in this book are based on the demonstrated principles of biomechanics coupled with chiropractic procedures. The clinical evidence supporting chiropractic care of spine related disorders, while not based on extensive experimental data, is supported by the survival and popularity of clinical chiropractic. Spinal manual therapy in the hands of the trained chiropractor has proven a safe and effective method of treating biomechanical disorders of the spinal column (1).

The scope of chiropractic practice has been defined by Vear (4) as follows:

Practice of Chiropractic means any professional service usually performed by a chiropractor, the aim of which is to restore and maintain health, and includes:

1. The diagnostics, treatment and prophylaxis of functional disturbances, pathomechanical states, pain syndromes and neurophysiological effects related to the statics and dynamics of the locomotor system, more particularly the spine and pelvis.

2. The treatment thereof by adjustment and/or manipulation of the spine and other anatomical structures.

3. The use of x-ray for diagnostic purposes.

4. The use of supportive measures including heliotherapy, thermotherapy, hydrotherapy, electrotherapy, mechanotherapy and patient hygiene, as required.

5. Nutrition: The combination of processes by which the living organism receives and utilizes the materials necessary for the maintenance of its functions and for growth and renewal of its components.

Local statues in some areas restrict use of the supportive measures outlined in paragraph 4, while others such as Oregon define a much broader scope of practice (see "Straights versus Mixers").

BEGINNING OF MANIPULATION

Manipulation as a form of therapy most likely predates most other procedures employed by the healing arts. It is easy to imagine prehistoric humans rubbing sore and aching muscles and tractioning painful joints. There appears to be no single origin of the art of manipulation, and as a form of therapy it is characterized by the universality of its concepts and empirical conclusions. Many early societies such as the ancient Chinese, Japanese, Polynesian, Indian, Egyptian, and Tibetan practiced this form of therapy. Therapeutic manipulation has been practiced by such diverse American Indian tribes as the Aztec, Toltec, Tarascan, Inca, Maya, Sioux, Winnebago, and Creek (5).

Hippocrates: The Father of Medicine (460–370 BC)

Hippocrates, recognized as the pioneer scientific investigator and researcher of medicine, was also a practitioner of manipulation (6). Two chapters in his monumental work the *Corpus Hippocrateum* deal with manipulative procedures. These chapters, entitled "Peri Arthron" (About Joints) and "Mochlikon" (The Lever), describe spinal manipulation with traction (extension) (7). With the patient prone and stretched in traction, Hippocrates suggests:

> Such extension would do no great harm, if well arranged, unless one deliberately wanted to do harm. The physician, or an assistant who is strong and not untrained, should put the palm of his hand on the hump, and the palm of the other on that, to reduce it forcibly, taking into consideration whether the reduction should naturally be made straight downwards, or towards the head, or towards the hip. This reduction method is also very harmless; indeed, it will do no harm even if one sits on the hump while extension is applied, and makes succussion by raising himself; nay, there is nothing against putting one's foot on the hump, and making gentle succussion by bringing one's weight upon it (8).

Even more effective according to Hippocrates was putting the end of a stout board in a cleft in a wall as a lever, which applied pressure on the hump beneath (9). While two assistants maintained traction, one or two others pushed the free end of the beam downward. While not to be considered sophisticated methods of manipulation, these procedures do outline the basic principle of spinal manipulation, that is, traction to the point of tension, at which point a thrust or pressure is applied to the vertebral lesion.

Galen: The Prince of Physicians (130–202 AD)

Galen was given the title "Prince of Physicians" after he relieved the paralysis of the right hand of Eudemas, a prominent Roman scholar (5). The paralysis, which was apparently the result of pressure on cervical nerves exiting the neck, was successfully relieved by manipulation of the cervical vertebrae.

Galen, who understood the relationship between the nervous system and spinal vertebrae, was greatly influenced by the works of Hippocrates (10). Eighteen of Galen's 97 extant commentaries relate to the works of Hippocrates, including the discourse on the joints (7). Galen's influence on the medical world lasted 1500 years, and his writing was characteristically based on his brilliant observations and wise therapeutic applications.

Bonesetters

During the Middle Ages and the Renaissance, the art of manipulation was practiced by bonesetters. This art was commonly handed down from generation to generation and was practiced in most communities in Europe, North Africa, and Asia by practitioners who learned their skills by apprenticeship.

Sarah Mapp

One of the best known of these bonesetters was an Englishwoman named Sarah Mapp. Because she was the subject of a number of humorous anecdotes, she may have been more infamous than famous. *London Magazine* for August 2, 1736 records the following tale:

> The Town has been surpriz'd lately with the Fame of a young woman at Epsom, who, tho' not very regular, it is said, in her Conduct, has wrought such Cures that seem miraculous in the Bonesetting way. The Concourse of People to Epsom on this Occasion is incredible, and 'tis reckon'd she gets near 20 Guineas a Day, she executes what she does in a very quick Manner . . . Her Strength makes the following Story the more credible. A Man came to her, sent, as 'tis supposed, by some Surgeons, on purpose to try her Skill, with his Hand bound up, and pretended his Wrist was put out, which upon Examination she found to be false; but to be even with him for his Imposition, she gave him a wrench, and really put it out, and bade him go to the Fools who sent him, and get it set again, or if he would come to her that Day Month, she would do it herself.

She was so popular that a play was written in her honor. The title "The Husband's Relief; or, The Female Bone-setter and the Worm Doctor" suggests that the medical man did not fare so well. There was also a song in her praise

> You surgeons of London who puzzle your pates,
> To ride in your coaches and purchase estates;
> Give over for shame, for your pride has a fall,
> The doctress of Epsom has outdone you all.

Once a week she drove up to London in a carriage drawn by four horses followed by footmen in gorgeous livery. On one occasion she was stopped by a mob when she was suspected of being one of the King's unpopular German mistresses. She put her head out of the window and shouted, "Damn your bloods, fools, don't you know me? I am Mrs. Mapp, the bone-setter." The crowd cheered her as she drove off. Later she moved her practice to Pall Mall, the most elegant part of London (7). Mrs. Mapp, who learned the art of manipulation from her father, became so successful that other bonesetters were encouraged to set up full-time practices as well (7).

Sir Herbert Barker

The best known of the English bonesetters was Sir Herbert Barker, who practiced in the early years of this century. He learned the art of bonesetting from his cousin and eventually practiced in London. In spite of being personally much maligned by the physicians and surgeons of the day, his work was characterized by success after success. Included among his patients were members of the royalty and nobility as well as members of Parliament. Paderewski, H. G. Wells, and John Galsworthy were among those who benefited from his expertise, but the forces of organized medicine relentlessly fought him, solely on the grounds of his lack of formal training.

It is clear that Barker was a man of integrity who was outstanding in his field. Finally, in July of 1936, he was called from retirement to demonstrate his techniques to an audience of more than 100 orthopaedic surgeons at St. Thomas Hospital in London. The *British Medical Journal* of August 1936, reporting on his performance, at last gave him great credit, stating: "He displayed in some cases remarkable dexterity and the warm thanks of the meeting for a most interesting demonstration was conveyed." Still, manipulation was denied medical respectability, and Barker, who was knighted in 1922 for his service to the public health, was considered an unorthodox practitioner and was never accepted by organized medicine (7).

OSTEOPATHY

Osteopathy had its beginnings in the teachings of Andrew Taylor Still (1828–1917). After losing three of his children from cerebrospinal meningitis, Still began a campaign against doctors' indiscriminate use of drugs. He became convinced that to function properly the body must be structurally sound, in order for natural recuperative powers to restore health. He referred to this power as the life force.

Concentrating his therapy around manipulation of the osteopathic (spinal) lesion, he believed that the treatment of structural and mechanical spinal derangements could relieve mechanical pressure on blood vessels and nerves. He felt that such abnormal pressure produced ischemia and eventual necrosis, which in turn obstructed the life force traveling along the nerves.

In 1892 he opened a school of osteopathy at Kirksville, Missouri. Osteopathy developed and flourished with a reported 13,000 practicing osteopaths in 1958. By 1968 the AMA had initiated the amalgamation of medicine and osteopathy. Currently, osteopaths receive full medical license to practice medicine in most American states (7). Many no longer employ manipulation as a method of therapy and through specialization have become almost indistinguishable from allopathic medical doctors.

CHIROPRACTIC

From the outset, chiropractic has had a turbulent history, beginning with the Palmer family (11). From humble beginnings at the close of the nineteenth century, chiropractic has grown to become the second-largest healing profession in North America.

D. D. Palmer (1844–1913)

Daniel David Palmer, in 1895, without the benefit of formal training, developed the principles upon which chiropractic theory is based. This self-styled magnetic healer, who had immigrated from Canada, is paradoxically recognized as a genius and an ec-

centric. His premise, that illness is essentially functional and becomes organic only as an end process, is finding wider acceptance today (12).

Whether Palmer was influenced in his thinking by Andrew Still is debatable (12), but it appears that at some time Palmer may have traveled to Kirksville, a distance of 200 miles from Davenport, Iowa, ostensibly to investigate Still's practice. However, it was Palmer who set up the first school of Chiropractic on Brady Street in Davenport in 1895 (12, 13). It was Palmer's contention that he had learned the art of manipulation from a Dr. Atkinson, who had also resided in Davenport (13) in the early 19th century. Palmer was apparently also knowledgeable about the use of manipulation by the ancient Greeks (11) and describes manipulation as follows:

> I have, both in print and by word of mouth repeatedly stated and now most emphatically repeat the statement, that I am not the first person to replace subluxated vertebrae, for this art has been practiced for thousands of years. I do claim, however, to be the first to replace displaced vertebrae by using the spinous and transverse processes as levers wherewith to rack subluxated vertebrae into normal position, and from this basic fact, to create a science which is destined to revolutionize the theory and practice of the healing art (13).

Following his imprisonment for practicing medicine without a license, the senior Palmer was to see the school in Davenport developed by his son, B. J. Palmer. The stormy relationship between father and son led D. D. Palmer to open the Palmer-Gregory College in Oklahoma in association with a medical doctor, Alva Gregory. Three months later, Palmer opened yet another school in Portland, Oregon, where he published his major work, *The Chiropractic Adjuster*, in 1910.

William Carver, who had served as the elder Palmer's attorney in Iowa, was also operating a chiropractic college in Oklahoma City at that time. For almost four decades, Carver was to engage in a bitter philosophical debate with both Palmers regarding the relative merits of the "tracto-thrust" and the "recoil thrust" in addition to Carver's "structuralist" approach to the spine (Chapter 13) as opposed to the Palmers' segmental focus. From these humble beginnings, chiropractic spread throughout North America, with numerous schools developing from the original teachings of D. D. Palmer.

B. J. Palmer (1891–1961)

According to Gibbons (12), Bartlet Joshua Palmer (D. D.'s son), commonly referred to as "B. J.", may have been the last great entrepreneur of folk medicine in the United States. He states:

> Taking over his father's fledgling infirmary and school when only 25, he built within a decade the country's largest nonmedical institution, assembled the world's largest osteological museum, started the nation's second commercial broadcasting station,

provided a forum for some of the greatest dissenters of the first quarter century, and established himself as a Prophet of Chiropractic, with the Iowa river town of Davenport as its Mecca. He was Elbert Hubbard, Titus Oakes, Baron Munchausen, and P.T. Barnum all rolled into one—yet to his research clinic at mid-century would come "hopeless" and terminal cases—some on referral from the Mayo and Cleveland clinics—to leave apparently cured.

STRAIGHTS VERSUS MIXERS

The progress and acceptance of chiropractic as a valid therapeutic modality has been impeded by an ongoing intraprofessional struggle between the so-called straights and mixers. The purists, or "straights," hold that true chiropractic is a "hands-only, spine-only" method of practice in which the chiropractor treats all ills with spinal manipulation alone. Eschewing diagnosis, the "straight" chiropractor simply analyzes subluxations of the spine and depends on the body's innate intelligence to cure any and all problems upon the reduction of such subluxations (11).

The "mixers," on the other hand, take a broader approach to the scope of practice of chiropractic, using a more inclusive range of diagnostic procedures to determine the patient's physiological status, as well as analyzing the biomechanical faults of the patient's spine. Treatment methods employed by these doctors utilize physical therapy and nutritional supplementation as adjuncts to manipulation. Chiropractors today, as primary care physicians, are required to diagnose in order to appropriately refer when necessary as well as treat disease in the majority of states and provinces in the United States and Canada.

LANDMARKS IN CONTEMPORARY CHIROPRACTIC HISTORY

In 1974, four major events signaled acceptance of the chiropractic profession in the United States (14). Of major importance was authorization by the United States Office of Education for the Council on Chiropractic Education (CCE) to establish an accrediting commission for chiropractic colleges, following nearly 40 years of effort on the part of chiropractic educators. In the decade following this recognition, the accrediting commission has continued to work diligently to raise the standards of education throughout chiropractic colleges.

Also in 1974, the last remaining state to establish licensing for chiropractors, Louisiana, did so. In the same year, Congress made provision for federal funds to be available to chiropractors for Medicare payments for services rendered to persons 65 years of age or older. In 1974 Congress also appropriated two million dollars to be used for the study of "the scientific basis of chiropractic." This was followed in 1975 by the historic conference at the National Institute for Neurological Disease and Stroke (NINCDS) of the U.S. Public Health Services, which focused on the more appropriate topic of "The scientific basis for spinal manipulative therapy" (23).

While the chiropractic profession has not received total acceptance in all quarters, it is no longer considered an "unscientific cult." The New Zealand Report of the Commission of Inquiry into Chiropractic in 1979 made the following comments in summarizing the principle findings of the commission (1):

- Chiropractors are the only health practitioners who are necessarily equipped by their education and training to carry out spinal manual therapy.
- General medical practitioners and physiotherapists have no adequate training in spinal manual therapy, though a few have acquired skill in it subsequent to graduation.
- Spinal manual therapy in the hands of a registered chiropractor is safe.
- The education and training of a registered chiropractor are sufficient to enable him to determine whether there are contra-indications to spinal manual therapy in a particular case, and whether the patient should have medical care instead of or as well as chiropractic care.
- Spinal manual therapy can be effective in relieving musculo-skeletal symptoms such as back pain, and other symptoms known to respond to such therapy, such as migraine.
- In a limited number of cases whether there are organic and/or visceral symptoms, chiropractic treatment may provide relief, but this is unpredictable and in such cases the patient should be under concurrent medical care if that is practicable.
- Chiropractors should, in the public interest, be accepted as partners in the general health care system. No other health profession is as well qualified by his general training to carry out a diagnosis for spinal mechanical dysfunction or to perform spinal manual therapy.

CHIROPRACTIC TERMINOLOGY
Subluxation

Traditionally, the chiropractic spinal lesion has been referred to as a subluxation. The conventional definition of subluxation is an incomplete or partial dislocation (15). D. D. Palmer redefined subluxation as "a partial or incomplete separation (of vertebrae), one in which the articulating surfaces remain in partial contact (13)." It is doubtful if there has been a more debated term in the healing arts, nor one that is more ambiguous. Since there is still no common agreement as to the exact meaning of this term in chiropractic, the following discussion is presented to lend an historical perspective to the issue.

With the prosecution of chiropractors for practicing medicine without a license, the need arose for a defense. While choosing to remain outside the medical mainstream, early chiropractors developed a separate terminology, which emphasized that they did not treat disease but rather promoted the healing of the body by focusing on the "innate intelligence" (13) or homeostasis of the body to heal itself. Stressing that the nervous system, the controlling system of the body, is interfered with by spinal lesions termed subluxations, these chiropractors thus developed a unique chiropractic terminology.

The reduction of subluxation became the primary goal of chiropractors, who employed "the chiropractic adjustment." It was stressed that the chiropractic adjustment differed from osteopathic manipulation in both the method and the intent or purpose of application (13). The chiropractic adjustment was seen as being more specific "using the vertebral processes as levers" (7), while the osteopathic manipulation was more general, utilizing a wide variety of manipulative and mobilizing procedures. Osteopathic manipulation tended to use long levers and slow, passive articular movements in contrast to chiropractic manipulation, which utilizes short levers and specific high-velocity forceful thrusts directed to specific articulations (3).

Perhaps the most significant point of differentiation between early chiropractors and medicine was the use of diagnosis. Palmer stated, "The allopath and osteopath agree on etiology and diagnosis, the only difference being that the latter tries to do with the hands what the former tries to do with drugs" (13). The chiropractor instead utilized "spinal analysis" to determine the site of subluxation, reducing only the subluxation, which in turn "adjusts causes of disease so that innate may correct abnormal functions and change morbid into normal structures" (13).

Modern Concepts of Subluxation

Because many attempts have been made to define and describe the chiropractic subluxation, this term has become exceedingly ambiguous. The concept most consistent with the observed facts emphasizes the disruption of the normal mechanical integrity of the vertebral motion segment (Chapter 1). If the rationale for manipulation is the restoration of biomechanical integrity of the vertebral motion segment, then the fixation subluxation is more accurate. This was defined by Drum (16) as "a vertebra . . . fixed in a position it could normally occupy during any phase of physiological movement."

Origin of the Concept of Joint Fixation

According to Dr. Budden, the term "fixation" was "common currency" as early as 1910, in both the osteopathic and chiropractic professions (17). Smith, Langworthy, and Paxson (18), in 1906 fought the idea of the little bone out of place or as they termed it the idea of the "displaced brick in the wall." In what appears to be the first textbook on chiropractic, they stated "A simple subluxed vertebra differs from a normal vertebra only in its field of motion and the center of its field of motion."

In 1923, in *Principles and Practice of Osteopathy*, Downing describes osteopathic spinal lesions as bony subluxations with ligamentous tension or shortening and muscular tension or contracture (19).

By 1930, Western States Chiropractic College in Oregon had adopted as its definition of subluxation "the fixation of a joint in a position of motion, usually at the extreme of such motion" (17).

In the early 1940s restricted motion in spinal joints became the focus of attention of chiropractors in both Europe and America. In Belgium, Leikans and the Gillet brothers (20), independently of Carver (21) and Vladeff (22) in America, were describing motion palpation as a method of detecting spinal "fixations." Henri Gillet has probably developed this art further than any other chiropractor. More recently Grice (23) in Canada and Faye (24) in the United States have enlarged upon Gillet's work through the Canadian Memorial Chiropractic College and postgraduate seminars.

The concept is based on the functional unit of the spine as composed of two adjacent vertebrae and their contiguous structures that form a complete set of articulations at one vertebral level. This three-joint complex is known as the vertebral motion segment (25) (Chapter 1). Vertebral motion segment dysfunction is clinically demonstrated manually by motion palpation and radiographically through range of motion studies and cineradiography (26).

ACA Classification of Subluxation (27)

The American Chiropractic Association, in response to the Medicare and Medicaid requirements, developed a classification of spinal subluxation demonstrated radiographically (Chapter 4). Their classification gives a broad perspective to the term subluxation. It encompasses many of the conditions treated by chiropractors, not solely by manipulation but also by adjunctive therapies.

EVOLUTION IN CHIROPRACTIC

Chiropractic has come a long way from its early beginnings in 19th century Iowa and has been perpetuated and developed through the chiropractic colleges. Initially chiropractic schooling was more "training in imparting the art of the adjustor, rather than any exposure to education in the biological sciences within a classical framework" (11). Through the years there has been a gradual evolution of didactic curriculum.

The standardization of chiropractic curriculums, expansion of libraries and laboratories, and the acquisition of top teaching faculties represent a long step from the limited educational experience in chiropractic in the decade following the death of the founder (11).

References

1. Inglis BD, Fraser B, Penfold BR: *Chiropractic in New Zealand: Report of the Commission of Inquiry.* Wellington, New Zealand, PD Hasselberg, Government Printer, 1979, pp 3–4.
2. Janse J, Houser RH, Wells BF: *Chiropractic Principles and Technic.* Chicago, National College of Chiropractic, 1947, p 3.

3. Leach RA: *The Chiropractic Theories: A Symposium of Scientific Research.* Mississippi, Mid-South Scientific Publishers, 1980, p 15.
4. Vear HJ: *Institutional Mission Policy.* Portland, Oregon, Western States Chiropractic College, 1978.
5. Shafer RC: *Chiropractic Health Care.* Des Moines, FCER, 1976, pp 10, 14.
6. Ligeros KA: *How Ancient Healing Governs Modern Therapeutics.* New York, GP Putnam's Sons, 1937, p x.
7. Schiotz EH, Cyriax J: *Manipulation Past and Present.* London, William Heinemann Medical Books, 1975, pp 5, 7–, 34–36, 45.
8. Hippocrates: *Hippocrates with an English Translation by Dr. E.T. Withington,* ed 3. Cambridge, Howard University Press, 1959, p 299.
9. Lomax E: Manipulative therapy: a historical perspective from ancient times to the modern era. In Goldstein M: *The Research Status of Spinal Manipulative Therapy.* Bethesda, NINCDS No. 15, DHEW, 1975, p 11.
10. Bendon GA: Galen; influence for 45 generations. In *A History of Medicine in Pictures.* Morris Park, NJ, Parke Davis, 1958.
11. Gibbons RW: Chiropractic history lost, strayed or stolen. *ACA J Chiro* 13(1):4, 13, 17, 18–24, 1976.
12. Gibbons RW: The evaluation of chiropractic: medical and social protest in America. In Haldeman S (ed): *Modern Principles and Practice of Chiropractic.* East Norwalk, CT, Appleton-Century-Crofts, 1979, p 5.
13. Palmer DD: *The Chiropractic Adjuster: The Science, Art and Philosophy of Chiropractic.* Portland, Oregon, Portland Printing House, 1910, pp 468,.
14. Wardwell WI: The present and future role of the chiropractor. In Haldeman S (ed): *Modern Principles and Practice of Chiropractic.* East Norwalk, CT, Appleton-Century-Crofts, 1979, p 31.
15. *Dorlands Illustrated Medical Dictionary,* ed 5. Philadelphia, WB Saunders, p 1488, 1974.
16. Drum DC: The nature of the problem. *N Engl J Chiro* 7(2):29, 1973.
17. Weiant CW: Comment on Dr. Gillet's article. *J Natl Chiro Assoc* 15(11):14, 1945.
18. Smith OG, Langworthy SM, Paxson MC: *Modernized Chiropractic.* Cedar Rapids, IA, Lawrence Press, 1906, vol 1, pp 22–26.
19. Downing CH: *The Principles and Practice of Osteopathy.* Kansas City, Williams, 1923, p 63.
20. Gillet H, Liekans M: A further study of spinal fixations. *Ann Swiss Chiro Assoc* 4:41–46, 1969.
21. Carver FJ: Postural adjusting to correct abnormalities of the pelvic inlet. *J Natl Chiro Assoc* 9(4):19, 44, 1940.
22. Vladeff T, Hardy M: The theory of the fixation points. *J Natl Chiro Assoc* 15(6):20–23, 1945.
23. Grice A: A biomechanical approach to cervical and dorsal adjusting. In Haldeman S (ed): *Modern Principles and Practice of Chiropractic.* East Norwalk, CT, Appleton-Century-Crofts, pp 331–358, 1979.
24. Faye LJ: Course lecture notes, Motion Palpation Institute, Box 6110, Huntington Beach, CA, 1981.
25. Gatterman MI: Lost in translation. *JCCA* 22:131, 1978.
26. Gatterman MI: Indications for spinal manipulation in the treatment of back pain. *ACA J Chiro* 19(10):51–63, 1982.
27. Swansen HE, Schafer RC: *Basic Chiropractic Procedural Manual,* ed 2. Des Moines, The American Chiropractic Association, pp VI, 54–60.

CHAPTER 1

Functional Anatomy
of the Spine

Table 1.1 Four Stages of Skeletal Axis Development

Nonsegmented axis (notochord)
Segmented mesoderm (somites, sclerotomes)
Chondrified vertebral elements
Ossified vertebral column

The functional unit of the spine is the three joint complex comprised of the intervertebral disc and two posterior facet joints known as the vertebral motion segment.

To successfully manipulate the joints of the spine, the doctor must have an extensive knowledge of articular anatomy and a thorough understanding of the basic unit of spinal function—the vertebral motion segment. An accurate understanding of the development of the spine from the embryonic period until growth ceases is also of great importance to the doctor of chiropractic. Spinal embryology is particularly valuable for the recognition and classification of variations and malformations that can occur in the spine during the developmental process. These variations have a profound effect on the biomechanics of the spine and can predispose the patient to biomechanical pain and joint locking in the spinal region (1).

SPINAL EMBRYOLOGY

The vertebrae of the spinal column are derived from mesenchyme, which subsequently undergoes chondrification and ossification (2). Before reaching its final condition the spinal column passes through four major stages (Table 1.1). The major embryological stages leading to the development of the spinal column and associated structures are diagramed in Figure 1.1.

The first stage is the formation of the nonsegmented notochord, a flexible rod of mesenchymal cells enclosed in a thick, membranous sheath. The notochord forms the axis around which the vertebral column develops. During the second stage other mesenchymal cells multiply rapidly, enclosing the notochord ventromedially as segmented scler-

otomes. Sclerotomic cells later migrate dorsally around the spinal cord, forming the neural arches. In the third stage the mesenchymatous models produce a cartilaginous vertebral column, which in the fourth stage of spinal development becomes ossified (2).

The segmental nature of the mature vertebral column reflects its origin from the mesenchymal somites of the early embryo. These somites are paired cubical masses that develop serially from the paraxial mesoderm surrounding the notochord, beginning around the third week of intrauterine life (3) (Fig. 1.2). During the fourth week the ventromedial wall of each somite separates into a mass of diffuse cells, forming the sclerotomes. From these sclerotomes develop the vertebrae and ribs (2). The cells of the dorsolateral part of the somite constitute the dermomyotome. The myotome or muscle plate is the forerunner of striated muscle, while the dermatome or skin plate lays the foundation for the dermis. This differentiation becomes clinically significant to sclerotomal and dermatomal pain patterns and their origin, corresponding to the development of the spinal nerves directly opposite their respective somites (see Chapter 11).

The sclerotomal cells from each somite pair are densely packed in the caudal region and loosely packed in the cranial region (Fig. 1.3A). As development proceeds, a scleratomic fissure separates these areas (Fig. 1.3B), and the component halves of adjacent sclerotomes reunite in new combinations (4) (Fig. 1.3B). The denser caudal section of each original sclerotome joins the looser cranial half of the ad-

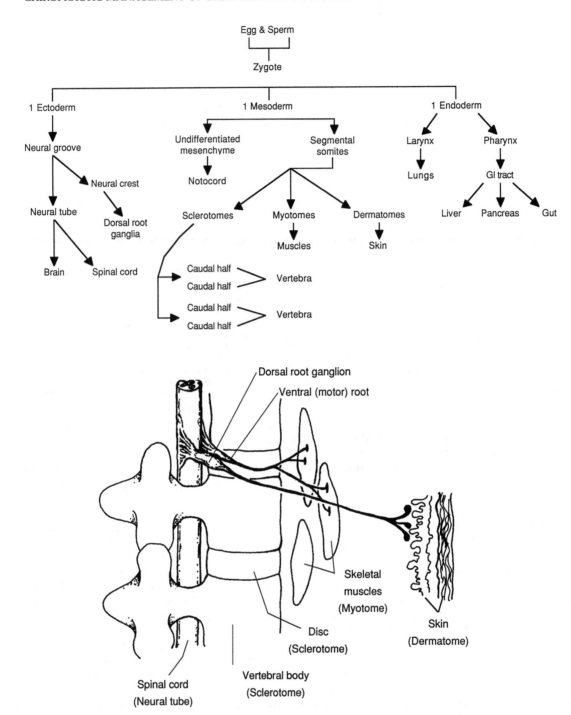

Figure 1.1. Major embryological stages leading to the development of the spinal column and associated structures. (Courtesy of Dr. Ron R. Goe.)

jacent caudal sclerotome (Fig. 1.3C). These recombinations then become the primordia of the vertebra. The cranial portion of the condensed caudal mass, which is farthest from the nutrition provided by the artery, remains undifferentiated as the precursor of the intervertebral disc. The poor vascularity of the early intervertebral disc is lost in adult life, when the nutritional demands of this tissue are met by diffusion from lymph.

The mesenchymal cells located between the cephalic and caudal portions of the original sclerotome segments fill the space between the two precartilaginous vertebral bodies as precursors of the intervertebral discs (5). Although the notochord regresses entirely in the region of the vertebral bodies, it persists in the region of the intervertebral disc until the second decade. Then it undergoes mucoid degeneration and forms the noncellular matrix of the

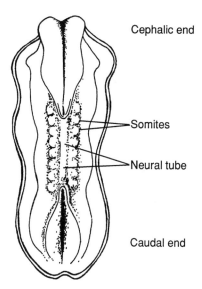

Figure 1.2. Mesenchymal somites develop from paired cubical masses lateral to the developing neural tube, beginning around the third week of intrauterine life. Development proceeds serially from the cephalic to caudal end.

Cephalic end

Somites

Neural tube

Caudal end

nucleus pulposus. The nuclear material after ten embryonic weeks is surrounded by the circular fibers of the annulus fibrosis, which is formed from fibroblastic cells. These two structures form the intervertebral disc, giving it a double origin. The central nucleus pulposus is derived from the notochord, and the annulus is derived from the fibroblastic extension of the vertebral bodies.

The rearrangement of the sclerotomes into definitive vertebrae causes the adjacent myotomes (which do not split) to overbridge the intervertebral disc, providing for movement of the spinal segments. The skeletal muscles develop from the dorsolateral or myotomal portion of the somite, which lies across the intervertebral joints setting them in a mechanical realationship to move the skeletal units (Fig. 1.3C). Thus are established the elements of the vertebral motion segments (i.e., two adjacent vertebrae and their bridging musculature with the intervening disc and neural and vascular structures). Because of recombination of the sclerotomal portions, the intersegmental arteries originally located between the sclerotomes eventually pass into the middle of the vertebral bodies (Fig. 1.3D).

The fibers of the ventral roots grow out from neuroblasts in the anterior and lateral parts of neural gray horn to supply the myotomes of the mesodermal somites. These fibers form the somatic and visceral motor efferents of the ventral nerve roots. The fibers of the dorsal roots are developed from the neural crest cells that form the spinal ganglia just medial to each primitive mesodermal somite and dorsolateral to the spinal cord. The spinal nerves eventually enter and exit through the intervertebral foramina.

Dorsal and lateral to the developing centra (body of the vertebra), the less dense portions of the scler-

otomes form the precartilaginous neural arches and transverse processes, while denser portions give rise to the intervertebral ligaments (2). Segmentation is induced by the notochord, which acts as an organizer in effecting the centrum. Segmentation proceeds in a craniocaudal direction. The neural crest cells that develop into the dorsal root ganglia act as organizers for vertebral arch segmentation. The clinical consequences of segmentation are discussed later.

The ribs develop from costal processes that extend from the primitive vertebral mass in the thoracic area (Fig. 1.4B). Costal processes become integral parts of the vertebrae in other areas of the spine. In the cervical vertebrae, the costal processes corresponding to the head and neck of each rib form that portion of the vertebra anterior to the foramen transversarium (Fig. 1.4A). In the lumbar area, the costal processes become the transverse processes of these vertebrae and the true transverse processes become much smaller accessory processes (Fig. 1.4C). The costal processes of the first two or three spinal segments fuse into the lateral masses of the sacrum forming the alae. (Fig. 1.4D). Costal processes are not normally found on the coccygeal vertebrae.

Ossification Centers

Ossification of the vertebrae involves both primary and secondary ossification centers.

Primary Centers of Ossification

Primary centers of ossification for each typical vertebra occur at three sites. The first centers appear in the two halves of each vertebral arch around the eighth embryonic week (Fig. 1.5) and in the vertebral body around the ninth embryonic week. Vertebral ossification begins in the lower thoracic region and upper lumbar region, rapidly extending cranially and less rapidly caudally (6). By the end of the fourth fetal month, ossification centers have appeared in all vertebral bodies.

Secondary Center of Ossification

At about the sixteenth year, secondary centers of ossification appear in the typical vertebra at the tips of the transverse processes, the tips of the spinous processes, and at the superior and inferior surfaces of the vertebral bodies (Fig. 1.6). The secondary centers of ossification do not fuse until the second decade of life.

Centers of Ossification of Atypical Vertebrae

The development of the atlas and axis from the embryological stage to adult life differs from that of other vertebrae because the first two cervical vertebrae are especially adapted to support the head and provide a wide range of head motion (7).

The atlas is normally ossified from three primary sites: one in each lateral mass, forming about the seventh embryonic week, and a third in the anterior arch (Fig 1.7), appearing around the time of birth.

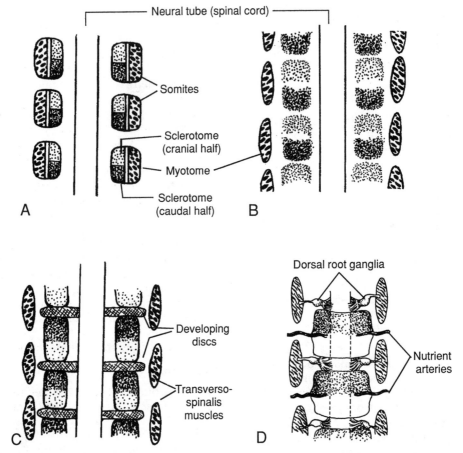

Figure 1.3. Recombination of the sclerotome occurs around a transverse split that forms the sclerotomic fissure. The denser caudal section of the sclerotome unites with the looser cranial half of the adjacent caudal sclerotome. The space between the recombined sclerotome segments is filled with mesenchymal cells that become the precursors of the intervertebral discs. The adjacent myotomes do not split with the sclerotome, thus the segmental muscles bridge the developing vertebrae. This bridging provides the mechanical relationship for the transversospinalis muscles to move the individual motion segments.

The axis is ossified from five primary sites (Fig 1.8) and two secondary sites. In addition to two centers in each arch and one in the centrum, two laterally placed primary centers appear about the sixth month. These lateral centers join in the midline to form the dens, and represent the centra of the atlas and axis. Two secondary sites of ossification appear on the axis anywhere from two to twelve years after birth, one in the apex of the odontoid process and the other at the bottom of the vertebral body. The lumbar vertebrae also have five centers of ossification, the three of a typical vertebra plus one extra center for each mamillary process (Fig. 1.9). The sacral vertebral segments ossify as a typical vertebra does. Each segment of the coccyx is ossified from one primary center. Ossification of the ribs begins from primary sites in parts of the rib adjacent to the vertebra.

Developmental Variations and Malformations of the Spine

Spinal developmental variations include differences in the number, arrangement, and morphology of the vertebrae. Most of these variations occur in the transitional areas of the spine (6), however, spinal malformations or anomalies can involve any vertebra.

Most commonly, variations occur in the occipitocervical or lumbosacral areas of the spine. Frequently, osseous anomalies of the spine are accompanied by soft tissue variations involving muscular, vascular, and neural tissues (7).

Variations in Number and Numerical Order of the Vertebrae

Approximately two-thirds of all humans have the typical number of regional vertebrae corresponding

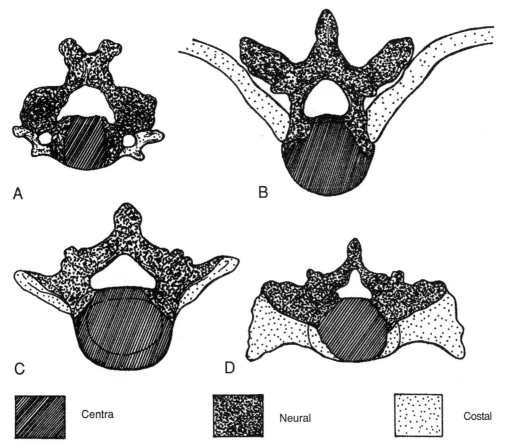

A

B

C

D

| | Centra | | Neural | | Costal |

Figure 1.4. The portions of the adult vertebrae derived from embryonic vertebra. The evolution of the vertebral anlage proceeds from the embryonic sclerotome flowing dorsally and ventrally around the notochord and the spinal cord like a mass of lava. (After Warwick R. Williams Ph: *Gray's Anatomy*, ed 35, British. Philadelphia, WB Saunders, 1973.)

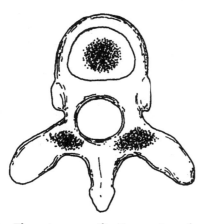

Figure 1.5. The primary ossification centers of each typical vertebra appear in the two halves of each vertebral arch and in the vertebral body.

to 7 cervical segments, 12 thoracic segments, 5 lumbar segments, 4 fused sacral segments and 3 fused coccygeal segments. Variations occur in one-third of the human population with either an increased or decreased total number of vertebrae (6). Of greatest significance to the chiropractor is a decreased number of segments in a given area, which limits mobility and increases biochemical stress in the area by transmitting the burden of motion to other levels of the column (6). An increase in the number of segments can also affect stability, with the stress falling primarily upon the soft tissue structures, which must check and limit motion (8). Variations in the costal processes may be manifest as costovertebral joints in the seventh cervical vertebra or as articulated ribs located at the level of the first lumbar vertebra. While technically not a variation in the typical number of segments, cervical ribs may produce clinically significant biochemical changes that affect the brachial plexus (9) (see Chapter 10).

Occipitocervical Malformation

The occasional failure of fusion of the occipital ossification centers may produce a persistent extra sclerotome. Fusion of the atlas to the occiput is more common than extra segmentation and is characterized by the absence of motion between the occiput and atlas. This may be verified by x-ray motion studies. Either a fusion of the occiput-atlas or an occipital vertebra can encroach upon the spinal cord

Figure 1.6. The secondary ossification centers of each typical vertebra appear at the tips of the transverse processes, the tips of the spinous processes, and at the superior and inferior surfaces of the vertebral bodies.

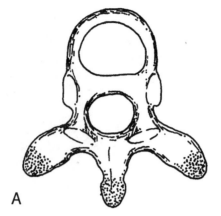

A

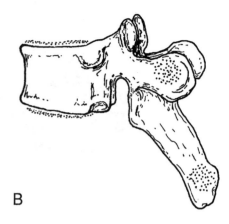

B

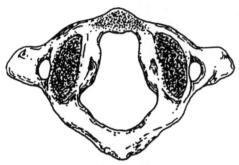

Figure 1.7. The atlas (C1) is normally ossified from three sites, one in each lateral mass and the third in the anterior arch. Ossification spreads from the lateral masses and anterior arch, joining by the eighth year.

due to osseous malformations about the foramen magnum (9).

Platybasia is an upward protrusion of the base of the skull into the posterior cranial fossa. This form of congenital anomaly should not be confused with basilar invagination, which is acquired and results from pathology such as Paget's disease, osteomalacia, or metabolic processes that cause softening of the base of the occiput. Platybasia allows the cervi-

cal spine to protrude upward, with the dens projecting into the skull. Diagnosis of platybasia and basilar invagination can be made from various linear measurements or a lateral radiograph including McGregor's line (10) (see Chapter 6).

Cervical Anomalies

Occasionally, failure of ossification of the posterior arch of the atlas occurs. The anterior arch may be defective as well. Minor defects may be asymptomatic, but more extensive architectural changes are associated with headaches, dizziness, and visual disturbances (11). Gentle manipulation may help to reduce the symptoms. Ossification of the posterior portion of the atlanto-occipital ligament (ponticulus posticus) is significant because it encloses the vertebral artery and the suboccipital nerve (Fig. 1.10). While the presence of this anomaly is not an absolute contraindication to any cervical manipulation, extension with rotation should be avoided, to reduce the risk of producing a vertebral artery syndrome (12) (see Chapter 4). Two additional anomalous conditions that may affect the atlas are a paramastoid process or bony column from the transverse process that articulates with the base of the skull at the jugular process and a paraoccipital pro-

Figure 1.8. The axis (C2) is ossified from seven ossification centers, five primary and two secondary. In addition to the two primary centers in each arch and one in the centrum, two laterally placed centers appear in the dens at about the sixth fetal month. The two secondary centers of ossification appear in the apex of the odontoid process and at the bottom of the vertebral body anywhere from two to twelve years after birth.

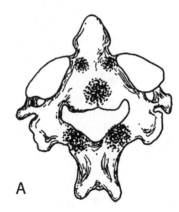

A

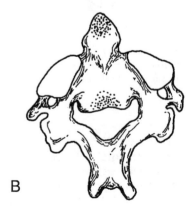

B

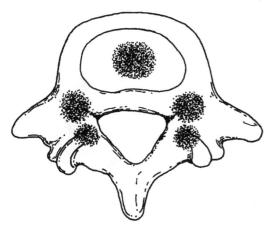

Figure 1.9. The normal lumbar vertebra has five primary ossification centers, three corresponding to the typical vertebra, plus one extra center for each mamillary process.

cess or bony connection between the occiput and transverse process of the atlas (9).

Anomalies of the Axis

Developmental anomalies of the odontoid process of the axis, while uncommon, present serious complications. The odontoid develops from the mesenchyme of the first cervical sclerotome, which would otherwise form the centrum of the first cervical vertebra. During early postnatal development the odontoid is separated from the body of the axis by a wide cartilaginous band.

Failure of fusion by the fifth or sixth year is referred to as os odontoideum, which is visible on radiographs as a wide radiolucent gap (12, 13) (Fig. 1.11). Os odontoideum can be further demonstrated by relative motion between the odontoid and the body of the axis in flexion-extension lateral radiographs (10). The os odontoideum cannot always be differentiated from fractures of the dens with subsequent displacement. None the less, the effect is the same. The AP, open-mouth, odontoid view with tomography is also useful in the evaluation of this condition. Trauma to the head may cause os odontoideum to become clinically manifest.

The deficient stability between the atlas and axis with this anomaly can produce luxation of the atlas either anteriorly or posteriorly, depending on the direction of force. In such cases of instability, manipulation of the upper cervical spine is definitely contraindicated (14). If the secondary center of ossification fails to fuse to the body of the odontoid as it should around the twelfth year, it is termed an ossiculum terminale. The consequences of an ossiculum terminale are often not as serious as those of an os odontoideum, and it may be considered an incidental finding on radiographs.

Block Vertebrae

Nonsegmentation of vertebral segments is relatively uncommon compared to many spinal anomalies such as tropism, spina bifida, and ponticulus posticus (see Fig 1.12). Failure of formation of the intervertebral disc results in adjacent provertebrae fusion when ossification occurs. Various degrees of nonsegmentation may occur, ranging from partial to total fusion of vertebral bodies, neural arches, and associated processes. Radiographic differentiation of a congenital block vertebra from an acquired fusion secondary to pathology can be made in several ways. Congenital block vertebrae tend to have a flat, smooth peripheral surface in the region of the missing intersegmental disc, while an acquired fusion appears prominent and irregular at the disc level.

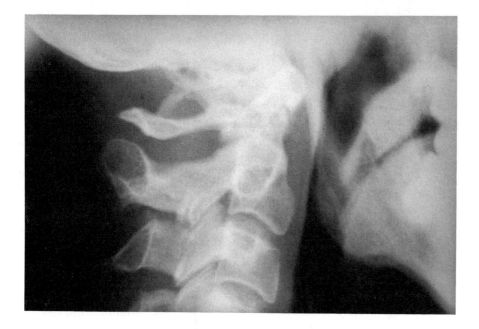

Figure 1.10. Ossification of the posterior portion of the atlantooccipital ligament (ponticulus posticus) is significant because it encloses the vertebral artery and suboccipital nerve in a bony ring that can potentially compromise vertebral artery flow when the neck is in extension.

Figure 1.11. Failure of fusion of the odontoid process to the body of the axis (os odontoideum) is demonstrated in the AP and lateral views.

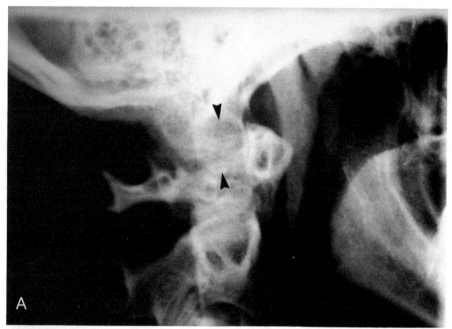

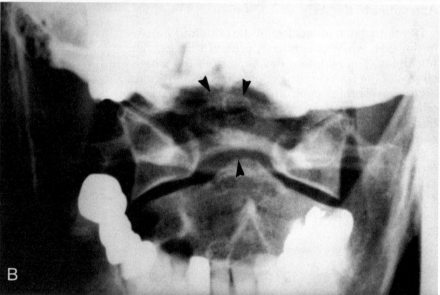

The AP diameters of congenital block vertebrae appear smaller than normal, with the intervertebral foramen appearing small, round, or oval. An acquired fusion will show a disrupted, renal-shaped foramen.

Klippel-Feil Syndrome

Congenital nonsegmentation of several cervical vertebrae is a major component of Klippel-Feil syndrome, along with a short neck, low hairline, rounded back, and limited painless movement of the back (Fig. 1.13). The syndrome is also characterized by prominent trapezius muscles, and frequently associated with undescended scapulae (Sprengle's deformity). Clinical symptoms depend on the severity of the deformity (9).

Hemivertebrae

The development of one lateral half of the ossification center with the failure of development of the opposite side results in a hemivertebra (Fig. 1.14). Seen on radiographs this gives the appearance of a triangular wedge inserted between two vertebrae whose upper and lower margins are deformed to correspond with the inserted wedge (9). Hemivertebrae in the cervical spine are frequently seen as part of the Klippel-Feil syndrome.

Cleft Spinous Processes (Spina Bifida)

Failure of fusion of the neural arches of one or more vertebrae is a common vertebral anomaly re-

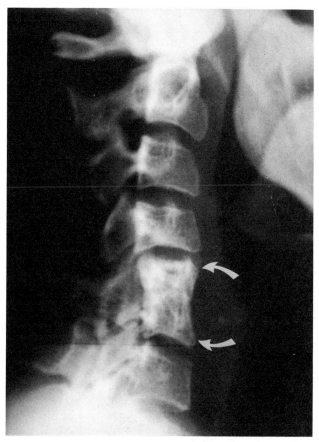

Figure 1.12. Nonsegmentation of vertebral segments produces a block vertebra seen at C5–6.

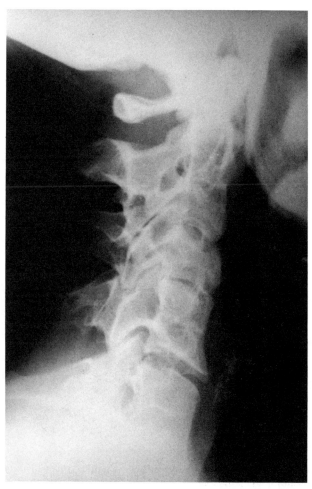

Figure 1.13. Klippel-Feil syndrome exhibits multiple block vertebrae of the cervical spine.

ferred to as spina bifida occulta (Fig. 1.15). It is often asymptomatic but can cause biomechanical prob-

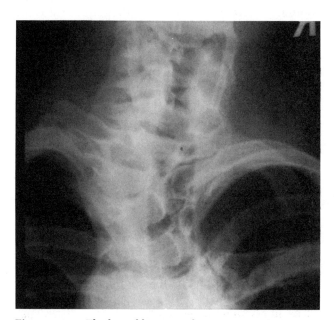

Figure 1.14. The lateral hemivertebra is seen on the AP radiograph as a triangular wedge.

lems because of anomalous soft tissue attachments that normally stabilize each vertebral motion segment. More extensive forms of spina bifida, along with anomalies of the associated meninges and spinal cord, can cause serious problems, and in the most severe cases are incompatible with life.

Cervicothoracic Transition and the Thoracic Spine

The most common and clinically significant anomaly in the cervicothoracic transition area of the spine is cervical ribs. This anomaly is a progressive development of the embryonic costal processes of C7. Appropriate radiographs can differentiate cervical ribs from an extended transverse process of C7 by demonstration of a costovertebral joint (15). The clinical effect of the cervical rib results from the compression it can produce upon the neurovascular bundle of the brachial plexus and subclavian artery (see Chapter 10). Radiographs visualize only the portion of the rib that is calcified. The structure may extend in a cartilaginous state or as a fibrous band, which can produce a compression syndrome. Cervical ribs are seen in a variety of anomalous configurations and are of-

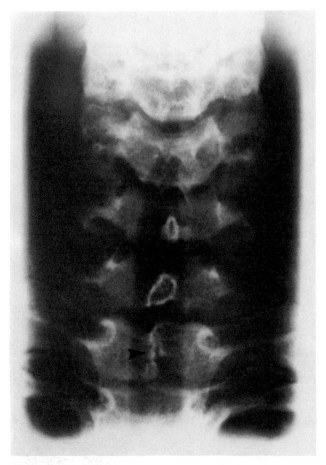

Figure 1.15. Failure of fusion of the neural arches (spina bifida) is visualized at T1.

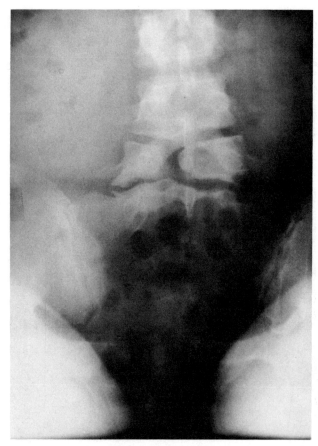

Figure 1.16. A butterfly vertebra (seen here as a sagittal cleft at L5) is produced when the sclerotomes fail to unite in the midline.

ten fused distally with the subjacent first ribs. Asymmetry of cervical ribs is common (15).

Thoracic Hemivertebrae

Unilateral hemivertebrae in the sagittal plane occur when there is a disturbance in the cartilage anlage or in the ossification of one half of the vertebral body. This can produce extensive spinal curvatures.

Dorsal and Ventral Hemivertebrae

Cases in which the dorsal or ventral part of the vertebral body fails to ossify in the coronal plane are much less common than hemivertebrae in the sagittal plane. The blood supply of each vertebral body develops progressively from posterior to anterior. If the blood supply fails to reach the anterior half of the vertebral body, the anterior ossification center fails to develop, producing a dorsal hemivertebra. This anomaly can produce a gibbus formation upon weightbearing (9).

Cleft Vertebrae

A cleft vertebra results when the notochord persists within the centrum of the vertebral body. The two lateral sclerotomes fail to unite, and ossification

produces a portion of the vertebral body on each side of the midline. This gives the appearance of a "butterfly vertebra" on an AP radiograph (Fig 1.16). Associated discs have a triangular (AP) appearance, compensating for the shape of the vertebra. The cleft is usually filled with cartilage. Biomechanically the anterior longitudinal ligament has weakened attachments that allow the segment to be displaced posteriorly, forming a kyphosis (9).

Thoracolumbar Transitional Area and the Lumbar Spine

Lumbar ribs, like cervical ribs in the cervicothoracic area, are the most common variation in the thoracolumbar area (Fig. 1.17).

Facet Tropism

Tropism is derived from the Greek word *trope*, which means turning. Facet tropism refers to asymmetrical facets in which one pair of facets faces in a more coronal plane while the contralateral faces in a more sagittal plane (16) (Fig. 1.18). This anomaly produces an asymmetric movement in which diminished mechanical effeciency makes these joints more susceptible to stress (1). The torque stress on the annulus

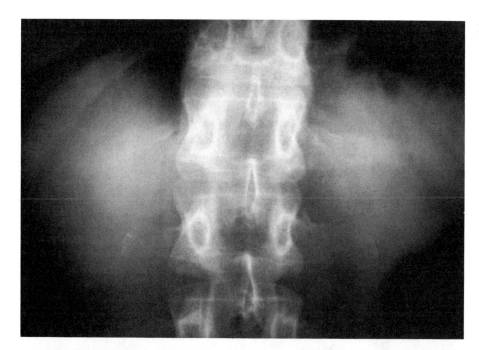

Figure 1.17. Lumbar ribs are visualized at L-1.

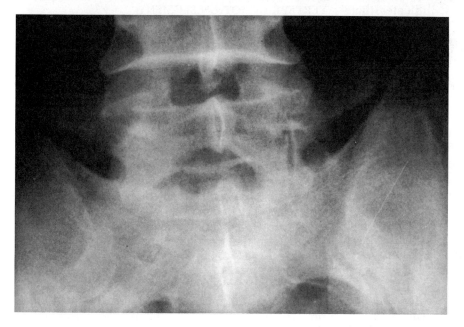

Figure 1.18. Tropism. Asymmetry of the facet joints (tropism) is commonly seen with one pair of facets oriented in the sagittal plane (seen as a vertical radiolucency) while the other pair are oriented in the coronal plane.

is thereby increased, which predisposes to facet joint locking because of the eccentric rotation and instability of the involved segments. This condition is characterized by painful limitation of passive rotation of the lumbar spine with loss of joint play on motion palpation. This condition is readily relieved by spinal manipulation (1) (see Chapter 8).

Lumbosacral Transitional Area

In addition to the high frequency of tropism found in the lumbar spine (17, 18), other anomalies of the lumbosacral transitional area suggest that this region is one of developmental instability.

Lumbarization and Sacralization

Failure of the first sacral segment to completely fuse to the remainder of the sacrum is termed lumbarization. Biomechanically this segment retains the characteristics of a lumbar segment with increased instability in the lumbar area. A lumbarized sacral segment tends to reduce tension on the posterior aspects of the intervertebral discs by distributing the normal lordosis over a greater number of mobile segments. Subsequently a greater than normal range of sagittal lumbar motion is produced, with resultant instability. The lumbosacral angle is increased, and the disc space is invariably decreased.

Figure 1.19. A transitional vertebra with an unilateral accessory joint at L5 produces asymmetric biomechanical stresses that can lead to degenerative changes.

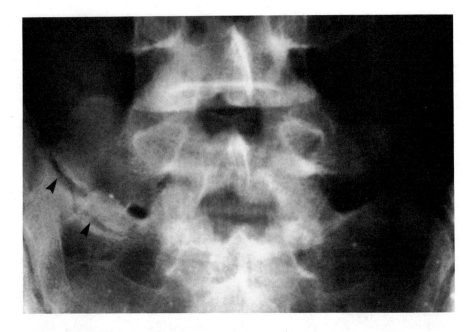

Sacralization, on the other hand, indicates that the last presacral segment shows unilateral or bilateral attachment to the lateral masses of the sacrum. When motion of the anomalous fifth lumbar segment is thus restricted, the lumbar lordosis must be accomplished in a shorter distance, which results in a greater compression of the posterior aspect of the annulus, especially of the fourth lumbar disc.

Bertolotti's syndrome (19) is characterized by herniation of the L4–5 disc in conjunction with a transitional lumbosacral segment. In this syndrome, the disc adjacent to the anomaly (L4) is affected, as instability is transferred upward. When lumbarization or sacralization is unilateral, the asymmetry of movement of the area restricts mobility while promoting contralateral hypermobility. This asymmetry of motion may also be transmitted to other levels of the spinal column (19).

Anomalies of the transverse processes are not uncommon in the lumbar spine and can take the form of elongated transverse processes, "butterfly" transverse processes, or spatulated transverse processes. These anomalies become most significant clinically when they produce an extra articulation in which the fifth lumbar segment contacts the ala of the first sacral segment and/or the ilium. This contact produces an accessory joint that is subject to degenerative changes including spur formation (Fig. 1.19).

Although this is not intended to be an exhaustive discussion of congenital anomalies, the more common conditions that alter spinal biomechanics have been outlined. Many of these anomalies and their clinical manifestations are discussed further in chapters dealing with specific areas of the spine.

VERTEBRAL MOTION SEGMENT

The functional unit of the spine is the three-joint vertebral motion segment (Fig. 1.20). This conceptual model has been defined as "two adjacent vertebrae and their intervening soft tissues" (20). The literal translation of the German *bewegunssegment*, popularized by Junghanns when referring to the functional unit of the spine, will be used in this text rather than the term "motor unit" as translated by Beseman (20). This is primarily because of the confusion produced by the prior use of "motor unit" by physiologists to refer to a single motor neuron and the group of muscle fibers that it innervates (20). The term vertebral motion segment (as opposed to motor unit), is gaining in popularity and usage throughout the chiropractic profession and other disciplines (21–27).

Typical Vertebral Motion Segment

The spinal column is made up of 23 typical vertebral motion segments from the C2-C3 segment to that of L5/S1 junction. Each segment is comprised of an intervertebral disc, two posterior spinal joints, neurological elements confined within the two lateral recesses and intervertebral foramina, plus all the connective and muscular tissues supporting and limiting intersegmental movement. The three major regions of the spine exhibit characteristic variations that distinguish these areas.

Variations in the lumbar spine occur in the mamillary processes, the iliolumbar ligaments, and the highly developed intertransverse ligaments. In the thoracic spine, the costovertebral articulations are unique. The joints of Luschka and the foramina transversarium for the vertebral arteries are peculiar to the cervical spine.

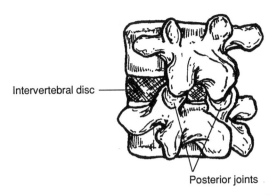

Intervertebral disc

Posterior joints

Figure 1.20. The vertebral motion segment is comprised of a three-joint complex. Motion at one site must reflect motion at the other two.

Atypical Vertebral Motion Segment

The two most cephalad articulations of the spinal column form atypical vertebral motion segments. No discs separate the anterior portions of these segments. The occipitoatlantal articulation (C0-C1) has the two paired condyles of the occiput, which fit into the concave articular surfaces of the atlas. The body of the atlas in the atlanto-axial (C1-C2) segment is replaced anteriorly with the peg-like odontoid process of the axis, which is bounded anteriorly by the anterior arch of the atlas and posteriorly by the transverse cruciate ligament. These two atypical vertebral motion segments allow a considerable amount of movement in the upper cervical region. C0-C1 allows for cervical flexion and extension, while C1-C2 accounts for 50% of the total cervical rotation (see Chapter 10).

A third atypical three-joint motion segment is formed by the pelvic ring. The paired posterior sacroiliac joints function similarly to the paired posterior joints of the typical vertebral motion segment, while the symphysis pubis allows the same type of movement as the intervertebral disc, due to the compressibility and elasticity of the amphiarthrodial interarticular material (see Chapter 7).

Components of the Vertebral Motion Segment

The vertebral motion segment as described by Junghanns (8) limits the components of this model to the soft tissue elements, including the intervertebral disc, the anterior and posterior longitudinal ligaments, the apophyseal joints, the ligamenta flava, the contents of the spinal canal and intervertebral foramina, and the ligaments and muscles joining the segment. Kapandji (28) separates the motion segment into an anterior static component and a posterior dynamic component, based on function. Parke and Schiff (29) include the adjacent superior and inferior halves of each vertebra, which corresponds to the embryologic somite.

This makes possible the study of these models on radiographs, even though the radiolucent soft tissue

elements most responsible for joint fixation and hypermobility are not visualized on the radiograph. These soft-tissue structures are the elements most often affected by spinal manipulation, and they most frequently form the holding elements of joint fixation (16, 30–33). In addition, it is these soft-tissue structures that may be further stretched by forceful manipulation following a sprain or strain. This further damage may be prevented by careful evaluation of motion by both x-ray motion studies (34–41) and palpation (23, 26, 42–53).

This concept is supported by Lewit (50), who states, "We know and teach that manipulation is effective only a) if we find some passive movement restriction and b) if we achieve normalization of mobility."

He cautions that it is essential for every student of manipulative therapy to learn to diagnose movement restriction. "If, for example, there is pain and normal or even exaggerated mobility, manipulation is futile or even harmful. This in itself is good evidence that manipulation acts on joint mobility."

Evaluation of the unstable hypermobile joint must therefore consider the soft tissue elements of the vertebral motion segments. Manipulation that forces further movement on an already hypermobile articulation may increase nerve and other soft-tissue irritation and is contraindicated.

Intervertebral Disc

There has been such a proliferation of published material in the last 40 years implicating the invertebral disc as the etiological factor in the production of back pain, that this period has been referred to as "the dynasty of the disc." Lesions of the discs are commonly involved in pathomechanical states of the spine, but frequency of failure of disc surgery indicates that this is not the only element causing back pain (51).

The intervertebral disc is a fibrocartilaginous coupling that forms the articulation between the bodies of the vertebrae. It serves both to unite the adjacent vertebral bodies and to hold them apart by means of the hydrostatic pressure of the centrally located nucleus pulposus. The viscid fluid of the nucleus under axial pressure supplies a shock-absorbing component to the spine. The nucleus exhibits considerable elastic rebound and allows the disc to assume its original physical state upon release of pressure. The intervertebral disc while serving both to unite and to separate the vertebral bodies, also allows the universal movements characteristic of the typical vertebral motion segment. In addition, this anterior component of the functional unit of the spine is normally the primary weight-bearing part of the spinal column, and as such it is subjected to an enormous compressive force. The harmful effects of axial compression are magnified by the stress of motion, which adds shearing and torsional forces to the disc.

It is little wonder that the pathomechanical state resulting from disc degeneration that occurs with the aging process has such a devastating effect on spinal motion. The vicious cycle is established because the nutrition of the disc is dependent on imbibition from surrounding tissues that in turn are affected by spinal motion for normal distribution of tissue fluid (54). Joint locking and consequent restriction of motion in one or both of the posterior joints can therefore have a detrimental effect on the health of the disc and be a contributing factor to disc degeneration.

Posterior Spinal Articulations

The posterior spinal articulations, commonly referred to as the zygapophyseal joints, are true diathrodial joints with characteristics similar to those of peripheral diathrodial joints. They have articular cartilage, a loose capsule lined with synovial membrane, reinforcing ligaments, and related muscles. The joints are well supplied with sensory nerve fibers and can be a source of referred back and leg pain as well as considerable proprioceptive information.

The shape and the orientation of the posterior spinal articulations vary according to their location in the spinal column. Spinal movement is determined by the direction of the facet planes, resulting in the different movement patterns in the various spinal areas. These posterior articular processes also add stability to the vertebral motion segment and, depending on the area of the vertebral column and spinal posture, may carry up to 30% of the weight placed upon the spinal column. In addition to locking or fixation of the posterior articulations, zygapophyseal joints are also subject to pathological changes such as spondylarthrosis (degenerative joint disease) (48, 55–60). The interaction between the posterior spinal articulations and the intervertebral disc articulations forming the three-joint complex must be emphasized. If primary disc degeneration has occurred and abnormal movement has developed subsequently within the vertebral motion segment, the reduction of the secondary zygapophyseal joint fixation does not protect the patient from a recurrence of facet subluxation (31).

Spinal Ligaments

The ligaments of the spine are arranged so as to provide postural support between vertebrae, with a minimum expenditure of energy, while at the same time allowing for adequate spinal motion. They must also restrict motion within physiological limits in order to protect the neural elements of the spine. They are designed to resist tensile forces acting parallel to the direction in which the fibers run. These vertebral ligaments may be classified as long spinal ligaments and short intersegmental ligaments. The long spinal ligaments are continuous supporting bands running the entire length of the spine, while the intersegmental bands connect adjacent vertebrae (Fig. 1.21).

The long spinal ligaments include the anterior and posterior longitudinal ligaments and the supraspinous ligament. The intersegmental ligaments include the ligamenta flava, the interspinous, intertransverse, and capsular ligaments. In addition there are regional accessory ligaments and the inconstant ligaments of the intervertebral foramina.

The anterior longitudinal is a broad fibrous network attached to the anterior surfaces of the vertebral bodies. It forms a strong bond from the sacrum to the basiocciput. The width of the anterior longitudinal ligament is diminished at the level of each intervertebral disc, and the ligament is not firmly attached to the annular fibers of the disc. The posterior longitudinal ligament, unlike the anterior longitudinal ligament, is wider at the level of the intervertebral disc where it is interwoven into the annular fibers. It runs inside the spinal canal from the sacrum to the body of the axis. It attaches to the posterior superior and posterior and inferior margins of the vertebral bodies. The upward extension of the posterior longitudinal ligament is the membrane tectora, which continues cephalward as a strong broad band also attached to the basilar part of the occiput. In the area between the posterior longitudinal ligament's vertebral attachments lie venous sinuses that may produce pressure on the ligament. This may be a contributing factor in back pain upon arising which results from increased abdominal pressure or central venous pressure (31).

The supraspinous ligament extends from the sacrum, along the tips of the spinous processes, to the ligamentum nuchae. It is a strong fibrous cord, thicker and broader in the lumbar region than in the thoracic region. It is much expanded in the cervical region as the ligamentum nuchae, which extends to the occiput.

These three long spinal ligaments have superficial fibers that extend over three or four vertebrae, forming continous supporting bands the entire length of the spinal column.

Mechanically the ligaments deform in response to the separation between vertebrae. In addition, the posterior and anterior longitudinal ligaments can be stretched by bulging of the disc. Excessive traction at the attachment points of these two ligaments causes spur formation, which can be visualized radiographically (Fig. 1.22).

The ligamenta flava extend from the anterior superior borders of the laminae to the anterior inferior borders of the laminae above. They connect adjacent vertebrae from the sacrum to the axis bridging the posterior elements of the spinal canal (22). These fibroelastic structures permit separation of the lamina in flexion and at the same time brake the movement, so that its limit is not reached abruptly (2).

The elastic property of these ligaments assists in the restoration of the vertebral column to the neutral

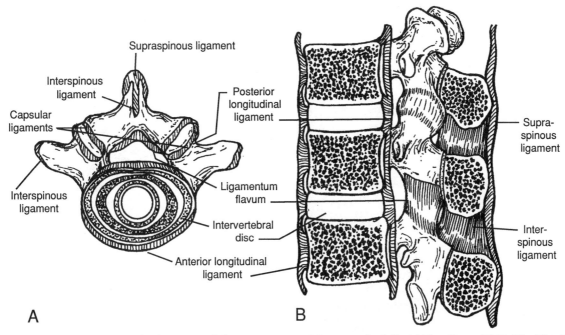

Supraspinous ligament

Interspinous ligament

Capsular ligaments

Interspinous ligament

Posterior longitudinal ligament

Ligamentum flavum

Intervertebral disc

Anterior longitudinal ligament

Supra-spinous ligament

Inter-spinous ligament

A

B

Figure 1.21. Spinal ligaments. The long spinal ligaments (*anterior* and *posterior longitudinal ligaments*) are continuous supporting bands running the entire length of the spine. The short intersegmental ligamentous bands (*interspinous, intertransverse,* and *capsular ligaments, ligamentum flavum,* and *intervertebral disc*) (After Kapandji IA: *The Physiology of the Joints the Trunk and Vertebral Column,* ed 2. Edinburgh, Churchill Livingstone, 1974, Vol 3.) connect adjacent vertebrae.

position following flexion. Additionally it protects the spinal cord from impingement by folding, which would occur with a nonelastic structure. It may also protect the discs from injury (2). The ligamenta flava form the medial and anterior aspects of the capsular ligaments, which may mean that the posterior joints of the spine are not as strong as other joints and are predisposed to subluxation and degenerative change (2). It has also been suggested that the shortening and lengthening of the ligamenta flava with spinal motion results in small, frequent, repetitive movements that assist in the nutrition of the posterior joint cartilage, the nucleus pulposus, and the cartilage plates of the disc, a function that would be expected to be absent or impaired by joint fixation.

The interspinous ligaments are thin and almost membranous. They connect adjacent spinous processes, and their attachments extend from the root to the apex of each process, meeting the supraspinous ligament at the back and the ligamenta flava in front. They are broad and thick in the lumbar region, becoming narrow and elongated in the thoracic region. They are only slightly developed in the neck, as part of the ligamentum nuchae. The interspinous ligaments add stability to the spine by checking excessive flexion (2). The intertransverse ligaments connect the ipsilateral transverse processes of adjacent vertebrae. In the lumbar region they are thin and membranous, while in the thoracic region they are rounded cords, intimately connected with the deep muscles of the back. They are largely replaced by in-

tertransverse muscles in the cervical region and consist of a few scattered fibers in this area.

The capsular ligaments are attached immediately peripheral to the lateral margins of the articular facets joining adjacent articular processes. As stated previously, medially and anteriorly the joint capsule is formed by a lateral continuation of the ligamentum flavum. Posteriorly the capsule is much thinner and loosely attached (61). Laxity of the capsule posteriorly and inferiorly, in addition to the elastic properties of the medial and anterior fibers, allows considerable range of movement in different directions. Disc degeneration leads to telescoping or imbrication of the facets, with destruction of the articular cartilage as the posterior joints increasingly bear weight.

Regional accessory ligaments, such as the iliolumbar ligaments at the lumbosacral junction, the radiate ligaments of the thoracic spine, and the ligaments of the atypical vertebral motion segments will be discussed when these specific areas of the vertebral column are considered.

Inconstant ligaments of the spine are also important to the practitioner of spinal manipulation. Commonly found in the lumbar spine, these sturdy ligaments transverse the intervertebral foramina and diminish the space available for the passage of the nerve root. The clinical significance of these ligaments has not yet been explored. They may well be a source of pathological nerve root entrapment (see Chapter 8).

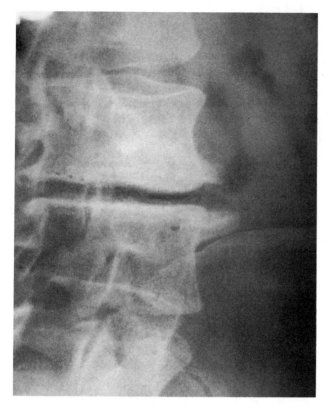

Figure 1.22. Traction at the attachment points of the anterior longitudinal ligament due to disc degeneration leads to spur formation.

Intersegmental Spinal Muscles

The transversospinal muscles that extend only between adjacent vertebrae act as dynamic ligaments and adjust small movements of the vertebral column. It is thought that these deep muscles function as postural muscles and insure the efficient action of the long superficial muscles. The vertebral column is made up of a series of small elements joined in series, and such a mechanical arrangement would buckle under compressive forces without a stablizing mechanism.

The deep transversospinal muscles are the multifidus and the rotatores. Only the deepest fibers of the multifidus muscles are thought to span contiguous vertebrae. They run obliquely upward, attaching to the entire length of the spinous process of the vertebrae above. In the sacral region they attach to the back of the sacrum; in the lumbar region from the mamillary processes; in the thoracic region from the transverse processes; and in the cervical region from the articular processes. The fasciculi vary in length. The most superficial fibers may span three or four vertebrae. They fill in the groove at the side of the spinous processes from the sacrum to the axis (2) (Fig. 1.23).

The rotatores lay deep to the multifidus. They are best developed in the thoracic region, where they

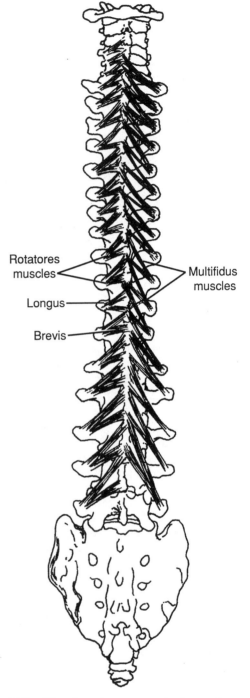

Figure 1.23. The deep transversospinal muscles run obliquely upward between vertebrae. (After Warfel J.H.: *The Head, Neck, and Trunk Muscles and Motor Points;* ed 4. Philadelphia, Lea & Febiger, 1973.)

connect the upper and posterior part of the transverse process of the vertebrae to the lower border and lateral surface of the laminae of an adjacent superior vertebra. In the lumbar and cervical regions the rotatores are irregular and variable, with attachments similar to those of the rotatores in the thoracic region (Fig. 1.23).

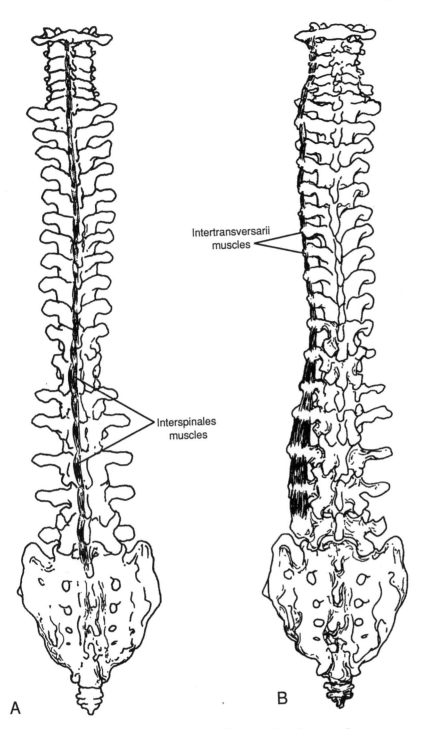

A

B

Figure 1.24. The *interspinales* and *intertransversarii muscles* run between adjacent vertebrae, best represented in the cervical and lumbar region. (After Warfel JH: *The Head, Neck, and Trunk Muscles and Motor Points*, ed 4. Philadelphia, Lea & Febiger, 1973.)

The interspinales are short, paired muscular fasciculi between the spines of adjacent vertebrae, one on each side of the interspinous ligament (2). They are not constant in the thoracic spine (Fig. 1.24A).

The intertransversarii are small muscles between the transverse processes of the vertebrae (Fig. 1.24B). They are best developed in the cervical region where they consist of anterior and posterior slips separated by the rami of the spinal nerves. In the thoracic region they consist of single muscles, which are found between the transverse processes of the last three thoracic vertebrae only and between the transverse processes of the twelfth thoracic and the first lumbar vertebrae. Two sets of intertransversarii muscles are found in the lumbar region. The intertransversarii mediales connect the accessory process of one vertebra with the mamillary process of the next. The intertransversarii laterales has two slips. The ventral slip connects the transverse processes (costal elements) while the dorsal slip connects the accessory process to the mamillary process of the subjacent vertebrae (2).

Theoretically the action of these muscles produces extension (multifidus and intertransversarii)

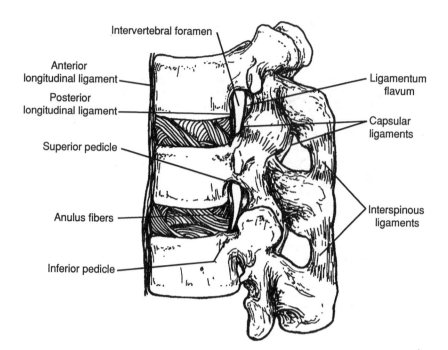

Intervertebral foramen

Anterior longitudinal ligament

Posterior longitudinal ligament

Superior pedicle

Anulus fibers

Inferior pedicle

Ligamentum flavum

Capsular ligaments

Interspinous ligaments

Figure 1.25. The *intervertebral foramen* is bounded superiorly and inferiorly by the pedicles of the adjacent vertebrae, anteriorly by the dorsum of the intervertebral disc covered by the *posterior longitudinal ligament*, and posteriorly by the articular capsules of the posterior facet joints and the *ligamentum flava*.

and rotation (multifidus and rotatores), but their detailed activity patterns have not been demonstrated, because of the complexity of the vertebral motion segment mechanism and the inaccessibility of these muscles.

Vertebral motion segment immobility may be the result of primary muscle spasm in an otherwise normal segment or occur as a secondary compensatory mechanism in an attempt to stabilize a hypermobile segment. This muscle activity may be the variation in the pattern seen as paradoxical activity on electromyography of deep muscles. Clinical evaluation must await further studies of the complex arrangement of muscle bundles acting on the multitude of equally complex joints (63).

Intervertebral Foramen

The intervertebral foramen is a short, elliptical canal forming an aperture for the exit of the segmental spinal nerves and the entrance of blood vessels and nerve branches that supply the structures of the vertebral canal (Fig. 1.25). It is bounded superiorly and inferiorly by the respective pedicles of the adjacent vertebrae. The anterior portion is formed by the dorsum of the intervertebral disc covered by the posterior longitudinal ligament. The articular capsules of the posterior joints and the ligamenta flava contribute to the posterior aspect of the foramen. This opening provides a margin of safety in the healthy spine with the caliber of the canal larger than the collective size of the structures that pass through it. The remaining space is occupied by loose areolar tissue and fat, to accommodate the relative motions of the canal contents.

However adequate the canal size may appear, the bore is readily affected by anomalies and pathological and pathomechanical changes. Anomalous development may take the form of lateral recess steno-

sis or the presence of transforaminal ligaments (62). Pathological changes affecting foraminal size can include degenerative disc disease, the most serious form of which is frank disc herniation and osteoarthric outgrowths from the posterior joints. Pathomechanical changes may be secondary to loss of disc height with facet imbrication and subluxation (46) or the result of displacement due to joint locking.

Any of these conditions have the potential to diminish the size of the intervertebral foramen and may be a source of interference with normal neurological function. Problems related to specific areas of the spine are further discussed with the unique characteristics of regional spinal dynamics.

Neurovascular Components

One of the most basic and important functions of the spinal column is protection of the spinal cord. The vertebral canal affords this protection and is occupied by the spinal cord, the meninges, and associated vessels. The combined vertebral motion segments form a hollow, flexible pillar comprised of the vertebral bodies anteriorly and the posterior vertebral arches made up of the pedicles and laminae. Passing through this canal from the brain stem to the conus medullaris is the spinal cord, housed in a bony, protective casing.

The spinal nerves formed by the union of the dorsal and ventral roots exit through the respective intervertebral foramina of each vertebral motion segment, protected by the dural root sleeve (Fig. 1.26). Passing back through the intervertebral foramen are the tiny sinuvertebral nerves formed by the union of a spinal afferent and a sympathetic postganglionic root. This recurrent branch innervates the articular connective tissues of the vertebral canal (Fig. 1.27). The sinuvertebral nerve

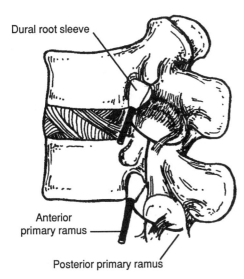

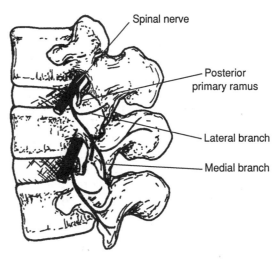

Figure 1.26. The spinal nerves are formed by the union of the dorsal and ventral roots. They exit through the intervertebral foramina, protected by the dural root sleeve.

Figure 1.28. Innervation of the posterior articulations and muscles is derived from the posterior rami of the spinal nerves. Each intervertebral joint is innervated by two spinal nerves. (After Lewin T: *Actu Orthop Scand*, Suppl. 73. 1964)

originates just distal to the dorsal root ganglion, where it unites with the autonomic fibers from the gray ramus communicans. It curves upward around the base of the pedicle and divides into a superior and inferior branch. Numerous filaments are distributed to the periosteum, the posterior longitudinal ligament, the dura, and the epidural vessels. Branches from each level anastomose with an overlapping consistent with the mutual overlapping of the segmental sensory nerve distribution, suggesting that discogenic pain from a single level may involve more than one recurrent branch of the spinal nerves (Fig. 1.27B).

Innervation of the posterior articulations and muscles is derived from the posterior rami of the spinal nerves (Fig. 1.28). These branches supply the articular capsules of the facets, the ligamenta flava, and the interspinous ligaments. Each intervertebral joint is innervated by two spinal nerves, a consequence of its embryonic origin from two vertebral (sclerotomal) segments, and in agreement with Hilton's law, since these are the nerves which supply the muscles acting on the joint.

A close relationship exists between the extensive and abundant blood supply of arterial branches that form the anterior lateral and posterior spinal arteries of the spinal cord. They also send anastomosing

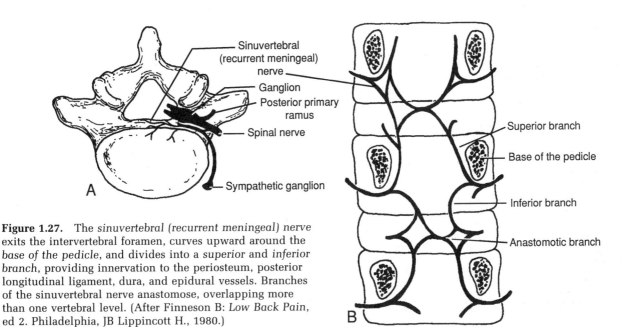

Figure 1.27. The *sinuvertebral (recurrent meningeal) nerve* exits the intervertebral foramen, curves upward around the *base of the pedicle*, and divides into a *superior* and *inferior branch*, providing innervation to the periosteum, posterior longitudinal ligament, dura, and epidural vessels. Branches of the sinuvertebral nerve anastomose, overlapping more than one vertebral level. (After Finneson B: *Low Back Pain*, ed 2. Philadelphia, JB Lippincott H., 1980.)

branches that supply the meninges, the vertebral bodies, and the posterior joints. There is an extensive venous plexus draining the spinal column, meninges, and spinal canal. Venous stasis that results in retrograde venous pressure can expand this plexus and cause pain due to impingement of spinal nerve roots at the cord itself. This offers a direct channel for the extension of inflammation, infection, or metastatic disease from the pelvic organs into the spinal column and even into the skull.

In the cervical region, vertebral arteries extend upward through the transverse foramina from the sixth cervical vertebra along the uncovertebral joints, a common site of degenerative arthritic changes. These arteries loop over the posterior arch of the atlas and continue through the foramen magnum. Anomalous development and pathological changes in this area may precipitate the most serious contraindication to spinal manipulation, vertebral-basilar syndrome (13) (see Chapter 4).

The functional approach to spinal disorders requires a thorough understanding of the concept and components of the vertebral motion segment. The interaction and movement between vertebral motion segments is also of great importance to spinal function. Aberrant motion of one element of the motion segment can affect other elements of the same motion segment, as well as affecting adjacent segments. This must be considered along with the soft-tissue pathology that can accompany biomechanical dysfunction of the spine.

References

1. Helfet AJ, Gruebel Lee, DM: *Disorders of the Lumbar spine.* Philadelphia, JB Lippincott, 1978, pp 21, 161.
2. Warwick R, Williams, PL: *Gray's Anatomy,* ed 35, British. Philadelphia, WB Saunders, 1973, pp 110–111, 413, 511–513
3. Carlson BM: *Patten's Foundations of Embryology,* ed 4. New York, McGraw-Hill, 1981, p 270.
4. Arey LB: *Developmental Anatomy: A Textbook and Laboratory Manual of Embryology,* ed 7. Philadelphia, WB Saunders, 1974, p 406.
5. Sadler TW: *Langman's: Medical Embryology.* Baltimore, Williams & Wilkins, 1984, p 144.
6. Schmorl G, Junghanns H: *The Human Spine in Health and Disease,* ed 2, translated by Beseman EF. New York, Grune & Stratton, 1971, pp 3–4, 55–56
7. Garber JN: Abnormalities of the atlas and axis vertebrae—congenital and traumatic. *J Bone Joint Surg* 46-A:1782–1791, 1964.
8. Steindler A: *Kinesiology of the Human Body Under Normal & Pathological Conditions.* Springfield, IL, Charles C Thomas, 1973, p 163.
9. Phillips RB: Clinical and roentgenographic considerations of spinal congenital anomalies important to the chiropractor. *ACA J Chiro* 11:S-141-S-150, 1974.
10. Turek SL: *Orthopedic Principles & Their Application,* ed 3. Philadelphia, JB Lippincott, 1977, pp 783, 785
11. Childers JC, Wilson FC: Bipartate atlas. *J Bone Joint Surg* 53A:578–582, 1971.
12. Gatterman MI: Contraindications & complications of spinal manipulative therapy. *ACA J Chiro,* 15:575–586, 1981.
13. Hensinger RN, Fielding JW, Hawkins RJ: *Congenital Anomalies of the Odontoid Process Symposium on the Upper Cervical Spine. The Orthopedic Clinic of North America.* Philadelphia, WB Saunders, 1976, p 903.
14. Kleynhans AM: Complications of and contraindications to spinal manipulations therapy. In Haldeman S (ed): *Modern Developments in the Principles and Practice of Chiropractic.* East Norwalk, CT, Appleton-Century-Crofts, 1979, p 373.
15. Epstein BS: *The Spine: A Radiological Text and Atlas,* ed 4. Philadelphia, Lea & Febiger, 1976, p 25.
16. Finneson BD: *Low Back Pain.,* Philadelphia, JB Lippincott, 1980, pp 69–70.
17. Cox JM: Statistical data on facet facings of the lumbar spine. *ACA J Chiro* 14:SZ39, 1977.
18. Farfan JF: *Mechanical Disorders of the Low Back.* Philadelphia, Lea & Febiger, 1973, p 33.
19. Keim HA, Kirkaldy-Willis WH: Low back pain clinical symposia. *CIBA* 32:8, 1980.
20. Gatterman MI: Lost in translation. *JCCA,* 22:131, 1978.
21. Cassidy JD: Report on the international society for the study of the lumbar spine. *JCCA* 22:140, 1978.
22. White AA, Panjabi MM: *Clinical Biomechanics of the Spine.* Philadelphia, JB Lippincott, 1978, p 63.
23. Grice A: A biomechanical approach to cervical and dorsal adjusting. In Haldeman S (ed): *Modern Developments in the Principle and Practice of Chiropractic.* East Norwalk, CT, Appleton-Century-Crofts, 1979, pp 331–358.
24. Kulak RF, Shultz AB, Belytschko, Galanto, J: Biomechanical characteristics of the vertebral motion segments and the intervertebral discs: Symposium on the lumbar spine. *Orthop Clin North Am* 6:121–133, 1975.
25. White AA, Panjabi MM: The basic kinematics of the human spine: a review of past and current knowledge. *Spine* 3:12–20, 1978.
26. ACA Council on Technique Conference on the Biomechanics of the Pelvis, ACA Denver, Colorado, June, 1980.
27. Anderson GB: Biomechanics of the lumbar spine. In Grahman R (ed): *Clinics in Rheumatic Diseases.* London, WB Saunders, 1980, p 37.
28. Kapandji IA: *The Physiology of the Joints. The Trunk and Vertebral Column,* ed 2 (translated by Honore) Edinburgh & London, Churchill Livingstone, 1974, vol 3, p 24.
29. Parke WW, Schiff DC: The applied anatomy of the intervertebral disc. *Orthop Clin North Am* 2:320, 1971.
30. Grecco MA: *Chiropractic Technique Illustrated.* New York, Jarl, 1953. p 22.
31. Drum DC: The vertebral motor unit and intervertebral foramen. *JCCA,* June 1975, pp 23–30.
32. Fisk JW: *The Painful Neck and Back: Diagnosis Manipulation Exercises, Prevention.* Springfield, IL, Charles C Thomas, 1977, p 141.
33. Farfan HF: The scientific basis of manipulative procedures. In Graham R (ed): *Rheumatic Diseases: Low Back Clinics.* London, WB Saunders, 1980, p 167.
34. Fielding JW: Cineroentgenography of the normal cervical spine. *J Bone Joint Surg* 39-A:1280–1288, 1957.
35. Hviid H: Functional radiography of the cervical spine. *Ann Swiss Chiro Assn* 3:37–65, 1965.
36. Conley RN: Stress evaluation of cervical mechanics. *J Clin Chiro* I:46–62, 1974.
37. Sandoz R: Classification of fixation, subluxations, and luxations of the cervical spine. *Ann Swiss Chiro. Assn.,* Geneva, 6:219–276, 1976.
38. Grice A: Preliminary evaluation of 50 sagittal cervical motion radiographic examinations. *JCCA* 21:133, 1977.
39. Jackson R: *The Cervical Syndrome,* ed 4. Springfield, IL, Charles C Thomas, 1977, p 215.
40. Penning L: Normal movements of the cervical spine. *Am J Roentgenol* 130:317–325, 1978.
41. Mannen EM: The use of cervical radiographic overlay to assess response to manipulation: a case report. *JCCA* 24:108–110, 1980.
42. Carver FJ: Postural sacro-iliacs: tests aid in determining type of distortion. *Natl Chiro J* 10:16, 1941.

43. Vladeff T: The theory of the fixation points. *Natl Chiro J* 15:20–23, 1945.
44. Gillet H: The evolution of a chiropractor. *Natl Chiro J* 15:15–21, 1945.
45. Hviid H: A consideration of contemporary theory. *J. Natl Chiro Assn* 25:17–18, 68, 1955.
46. Gillet H, Liekans: A further study of spinal fixations. *Ann Swiss Chiro Assn*, Geneva IV: 41, 1967.
47. Droz JM: Indications and contraindications of vertebral manipulation. *Ann Swiss Chiro Assn*, V:81–92, 1971.
48. Sandoz R: Newer trends in the pathogenesis of spinal disorders. *Ann Swiss Chiro Assn*, V:93–180, 1971.
49. Mennel JM: *Back Pain: Diagnosis and Treatment Using Manipulative Technique.* Boston, Little Brown & Co., 1960, p 18.
50. Lewit K: The contribution of clinical observation to neurobiological mechanism in manipulative therapy. In Korr IM (ed): *The Neurobiological Mechanisms in Manipulative Therapy.* New York, Plenum, 1977, p 4.
51. Kirkaldy-Willis WH, Hill RT: A more precise diagnosis for low-back pain. *Spine* 4:102–109, 1979.
52. Gittleman R: A chiropractic approach to biomechanical disorders of the lumbar spine and pelvis, In Haldeman S (ed): *Modern Developments in the Principles and Practice of Chiropractic.* Norwalk, CT, Appleton-Century-Crofts, 1980, pp 297–330.
53. Wiles MR: Reproducibility and interexaminer correlation of motion palpation findings of the sacro-iliac joints. *JCCA* 24:59–69, 1980.
54. Drum DC: Disc regeneration: the rationale for a therapeutic approach. *JCCA* 13:18–23, part I, 1969, *JCCA* 14:9–15, part II, 1970.
55. Badgley CE: The articular facets in relation to low back pain and sciatic radiation. *J Bone Joint Surg* 23:481–495, 1941.
56. Hadley LA: Intervertebral joint fixation, bony impingement and foramen encroachment with nerve root changes. *J Bone Joint Surg* 65:377, 1954.
57. Hadley LA: Anatomico-roentgenographic studies of the posterior spinal articulations. *J Bone Joint Surg* 86:270–276, 1961.
58. Hussar AE, Gullen EJ: Correlations of pain and the roentgenographic findings of spondylosis of the cervical and lumbar spine., *Am J Med Sci* 232:518, 1956.
59. Lewin T: Osteoarthritis in lumbar synovial joints: a morphological study. *Acta Orthop Scand* I suppl 73, 1964.
60. Shealy CN: The role of the spinal facets in back and sciatic pain. *Headache* 14:101–104, 1974.
61. Yong-Hing K, Reilly J, Kirkaldy-Willis WH: The ligamentum flavum. *Spine* 1:226–234, 1976.
62. Golub BS, Silverman B: Transforaminal ligaments of the spine *J Bone Joint Surg* 51-A:947–956, 1969.
63. Donisch EW, Basmajian JV: Electromyography of deep back muscles in man. *Anatomy* 133:25–36, 1972.

CHAPTER 2

Basic Kinesiological and Biomechanical Principles Applied to the Spine

The spine is a multilinked mechanical system.

The spine is a multilinked mechanical system that combines weightbearing with physiological movement (1) (Fig. 2.1). The opposite characteristics of stability and mobility are combined in a central axis, which provides a stable attachment for muscles. They then contribute to spinal stability as well as provide for spinal movement. In addition, the spinal column protects the neural elements of the spinal cord and exiting spinal nerves. To adequately understand spinal function, one must have not only a knowledge of spinal anatomy but also a working knowledge of basic kinesiological and biomechanical principles as they apply to the spine.

Kinesiology refers to the study of movement, in this case movement of the vertebrae at the spinal joints. The study of human movement includes the means by which it is faciliated or restrained: the physical laws governing all motion, the mechanics of the joints, and the forces generated by the paravertebral muscles.

Biomechanics is a branch of kinesiology which applies mechanical laws to biological tissues and includes two basic areas, statics and dynamics. Statics deals with the study of bodies remaining at rest or in equilibrium as a result of forces acting upon them, while dynamics involves the study of moving bodies.

Dynamics is further subdivided into kinematics and kinetics. Kinematics is that phase of mechanics concerned with the study of motion of particles and rigid bodies, in this case bones, with no consideration of the forces involved. It deals with the relationships that exist between displacements, velocities, accelerations, and decelerations in translational or rotational motion. Spinal kinematics describes the movement of the vertebral motion segments in all planes including flexion/extension, lateral flexion, rotation, and distraction. Kinetics deals with moving bodies and the forces that act to produce the motion, including analysis of the muscle action as well as the opposite forces of gravity and disc pressure (2).

While the practitioner may not need exact biomechanical computations of the many forces involved in human motion, an understanding of the mechanical principles used in the study of human kinesiology is helpful. Such factors as lever action and muscle force should be understood, since manual muscle testing depends on the skill of the clinician in applying these principles. The significance of the lever arm lengths involved in muscle tests is as important as the force applied. The concept of the center of mass of the body and its component parts and their relation to the base of support in stance and locomotion is equally important to the understanding of the functioning of the musculoskeletal system.

Postural evaluation is based on the mechanical principles involved while the patient is standing, sitting, lifting, and carrying objects. Evaluation and treatment of gait abnormalities also requires a working knowledge of biomechanical principles. Evaluation of exercise programs should be based on the mechanical analysis of forces in order to avoid the harmful effects of inappropriate exercises, which may develop stresses that can damage joints and soft tissues of the body.

An understanding of the exact mechanism of injury is essential when dealing with the trauma patient. The tissues involved are more easily located, the extent of the injury can be better evaluated, and more specific treatment can be planned when the doctor understands the mechanics involved in producing the injury. Fractures, strains, and sprains are

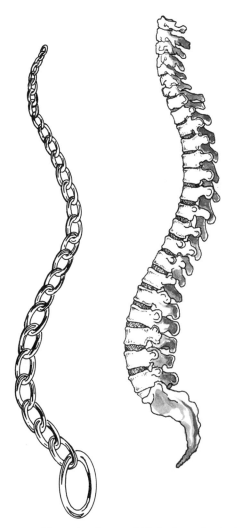

Figure 2.1. The spine is a multilinked mechanical system.

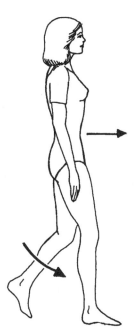

Figure 2.2. Translational and rotational movement. The human body translates as a unit (moves in a straight line) during gait, while the leg rotates (moves in an arc).

all caused by forces that can be analyzed to determine the exact nature of injury.

Perhaps the most useful application of biomechanical principles for the chiropractor is a knowledge of the planes of motion of various joints. Then the manipulative thrust may be delivered in the most efficient manner, with a minimum amount of trauma to the patient. General biomechanical principles are discussed in this chapter in order that they may be applied more specifically in succeeding chapters that discuss the biomechanics of each spinal region.

MOTION

Motion is defined as a continuous change of position of a body. This change may be translational, rotational, or curvilinear motion. Translational or linear motion is defined as the motion of a rigid body in which a straight line in the body always remains parallel to itself. The units of measure for translational motion are meters or feet. The human body translates as a unit during gait (Fig. 2.2). Rotational

or angular motion is defined as movement about an axis. Swinging the leg in an arc during gait is an example of rotational movement (Fig. 2.2). Rotational motion is described in units of radians or degrees (3).

Rotatory and translatory motions frequently combine to produce curvilinear motion. Curvilinear motion is produced in the human body when rotation of bones around a joint axis is accompanied by a sliding of bone surfaces such as at the knee and in the temporomandibular joint. MacConail has applied the fundamentals of geometry to the joint surfaces, utilizing the terms slide, roll, swing, and spin to describe the various types of articular movement. (4–7).

Planes Of Motion

The standard position of reference in anatomy texts is the anatomic position, with the body facing forward, hands at sides with palms facing forward, and feet straight ahead (Fig. 2.3A). A variation of this position is referred to as the fundamental standing position with the palms facing the body (Fig. 2.3B). The fundamental standing position is usually the starting point for describing human motion.

Coordinate System

To facilitate the description of motion, kinesiologists have adopted the three-dimensional, rectangular coordinate system used in solid geometry. This

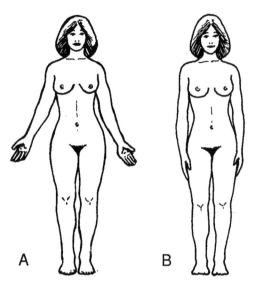

Figure 2.3. Standard body positions. **A,** The anatomic position with the erect body facing forward, hands at the sides with the palms facing forward, and feet straight ahead is the position usually depicted in anatomy textbooks. **B,** The fundamental standing position is similar to the anatomic position with the feet slightly apart and the arms hanging easily at the sides with the palms facing the body. This is the position usually described as the starting point for analyzing human motion.

into four quadrants, with the center of these quadrants known as the origin or 0. This is located at the junction of the perpendicular lines. These lines are generally termed the abscissa or X-axis running vertically and the ordinate or Y-axis running horizontally (Fig. 2.4A). Movement can then be plotted and expressed in X units and Y units.

Movement along the Y-axis and below the origin and movements to the left of the origin along the X-axis are given negative values. The location of the end point of motion can then be assigned X and Y unit values. The two numbers that determine the point location are referred to as the coordinates of the point. When point A is found 2 units to the right of the abscissa and 3 units above the ordinate, its location can be expressed as X = 2 and Y = 3. (Fig. 2.4C). A point B expressed as X = −4 and Y = 1 is found 4 units to the left of the origin and one unit above. (Fig. 2.4D).

To describe motion in three dimensions, a third axis must be introduced. This axis is usually termed the Z-axis and is perpendicular to the X-Y axes. The points in front of the original X-Y axes are expressed as positive values, while those behind are given negative values (Fig. 2.4B).

This coordinate system can be used to describe whole body motion by placing the origin at the center of mass of the body (which lies approximately 2 cm anterior to the second sacral vertebra) or on a point in the body from which movement can then be defined (Fig. 2.5).

In describing segmental spinal motion, the origin is commonly placed at the center of the body of the superior vertebra of the vertebral motion segment,

system makes it possible to define motion or forces acting along any combination of the X, Y, and Z axes.

Using this 90° angle coordinate convention, we can exactly define any point in space. If a two-dimensional description is used, the plane is divided

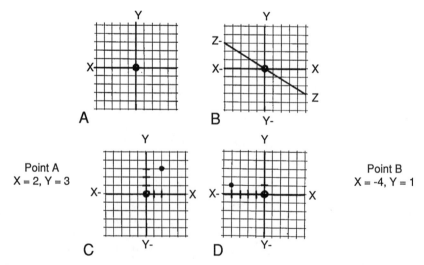

Figure 2.4. The right-handed coordinate system. **A,** The two-dimensional coordinates system divides the plane into four quadrants by means of two perpendicular lines or axes. The horizontal axis is labeled the X-axis (abcissa), while the vertical line is labeled the Y-axis (ordinate). The center of these quadrants is the origin with O. **B,** Addition of a third axis, labeled the Z-axis, permits the location of points in space, with movement described in relation to the origins of the three coordinates. **C,** Movement to the right and upward is plotted along the X and Y axes, where the end point is described as X = 2, Y = 3. **D,** Movement to the left along the X-axis and upward along the Y-axis is described as X = −4, Y = 1.

Table 2.1 Axes and Planes of Motion

Plane	Axis of Rotation	Coordinate of Translation	Motion
Sagittal (YZ)	X	Z	Flexion/extension
Frontal/coronal (XY)	Z	Y	Lateral bending
Horizontal (XZ)	Y	X	Rotation

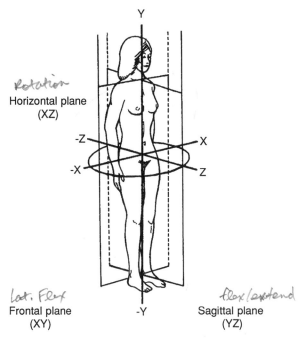

Rotation

Horizontal plane
(XZ)

Lat. Flex

Frontal plane
(XY)

flex/extend

Sagittal plane
(YZ)

Figure 2.5. The right-handed coordinate system can be used to describe whole body motion by placing the origin at the center of mass of the body, anterior to the second sacral tubercle. The origin is the zero point. Forward translation is + Z, up is + Y, and to the right is + X. Backward is − Z, down is − Y, and to the left is − X. The three cardinal planes correspond to the coordinate system as follows: sagittal plane (Y,Z), frontal plane (X,Y), and horizontal plane (X,Y).

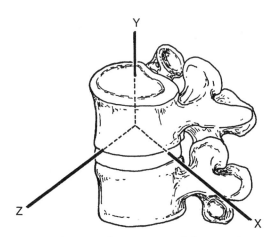

Figure 2.6. The spatial orientation of the superior vertebra relative to the inferior vertebra can be plotted by placing the origin at the center of the superior vertebra. Motion can then be described in relation to translation along any of the three axes or rotation around any of the three axes. These six components of vertebral motion give six degrees of freedom to the vertebral motion segment.

with the lower vertebra regarded as the fixed element. The spatial orientation of the superior vertebra on the inferior vertebra can then be plotted. The

movement of each vertebral motion segment can thus be described in terms of any combination of translation and rotation (Fig. 2.6).

By combining data relative to the physical properties of the individual elements of the vertebral motion segments with an accurate description of their motions, it is possible to simulate by computation, movement of any spinal region or of the entire spine (8, 9). These mathematical models can simulate the behavior of the human spine in situations where other means of investigation are not feasible, since clinical investigations are restricted to studies where the human subjects are not endangered, and animal models are limited by the anatomical differences between the animal and the human spines.

Some authors have suggested that the right-handed Cartesian orthogonal system provides a more exact listing method for describing vertebral fixation. While the use of this system allows an accurate description of vertebral segmental motion by describing the spatial orientation, it is still a static description. For research purposes it gives a more accurate description for plotting vertebral displacement, but it offers little advantage to the clinician in determining the application of manipulation over conventional kinesiological terms such as flexion, extension, lateral flexion, and rotation (10–12) (Table 2.1).

Degrees Of Freedom

When the motion of a rigid body has the potential for translation along the three perpendicular lines and rotation around the three perpendicular axes, it is said to have six degrees of freedom. The motion of a rigid body has six degrees of freedom: three translations along the linear coordinates and three rotations around the angular coordinates.

The typical vertebral motion segment can be considered to have six degrees of freedom, because the upper vertebra has the capability of translating along each of the X, Y, and Z coordinates and of rotating around these coordinates (Fig. 2.6). These six degrees of freedom are possible because of the unique arrangement of the intervertebral discs separating the vertebral bodies, which allows the shearing action along the X and Z coordinates in addition to compression and distraction along the Y-coordinate. Rotation around these 3 axes, while generally restricted by the planes of the articular facets, is allowed in some measure in each segment (2) (Fig. 2.6).

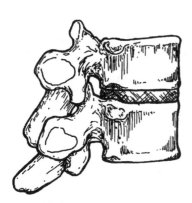
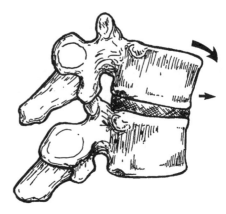

Figure 2.7. Coupled motion during flexion combines rotation around the X-axis with rotation around the Y-axis.

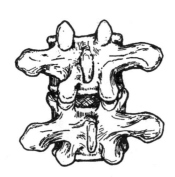
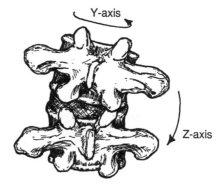

Figure 2.8. Coupled motion occurs during lateral flexion and rotation, with rotational movement occurring around both the Y and X axes.

Coupling

Coupling of more than 1 degree of freedom occurs, in which rotation or translation of the vertebra about one axis is consistently associated with rotation or translation of that same vertebra about another axis. Coupling of motion occurs in the spinal column during flexion, with translation of the vertebra occurring along the Z-coordinate while rotation occurs around the X-axis (Fig. 2.7). Another example of coupled spinal motion occurs during lateral flexion and rotation. Here rotational motion occurs around both the Y and Z axes (Fig. 2.8).

With coupled motion, a change in the axis of rotation occurs, which can be computed as the instantaneous axis of rotation (2). Changes in the instantaneous axis of rotation in the lumbar spinal motion segments with reduction of aberrant motion has been noted following manipulation. This has been demonstrated by plotting pre- and postmanipulation motion on lateral bending x-rays using the orthogonal coordinate system (10).

The X, Y, and Z axes can be related to the three cardinal planes of the body (Table 2.1). The conventional physiologic patterns of motion are flexion and extension in the sagittal plane, lateral flexion in the frontal or coronal plane, and rotation in the horizontal or transverse plane (2) (Fig. 2.9).

FORCE

Force may be defined as any action that tends to change the state of either rest or motion of a body to which it is applied. Force may be applied as a push or pull. In the human body, muscles can only pull, which produces a force that causes the affected body part to push against some resistance. The relation of force to motion can be summarized by Newton's three laws.

The first law, the law of inertia, states that a body remains at rest or in uniform motion until acted upon by an unbalanced or outside set of forces. This law is familiar to patients suffering a head-on collision. As the car stops abruptly, the passenger continues in motion until stopped by the seatbelt or windshield.

The second law, or the law of acceleration, states that the acceleration of a particle is proportional to the force acting upon it and inversely proportional to the mass of the particle. Acceleration is the change in velocity from a given time unit to a greater time unit. A large force acting on a small

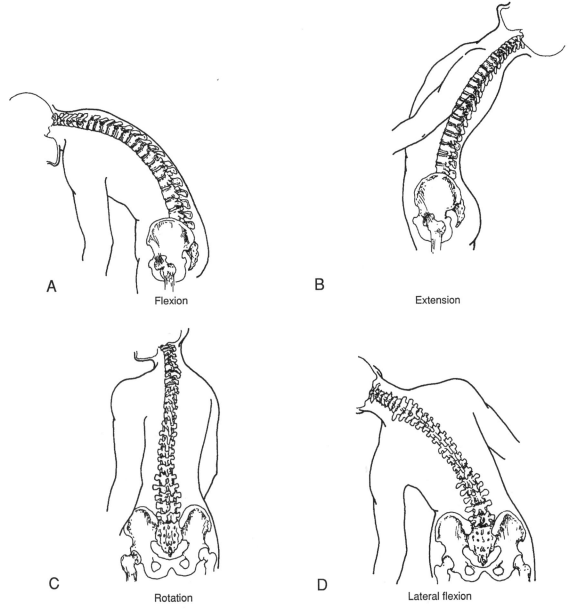

Figure 2.9. Conventional physiological motion of the spine corresponds to **A**, flexion and **B**, extension in the sagittal plane, **C**, rotation in the horizontal plane, and **D**, lateral flexion in the coronal plane.

object will cause rapid acceleration, while a small force acting on a large object will cause slower acceleration.

Newton's third law, or the law of reaction, states that for every action, there is an equal and opposite reaction. When force is applied to an object, that object reacts or pushes back. This reciprocity is central to the explanation of how movement is produced.

Biomechanical forces can be classed as either external or internal. Gravity is a constant external force affecting the human body, while internal forces are created by the pull of muscles and resistance of ligaments on bones.

Characteristics of Force

The four factors that characterize force are magnitude, action line, direction, and point of application. Magnitude is a scalar quantity like speed, length, and temperature, and as such has no direction. Force is a vector quantity that expresses direction as well as magnitude.

The magnitude of a vector force may be illustrated by the length of the lines representing the individual forces. An action line and direction, indicating a pull toward the source or push away from the source, is shown by arrows along the line of action. The point of application indicates the site where the

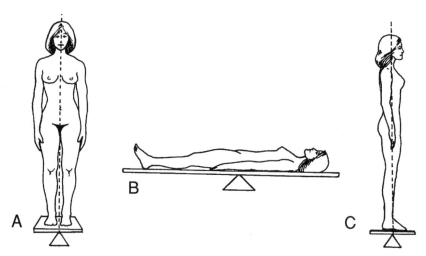

Figure 2.10. The center of gravity of the body can be determined by balancing the body in the three cardinal planes and noting the intersection of the three balance points.

force is applied. Quantification of distance, mass, velocity, acceleration, and time are required for a precise description of the motion of an object. The basic units involved are distance and time, since velocity is defined as the change of distance per unit time. Acceleration is defined as the rate of change of velocity (13).

Gravitational Forces

Gravity is a constant force acting on all objects on the earth's surface. It is the most constant force encountered by the human body and acts in a predictable and describable manner. Since it is a vector quantity, it can be described by its point of application, action line, direction, and magnitude. While gravity acts on all points of an object, its point of application is given as the center of gravity (C of G) of the object.

The C of G of an object can be determined by suspending or balancing the object in one plane, to locate the action line of the force of gravity with respect to that plane. The object must then be rotated 90° and balanced in the other two planes to find their action lines. Then, by determining the intersection of these three lines of gravitational force, it is possible to determine the center of mass (or center of gravitational pull) of the object (Fig. 2.10).

The center of gravity of the human body has been located between 53 and 59% of the total height of the body from the soles of the feet to the top of the head. The location varies with individual body build and is comparatively lower in women because of their wider pelvic girdle and narrower shoulders. It is located 2–3 cm anterior to the second sacral vertebra in the average upright human body (14).

The center of gravity shifts anteriorly in the obese patient, which increases the rotational forces that tend to pull the body forward. The compensatory forces opposing the shift in the C of G tend to accentuate the already existing curves of the spine and to cause an increase in the lumbar lordosis. This in turn increases the stress in the lumbosacral junction. In the thoracic region, there is a tendency for the spine to collapse in forward flexion and crowd the viscera.

Line of Gravity

The action line of gravity of the body in the upright positon is commonly used to evaluate posture (Fig. 2.11). As the center of gravity of the body shifts, so does the line of gravitational change, which creates various postural problems (see Chapter 13).

Intrinsic Equilibrium

The intrinsic forces that make the healthy spine a comparatively stable and rigid mechanical unit are vested in the elastic properties of the noncontractile structures of the spine. These forces acting on the typical vertebral motion segment include the axial pressure of the nucleus pulposus against the vertebral endplates (which resist compression and separate adjacent vertebrae) and the tension exerted by the ligaments holding each segment together (Fig. 2.12). These forces form an intrinsic equilibrium that depends on the turgor of the nucleus pulposus and the integrity of the intervertebral ligaments, which form a delicate balance mechanism maintaining erect posture with relatively little muscular force (15). When the intervertebral disc degenerates, this intrinsic balance mechanism is disrupted. With reduced turgidity of the nucleus, segmental instability results because the balancing ligaments cannot take up the slack, and mechanical derangement of the three-joint complex occurs (see Chapter 8).

Muscle Force

The balance or equilibrium of the upright human body, including the articulated parts of the vertebral column, depends on a fine neutralization of the

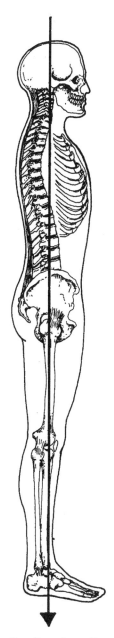

Figure 2.11.   The action line of gravity relative to the body in the upright position is commonly used to evaluate posture.

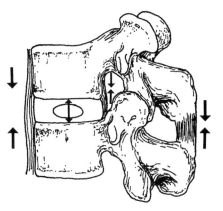

Figure 2.12.   The ease with which the normal human spine can be held erect with a relatively small amount of muscle force is due to the intrinsic equilibrium of each vertebral motion segment. The hydrostatic pressure of the nucleus pulposus present in the healthy disc separates the vertebral bodies and resists compression, while spinal ligaments produce tension, holding the vertebrae together. These opposing forces provide an elastic buffer, which absorbs pressure stresses and stabilizes the vertebral column.

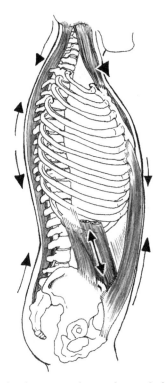

Figure 2.13.   The long spinal muscles and the abdominal muscles stabilize the spine as a unit.

forces of gravity by counterforces. These counterforces are produced by muscle activity. In the upright, well-balanced stance of the human subject, minimal muscle power is required to maintain standing posture. The long spinal muscles and the abdominal muscles stabilize the spine as a unit (Fig. 2.13).

An increased pull of gravity is counteracted by increased activity in one set of muscles of either the back or anterior abdominal wall. These antigravity muscles become much more active when called upon to produce the powerful movements necessary for major postural changes, from lying to sitting to standing (16). The short spinal muscles produce stabilizing forces that increase the efficiency of the long muscles (17). Without the stabilizing effect of these short spinal muscles, the vertebral column would tend to collapse under compressive forces.

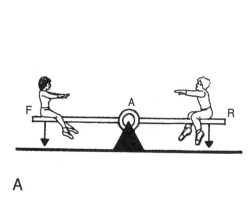

A

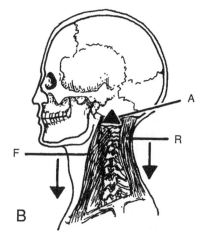

B

Figure 2.14. **A**, A first-class lever is designed for balance and conservation of energy, like a teeterboard. **B**, The head is balanced on the atlas, minimizing the amount of muscle force

necessary to maintain the head in the upright position. The axis of rotation is placed between the force point and the resistance point in a first-class lever.

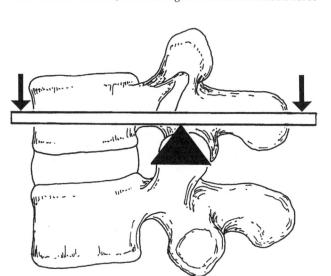

Figure 2.15. The typical vertebral motion segment functions as a first-class lever, with the axis at the posterior articulations.

LAWS OF LEVERAGE

A lever is a rigid bar turning about a fixed point or axis. In human motion, bones serve as the lever arms, with muscles providing the force to move these levers about the axis or joints. A lever requires three points for movement to occur. The relative position of each of these three points, the axis, force point, and resistance point, determines which of the three classes of levers we are dealing with and subsequently what type of mechanical advantage we can employ. These three points may be abbreviated as follows:

1. Axis of rotation, or the joint = A
2. Force point, or point of muscle attachment = F

3. Resistance point, or center of resistance = R

We obtain the three classes of lever, therefore, by changing the relative position of these three points.

A first-class lever is designed for balance and has the axis between the force point and the resistance point. There are many clear examples of first-class levers in the human body, such as the head balanced on the atlas like a teeterboard (Fig. 2.14A). The action of the anterior and posterior muscle groups pulls the head either forward or backward, with a minimum expenditure of energy required to balance the head in normal posture (Fig. 2.14B). According to Kapandji (18), the typical vertebral motion segment functions as a first-class lever, with the disc allowing for the absorption of axial compression and the spine balanced for minimal muscle force expenditure (Fig. 2.15).

The second-class lever saves force by having the resistance point between the axis and the force point. The wheelbarrow is an example of a second-class lever, with the axis at the wheel on one end, the weight (or resistance) in the center, and the force applied at the handles on the other end (Fig. 2.16A). The mechanical advantage here is that a large weight (resistance) can be moved with minimal force.

The existence of a second-class lever in the body is controversial. The action of the ankle, when one stands on the toes is the example most frequently used (Fig. 2.16B). In this case, the axis is within the metatarsal joint, the resistance is the weight of the body in the center, with the force provided by the plantar flexors as they raise the body upward. This situation is only momentary, since the center of gravity shifts to the anterior of the metatarsal heads in order to maintain balance, thereby moving the resistance in front of the axis and creating a first-class lever (Fig. 2.16C).

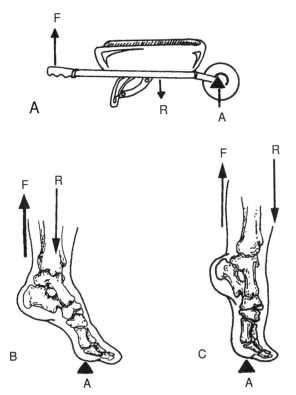

Figure 2.16. **A**, A second-class lever saves force by having the resistance point between the axis and the force, such as in a wheelbarrow. **B**, The presence of a second-class lever in the body is commonly debated, the most frequent example being the action of the ankle when one stands on the toes. In this case the axis is within the metatarsophalangeal joint, the resistance is the weight of the body in the center, with the force provided by the posterior plantar flexors. This example is only momentary, however, since the center of gravity shifts to the anterior of the metatarsal heads in order to maintain balance. **C**, Moving the resistance in front of the axis creates a first-class lever.

The action of the third-class lever increases speed and range of movement at the expense of power. In this case, the force point is between the axis and resistance point (Fig. 2.17A). Many of the lever systems in the body are third-class levers. The biceps muscle as it flexes the forearms is an example (Fig. 2.17B). The resistance in this case may be extrinsic (e.g., a book held in the hand) or intrinsic (e.g., the weight of the arm or forearm). The axis of rotation in this case is the elbow joint (19).

The major principle of leverage states that a lever of any class will balance when the product of the force and the force arm equals the product of the resistance and the resistance arm. Mathematically, $F \times fa = R \times ra$.

In order for a lever to become a factor in motion, the force must be strong enough to overcome the resistance. For example, in order to balance a resistance of 2 pounds with a resistance arm of 50 inches and a force arm of 5 inches, a force of 20 pounds is needed. This is easily demonstrated on the teeter-

board. If one partner weighs less than the other, then the heavier person must move closer to the axis in order to balance the board. By shortening th resistance arm on the patient, the doctor is less apt to overpower the patient. For example, when testing the deltoid muscle, you are less apt to apply too much force if you apply pressure above the elbow rather than at the wrist (Fig. 2.17A&B).

Leverage, when applied in a practical situation, demonstrates that the position of the head causes a greater expenditure of energy if the head is displaced forward (Fig. 2.19). This is a common postural fault known as "poked head." If the weight of the head is 10 pounds and the resistance arm (or distance from the center of the weight to the axis of rotation) is 6 inches, then a force of 15 pounds is required to balance the head if the distance from the center of rotation to the muscle insertion is 4 inches. If the head is held forward, increasing the distance from the center of the weight of the head to the axis of movement to 8 inches, then a force of 40 pounds is required to balance the head. This is not only fatiguing but also acts as an added compressive force on the soft tissues, including the disc.

This type of pathomechanics can be seen in the fatigue slump, since gravity pulling the weight of the body forward must be overcome by the spinal extensors. It is not surprising to find patients with hypertonicity in the paraspinal muscles suffering from tension headaches and low back pain, especially following periods of prolonged reading. The patient with a pendulous abdomen and a woman in the later stages of pregnancy have longer resistance arms anterior to the spine, which places strain on the muscles of the low back (Fig. 2.20). By the same principle, women with large breasts have a tendency to develop excessive kyphosis, with resultant symptoms in the thoracic area.

In angular or rotatory movements, speed and range of movement are interdependent. For instance, if two levers of different lengths move through a 40° angle at the same angular velocity, the tip of the longer lever will be traveling a greater distance, or covering a greater range of movement, than the tip of the shorter lever. The tip of the longer lever will also be moving faster than the tip of the shorter lever, since it covers a greater distance in the same time. This may be illustrated by superimposing a shorter lever arm on a longer one (Fig. 2.21).

This principle applies to the human body, where a skeletal muscle contracts over a very short distance while the bone forming the long resistance arm of the extremity moves through a wide arc of movement. Many of the longer resistance arms of the body require a large muscle force to overcome the resistance; but according to the law of conservation of energy, that which is lost in force is gained in speed and range of movement. With few exceptions, the force arm is shorter than the resistance arm in

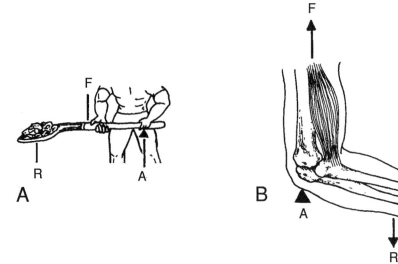

Figure 2.17. **A,** A third-class lever is designed to increase speed and range of movement, with the force point between the axis and the resistance point. **B,** Movement of the forearm at the elbow joint by the biceps muscle is an example of a third-class lever.

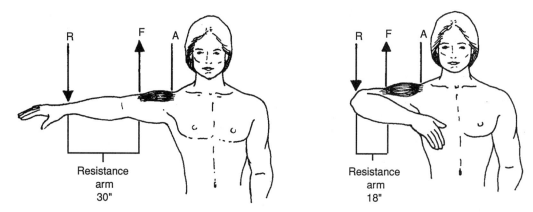

Figure 2.18. The laws of leverage can be applied to muscle testing. By shortening the resistance arm, there is less chance of overpowering a patient.

skeletal levers, thus anatomic levers tend to favor speed and range of movement at the expense of force. The amplification of movement by a long lever arm is the mechanism whereby minute movement at the sacroiliac joint can be palpated at the posterior superior iliac spine with the ilium acting as the lever arm (Fig. 2.22).

KINEMATIC CHAINS

In 1875, Reuleaux introduced the term "kinematic chain" in reference to a mechanical system of links. This engineering concept was applied in 1955, by Dempster, to kinetic and kinematic problems involving movements of the human body (20). While Dempster's work is significant, he did not apply this principle to the human spine. He treated the trunk as a single unit as opposed to a multilinked mechanical system (Fig. 2.1).

Open and Closed Kinematic Chains

In an open kinematic chain, the distal segment terminates in free space, and as such, the cervical spine qualifies as an open kinematic chain. This becomes most significant in the patient suffering a whiplash injury, since the terminal link in the chain supports the weight of the head, which makes the neck more vulnerable to impact in all directions.

In a closed kinematic chain, the end segments are united to form a ring or closed circuit, with motion of one link having determinate relations with every link in the system. The pelvic girdle is considered a closed kinematic chain that is made up of three bony segments, united at the two sacroiliac joints and at the symphysis pubis. Sacroiliac fixation at one joint in this closed chain can affect the mechanics of the entire chain, with hypermobility usually being exhibited in the contralateral articulation.

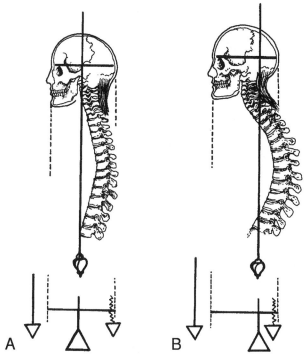

Figure 2.19. Through the application of the laws of leverage, it can be seen that a common postural fault, "poked head," requires a greater expenditure of energy when the head is protruded. In this case, the cervical muscles must provide more force to balance the head. **A**, For example, if the weight of the head is 10 lbs, and the resistance arm is a distance of 6″ from the center of the weight to the axis of rotation, then a force of 15 lbs is required to balance the head, if the distance from the center of rotation to the muscle insertion is 4″ (4 × 15 = 10 × 6). **B**, When the head is held forward, increasing the distance from the center of weight of the head to the axis of movement to 8″, a force of 40 lbs is required to balance the head (2 × 40 = 10 × 8). (After Calliet R: Neck and Arm Pain Philadelphia, FA Davis, 1978.)

Compensatory hypermobility is also a common finding with fixations of the spine. This may take the form of eccentric mobility on the hypermobile side of a vertebra when the contralateral posterior joint is fixated, or may be found as compensatory hypermobility in joints adjacent to locked vertebral motion segments. This chain-link concept of spinal dynamics is of utmost importance to the chiropractor who seeks to treat the area of hypomobility or joint fixation while avoiding areas of compensatory hypermobility.

LOADS AND STRESSES

The human body is constantly subjected to mechanical forces. These forces, as we have said, may be external or internal. External forces are referred to as loads and include such forces as gravity, inertia, muscle action, and ground reaction.

The internal forces reacting to these loads are referred to as stresses. Stress can be defined as the internal resistance of a material that reacts to an exter-

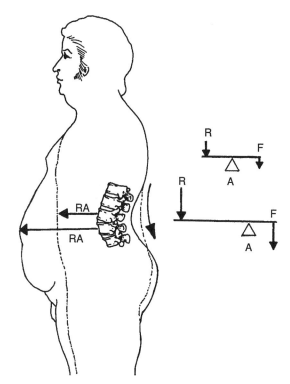

Figure 2.20. The obese patient with a pendulous abdomen has a longer resistance arm anterior to the spine, which places increased strain on the muscles of the low back.

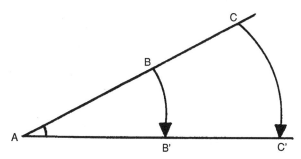

Figure 2.21. The shorter lever, AB, has been superimposed on the longer lever, AC. As the levers move from the diagonal to the horizontal position, point C travels to position C′ in the same time that it takes point B to travel to position B′. Point C obviously moves faster than point B. This principle applies to the human body, where a skeletal muscle contracts over a very short distance while the bone forming the long resistance arm of the extremity moves through a wide arc of movement.

nally applied load (3). In the spine we have loads producing deformation, which are resisted by bone and soft tissue (1). Mechanical failure when loads become too great can be predicted when the functions of the individual structural members are understood relative to the whole structure. Knowledge of the mechanical behavior of each member allows the site of failure to be predicated and generates a

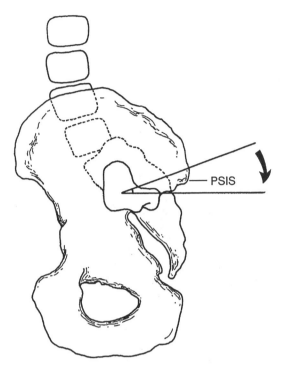

Figure 2.22. Movement at the sacroiliac joint is amplified through the extension of the lever arm (ilium), which may be palpated at the posterior superior iliac spine (*PSIS*).

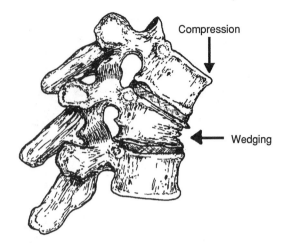

Figure 2.23. Severe *compression* of the spine results in a compression fracture of the anterior body and can cause *wedging* of the vertebral body.

clearer understanding of the mechanism of biomechanical injuries (21). The loads to which an object can be subjected are combinations of tension, compression, torsion, and shear. These loads are defined in terms of the movement they produce (Table 2.1). Mechanical structures fail because they are unable to support the stresses induced by the loads applied to them.

Compression (Axial Loading)

Under a compressive load the most vulnerable elements in a vertebral motion segment with a normal disc are the cancellous bone and the endplate adjacent to the nucleus space (22). This correlates with the frequent occurrence of Schmorl's nodes in nondegenerated herniated discs. In a degenerated discs, however, the most vulnerable element is the annulus, which must withstand great radial tensile strain. This correlates with the occurrence of circumferential clefts in degenerated discs.

Compression of the spine to the breaking point results in fracture of the endplate with loads greater than 500 to 600 psi (23). Breaking strength is related to strain rate, and as strain rate increases breaking strength increases (24). Spinal injuries due to compression usually result from off-center loading, producing a combination of axial loading and hyperflexion. Such a force can result in a compression fracture of the anterior body. These fractures occur most frequently in the lower thoracic and upper lumbar regions (25) and cause wedging of the vertebral body (Fig. 2.23).

In pure vertical loading of a vertebral motion segment, the posterior elements bear a significant portion of the load. In a fracture from predominantly vertical compression, the posterior elements should be subjected to careful radiographic evaluation. A more common cause of back pain is facet loading from compression forces. This hypothesis is consistent with clinical and anatomic evidence that indicates that the lumbar facets are possible sites for low back pain. Yang and King found (26) that normal lumbar facets carry 3–25% of the axial load, with the arthritic joint carrying as much as 47%. Axial loading of the facets varies with posture and is greatest upon trunk extension. This accounts for the increase in pain during hyperextension in the patient suffering from a lumbar facet syndrome. A Jefferson fracture or comminuted fracture of the ring of the atlas is a classical compression injury (Fig. 2.24 A&B), usually due to a blow to the vertex of the head.

Distraction (Tension)

Distraction, or tension, is uncommon as an isolated force affecting the spine, but it can occur on sudden deceleration opposite to an area under compression, when distraction is combined with hyperflexion or hyperextension. With hyperflexion injuries, a compression fracture to the anterior vertebral body will be accompanied by distraction or tension of the interspinous ligament complex (Fig. 2.25). A more isolated distraction injury can occur with injuries produced by a seat belt, where an axis around which flexion occurs is located in the abdominal wall, and the entire vertebral body and the neural arches are exposed to tensile stress.

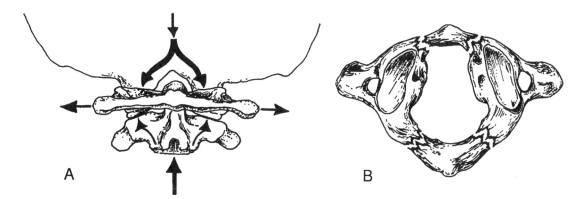

Figure 2.24. A Jefferson fracture can result from a direct caudad blow to the vertex of the head. **A,** Seen from the posterior. **B,** Viewed from above.

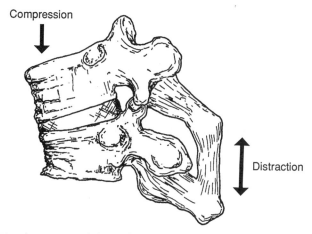

Figure 2.25. With hyperflexion injuries, a compression fracture to the anterior vertebral body will be accompanied by distraction of the interspinous ligament complex.

Translation (Shear)

The vertebral motion segment is subjected to shearing forces most commonly when the body leans forward. In shear loading, the load is conceived to be applied at a right angle to an axis in such a way that no rotational movement is applied. Translation, or shearing, rarely occurs in isolation but may be the dominant force in combination with other forces. Such forces may produce a fracture dislocation, most commonly in the thoracolumbar region of the spine (1).

Flexion (Bending)

Bending forces also are rare without accompanying compressive forces. Forceful hyperflexion of the neck, which occurs as the body is decelerated suddenly, may tear or stretch the nuchal ligaments, the posterior longitudinal ligaments, the interlaminar ligaments, and the capsular ligaments of the lateral interbody joints and the posterior joints. It is not unusual to have compression fractures of the anterior vertebral bodies (21). Forced hyperflexion combined with hyperextension is the mechanism of the "whiplash" injury. If the posterior ligaments have been damaged by bending forces, the possibility of clinical progression of deformity or instability is significantly greater.

Extension (Bending)

Hyperextension of the neck, which occurs when the body is accelerated forward as during a rear-end collision, places traction on the anterior longitudinal ligament. However crush fractures of the neural arch generally occur first, due to accompanying compressive forces (1). Fractures of the spinous processes may also occur, and in some instances the articular facets may be fractured. This can produce subsequent excessive mobility in the vertebral motion segments. The vertebral arteries may suffer trauma, or they may be pulled backward against the posterior wall of the bony rings (foramina) which they transverse. If the vertebrae are forced into an extremely lordotic position, the superior articulations displace inferiorly to an extreme degree, and the capsular ligaments are stretched (27).

Lateral Flexion (Bending)

Forced lateral flexion of the neck also combines distraction force with compression forces. Compression to the structures on the side of the lateral flexion may result in contusion injuries of the vertebral arteries in the transverse foramen as well as compression of all the structures within the intervertebral canals (intervertebral foramina), producing nerve root irritation. Tension produced by the distraction of contralateral structures may produce actual tears in the supporting muscles and ligaments (21).

Rotation (Torsion)

The vertebral motion segment is far more resistant to compression, distraction, and bending than it is to rotation (1). Especially when coupled with flexion, rotational forces produce deformation and disruption of the posterior ligaments and joint capsules, and permit dislocation. Torsional stresses are responsible for the small circumferential tears that appear at the onset of disc degeneration. As the lesion advances, these tears enlarge and coalesce, until they become radial tears, which may ultimately result in disc herniation. These rotational lesions are comon, causing changes in both the posterior joints and in the disc. Rotational strain to one side leads to tension in the joint capsule, while the approximation of the contralateral posterior joint surfaces is effected by compression forces. Spinal manipulation has proven effective in dealing with these torsional lesions.

The occurrence of asymmetry of the apophyseal joints produces diminished mechanical efficiency and makes these joints more vulnerable to torsional forces on the side of the more oblique or coronal facet. Such tropism in the lumbosacral region often produces a lesion readily relieved by manipulation (28). It is hypothesized that the external forces applied to specific vertebral motion segments during spinal manipulation serve to restore motion to vertebral and extravertebral articulation in which mobility is restricted. Successful manipulation should apply a mobilizing force to the areas of the spine that are stiff or hypomobile, while avoiding areas of hypermobility and instability (29).

The effect of external forces varies in various segments of the spinal column, because of anatomical differences in the particular region. Except under experimental conditions, a single applied force in one plane rarely occurs; rather one or the other of the described forces is dominant, coupled with secondary forces.

The unsupported vertebral column is unable to sustain the loads frequently applied to it, but through the additional support of the trunk musculature and intrathoracic and intraabdominal pressure, greater loads to the spine can be sustained (see Chapter 13). A fundamental knowledge of spinal biomechanics is necessary to treat patients with manipulable lesions. With a further understanding of spinal mechanics, prevention of pathomechanical states affecting the human spine can be significantly enhanced.

References

1. Gonza ER, Harrington IJ: *Biomechanics of Musculoskeletal Injury.* Baltimore, Williams & Wilkins, 1982, p 165.
2. White AA, Panjabi MM: The basic kinematics of the human spine: a review of post and current knowledge. *Spine* 3:12–20, 1978.
3. Le Veau B: *Williams and Lessner: Biomechanics of Human Motion,* ed 2. Philadelphia, WB Saunders, 1977, pp 4, 6.
4. MacConail MA: The geometry and anatomy of articular kinematics. *Bio-medical Engineering I* pp 205–212, 1966.
5. Warwick R, Williams PL: *Gray's Anatomy,* ed 35. WB Saunders, 1973, pp 398–407.
6. MacConail MA, Basmajian JV: *Muscles and Movements: A Basis For Human Kinesiology,* ed 2. Huntington, NY, Krieger, 1977, pp 13–30.
7. Scull ER: Joint biomechanics and therapy: contribution or confusion? In Glasgow EF, Tomey LT, Scull ER, Kleynhans AM, Idczak RM: *Aspects of Manipulative Therapy,* ed 2. New York, Churchill Livingstone, 1985, pp 3–15.
8. Belytyschko T, Andriacchi T, Shultz AB, Galante J: Analog studies of forces in human spine: computational techniques. *J Biomech* 6:361, 1973.
9. Hong SW, Suh CH: A mathematical model of the human spine and its application to the cervical spine. Proceedings of the 6th Annual Biomechanics Conference, University of Colorado, 1975.
10. Carrick FR: Treatment of pathomechanics of the lumbar spine by manipulation. *JMPT* 4:173–178, 1981.
11. Gilford SR, Dano CJ: Let's speak the same language. *Dynamic Chiropractic,* MPI, Nov, pp 35–36, 1985.
12. Simmon J: A more precise listing system—the "international." *J ACA,* 23:62, 1986.
13. Nave CR, Nave BC: The description of motion. In Nave CR, Nave BC, *Physics for the Health Sciences,* ed 2. Philadelphia, WB Saunders, 1980, pp 5–10.
14. Scott MG: *Analysis of Human Motion,* ed 2. East Norwalk, CT, Appleton-Century-Crofts, 1963, p 162.
15. Steindler A: *Kinesiology of the Human Body under Normal & Pathological Conditions.* Springfield, IL, Charles C Thomas, 1973, pp 141–142.
16. Basmajian JV: *Muscles Alive.* Baltimore, Williams & Wilkins, 1978, p 178.
17. Donisch EW, Basmajian JV: Electromyography of deep back muscles in man. *Anatomy,* 133:25–36, 1972.
18. Kapandji: *The Physiology of the Joints,* ed 2, translated by Honore LH. Edinburgh, Churchill Livingstone, 1974, vol 3, p 24.
19. Wells KF, Luttzens K: *Kinesiology Scientific Basis of Motion,* ed 6. Philadelphia, WB Saunders, 1976, p 311.
20. Brunnstrom S: *Clinical Kinesiology,* ed 3. Philadelphia, FA Davis, 1979, p 11.
21. Farfan HF: Biomechanics of the lumbar spine. In Kirkaldy-Willis WH: *Managing Low Back Pain.* New York, Churchill Livingstone, 1983, p 21.
22. Shirazi-ADL SA, Shrivastava SC, Ahmed AM: Stress analysis of the lumbar disc body unit in compression. *Spine,* 9:120–134, 1984.
23. Farfan, HF: *Mechanical Disorders of the Low Back.* Philadelphia, Lea & Febiger, 1973, p 165.
24. Kazarian L, Graves GA: Compressive strength characteristics of the human vertebral centrum. *Spine,* 2:1–14, 1977.
25. White AA, Panjabi MM: *Clinical Biomechanics of the Spine.* Philadelphia, JB Lippincott, 1978, p 170.
26. Yang KH, King AI: Mechanism of facet load transmission as a hypothesis of low-back pain. *Spine,* 9:557–565, 1984.
27. Turek SL: *Orthopedics Principles and Their Application,* ed 3. Philadelphia, JB Lippincott, 1977, p 740.
28. Helfet AJ, Gruebel Lee DM: *Disorders of the Lumbar Spine.* Philadelphia, 1978, p 161.
29. Cassidy JD, Potter GE: Motion examination of the lumbar spine. *JMPT* 2:3, 1979.

CHAPTER 3

Principles of Chiropractic

One question was always uppermost in my mind in my search for the cause of disease. I desired to know why one person was ailing and his associate, eating at the same table, working in the same shop, at the same bench was not. D. D. Palmer

The principles upon which chiropractic are based were Daniel David Palmer's answer to the question above (1). His questions and conclusions are not dissimilar to those outlined by Hans Selye (2). Selye noted that the patients whom he observed as a young medical student all exhibited the same characteristics of illness, which he termed the "syndrome of just being sick." Palmer concluded that disease was due to interference with the nervous system, primarily at the site where the spinal nerves exit the intervertebral foramen. He attributed interference with normal nerve function to approximation of vertebrae, which he termed subluxation (1). Selye, half a century later, explored the body's response to stress, determining that failure of the immune system through the mediating effects of the neuroendocrine system is responsible for disease.

The nervous system and the endocrine system both play important roles in the body's resistance to disease. While the relationship of biomechanical lesions of the spine to the function of these two mediating systems has not been adequately studied, recent research (3) has demonstrated the profound effect that the nervous system has on the body's ability to fight disease, primarily through the immune response.

Traditional chiropractic theories center on the overriding effect of the nervous system in maintaining health. Health is seen by chiropractors as a continuously active homeostatic process that maintains a disease-free state. Palmer (1) has defined health as "that condition of the body in which all the functions are performed in a normal degree," and he stressed the importance of the nervous system in "running the bodily functions" (1).

The role of the nervous system and its interplay with the endocrine system in maintaining homeostasis is universally recognized. Selye (2) defined homeostasis as "the body's tendency to maintain a steady state despite external changes; physiologic stability." This fight of the body to maintain stability was described by Hippocrates as *ponos*, that is, the attempt of the body to restore itself to normal. It was understood as *vis medicatrix naturae*—the healing force of nature, which cures from within. This concept is the underlying theme in Palmer's emphasis on the "innate intelligence" of the body and its ability to maintain health.

Body homeostasis was popularized by Bernard, the French physiologist, during the second half of the nineteenth century. He stressed that one of the most characteristic features of all living things is the ability to maintain the constancy of their internal milieu, despite changes in their surroundings. This power to maintain constancy was subsequently termed homeostasis by Cannon, a Harvard physiologist. Disease then is not just suffering but a battle to maintain the homeostatic balance of tissues despite damage (2).

The concept of holistic health care that is based on the body's power of self-regulation and the coordination of organs and functions is becoming increasingly popular (4–6). The current prevailing model, based on the germ theory popularized by Pasteur, is in contrast to this approach. Throughout the history of medicine there has been controversy concerning the internal versus the external determinants of health and disease. This problem was pivotal to D. D. Palmer's model of chiropractic.

The answer to Palmer's question above is related to the host's resistance. This resistance is dependent upon the immune response, mediated through the neuroendocrine system. Recent investigations have focused upon the psychophysiological interactions that are thought to be responsible for the observed individual variability in susceptibility to disease. Among the most pressing issues in current research and clinical practice is how excess emotional stress induces disease, and why the same stress triggers different disorders in some individuals, while others remain totally unaffected and healthy.

It appears now that the role played by the nervous system in the prevention of disease was not overstated by Palmer's challenging concepts. If the human body is to operate at its full potential, the nervous system must function effectively to control and coordinate every cell, organ, and structure in the body, in order to adapt the organism to its environment. There is no part of the human body that is not in some way interrelated neurohumerally with every other part of the body. The individual's ability to deal with stress is contingent upon an intact neuroendocrine system regulating the host's immune response.

The major factors in holistic, preventative medicine are appraisals of health status, life-style change, and management of stress, diet, and exercise. These factors work to support the life force (i.e., Palmer's "innate intelligence") and to promote patient health, as opposed to the traditional role of medicine, working to cure disease. This essence of holistic health care is the position strongly advocated by the chiropractic profession. Holistic health care does not rely on technological intervention but rather seeks to promote the body's innate ability to heal itself. The chiropractor promotes this through normalization of nervous system function through spinal manipulative therapy, in addition to modification of the patient's life-style.

SELYE'S STRESS THEORY

Selye discussed the generalized and localized effects of stress on the body. He saw stress (2) as anything that causes marked deviation from the normal resting state in the active organs. He stated that by stress "the physician means the common results of exposure to anything." This includes "nervous tension, physical injury, infection, cold, heat, x-rays and anything else" (2).

Palmer (1) similarly concluded that "direct traumatism, poisons or auto-suggestion" resulted in vertebral displacements, which lead to disease. Selye's model for the general response of the body to stress he called the "general adaptation syndrome" (GAS). He described three stages of response to stress. Regardless of the type of stress involved, the body responds in the same manner with adrenocortical enlargement, thymicolymphatic involution, and intestinal ulcers. He further stated that the body reacts to stress in a triphasic response (2) beginning with the alarm reaction, followed by the stage of resistance, and finally, if the body's resistance becomes depleted, by the stage of exhaustion. He outlined the part played by the nervous system and the endocrine system in the maintenance of resistance during stress. The "general adaptation syndrome" includes many and diverse physiological reactions to various stressors (2). The localized response of a body part to stress he termed the "local adaptation syndrome" (2), which also develops in three stages. These stages are characterized mainly by inflammation, degeneration, and death of cell groups in the directly affected part.

A primary concept in Selye's stress theory is that of adaptation energy (2). He believed that the body possesses hidden reserves of adaptability. When local reserves of adaptation energy have been depleted, local exhaustion begins and activity of the area ceases. He saw this as a protective mechanism in which more adaptation energy can be made available, either from less readily accessible local stores or from reserves in other parts of the body. Only when all of the adaptability is depleted does irreversible general exhaustion and death follow.

PSYCHONEUROIMMUNOLOGY

The idea that mental states influence the body's susceptibility to and recovery from disease has long been recognized, if not by organized medicine, certainly by the practitioners of folk medicine. From the witch doctor's exorcism to the well-publicized recovery of Norman Cousins through laughter and the use of vitamin C, there is empirical evidence that the mind effects healing (7).

Factors in the Immune Response

The first line of defense against bacteria and viruses, when the skin is breached, is the phagocyte. These scavenging white blood cells literally devour the transgressor. The phagocyte acts in a general manner, indiscriminately scavenging the invader.

A more specialized type of defense involves highly specific chemical counterattacks. The basic functional units of this immunity are the lymphocytes, which are found in the reticuloendothelial system, lymph, and blood. There are two types of lymphocytes, both of which are derived from bone marrow. Those that remain in the marrow until they reach full maturity are designated B cells, while others migrate to the thymus early in their development, becoming T cells. Both types of lymphocytes circulate through the blood stream before they are stored in the lymphoid tissue of the spleen, tonsils, and adenoids, where they remain inactive until exposed to any one of thousands of antigens such as viruses, bacteria, toxins, and even organic waste.

When exposed to a particular antigen, the B cells synthesize and release proteins known as antibodies, which are designed specifically to destroy that antigen. The T cells respond to antigens as support cells, by releasing lymphokines, chemicals that assist the B cells in producing antibodies. Other T cells directly attack antigens by releasing chemicals that are lethal to the antigens. Some become suppressors, protecting the body's tissue from being ravaged by its own immune response. Failure of the suppressor T cells leads to autoimmune diseases in which the body literally attacks itself.

In addition to these functions, the T cells become chemical mediators, which release histamine. Histamine dilates blood vessels in preparation for the invasion of lymphocytes and complement proteins, which creates an increase in temperature. This action causes inflammation, which is inhospitable to foreign substances. Prostaglandins and leukotrienes are also released, which control the function of the T cells and other phagocytes called macrophages.

The complexity of the immune response is now known to be heavily influenced by the central nervous system via the neuroendocrine response and the autonomic nervous system. These biochemical pathways are controlled by the hypothalamus, which directly affects the pituitary and adrenal glands.

The neurotransmitters that carry the electrical impulses between the nerve cells in the brain mediate the hypothalamic-pituitary-adrenal axis. These compounds, including serotonin, acetylcholine, and norepinephrine regulate the secretion of corticotropin-releasing factors from the hypothalamus. These same neurotransmitters control the immune system through the autonomic nervous system. Branches of the autonomic nervous system which secrete norepinephrine and acetylcholine directly affect lymphatic tissue. Autonomic fibers also occur in the spleen, bone marrow, lymph nodes, and thymus. These neural fibers follow blood vessels into the glands and radiate into fields profuse with T cells. Adrenalin, norepinephrine, and acetylcholine receptors have been identified on the surfaces of lymphocytes.

Immunotransmitters provide a feedback loop through the hypothalamic-pituitary-adrenal axis. This mechanism is mediated through the influence of adrenocorticotrophic hormone and β-endorphin, an internally manufactured opiate; lymphokines and cytokines, the chemical products of macrophages; and the hormones such as thymosins, which are synthesized in the thymus (8). Psychosocial stresses have been examined through the chemical links between emotions and the immune response (9, 10).

Leach (11) has recently outlined the current research supporting the neurodystrophic hypothesis, which holds that immunity is influenced directly by neuroendocrine factors as well as by direct neural modulation. He asks "If psychosocial stresses can influence immunological competence by acting through neuroendocrine or direct neural mecha-

nism, why couldn't the intervertebral subluxation?" His conclusion is that "there is overwhelming evidence to support the chiropractic neurodystrophic hypothesis, but there is scant evidence to directly link the vertebral lesion with immunologic competence in human clinical studies." Much work remains to conclusively demonstrate if such a link exists. However, research is increasingly supportive of the Palmer theory that a sound nervous system is a major factor determining health. In the final analysis, it appears highly likely that the subluxation complex, through its effect on the nervous system, does play a role in immunological competence.

SUBLUXATION COMPLEX

Homewood, (12) in the classic chiropractic text *The Neurodynamics of the Vertebral Subluxation*, has described the mechanism by which the disrelationship of vertebral segments and other articulations may result in widespread functional derangement and the tissue changes of disease. Expanding on Palmer's theory on the causes of disease: traumatism, poison and autosuggestion, Homewood discusses these causes as mechanical, chemical, and mental stresses; which create the structural distortions that interfere with nerve supply and result in altered function to the point of demonstrable cellular changes known as pathology (12).

Under mechanical causes of subluxation he includes direct trauma such as falls, strains from lifting, postural stresses, occupational distortions, and automobile accidents. He states, "The site of the actual subluxation is likely to be pre-ordained by the structural weakness, of post-history of injury, postural, occupational, or recreational abuses which may have produced frank trauma or merely microtraumata which tend to summate, or by mechanical force being concentrated upon a localized area" (12).

Chemical irritants or poisons he describes as producing subluxation through viscerosomatic reflexes. Such chemicals, entering through the gastrointestinal system and respiratory tracts, etc., and those produced by faulty metabolism or microorganisms produce an irritability of the patient's nervous system, which causes viscerosomatic irritability and subluxation (12).

Mental stresses are seen to produce muscular tension of a psychogenic nature, creating localized subluxations in the regions of the spine under greatest total strain. The upper cervical postvertebral tension and the headache occasioned by worry, prolonged concentration, or the stress of a protracted meeting in a supercharged atmosphere of unpleasant emotion and cigarette smoke are given as examples (12).

He concluded that "the chiropractic physician, through his most astute structural analysis, may locate the problem and with great skill restore the function of an articular kinetic aberration, but the response of the nervous system is beyond his power

Table 3.1 The Subluxation Complex[a]

Subluxation Complex → Kinesiopathology → Neuropathophysiology → Patholody

Axiom—manipulation (adjustment) of a subluxation normalizes vertebral motion segment fixation, optimizes physiological processes and homeostasis, and thus reverses pathology.

Kinesiopathology
    Joint fixation—Hypomobility
                    —Compensation (change in axis of rotation)
                    —Adjacent hypermobility (pain-spasm-pain)
Neuropathophysiology
    Neural irritation   Ant. horn—muscle hypertonicity
    (facilitation)   Lat. horn—sympathetic vasomoter changes
                        Post. horn—sensory changes
    Neural pressure   Ant. horn—muscle atrophy (weakness)
    (inhibition)   Lat. horn—sympatheticotonia
                        Post. horn—sensory loss (numbness)
Histopathology
    Biochemical changes—LAS
        Inflammation (histamines, kinins, prostaglandins)
        Degeneration
        Death of cell groups
    GAS and neuroimmune responses
        Alarm—endorphin release, neuroimmune response
        Resistance—hypothalamo-pituitary-adrenal activators
        Exhaustion—systemic dysfunction

Chiropractic Therapeutic Approach
  Manipulation and other forms of manual therapy are used to reverse kinesiopathology. Adjunctive procedures are used to reduce inflammation and reverse the histopathology. Life-style changes are recommended to prevent reccurance of the subluxation complex. Management of emotional and occupational stress, diet, and exercise are promoted. Regular motion palpation examinations are recommended to discover early aberrant motion, especially fixations to prevent the subluxation complex from developing. The patient's prognosis will depend on the reversibility of the pathology and the restoration of normal physiology through reduction of the kinesiopathology of the neuromusculoskeletal system.

[a]Modified from. Faye LJ: Spinal motion palpation and clinical considerations of the lumbar spine and pelvis. Lecture notes, Motion Palpation Institute, Huntington Beach, CA, 1986, p 2.

to influence in the manner desired, and the end-result rests exclusively with the neural response" (12).

Building on Homewood's work, Faye (13) has formulated a model based on the scientific principles of chiropractic, which he has termed the subluxation complex (Table 3.1). The rationale for this model is that chiropractic manipulation (adjustment) restores normal physiological motion to joints that have been fixed and their adjacent tissues compromised. This is in contrast to the static concept developed by B. J. Palmer that the adjustment realigns a bony misalignment that has caused nerve compression (11).

The subluxation complex encompasses elements of the kinesiopathology of joints and muscles, neuropathophysiology, and the biochemical effects of histopathology. The prognosis for the patient depends upon the reversibility of the pathophysiological elements of the subluxation complex. This holistic approach emphasizes the totality of each individual patient, as opposed to the simplistic and unrealistic view of the patient with "a bone out of place."

The rationale for the application of chiropractic manipulation goes beyond the simple restoration (normalization) of joint movement. This rationale also implies that the subluxation complex leads to pathophysiology, which in turn leads to pathology.

This theory of the neurobiological mechanism of manipulative therapy is outlined in the following postulate elucidated by Haldeman (14).

Manipulative therapy →	Change in the musculoskeletal system →	Change in the nervous system →	Effect on organ dysfunction, tissue pathology, or symptom complex

While the evidence to support this sequence is not conclusive, the reflex connections have been documented from somatic and visceral nerve stimulation (15–16). What remains to be tested is the influence that manipulation has on these reflexes.

Components of the Subluxation Complex

Neuropathophysiology

The subluxation complex is based on the model that spinal joint fixation compromises neural elements, which produces irritation and/or compression of these structures. Nerve irritation results in increased neuronal activity through facilitation, while pressure that produces nerve compression leads to tissue degeneration. Both nerve pressure and facilitation may have far-reaching effects, by chronic and excessive activation of the sensory, motor, and autonomic neurological mechanism.

Nerve Irritation.   Korr (17–26) has written extensively on the clinical significance of the facilitated state. His hypothesis is that the spinal cord segments adjacent to the fixed vertebral motion segment have at least some of the neurons mediating sensory, motor, and autonomic function maintained in a state of hyperexcitability. This facilitated state thereby produces exaggerated activity, which influences the tissues that are innervated by the neurons.

Facilitation of the anterior horn cells effects motor outflow, leading to sustained muscular tensions, postural asymmetries, and limited and painful motion. The richly innervated muscles, tendons, ligaments, and joint capsules may subsequently produce intense and exaggerated streams of afferent impulses with resultant pain. This facilitation of posterior horn cells expedites impulses to the central nervous system, including the higher center, magnifying noxious or painful stimuli. Pain impulses may refer locally to perpetuate muscle spasm or ascend via secondary interneurons to the brainstem reticular formation, which projects back to the fusimotor neurons. Some impulses continue to ascend to the thalamus, where they are relayed to the primary somatosensory cortex and the associated areas of the cortex, where they are then interpreted and characterized as pain. This disproportionate neurological activity ultimately produces a functional pathology, which frequently manifests as myofascial trigger points, painful muscle spasm, and restricted motion.

Facilitation of the lateral horn cells effects autonomic outflow, which may have deleterious effects on target tissues including the viscera, blood vessels, and glands. Korr (26) has summarized the large body of clinical and experimental literature on the significance of chronic hyperactivity of the innervating sympathetic pathways that produce a variety of syndromes. Chronic hyperactivity of the innervating sympathetic nervous system seems to be a prevailing theme in many clinical conditions involving many organs and tissues. Areas of sympathetic hyperactivity correlate well with segmental distribution and existing musculoskeletal strain, trauma, deep and superficial tenderness, and electromyographic activity of paraspinal muscles.

Similar signs of sympathetic activity have been found to be associated with visceral pathology, apparently in areas of referred pain and tenderness segmentally related to visceral pathology (26). A classic example of sympathetic hyperactivity that produces a pathophysiological state is vasospastic hypertension. Iriuchijima's (27) studies indicated a much higher efferent impulse traffic in the splanchnic nerves of hypertensive rats than in normotensive rats. Sympathetic hyperactivity caused by irritative factors of the subluxation complex may result in tissue and organ pathology (Chapter 14).

Nerve Compression.   More commonly recognized than nerve irritation, within the chiropractic profession, has been the hypothesis that subluxation causes nerve compression (11). This concept while not original to D. D. Palmer, has been discussed by him as follows: "When a nerve is interfered with by pressure or other injury, sooner or later its expression becomes abnormal, manifesting in disease" (1).

While Palmer espoused the idea that subluxed vertebrae can cause nerve pressure, he was under the impression that nerve compression caused both facilitation and degeneration. This theme prevails in his writing.

> Pressure on nerves usually excites, irritates, thereby creating too much an excess of nerve force at the peripheral nerve endings.
> Pressure upon any portion of the nervous system, whether of the brain, spinal cord or its nerve branches increases or impairs its carrying capacity of impulses, deranging the sensory nerve, or causing too much or not enough functionating. [sic] An organ so delicate and sensitive refuses to perform its function properly when encroached upon.

Nerve root pressure caused by bony impingement at the intervertebral foramina was understood by Galen in the second century. This concept was emphasized by Sunderland (28).

> In accord with Galen's dictum, attention will first be directed to those normal anatomical features of intervertebral foramina which constitute an essential background for the subsequent consideration in this region which disturb spinal nerve and nerve root function.

While it is generally considered that neural structures normally have ample room as they exit the intervertebral foramina (IVF), being protected and well cushioned by loose areolar tissue and adipose tissue, several factors may compromise this margin of safety. The most widely acknowledged cause of nerve compression at the IVF has been intervertebral disc pathology, including disc bulge, disc protrusion, and frank herniation with or without sequestration. This theory has been so popular that for over 40 years since Mixter and Barr (29) wrote their classic paper, disc herniation has been considered to be the primary cause of sciatica. This emphasis on the disc as the etiological factor in low back and lower extremity pain has become legendary as the "dynasty of the disc" (30).

While disc herniation can and does produce sciatica, much back and leg pain results from apophyseal subluxation (facet syndrome) produced by narrowing of the intervertebral disc. Disc narrowing allows the inferior articular process of the superior vertebra above to move inferiorly toward the pedicle of the vertebra below, reducing the dimensions of the IVF. As the medial (superior) articular pedicle is displaced downward, it stretches the capsule and presses directly on the nerve. Inflammation and osteophytic formations on the apophyseal joints may significantly alter the size of the IVF and entrap the nerve. Soft tissue compromise of the intervertebral foramen can also be produced by hypertrophy of the ligamentum flavum or by transforaminal ligaments, both of which narrow the aperture of the IVF.

The earliest neurological signs and symptoms are probably due to venous congestion, because the veins are the primary structures passing in the IVF which are to be affected. Venous congestion with impaired return of venous blood then interferes with neural transmission. Lateral recess entrapment, as the nerve root passes through an osseous-fibrous tunnel before exiting the IVF, is also a potential site of nerve pressure following pathological changes (31).

Compression affects nerve fibers both directly and indirectly. Characteristically, compression directly affects the nerve by physical deformation of nerve fibers. In extreme cases, deformation progresses to the total destruction of the compressed section of the nerve. Indirectly, nerve pressure disturbs nerve conduction by interfering with the blood supply to the nerve fibers (28). Sharpless (32) has demonstrated that dorsal nerve roots are more susceptible to compression block than peripheral nerves. It is thought that pressure due to mechanical deformation blocks longer nerve fibers first, while anoxia-producing ischemia affects small fibers first.

Effects of Nerve Compression. While nerve irritation and subsequent facilitation leads to pain, nerve pressure leads to decreased axoplasmic flow and resultant Wallerian degeneration. Clinically, we see this manifested as areflexia, motor weakness, and muscle atrophy, with sensory loss producing numbness and paresthesia. Chiropractors have long theorized involvement of the somatoautonomic reflex as a result of nerve compression (1, 33–39). Sympathetic atonia from somatovisceral reflexes appears to be a valid assumption based on the work of a number of authors including Coote (40, 41) and Sato (42) (Chapter 15).

Nonelectrical Neuronal Functions. Nonelectrical neuronal functions include axonal transport and neurotrophic phenomena. These influences are essential for the development, growth, and survival of the target cells, as well as the integrity of the neurons.

Axoplasmic transport occurs bidirectionally. Anterograde movement (transport away from the cell body) is faster than retrograde movement (toward the cell body). Anterograde volume also significantly exceeds retrograde transport in volume. The anterograde molecular materials include proteins, phospholipids, enzymes, glycoproteins, and neurotransmitter precursors. Axoplasmic transport depends primarily on the integrity of the intracellar microtubular system, which can be compromised by mechanical deformation. If the target organs, muscles, and glands are deprived of the neurotrophic substances, they atrophy and die. When target cells are deprived of their neuronal contact, they become hypersensitive to their usual neurotransmitter substance, resulting in hypersensitivity.

When mechanical impingement on a neuron interferes with axoplasmic transport, deprivation of the molecular materials to the target organ leads to a loss of organ function and concomitant restriction of the retrograde trophic supply to the neural cell body. The works of Korr (25) show that deformation of nerves and roots (compression, stretching, angulation, and torsion), which are known to occur all too commonly in the human, are likely to disturb the intraaxonal transport mechanisms, intraneural microcirculation, and the blood-nerve barrier. He postulates that neural structures are especially vulnerable in their passage over highly mobile joints, through bony canals, intervertebral foramina, fascial layers, and tonically contracted muscles (e.g., the posterior rami of spinal nerves and spinal extensor muscles). He concludes that many of these biomechanically induced deformations are subject to manipulative amelioration and correction.

Kinesiopathology

If the rationale for chiropractic manipulation is the restoration of joint mobility, then the fundamentals of kinesiopathology must be thoroughly understood. Chiropractic manipulation has been defined as a passive maneuver in which specifically directed manual forces are applied to vertebral or extravertebral articulations of the body, with the object of restoring mobility to restricted areas (43). Following this line of thinking, manipulation should apply a mobilizing force to areas of the spine that are fixed or hypomobile (44). The successful manipulation thus restores restricted mobility while avoiding areas of hypermobility or instability (45) (Table 3.2).

Definition of Joint Fixation. Gillet has defined a spinal fixation as "the element which in a subluxation holds the vertebra in its abnormal placement and hinders its normal movement" (46). He considered joint fixation not only as the element that produces the displacement, but also as the factor that the manipulative thrust eliminates, permitting the vertebra to regain its normal resting position. Sandoz (47) has stated "by fixation we mean a state whereby a vertebra or a pelvic bone has become temporarily immobilized in a position which it may normally occupy during any phase of a physiological spinal movement." While Sandoz classifies a fixation as a type of subluxation, Illi (as quoted by Sandoz), equates the term subluxation with joint fixation. He defines a subluxation, therefore, as "the immobilization of a vertebra in a position of movement when the spine is at rest, or in a position of rest when the spine is in movement."

With the ambiguity surrounding the term subluxation, the ACA classification of subluxation (48), with fixation forming a category within that classifi-

Table 3.2 A Model for Spinal Kinesiology[a]

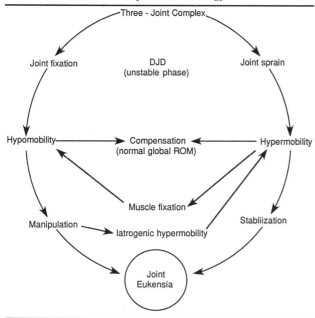

[a]The successful manipulation restores restricted mobility while avoiding areas of hypermobility. (Gatterman, Goe, Panzer)

Table 3.3 American Chiropractic Association Classification of Subluxation[a]

Static intersegmental subluxations
1. Flexion malposition
2. Extension malposition
3. Lateral flexion malposition
4. Rotational malposition
5. Anterolisthesis (spondylolisthesis)
6. Retrolisthesis
7. Lateral listhesis
8. Altered interosseous spacing (decreased or increased)
9. Osseous foraminal encroachments
Kinetic Intersegmental Subluxations
1. Hypomobility (fixation subluxation)
2. Hypermobility (loosened vertebral motion segment)
3. Aberrant motion
Sectional Subluxation
1. Scoliosis and/or alterations of curves secondary to muscular imbalance
2. Scoliosis and/or alterations of curves secondary to structural asymmetries
3. Decompensation of adaptational curvatures
4. Abnormalities of motion
Paravertebral subluxations
1. Costovertebral and costotransverse disrelationships
2. Sacroiliac subluxations

[a]This classification of subluxation is based on the internal disrelationship of the vertebral motion segement.

cation, is more useful (Table 3.3). This allows the chiropractor the freedom to treat a variety of subluxations with various types of therapy, reserving spinal manipulation for the correction of joint fixations. The aim of manipulative therapy is not to reposition a displaced vertebra, but to remove the

obstacle that prevents normal movement at that vertebral motion segment.

Causes of Joint Fixation. A number of theories about the cause of joint locking or fixation have been discussed. Gillet (46) suggests that there are three stages of joint fixation, which begins with muscular hypertonicity, progresses to ligamentous shortening, and results in articular adhesions. Other authors have suggested mechanical joint locking, disc displacement, and intraarticular jamming of various tissues as the mechanism for blockage of articular movement.

Fixation Due to Muscle Hypertonicity. The concept that restricted segmental movement can be caused by hypertonicity of the short spinal muscles has been popular with a number of authors (47, 49–57). Indeed, Smith, Langworthy and Paxson (49), in 1906, discussed the change in the field of vertebral motion when there is a change from normal muscle tonicity. Downing (50), in 1923, described the palpatory consistency of the muscles of the vertebral lesions as having a doughy, inelastic quality, with areas of firmer or "knot-like" contractural masses within the muscles. He describes these areas as being exquisitely hypersensitive. This description is consistent with the trigger points described more recently by Nimmo (58), Mennell (59), and Travell and Simons (60) (Chapter 12).

Role of Muscle in Joint Stabilization. While the primary function of muscles is to produce movement, muscles can also effectively restrict motion, and the same contractile forces that produce movement can also oppose it. A swinging limb is thus controlled by muscle force that regulates, resists, retards, and arrests motion. The energy-absorbing capabilities of skeletal muscle is no less important to the control of motion than its energy-imparting function, both of which depend on muscle contraction.

Coordination between agonists and antagonists is the result of reciprocal innervation. This reciprocal reflex mechanism provides the fine muscle coordination necessary to prevent joint damage, especially during fast movement. At the end of fast movement, the active inhibition of the antagonist changes to rapid facilitation and contraction in order to slow movement and prevent injury (55).

Voluntary movement of the spine is produced by the long spinal muscles (Chapter 1), which provide the force necessary for the global movements of spinal flexion, extension, lateral flexion, rotation, and circumduction. Movement at the segmental level is produced by short intersegmental muscles, the interspinales, intertransversarii, rotatores, and deep fibers of the multifidus. These intersegmental muscles cannot be controlled voluntarily. They appear to serve as vertebral motion segment stabilizers during spinal motion (61) and have been implicated by a number of authors as factors in spinal articular blockage. Grice (53) has demonstrated decreased muscle activity following manipulation, which supports this theory.

Two reflex systems have been suggested as mechanisms whereby the muscle hypertonicity that produces restricted motion of a joint is relieved by manipulation. The first is the stretch reflex, which involves the muscle spindle of the intersegmental muscles. The second implicates the arthrokinetic reflex and involves both the joint receptors and the intersegmental muscles.

Muscle Spindle–Muscle Spasm Cycle. Korr (54) attributes the intersegmental muscle spasms and fixation of joints to aberrant muscle-spindle activity. He concludes that the muscle spindle as the coordinator of muscle activity may increase or decrease muscle contraction. Accordingly, if the vertebral attachments of the short spinal muscles are approximated by unguarded movement and silence annulospiral receptor activity, the lack of input to the CNS then results in a turning up of the γ-motoneuron "gain," increasing the intensity of the muscle contraction producing the muscle spasm. Due to this contraction, the vertebral attachments cannot resume their normal positon, and the muscle spasm is perpetuated. Sandoz (56) points out that unlike a spasm in the calf muscle these involuntary muscles cannot be stretched by voluntary contraction of the antagonists, which in the leg can place the spastic muscle under stretch.

Both Korr (54) and Sandoz (56) have theorized that the Golgi tendon end organs (GTO) may provide the mechanism whereby muscle spasm–producing joint fixation is relieved by manipulation. These GTO receptors act as brakes and limit excessive joint movement by initiating a reflex inhibition of motor activity in muscles operating over the joint. It is feasible that a high-velocity manipulative thrust performed at the extreme of the restricted joint's motion activates the Golgi tendon organs inhibiting muscle activity, thereby reducing muscle spasm.

Arthrokinetic Reflex. Wyke (62) has determined that the mechanoreceptors located in the spinal joints are major contributors to postural and kinesthetic sensations, along with input from the labyrinth, eyes, and skin. He refers to this joint regulation of postural muscle tone as the arthrokinetic reflex. The intersegmental spinal muscles are capable of reacting individually to nociceptor and mechanoreceptor stimuli arising in individual vertebral motion segments. The crucial point of Wyke's theory is that afferent input from the nociceptors (type IV receptors) is inhibited by static and dynamic mechanoreceptors (type I and II receptors). This inhibition may be a form of presynaptic inhibition. If stimulation of type I and/or type II receptors yield inhibition of the type IV nociceptors, stretching of the apophyseal joint would reduce the nociceptive input at the anterolateral spinothalamic tract and thereby reduce pain (Table 3.4).

Joint Sprain–Muscle Spasm Cycle. It is essential that we distinguish movement restriction due to primary muscle spasm from tonic protective reflexes, which are designed to protect sprained (hypermobile) joints. This distinction can be determined clinically by patient response to manipulative therapy (63).

Joint fixation due to primary muscle hypertonicity responds rapidly to spinal mainipulative therapy and requires relatively few treatments. If a patient fails to respond favorably to manipulation in 12 visits or less, then one should consider the possibility that joint restriction is due to a tonic protective reflex, which minimizes nociceptor activity in joints that have been sprained. Repeated manipulation of hypermobile joints is contraindicated, even though manipulation brings temporary relief from pain. While this relief may last up to several hours, the patient will be worse in the long run, becoming increasingly dependent on palliative care that in itself worsens the hypermobility through the continued stretching of joint capsules. These sprained joints must then be chronically protected by further reflex muscle spasm, which perpetuates the pain-spasm-pain cycle.

Lewit (44) reminds us that "the motor system constitutes not only the greatest part of the human body" but also "the great majority of pain patients treated in pain centers by anaesthesiologists and psychiatrists i.e. pharmacologically and psychologically have undiagnosed problems of the motor system." Unfortunately this failure to recognize and diagnose muscle syndromes is all too common in the chiropractic profession as well.

It is essential that we distinguish movement restriction caused by muscle spasm due to the tonic reflexes that protect sprained hypermobile joints from restriction produced by muscle spindle and Golgi tendon organ interaction. Lewit (64) has demonstrated that segmental movement restriction is not caused solely by muscle spasm. He has found that restricted joint motion remained unaltered in the cervical spines of ten patients who were examined during narcosis with myorelaxants. In all cases the movement restriction remained unchanged and was even more easily recognizable.

If spinal articular blockage were due to muscle spasm alone, one would expect that many of the cases of acute joint fixation that respond to manipulation would respond equally well to muscle relaxants. Clinically this does not appear to be the case, since many patients ultimately seek relief through chiropractic manipulation following a prior course of treatment with myorelaxants. Although muscle spasm is universally acknowledged as a factor in the genesis of back pain, it must be determined if it is the cause or the result of joint dysfunction and articular blockage.

Table 3.4 Articular Neurology[a]

Type	Site	Function
I	Outer layers of joint capsule	Static and dynamic mechanoreceptors responding to small increments of tension in the joint capsule, slow adapting
II	Deeper subsynovial layers of joint capsule articular fat pads	Dynamic mechanoreceptor that responds at the moment of increased tension, inactive in immobile joints, rapidly adapting
III	Surface of collateral and intrinsic joint ligaments	Responds only to high tension (activated by forceful manipulation and/or high-traction forces)
IV	Joint capsule articular fat pads, adventitial sheath of articular blood vessels and collateral and intrinsic joint ligaments	High-threshold, nonadapting nociceptors irritated by the development of abnormal mechanical or chemical (inflammatory) changes

[a]Modified from Wyke BD: Articular neurology and manipulative therapy. In Glasgow EF, Twomey LT, Scull ER, Kleynhans AM, Idczak RM (eds): *Aspects of Manipulative Therapy*, ed 2. New York, Churchill Livingstone, 1985

Joint Fixation due to Ligamentous Shortening

As previously stated, Gillet (46) discusses the etiology of joint immobility as a progressive degenerative process, with ligamentous shortening occurring in the wake of long-standing muscular hypertonicity, in which the contiguous parts of adjacent vertebrae are pulled together. Smith, Langworthy, and Paxson (49) also consider the inequality of tension in ligaments as a factor in subluxations, particularly in the upper cervical region. Downing (50) discussed the osteopathic lesion as a bony subluxation with ligamentous tension or shortening as well as muscular tension or contractures. Grice (52) suggests that if ligaments are involved with contracture, then mobilizing procedures and dynamic stretch techniques are indicated, because the tensile strength of ligamentous tissue is considerably greater than that of bone; therefore, a short, sharp thrust of uncontrolled amplitude may be more apt to produce an avulsion fracture than the desired stretch.

Articular Adhesion. Gillet (46), in his discussion of the degenerative process, suggests that the continued retraction of shortened ligaments progresses to the point at which the restrictive element is probably "one or several adhesions" in the interarticular space. Mennell (65) also discusses therapeutic manipulation to break intraarticular joint or capsular adhesions.

Stoddard (66) feels that the concept of joint lesion (as distinct from a bone displacement) is much more valid. He attributes the joint lesion to adhesions that form following a joint sprain, with unilateral restriction of bending toward one side and ligamentous shortening affecting apophyseal joints. He describes the adhesions as factors that hold vertebrae more to one side, which gives rise to positional variations. Adhesive capsulitis results from an acute inflammation of the synovial membrane, with exudation and subsequent formation of adhesions between folds of synovium, its connective tissue, bone, and the capsule.

Fibrous adhesions may result from both trauma and immobilization. Adhesions due to trauma result from inflammation and subsequent repair, with an increase in collagen leading to the formation of "scar tissue" or fibrosis. This process is consistent throughout the connective tissue of the body (67).

Articular adhesions that occur following joint immobilization are due to a reduction in glycosaminoglycans, a decrease in water content, and an increase in the intermolecular cross-links in the collagen fibers (68). It is possible that manipulation of joints fixed by articular adhesions severs the cross-links formed during immobilization, without a resultant inflammatory reaction that would only lead to further articular adhesions.

Fisk (69) feels, however, that it is most unlikely that manipulation breaks adhesions, since this would be a very painful procedure. He states rather that manipulation works in relieving something that is trapped, jammed, or blocked.

Joint Fixation Due to Intraarticular Jamming

Meniscoid fragments or small discs that become incarcerated in the apophyseal joints, or villi of synovial membrane which project into the articular space, are considered the etiological factor in facet joint locking by Schmorl and Junghans (70). They describe a disc-like tissue in the joint space, similar to menisci in other places of the body.

Meniscoids are wedge-shaped, intraarticular structures, attached by their base to the capsule, with their free border directed toward the inside of the joint cavity. They vary in size, and this variation appears to be related to the degree of mobility of the joint, with the greatest development of meniscoids in joints with much mobility. Histologically, meniscoids consist of synovial tissue with adipose backing at the base, and they appear to increase the congruence of the articular surfaces during movements.

Kraft and Levinthal (71) described redundancy of the capsule, particularly accompanying coronal-facing facets, in which the synovial tissue becomes pinched as analogous to the pinched infrapatellar fat pad that causes derangement of the knee. Putti, quoted by Badgley (72), described degenerative changes in the facet joints with hypertrophic villi of three to four times normal size, chondrification and ossification occasionally in the villi, detached chondral bodies, and ulcerative areas with complete loss of cartilage. Badgley also postulates that these changes in the synovial membrane and the free bodies in the joint might conceivably produce symptoms similar to those of knee joint derangement. Hadley (73) describes tabs of synovial tissue projecting inward from the facet joint margins. He suggests that "pinching of soft tissue structures between the articular surfaces would seem to be a factor in producing the 'sudden catch' spontaneous type of localized back pain."

Bogduk and Engel (74) have described zygapophyseal meniscoids as fibrous invaginations of the dorsal and ventral capsule, which probably arise as a result of mechanical stress. They conclude that the theory of meniscus entrapment has been overstated as a cause of the "acute locked back" that responds to manipulation.

Giles (75) has added support to the theory that meniscoids can become entrapped leading to blocked articular motion. He has recently demonstrated small myelinated nerves (0.6 to 12 μm) coursing through the synovial folds not in association with blood vessels, suggesting that these nerves are nociceptive. He postulates that should the synovial folds become pinched between the articulating facet surfaces of the zygapophyseal joint, they might have clinical importance as a source of back pain (76–78).

Small fragments of articular cartilage and underlying bone may be broken off the joint surface and form loose bodies, according to Harris and Macnab (79), causing recurrent or chronic pain. Further pathology affecting the posterior joints may include uneven compression of joint surfaces, with damage to the articular cartilage leading to small subchondral fractures that distort the joint surfaces permanently (80). These uneven surfaces may also be a source of joint catching.

It is debatable whether intraarticular jamming can be caused by a small fragment of incarcerated villi of synovial membrane, a meniscoid, or a fragment of articular cartilage or bone, since it has not been demonstrated that any of these structures are capable of mechanically restricting a joint. It is possible, in the case of meniscoid structures, that aberrant receptor feedback involving the arthrokinetic reflex produces muscle spasm, an additional theory on the mechanism of muscular fixation of a joint.

Joint Fixation due to Disc Displacement

Perhaps the most vocal proponent of disc displacement as the cause of spinal joint dysfunction has been Cyriax (81). He states that not all small disc displacements respond to manipulation, but that manipulation can nearly always reduce a small cartilaginous displacement. He feels that pulpy protrusions are rarely affected; however "small and very recent nuclear herniations sometimes respond, provided that the technique of manipulation is changed from the jerk to sustained pressures."

Maigne (82) alleges that the herniated disc acts as a wedge between the vertebral bodies, thereby modifying the reciprocal relationships of the posterior articulations and their functions, so that (a) they assume the position which they occupy in hyperflexion movement (the position of maximum divergence when the hernia is posterior and central) or (b) they assume an asymmetric position, which they occupy in a movement of lateroflexion (when a hernia is posterolateral). This, he states, leads to "one joint in maximum convergence the other in maximum divergence," with the discal block perpetuated by muscle spasm, which may outlast the cause of the disorder. He proposes that most of the minor vertebral derangements are due to a fragment of the nucleus pulposus, blocked in a fissure that occurs in the annulus fibrosis (dorsally, ventrally, or laterally). He feels that the blocked fragment is liberated by manipulation, which permits restoration of normal functioning to one segment (82).

Sandoz (83) implicates the disc in joint fixation, referring to the stage of nuclear or sequestral impaction as internal derangement of the disc. Leading to this stage is degeneration of the nucleus pulposus, whereby vertical compression forces are transformed into horizontal forces as the nucleus loses its hydraulic shock-absorption capabilities (Chapter 8). When the nucleus tends to become pushed toward the periphery of the disc, a simple protrusion may occur. As the vertebrae tend to shift horizontally, a shearing stress is exerted on the fibers of the annulus fibrosus, which predisposes them to tearing. He postulates that a person may suddenly change positions in such a way that a fragment of the nucleus is forced into a weakened portion of the annulus and becomes sequestered. This sequestered fragment can produce both a mechanical barrier and a nociceptive reflex muscle spasm leading to joint fixation. Manipulation frees the incarcerated nucleus sequestrum by aspirating it centripetally (84).

Reduction of lumbar disc prolapse by manipulation has been demonstrated in one study with repeated epidurography by Mathews and Yates (85). In this study, treatment by manipulation relieved the symptoms of lumbago, with reduction in the size of the visualized disc material. Cox (86), in America, and Kuo and Loh (87), in China, have more recently claimed success in treating disc lesions with spinal manipulation. Since manipulation is just as effective in atypical vertebral motion segments without discs (including the occipitoatlantal, atlantoaxial and sacroiliac joints), it appears that disc displacement is not the only obstacle in spinal joint blockage.

Mechanical Joint Locking

Coplans (88) suggests that tropism or asymmetry of the apophyseal joints causes diminished mechanical efficiency, leading to limitation of rotation, which may be readily relieved by manipulaton.

The geometrical contour of the facet joint may allow the articular facets to lock at the extreme of the physiologic position because of a sudden unguarded movement. The orientation of the articular facets in different regions of the spine varies considerably, with no facet exhibiting a truly planar surface. In addition to rotation, translation in these joints (due to the unique mechanics of the three-joint complex) allows for greater gapping than is found in the other diathrodial joints. This translation may allow the joints to separate or approximate in such a manner that they lock just slightly beyond the extreme of the normal range of motion or jam as a result of the discrepancy between the radius of the joint surface and the axis of movement (43). The concept that joint locking frequently occurs at the end point of range of motion has been formulated by other authors (46, 47, 82).

Multiple Causative Factors

Just as there are multiple causes of back pain, there may be multiple causes of articular blockage. The more commonly attributed etiological factors of joint fixation have been discussed above. Each of these theories deserves careful consideration as do other, yet undetermined, factors. Careful histological and pathological studies must be undertaken to evaluate a number of these elements. Other factors may be best determined by biomechanical analysis. Much investigation and exploration must be undertaken before the kinesiology of vertebral motion segments is understood.

Joint Hypermobility

Joint hypermobility can occur anywhere in the spine (47, 66, 89). It is commonly found in combination with hypomobility as a compensatory mechanism. In such cases the hypermobile state is secondary to joint fixation either in adjacent segments (47) or in the contralateral joint of the same vertebral motion segment (89).

Generalized (constitutional) hypermobility predisposes to joint sprains and is commonly seen in esthenic individuals who exhibit a general ligamentous laxity. Traction of the peripheral joints can be used to ascertain the individual's type of ligaments, and if all of the peripheral joints are extremely loose, then it is expected that spinal mobility will be above average (66). Such individuals typically exhibit greater than average global flexibility. Pregnancy also predisposes to physiological hypermobility, particularly in the lower lumbar and sacroiliac joints (66).

Etiology. Spinal joint hypermobility commonly results from disc degeneration (47, 66, 82) as well as ligamentous sprains. As the intervertebral disc degenerates, the adjacent vertebral bodies approximate, due to the loss of disc turgor. This produces a slackening of the ligaments, resulting in instability characterized by listhesis or slippage. This is the phase of disc instability described by Kirkaldy-Willis (90) (Chapter 8).

Vertebral joint sprain that produces segmental hypermobility is frequently the result of rapid hyperflexion and hyperextension of the neck. Common sites of hypermobility in these cases are found in the midcervical region, primarily at the C4–5 and C5–6 vertebral motion segments (91, 92) (Chapter 10). In the lumbar spine, severe hyperflexion injuries can lead to ligamentous sprain with resulting hypermobility.

Habitual ligamentous strain from faulty sitting posture, habitual standing on one leg, anatomical short leg, or repetitive movements that produce unilateral strain to one side of the body can also produce chronic ligamentous stretching (66). Hormonal change during pregnancy and the menstrual cycle also produces ligamentous stretching and joint hypermobility, primarily in the lower lumbar spine and sacroiliac joints (93–95). (Chapter 7). Repeated forceful manipulation of the same joint can lead to iatrogenic hypermobility (96), especially long-lever, nonspecific manipulation, which tractions the entire length of the spine, exerting stretch of the hypermobile, weak ligaments first (66).

Hypermobile joints should not be manipulated (43, 45, 95, 97) because this only aggravates the patient's pain (66). Gillet (98) has found that severe irritation is not caused by the actual fixation itself but by the abnormal and eccentric mobility of the hypermobile side of the vertebra. This was determined by comparing palpation with hypersensitive heat readings and vasomotor variations. He determined that forcing movement upon such hypermobile articulations invariably increased the signs of irritation. The rationale for using signs of nerve irritation as criteria for spinal manipulative therapy is therefore questionable. This also supports the theory that the temporary relief obtained by the manipulation of hypermobile segments results in an increase in the pain-spasm-pain cycle, which iatrogenically perpetuates the patient's chronic pain.

Symptoms of Joint Hypermobility. The pain of a hypermobile joint is typically a dull, diffuse ache (66), accompanied by sustained muscle spasm to protect the joint. The ligaments are tender if they are accessible to palpation, and pain is elicited through sustained stretching of the involved joint.

Palpatory findings of joint hypermobility, in addition to bilateral comparison of spinal and pelvic joints, include a boggy, squashy, unphysiological feel to joint motion. The amplitude of movement is greater than expected, and end-feel may not be encountered. Joint range of motion is greater than that on the contralateral side, which exhibits normal end-feel. Palpation of the hypermobile joint elicits a complaint of tenderness accompanied by excess motion.

Radiologic Findings of Joint Hypermobility. Plain films frequently show a vertebral listhesis, although this is not conclusive and may be due to joint fixation. Further evaluation of joint movement can be determined by stress films taken in the same plane at the ends of range of motion and then templated (43) (Chapter 6).

Treatment of Joint Hypermobility. Rather than repeated manipulation of the hypermobile joint, which offers temporary relief at best and creates a dependency on chiropractic care (Chapter 4), stabilization of the involved joint brings successful relief of symptoms. A support belt in the lumbar region (Chapter 8) and a cervical collar (Chapter 10) for the neck may be utilized. The patient should not be encouraged to become dependent on these supports. Hypermobility in the thoracic region (Chapter 9) may require a rib belt for stabilization, while sacroiliac hypermobility (Chapter 7) should be stabilized by use of a trochanteric belt. Stabilization should ideally restrict excessive motion only, while allowing normal motion. Treatment to reduce muscle splinting brings rapid results in most cases (Chapter 12). Weight loss and improved posture through exercise and habituation (Chapter 13) will improve spinal biomechanics and reduce instability.

The importance of not thrusting into hypermobile segments must be stressed. Adhering to the concept that manipulation replaces a displaced segment is fraught with danger, for it may be the hypermobile segment that appears malaligned on the static x-ray. While there is often complete relief of pain following manipulation of a hypermobile segment, this effect results from relaxation of protective muscle splinting. Hypermobile articulations must be identified and avoided when applying the manipulative thrust. Manipulation of the painful joint without due consideration of the status of mobility can perpetuate the pain produced by hypermobility. Temporary relief at hypermobile joints may occur because splinting muscles are tractioned and muscle spasm is removed, but it returns as motion is introduced into the hypermobile area. The source of the pain must be treated rather than the symptom itself; the cause of the problem, rather than the effect.

Zygapophyseal Arthrology

An understanding of the structure and function of the posterior spinal joints is of prime importance to chiropractors, since spinal manipulation is directed toward removal of reversible fixations of the zygapophyseal articulations. These spinal joints are not merely the meeting place of bones. They are essential to motor function, and they are richly innervated by both proprioceptive and nociceptive fibers (99) (Table 3.4) that provide essential kinesthetic and postural information as well as being the source of much back pain (100) (Chapter 11).

Movement between individual vertebral motion segments is slight, but the summation of all the spinal joints gives a wide range of trunk and neck motion. While the absence of motion at a single facet joint does not significantly affect global flexibility, it does have far-reaching reflexogenic effects influencing muscle tone and the excitability of stretch reflexes in all the striated muscles. Wyke (99) states that

> Since the articular mechanoreceptor afferent nerve fibers give off collateral branches that are distributed intersegmentally as well as segmentally throughout the neuraxis, manipulation of an individual joint not only affects motor unit activity in the muscles operating over the joint being manipulated, but also that in more remote muscles (including muscles on the opposite side of the body). It is through this mechanism that manipulation of joints by therapists gives rise to the reflex changes in muscle tone (involving both facilitation and inhibition of motor unit activity) that have long been empirically familiar to practitioners of manipulative therapy.

Grieve (101) presents an interesting analogy, likening the specialist in spinal manipulation to a telecommunications expert as opposed to the traditional medical view of the medical manipulator as a mechanical engineer. While the medical manipulator restores normal mechanics or function to the spinal vertebrae and associated muscles, the telecommunications engineer goes far beyond the mechanical engineer. The spinal joints are richly and extensively "wired up" to the whole body by the nervous system, and skilled spinal manipulation not only corrects local problems but also influences body functions and many disease states through reflex mechanisms. Mennell (65) furthers this notion, stating

> Pain from joint pathology may be appreciated in any distant structure which shares its nerve supply with the joint. Indeed, one may postulate interference with the function of viscera as a result of referred joint pain through a somatic/visceral reflex arc. I am certain that such phenomena occur.

Characteristics of the Zygapophyseal Joints

The posterior spinal articulations are diarthrodial (synovial) joints with curved articular surfaces covered with hyaline cartilage. Each joint is encased in a thin, loose, sleeve-like ligamentous capsule lined with synovial membrane, which secretes synovial fluid. The synovial fluid normally permits frictionless and pain-free movement. Immobility is the enemy of articular cartilage because it interferes with the furnishing of nutrition by the synovial fluid as well as the removal of waste products (102, 103).

Synovial fluid is viscous, elastic, and plastic, providing a substantial layer of lubricating fluid that enhances the gliding of the joint surfaces. Synovial joints are designed to last a lifetime, but become damaged by trauma and overuse. Since it is avascular, articular cartilage depends on the diffusion of low molecular weight nutrients either from the subchondral capillaries in the underlying bone or from the synovial fluid. Studies that show healing of articular cartilage with passive continuous motion suggest that the agitation of the fluid film on the cartilage surface during exercise, is a major factor that increases the flow of nutrients (104).

Equally damaging is continuous compression of articular cartilage, which can occur when a joint is fixed in an extreme position. Mechanical stress can result in damage and death of chondrocytes when cartilage is subject to high-impact loads or abnormal loading (104). Salter (105) has stated that disorders and injuries of joints constitute the greatest single physical cause of disability in civilized man. The reversal of immobility and the restoration of normal motion in blocked spinal joints by manipulation has been empirically demonstrated to significantly reduce this disability.

PRINCIPLES OF MANIPULATION

Chiropractic manipulation (adjustment) utilizes specific short levers to which a high-velocity thrust of controlled amplitude is directed, with the aim of restoring mobility to individual articulations. A wide variety of procedures have come under the umbrella of the term manipulation. The term manual therapy more aptly describes the various procedures by which treatment utilizing the hands is directed to the neuromusculoskeletal system. Manual therapy includes such procedures as nonspecific long-lever thrusts, mobilization techniques, traction, massage, and pressure techniques such as ischemic compression (Chapter 12) and reflex therapies (i.e., Logan basic) (Chapter 7).

This is not to say that chiropractors do not employ these various modes of manual therapy. Chiropractors should not view the subluxation as a nail with the only useful tool being the hammer of manipulation. Many other procedures are at times more appropriate in dealing with spinal disorders, and they are described in other chapters. Especially important is a thorough understanding of the contraindications to manipulation (Chapter 4). In many cases the patient may benefit from another form of manual therapy when manipulation is contraindicated.

Manipulation versus Mobilization

While manipulation and mobilization have been used synonomously in the scientific literature (106), a clear distinction exists in the effects of these procedures on synovial joints. Beyond the normal range of active movement of any synovial joint, there is a small buffer zone of passive mobility (84). This is the motion referred to by Mennell (65) as joint play and is not under the control of the voluntary muscles. Absence of joint play can only be restored by inducing normal movement. Palpation of this motion produces end-feel.

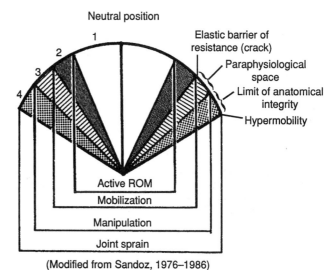

(Modified from Sandoz, 1976–1986)

Figure 3.1. Four stages of range of movement in diarthrodial joints: 1, Active range of movement (motion produced by muscular action). 2, Passive range of movement (motion produced by traction or springing the joint—joint play, up to the elastic barrier of resistance). Characterizes mobilization. 3, Paraphysiological range of movement (motion beyond the elastic barrier of resistance up to the limit of anatomical integrity produced by manipulation and accompanied by an audible release). 4, Pathological movement (motion beyond the limit of normal anatomical integrity, which damages ligaments and capsule, resulting in joint hypermobility). Manipulation that is too forceful may move the joint beyond the limit of anatomical integrity, creating or perpetuating joint instability.

End-feel is described by Lewit (63) as the springiness palpated in the final position of joint movement. This end position is never reached abruptly in a normal joint. A joint with restricted mobility has lost this springiness, and the end-feel is one of an abrupt barrier. The normal, spring-like end-feel is the result of negative or subatmospheric intraarticular pressure. This negative pressure acts to stabilize the joint surfaces in approximation. Mobilization is a passive movement that tractions the joint to the end point of this elastic barrier (the limit of end-feel).

Manipulation consists of forcing the joint beyond this elastic barrier, which produces a cracking noise as the articular surfaces suddenly move apart. The cracking noise is the result of a sudden liberation of the dissolved synovial gases (107). This liberation of gases is referred to as cavitation. Following the release of gases, there is a refractory period as the synovial gases are redissolved. During this period (approximately 20 minutes), the articular crack cannot be reproduced, and the joint has a tendency toward instability. Attempts at remanipulation during this period will not produce the familiar crack and are not recommended (84). Manipulation of the joint should be forceful enough to produce the articular

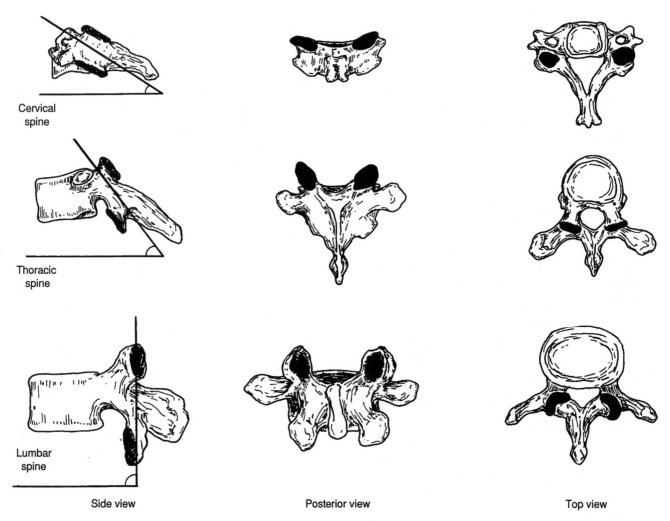

Cervical spine

Thoracic spine

Lumbar spine

Side view   Posterior view   Top view

Figure 3.2. Planes of motion of the articular facets.

crack but not so great as to separate the joint surfaces beyond their limit of anatomical integrity.

Sandoz (84) refers to the range of motion beyond the passive range and up to the limit of anatomical integrity as the paraphysiological space (Fig. 3.1). Carrying the joint movement beyond the limit of anatomical integrity results in sprain and, if extreme, dislocation. Repeated manipulations into the paraphysiological space are thought to lead to segmental instability (108).

Three physical events in manipulation that differentiate it from mobilization are (a) as the elastic barrier of the joint is passed the articular surfaces separate suddenly, (b) a cracking noise is heard, and (c) a radiolucent space appears within the joint. These findings were demonstrated by Rosten and Haines (109) in 1947. They studied the effects of a progressively increasing force taken beyond the elastic barrier in the metacarpophalangeal joint of the middle finger. The finger was first wrapped in adhesive tape and then attached to a spring dynamometer that measured the degree of tension applied to the finger. Radiographs were taken at intervals to record

changes in the joint space as the metacarpophalangeal joint was progressively tractioned. While the traction was provided by a machine rather than a manipulative thrust, the joint surfaces were separated until a cracking noise was heard. Simultaneously, a radiolucent space appeared within the joint.

It appears likely that the effects of manipulation differ significantly from those of mobilization, which may account for differences found in various studies where mobilization was used instead of manipulation (108). In evaluating the efficacy of manipulation, the patient must have truly received manipulation, not mobilization.

Indications for Chiropractic Manipulation

The primary indication for spinal manipulation is a reversible mechanical derangement of the intervertebral joint which produces a barrier to normal motion. This movement restriction has been referred to as joint fixation (12, 13, 43, 46, 47, 51, 52, 84, 86), joint locking (65, 66, 70) or joint blockage (65) that

Table 3.5 Hypothesized Effects of Intervertebral Subluxation

Primary			
		Intervertebral subluxation	
Secondary			
Somatic afferent bombardment	Spinal cord compression	Spinal nerve root compression	Vertebrobasilar arterial insufficiency
Tertiary			
Aberrant somatosomatic reflexes	Aberrant somatoautonomic reflexes		Axoplasmic aberration
Quaternary			
		Neurodystrophic phenomena	

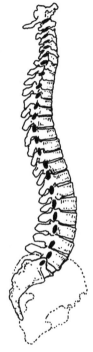

Figure 3.3. Plane line of the facet articulations changes from horizontal to coronal, to sagittal, to coronal, in a caudal direction.

can be determined clinically by motion palpation (Chapter 5) and stress radiographs (Chapter 6) (44).

Motion palpation is used to detect relative movement between palpable bony landmarks. An increase or decrease in the interspinous spaces, the intercostal spaces, or the spaces between the posterior superior iliac spines and the second sacral tubercle may be palpated. Increased resistance to joint movement can also be determined by springing or tractioning the joint. Tractioning a joint along its long axis is commonly used to determine movement restriction in extremity joints. Springing a spinal joint to test for end-feel can be done by pushing the spinous process through the three planes of motion.

Biomechanics of Manipulation

The biomechanical principles of leverage and force are utilized during chiropractic manipulation. A short lever arm, although it requires more force, is employed to mobilize a specific joint that is fixed. The lever arm should be as practical and comfortable as possible (110). Because hypermobility may be present anywhere in the spine, long-lever techniques should be avoided when possible. Any traction applied to the entire length of the spine will exert its stretch on the hypermobile and weak ligaments (66) before it releases the fixed joints.

The mechanical principles of force are utilized during the thrust phase of the manipulation. The amount of force necessary to release a locked joint can be minimized by first tractioning the joint to tension. If the joint is not tractioned until all of the slack is taken out, then much of the force will be absorbed by the soft tissue surrounding it. This can be quite painful to the patient, and it is one of the most common faults of the beginning manipulator.

The direction of force is along the plane lines of the joint (Fig. 3.2), which change from the near-horizontal plane in the cervical region to the coronal plane in the thoracic region, the sagittal plane in the upper lumbar region, and back to the coronal plane in the lower lumbar region (Fig. 3.3). A force directed perpendicular to the plane lines of the joint will only jam a locked joint further and is futile.

With enough force any joint can be gapped and a release obtained, but the more forceful the thrust, the greater the likelihood of creating iatrogenic hypermobility through ligamentous sprain. The amount of force therefore should be minimized (110). The more skilled the manipulator the less force is likely to be employed.

The amplitude of the thrust refers to the arc through which the lever is operated and determines the distance the thrust is set to travel. Obviously, if the amplitude should exceed the distance of the normal articular range of the joint, then substantial damage will result.

The velocity of the thrust refers to the speed of the applied force and is defined as the time rate of change of displacement. A high-velocity thrust is less apt to precipitate muscle guarding, and less force will be required. Biomechanical principles of leverage and force indicate that the high-velocity, low-amplitude manipulative thrust requires less force, and by employing a shorter lever contact, the thrust is more specific. It was Palmer's contention that while he was not the first to practice manipulation he was the first to utilize the spinous and transverse processes as levers, thereby making spinal manipulation safer and more specific (1).

CHIROPRACTIC HYPOTHESIS

Any therapy must be based on a theory. Chiropractic therapy is based on the hypothesis that reversible joint lesions of the spine produce far-ranging effects on the human body. This is summarized in Table 3.5. Chiropractors rely on spinal manipulation (adjustment) as their primary therapeutic tool in reversing the subluxation complex. Modern chiropractic does not claim to be a total therapy, but it does adhere to the idea that biomechanical dysfunction can have a profound effect not only on the musculoskeletal system but also on the other systems of the body. While the restoration and normalization of joint motion is the mechanism of chiropractic therapy, the ultimate goal is to promote homeostasis of the body. "Our facts must be correct. Our theories need not be if they help us to discover important new facts" (111).

References

1. Palmer DD: *The Chiropractor's Adjuster: The Science, Art and Philosophy of Chiropractic.* Portland, OR, Portland Printing House, 1910, pp 11, 18, 27, 36, 72, 141, 293, 571, 674.
2. Selye H: *The Stress of Life.* New York, McGraw-Hill, 1956, pp 3, 11–12, 16, 53, 65–66, 309, 311.
3. Brooks WH, Cross RJ, Roszman TL, Markesbery WR: Neuroimmunomodulation: neural anatomical basis for impairment and facilitation. *Ann Neurol* 12:56–61, 1982.
4. Nelson WA: The holistic concept. *ACA J Chiro* 15(10):19–22, 1978.
5. Yahn G: The impact of holistic medicine, medical groups, and health concepts. *JAMA* 242:2202–2205, 1979.
6. Brown MW: Holism and chiropractic. *ACA J Chiro* 17(3):24–26, 1980.
7. Hall NR, Goldstein AL: Thinking well: the chemical links between emotions and health. *The Sciences* 26(2):34–40, 1986.
8. Blalock JE, Smith EM: A complete regulatory loop between the immune and neuroendocrine systems. *Fed Proc* 44:108–111, 1985.
9. Macek C: Of mind and morbidity: can stress and grief depress immunity? *JAMA* 248:405–407, 1982.
10. Solomon GF, Amkraut AA: Psychoneuroendocrinological effects of the immune response. *Ann Rev Microbiol* 35:155–184, 1981.
11. Leach RA: *The Chiropractic Theories: A Synopsis of Scientific Research.* Baltimore, Williams & Wilkins, 1986, pp 16, 57, 153–184.
12. Homewood AE: *The Neurodynamics of the Vertebral Subluxation,* ed 3. St. Petersburg, FL, Valkyrie Press, 1977, pp 15, 54, 72–82, 89, 94, 299.
13. Faye LJ: Spinal motion palpation and clinical considerations of the lumbar spine and pelvis. Lecture notes, Motion Palpation Institute. Huntington Beach, CA, 1986, p 2.
14. Haldeman S: The clinical basis for discussion of mechanisms of manipulative therapy. In Korr IM (ed): *The Neurobiologic Mechanisms in Manipulative Therapy.* New York, Plenum, 1978, p 55.
15. Coote AB, Downman CB, Weber WV: Reflex discharges into thoracic white rami elicited by somatic and visceral afferent excitation. *J Physiol* 202:147–159, 1969.
16. Sato H, Schmidt RF: Somatosympathetic reflexes: afferent fibers, central pathways, discharge characteristics. *Physiol Rev* 53:916–947, 1973.
17. Denslow JS, Korr IM, Krens AD: Quantitative studies of chronic facilitation in human motoneuron pools. *Am J Physiol* 150:229–238, 1947.
18. Korr IM: Skin resistance patterns associated with visceral disease. *Fed Proc* 8:87, 1949.
19. Korr IM: The concept of facilitation and its origins. *J Am Osteopath Assoc* 54:265–268, 1955.
20. Korr IM: Clinical significance of the facilitated state. *J Am Osteopath Assoc* 54:277–282, 1955.
21. Korr IM, Thomas PE: Relationship between sweat gland activity and electrical resistance of the skin. *J Appl Physiol* 10:505–510, 1957.
22. Korr IM, Thomas PE, Wright HM: Patterns of electrical skin resistance in man. *Acta Neuroveg* 17:77–96, 1958.
23. Korr IM, Wright HM, Thomas PE: Effects of experimental myofascial insults on cutaneous patterns of sympathetic activity in man. *Acta Neuroveg* 23:329–355, 1962.
24. Korr IM, Wright HM, Chace JA: Cutaneous patterns of sympathetic activity in clinical abnormalities of the musculoskeletal system. *Acta Neuroveg* 25:589–606, 1964.
25. Korr IM: The spinal cord as organizer of disease processes: some preliminary perspectives. *J Am Osteopath Assoc* 76:89–99, 1976.
26. Korr IM: Sustained sympathicatonia as a factor in disease. In Korr IM (ed): *The Neurobiologic Mechanisms in Manipulative Therapy.* New York, Plenum, 1978, pp 229–268.
27. Iriuchijima J: Sympathetic discharge rate in spontaneously hypertensive rats. *Jap Heart J* 14:350–356, 1973.
28. Sunderland S: The anatomy of the intervertebral foramen and the mechanisms of compression and stretch of nerve roots. In Haldeman S (ed): *Modern Developments in the Principles and Practice of Chiropractic.* Norwalk, CT, Appleton-Century-Crofts, 1980, pp 45, 58.
29. Mixter WJ, Barr JS: Rupture of the intervertebral disk with involvement of spinal canal. *N Engl J Med* 211:210, 1934.
30. Anderson JE: Lumbar facet arthropathy and injection: a preliminary report. *Clin J Wash Chiro Assoc* 3(1):24–27, 1985.
31. Sunderland S: Traumatized nerves, roots, and ganglia: musculoskeletal factors and neuropathological consequences. In Korr IM (ed): *The Neurobiologic Mechanisms in Manipulative Therapy.* New York, Plenum, 1978, pp 159–160.
32. Sharpless SK: Susceptibility of spinal roots to compression block. In Goldstein M (ed): *The Research Status of Spinal Manipulative Therapy.* NINCDS Monograph no 15. Bethesda, MD, US Department of Health, Education and Welfare, 1975, p 160.
33. Janse J: History of the development of chiropractic concepts; chiropractic terminology. In Goldstein M (ed): *The Research Status of Spinal Manipulative Therapy.* NINCDS Monograph no 15. Bethesda, Maryland, US Department of Health, Education and Welfare, 1975, pp 25–40.
34. Palmer BJ: *The Science of Chiropractic: Its Principles And Philosophies,* ed 4. Davenport, IA, Palmer School of Chiropractic, 1920, vol 1, p 11.
35. Carver W: *Carver's Chiropractic Analysis of Chiropractic Principles as Applied to Pathology, Relatology, Symptomology, and Diagnosis,* ed 3. Oklahoma City, Paul O Parr, 1921, vol 1, p 5.
36. Beatty HG: *Anatomical Adjustive Technique,* ed 3. Ft. Worth, Parker Chiropractic Research Foundation, 1983, p 102.
37. Weiant CW, Goldschmidt S: *Medicine and Chiropractic,* ed 4. New York, CW Weiant, 1966, pp 40–45.
38. Hviid H: A consideration of contemporary chiropractic theory. *J Natl Chiro Assoc* 25(1):17–18, 1955.
39. Haldeman S, Drum D: The compression subluxation. *J Clin Chiro Arch Ed* 1:10–21, 1971.
40. Coote JH, Sato A: A role for a descending sympathoinhibitory pathway in the ventral part of the spinal cord. *J Physiol* 252:21–27, 1975.

41. Coote JH: Somatic sources of afferent input as factors in aberrant autonomic, sensory, and motor function. In Korr IM (ed): *The Neurobiologic Mechanisms in Manipulative Therapy*. New York, Plenum, 1978, p 103.

42. Sato A: The somatosympathetic reflexes: their physiological and clinical significance. In Goldstein M (ed): *The Research Status of Spinal Manipulative Therapy*. NINCDS Monograph No 15. Bethesda, Maryland, US Department of Health, Education and Welfare, 1975, pp 163–172.

43. Gatterman MI: Indications for spinal manipulation in the treatment of back pain. *ACA J Chiro* 19(10):51–66, 1982.

44. Lewit K: Manipulation-reflex therapy and/or restitution of impaired locomotor function. *Manual Med* 2:99–100, 1986.

45. Cassidy JD, Potter GE: Motion examination of the lumbar spine. *J Manip Physiol Ther* 2:151–158, 1979.

46. Gillet H: The anatomy and physiology of spinal fixations. *J Natl Chiro Assoc* 33(12):22–24, 63–66, 1963.

47. Sandoz R: A classification of luxations, subluxations and fixations of the cervical spine. *Ann Swiss Chiro Assoc* 6:248–249, 256, 1976.

48. Schaefer R: *Basic Chiropractic Procedural Manual*, ed 2. Des Moines, American Chiropractic Association, 1977, pp 11–18.

49. Smith OG, Langworthy SM, Paxson MC: *Modernized Chiropractic*. Cedar Rapids, Lawrence Press, 1906, vol 1, p 26.

50. Downing CH: *The Principles of Osteopathy* 1923, p 63.

51. Gillet H: The evolution of a chiropractor. *J Natl Chiro Assoc* 15(11):15–19, 54–55, 1945.

52. Grice AS: A biomechanical approach to cervical and dorsal adjusting. In Haldeman S (ed): *Modern Developments in the Principles and Practice of Chiropractic*. East Norwalk, CT, Appleton-Century-Crofts, 1979, pp 331–358.

53. Grice AS: Muscle tonus change following manipulation. *J Can Chiro Assoc* 18(4):29–31, 1974.

54. Korr IM: Proprioceptors and somatic dysfunction. *J Am Osteopath Assoc* 74:638–650, 1975.

55. Janda V: Muscles, central nervous motor regulation, and back problems. In Korr IM (ed): *The Neurobiologic Mechanisms in Manipulative Therapy*. New York, Plenum, 1978, pp 27–41.

56. Sandoz RW: Some reflex phenomena associated with spinal derangements and adjustments. *Ann Swiss Chiro Assoc* 7:60, 1981.

57. Lewis M McD: Muscle spindles and their functions: a review. In Glasgow EF, Twomey LT, Scull ER, Kleynhans AM, Idczak RM (eds): *Aspects of Manipulative Therapy*, ed 2. New York, Churchill Livingstone, 1985, pp 55–58.

58. Nimmo RL: *The Receptor*. Grandbury, TX, I:1–6, 1971.

59. Mennell JM: The therapeutic use of cold. *J Am Osteopath Assoc* 74:1146–1158, 1975.

60. Travell JP, Simons DG: *Myofascial Pain and Dysfunction. The Trigger Point Manual*. Baltimore, Williams & Wilkins, 1970, p 4.

61. Donish EW, Basmajian JV: Electromyography of deep back muscles in man. *Anatomy* 133:25–36, 1972.

62. Wyke B: The neurology of joints. *Ann R Coll Surg Engl* 41:25–58, 1967.

63. Lewit K: The muscular and articular factor in movement restriction. *Manual Med* 1:83–85, 1985.

64. Lewit K: The contribution of clinical observation to neurobiological mechanisms in manipulative therapy. In Korr IM (ed): *The Neurobiologic Mechanisms in Manipulative Therapy*. New York, Plenum, 1978, p 5.

65. Mennell JM: *Back Pain: Diagnosis and Treatment, Using Manipulative Techniques*. Boston, Little, Brown & Co., 1960, pp 16, 18, 25, 211.

66. Stoddard A: *Manual of Osteopathic Techniques*. London, Hutchinson, 1959, pp 44, 62, 77, 82–83, 120, 123, 129, 218.

67. Perez-Tomayo R: *Mechanism of Disease: An Introduction to Pathology*, ed 2. Chicago, Year Book, 1985, p 222.

68. Aheson WH, Amiel D, Woo SL: Immobility effects on synovial joints: the pathomechanics of joint contracture. *Biorheology* 17:95–110, 1980.

69. Fisk JW: *A Practical Guide to the Painful Neck and Back: Diagnosis, Manipulation, Exercises, Prevention*. Springfield, IL, Charles C Thomas, 1977, p 141.

70. Schmorl G, Junghans H: *The Human Spine in Health and Disease*, ed 2. New York, Grune & Stratton, 1971, pp 221–223.

71. Kraft GL, Levinthal DH: Facetal synovial impingement. *Surg Gynecol Obstet* 93:439, 1951.

72. Badgley CE: The articular facets in relation to low back pain and sciatic radiation. *J Bone Joint Surg* 23:481, 1941.

73. Hadley LA: *Anatomico-Roentgenographic Studies of the Spine*. Springfield, IL, Charles C Thomas, 1979, p 181.

74. Bogduk N, Engel R: The menisci of the lumbar zygapophyseal joints: a review of their anatomy and clinical significance. *Spine* 9:454–460, 1984.

75. Giles LGF: Lumbar apophyseal joint arthrography. *J Manip Physiol Ther* 7:21–24, 1984.

76. Giles LGF, Taylor JR, Cochson H: Human zygapophyseal joint synovial folds. *Acta Anat* 126:110–114, 1986.

77. Giles LGF, Taylor JR: Innervation of lumbar zygapophyseal joint synovial folds. *Acta Orthop Scand* 58:43–46, 1987.

78. Giles LGF: Lumbo-sacral and cervical zygapophyseal joint inclusion. *Manual Med* 2:89–92, 1986.

79. Harris RI, Macnab I: Structural changes in the lumbar intervertebral discs: their relationship to low back pain and sciatica. *J Bone Joint Surg (Br)* 36B:304–322, 1954.

80. Reilly J, Yong-Hing K, MacKay RW, Kirkaldy-Willis WH: Pathological anatomy of the lumbar spine. In Helfet AF, Gruebel Lee DM (eds): *Disorders of the Lumbar spine*. Philadelphia, JB Lippincott, 1978, p 28.

81. Cyriax J: *Textbook of Orthopedic Medicine. Vol I: Diagnosis of Soft Tissue Lesions*, ed 8. London, Bailliere Tindall, 1982, p 308.

82. Maigne R *Orthopedic Medicine: A New Approach to Vertebral Manipulations*, translated by Liberson WT: Springfield, IL, Charles C Thomas, 1972, pp 24, 33.

83. Sandoz R: Newer trends in the pathogenesis of spinal disorders: a tentative classification of the functional disorders of the intervertebral motor unit. *Ann Swiss Chiro Assoc* 5:93–180, 1971.

84. Sandoz R: Some physical mechanisms and effects of spinal adjustments. *Ann Swiss Chiro Assoc* 6:91–141, 1976.

85. Mathews JA, Yates DAH: Reduction of lumbar disc prolapse by manipulation. *Br Med J* 3:696–697, 1969.

86. Cox JM: Mechanism, diagnosis and treatment of lumbar disc protrusion and prolapse. *ACA J Chiro* II(11):S167-S172, 1974.

87. Kuo PPF, Loh ZC: Treatment of lumbar intervertebral disc protrusions by manipulation. *Clin Orthop* 215:47–55, 1987.

88. Coplans CW: The conservative treatment of low back pain. In Helfet AJ, Gruebel Lee DM (eds): *Disorders of the Lumbar Spine*. Philadelphia, JB Lippincott, 1978, p 161.

89. Grieve GP: The sacroiliac joint. *Physiotherapy* 62:384–400, 1976.

90. Kirkaldy-Willis WH: Five common back disorders: how to diagnosis and treat them. *Geriatrics* 33:32–33, 37–41, 1978.

91. Hviid H: Functional radiography of the cervical spine. *Ann Swiss Chiro Assoc* 3:37–65, 1965.

92. Hviid H: The influence of the chiropractic treatment on the rotary mobility of the cervical spine—a kinesiometrical and statistical study. *Ann Swiss Chiro Assoc* 5:31–44, 1971.

93. Goldthwait SE, Osgood RB: A consideration of the pelvic articulations from an anatomical, pathological and clinical standpoint. *Boston Med Surg J* 152:593–634, 1905.

94. Ohlsen H: Moulding of the pelvis during labor. *Acta Radiol Diagn* 14:417–434, 1973.

95. Sandoz RW: Structural and functional pathologies of the pelvic ring. *Ann Swiss Chiro Assoc* 7:101–160, 1981.

96. Grieve GP: Lumbar instability. *Physiotherapy* 68:2–9, 1982.

97. Gatterman MI: Contraindications and complications of spinal manipulative therapy. *ACA J Chiro* 18(9): S75-S86, 1981.

98. Gillet H, Liekens M: A further study of spinal fixations. *Ann Swiss Chiro Assoc* 4:41–46, 1969.

99. Wyke BD: Articular neurology and manipulative therapy. In Glasgow EF, Twomey LT, Scull ER, Kleynhans AM, Idczak RM (eds): *Aspects of Manipulative Therapy*, ed 2. New York, Churchill Livingstone, 1985, p 72.

100. Lora J, Long D: So called facet denervation in the management of intractable back pain. *Spine* 1:121–126, 1976.

101. Grieve G: *Mobilization Of The Spine: Notes on Examination, Assessment and Clinical Method*, ed 4. New York, Churchill Livingstone, 1984, p 218.

102. Amiel D, Abel MF, Kleiner JB, Lieber RL, Akeson WH: Synovial fluid nutrient delivery in the diathrodial joint: an analysis of rabbit knee ligaments. *J Orthop Res* 4:90–95, 1986.

103. Salter RB, Hamilton HW, Wedge JH, Tile M, Torode IP, O'Driscoll SW, Murnaghan JJ, Saringer JH: Clinical application of basic research on continuous passive motion for disorders and injuries of synovial joints: a preliminary report of a feasibility study. *J Orthop Res* 1:325–342, 1984.

104. Lowther DA: The effect of compression and tension on the behavior of connective tissues. In Glasgow EF, Twomey LT, Scull ER, Kleynhans AM, Idczak RM (eds): *Aspects of Manipulative Therapy*, ed 2. New York, Churchill Livingstone, 1985, pp 16–22.

105. Salter RB: *Textbook of Disorders and Injuries of the Musculoskeletal System: An Introduction to Orthopedics, Rheumatology, Metabolic Bone Disease, Rehabilitation and Fractures*. Baltimore, Williams & Wilkins, 1970, p 22.

106. Ottenbacher K, Difabio RP: Efficacy of spinal manipulation/mobilization therapy: a meta-analysis. *Spine* 10:833–837, 1985.

107. Unsworth A, Dowson P, Wright V: Cracking joints: a bioengineering study of cavitation in the metacarpophalangeal joint. *Ann Rheum Dis* 30:348–358, 1971.

108. Meal GM, Scott RA: Analysis of the joint crack by simultaneous recording of sound and tension. *J Manip Physiol Ther* 9:189–195, 1986.

109. Rosten JB, Haines RW: Cracking in the metacarpo-phalangeal joint, *J Anat* 81:163–173, 1947.

110. Blackman J: Manipulation: a personal view. In Grieve GP (ed): *Modern Manual Therapy of the Vertebral Column*. New York, Churchill Livingstone, 1986, p 657.

111. Selye H: *The Physiology and Pathology of Exposure to Stress*, ed 1. Montreal, Acta Incorporated Medical Publishers, 1950, frontispiece.

CHAPTER 4

Complications of and Contraindications to Spinal Manipulative Therapy

Primum non nocere Hippocrates

"Primum non nocere" (First, do no harm) (1). Hippocrates admonished us "as to disease, make a habit of two things—to help, or at least to do no harm." Spinal manipulation is not a totally innocuous procedure.

The reported frequency of severe adverse reactions and complications following spinal manipulation is very low, with a mortality rate estimated by Maigne to be less than one death per tens of millions of manipulations (2). This estimate is contrary to inferences that the risk is actually much greater (3). The benefits of spinal manipulation far outweigh the risks of complication, and with careful patient screening, the low incidence of adverse reactions following manipulation can be reduced even further.

It is imperative that careful diagnostic procedures be utilized and that skilled and precise manipulative techniques be employed. Treatments can be modified to minimize the occurrence and the undesired effects of adverse reactions. These are discussed relative to specific spinal areas in chapters 7 through 10.

VASCULAR COMPLICATIONS

Vascular accidents are generally considered to be the most serious of all complications of spinal manipulative therapy (2–27). The extension-rotation test suggested by Smith in 1962 (8) can help in identifying high-risk patients and provide precaution. A ponticulus posticus viewed on cervical radiographs has been considered an insignificant finding by some, but may be a complicating factor in the compromise of vertebral artery flow (28). Aneurysm involving a major blood vessel is an absolute contrain-

dication to spinal manipulation. The chiropractic physician has the responsibility of recognizing aneurysms visualized on radiographs, palpated as pulsating masses, or detected by auscultation. Prompt referral for a vascular evaluation is essential in these cases.

Vertebral Artery Syndrome

Compromise of the vertebral arteries that causes interruption of the blood supply into the basilar area of the brain can result in a number of symptoms and in the most serious cases can lead to death (29). The mechanism by which this occurs and the clinical implications are discussed below.

Incidence of Vertebral Artery Syndrome

Of the 45 cases of vertebral artery syndrome following cervical manipulation reviewed by Jaskoviak (29) in 1980, 11 had died as a result of the complications. Of the remainder, 24 had some residual symptoms, including 9 with some form of paralysis or quadriplegia. In the remaining 11 patients, the symptoms abated without serious consequences. While there are doubtless some cases that go unreported in the literature, it is apparent that the incidence of vertebral artery syndrome is not high.

Signs and Symptoms

The most common symptoms of vertebral artery syndrome are transient attacks of dizziness, nausea, vomiting, visual disorders, or headaches (29). Less common are postural collapse resulting from interference with the mechanism regulating postural extensor tone (30), ataxia, and paresis of a limb or limbs (29). Visual disorders include diplopia, blurred vision, and nystagmus (28). In some cases Horner's syndrome has been produced with blepharoptosis, enophthalmos, and miosis. Dysarthria and cranial palsies have also been reported in several cases (29) (Table 4.1).

Table 4.1 Vertebral Artery Syndrome

Symptoms
  Dizziness
  Vertigo
  Blurred vision
  Ataxia
  Drop attack
  Headaches
  Nausea
  Tinnitus
Signs
  Nystagmus
  Blanching or cyanosis surrounding the mouth
  Ocular signs
  Horner's syndrome
  Dysarthria
  Dysphagia
  Palsies
  Paresis
  Syncope
  Opisthotonus
  Vomiting
Tests
  Extension-rotation
  Doppler
  Angiography
  X-ray
Treatment
  Anticoagulants (aspirin, dicumarol, heparin)
  Cervical immobilization
  Bed rest
  Surgical immobilization of the neck or decompression of
    transverse foramina

Anatomical Relationships of the Vertebral Arteries

Vertebral artery syndrome occurs when sudden head movements that result in extension and rotation of the neck interfere with the normal blood flow supplied by the vertebral and basilar arteries. This decreased blood flow subsequently produces ischemia of the brain stem, cerebellum, and occipital cortices, which produces neurological findings (30).

The vertebral arteries ascend through the foramina of the transverse processes of the first six cervical vertebrae, passing upward and outward from the foramina in the axis, to reach the foramina in the atlas (Fig. 4.1). After their exit from the transverse foramina, the vertebral arteries pass over the posterior arch of the atlas, forming grooves called the vertebral artery sulci (Fig. 4.2). These sulci are situated in the posterolateral region of the posterior arch of the atlas, vary in size, and in some instances are very deep.

The posterior occipital ligaments are attached inferiorly to the posterior arch of the atlas and are connected above to the posterior margin of the foramen magnum. These ligaments are broad but thin membranous sheets, intimately blended with the dura. The lateral divisions are known as the oblique atlantooccipital ligaments. These ligaments are incomplete at their inferior margins, allowing an opening for the passage of the vertebral artery and suboccipital nerve into the foramen magnum (31).

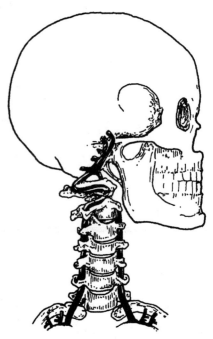

Figure 4.1. The vertebral arteries ascend through the foramina of the transverse processes of the first six cervical vertebrae, passing upward and outward from the foramina of the axis, to reach the foramina of the atlas. These arteries are well protected in their passage through the transverse foramina, but they are vulnerable to distortion, particularly on extension and rotation, as they pass into the foramen magnum.

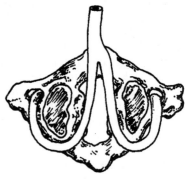

Figure 4.2. The vertebral arteries lie in sulci on the posterior arch of the atlas. On extension-rotation of the neck these arteries are subject to stretching and subsequent decreased blood flow that can cause brain stem ischemia leading to vertebral basilar syndrome.

Inside the skull, the two arteries run forward along either side of the medulla to the lower border of the pons, where they join to form the midline artery. As they ascend through the vertebral transverse processes, the vertebral arteries are well protected, but they are relatively unprotected in their passage from the atlas into the skull. There is considerable laxity of the vessels as they course between C1 and C2, which allows them to move freely with movement of the cervical spine and head (30).

Kinking of the contralateral artery as it exits from the transverse foramen of the axis occurs with 30° of

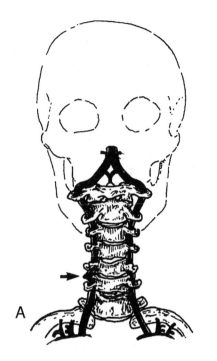

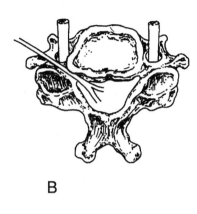

Figure 4.3. The most common site of degenerative change with osteophyte formation is lateral to the uncinate processes between C4–5 and C5–6, which can compromise both the vertebral artery and/or the cervical nerve.

A

B

rotation and becomes greater as the the angle of rotation increases to 45°. Past 45°, kinking occurs in the ipsilateral vertebral artery (32). Rotation of the atlas on the axis reduces the flow in the contralateral vertebral artery as it is stretched. The decrease in flow is proportional to the amount of rotation.

Significant rotation will also cause a decrease in the flow in the ipsilateral artery. The reduction of flow in the contralateral artery is caused by forward movement of the contralateral lateral mass of the atlas and the stretching of the artery at its exit from the transverse foramen of the axis (Fig. 4.3). The backward movement of the ipsilateral lateral mass of the atlas beyond 45° causes a stretching that decreases flow in the ipsilateral artery.

Pathological and Anomalous Variations

Giles (30) lists the following conditions that should be carefully considered before spinal manipulation is undertaken.

1. Abnormal vascular pattern such as
   a. Tortuosity of one or both vertebral arteries with destructive bone changes;
   b. The presence of only one vertebral artery;
   c. The presence of only one effective vertebral artery that constitutes the major blood flow into the basilar system;
2. Vascular disease such as atherosclerosis;
3. Abnormal bony structures in apposition to the vertebral arteries by virtue of degenerative changes such as osteophytic proliferation in the vertebral artery or congenital malformations.

The most common sites of osteophyte formation are between C4 and C5, and between C5 and C6 (Fig. 4.3). They can project anteriorly from the facetal joint or, more commonly, laterally from the intervertebral joint (uncinate processes, Fig. 4.3*B*) to displace the vertebral artery. If retrolisthesis is present due to disc degeneration, the superior articular facet of the vertebra below can compromise the vertebral artery when the cervical spine moves into extension. Shortening of the cervical spine resulting from disc degeneration can lead to sinuosity and compression of the artery, even in the absence of bony degenerative changes.

Calcification of the atlantooccipital ligaments known as the ponticulus posticus and posticulus lateralis (Fig. 4.4) may also be a factor that produces symptoms of vertebral artery syndrome by compromising these arteries during extension and rotation (28). These anomalous ossification centers bridge the vertebral artery sulci, forming bony arches enclosing the foramen arcuale. The complex has been called Kimerle's anomaly (33). When ossification occurs in the posterior portion of the posterior atlantooccipital ligament, it is referred to as the posticulum ponticus. The posticulum lateralis occurs with ossification of the oblique atlantooccipital ligaments (34).

Seen on lateral cervical radiographs (Fig. 1.10), the posticulum ponticus may be unilateral or bilateral. Pyo and Lowman (31) found an incidence of 12.6% in a study of 300 normal cervical radiographs. They described a wide range of anatomic variation with respect to size, configuration, and position. Dissections have revealed a variable degree of

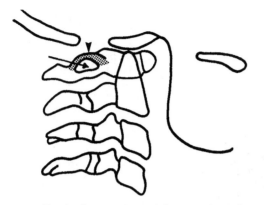

Figure 4.4. Ponticulus posticus. A bony arch encloses the vertebral artery when anomalous ossification of the posterior atlantooccipital ligament occurs (*arrowhead*). This forms an arcuate foramen (*arrow*). (see Fig. 1.10.) (Courtesy Yokum TR and Rowe L: *Essentials of Skeletal Radiology*. Baltimore, Williams & Wilkins, 1987, p 101.

atlantic ponticles in 33% of cases with either an incomplete or a complete ring noted (23).

Four of the five patients with symptoms of vertebral artery syndrome produced by the extension-rotation test, in 2000 patients tested, show a posterior ponticulus on radiographs. The fifth patient previously had ligation of one of the carotid arteries, which was subsequently repaired surgically. Following surgery, there was a complete remission of the patient's symptoms, which included horizontal nystagmus on cervical extension and rotation.

Vertebral basilar insufficiency following cervical manipulation with the neck or back in extension and rotation may also be produced in patients predisposed to arteriospasm (13).

Identification of Risk Patients

Identification of patients with a high risk of developing the vertebral artery syndrome is by no means conclusive. A number of screening tests may be used as part of the premanipulation evaluation.

The extension-rotation test can be more effectively performed with the patient in the supine position with the head and neck extended beyond the end of the table. The head is then slowly and actively rotated to each side, maintaining the extended position. It is important that the patient rotate the head to the extreme range of motion and that the eyes remain open. If there are signs of blanching, nystagmus, or cyanosis around the mouth, or if the patient complains of dizziness or nausea, manipulation in this position is contraindicated.

The test has been described in the chiropractic literature by Houle (35) in Canada and George (36) in the United States and has been designated as both Houle's test and George's test. Since descriptive names for tests are less confusing than eponyms, this test will be referred to as the cervical extension and rotation test to determine patency of the verte-

bral arteries. Fisk (37) has stated that the cervical extension-rotation test should be known to all that have the temerity to manipulate necks. He also noted that those at high risk include mid-30 females on birth control pills, particularly if they smoke, and women immediately following the postpartum period.

Radiographs should be carefully evaluated for osteophytic proliferation, particularly of the uncovertebral joints (38–39), atherosclerosis, and the presence of a posterior ponticulum. Retrolisthesis due to disc degeneration should also be carefully evaluated to determine if it is due to joint instability or articular fixation. Follow-up angiography can provide second-stage identification of patients with increased risk of vertebral artery syndrome following the posterior extension-rotation test (23, 25). Doppler flow and imaging techniques provide a noninvasive procedure for evaluating vascular adequacy (40–41).

Management

In those unfortunate cases where vertebral artery syndrome occurs as a result of therapeutic or spontaneous extension and rotation of the neck, appropriate management can minimize adverse sequelae. Immediate medical treatment with anticoagulant therapy (27, 30) can reduce the risk of thrombus formation and subsequent embolization. The patient's immediate response and specific adverse signs should be noted, and the patient referred for prompt and appropriate evaluation and management. Limitation of neck movement with a cervical collar should precede movement and transportation of the patient. In severe cases, surgical immobilization of the neck or decompression of the transverse foramina may be necessary (39).

Since manipulation has not been positively identified as the primary cause of a subsequent stroke, its role must be considered in each individual case (23). Although it has been demonstrated that manipulation of the neck in extension and rotation can significantly narrow the lumen of the vertebral artery, susceptibility to vertebrobasilar accidents may depend on an abnormal vascular supply to the basilar system due to vessel asymmetry, atherosclerosis, arteriospasm, or spondylotic or congenital impingement. The relative rarity of such accidents, in a view of the large number of cervical manipulations, further suggests that the predisposed patient has an abnormal vertebral artery blood supply (7, 23, 27).

Aneurysms

Aneurysms involving a major blood vessel are an absolute contraindication to manipulation (42). Because abdominal aortic aneurysm can cause severe back pain, it is imperative that abdominal palpation be included in the premanipulation examination (42). When examining the abdomen, the aorta can usually be palpated in the midline, and by examin-

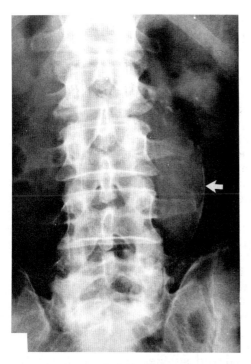

Figure 4.5. AP view of abdominal aortic aneurysm.

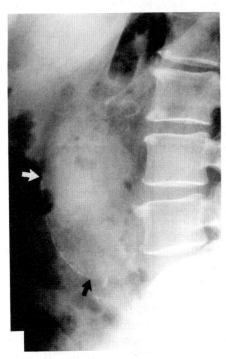

Figure 4.6. A calcific outline of the abdominal aorta (lateral view) shows bulging aneurysm. (Courtesy Yokum TR, Rowe L: *Essentials of Skeletal Radiology*. Baltimore, Williams & Wilkins, 1987, p 1022.

ing from the midline outward, the size of the aorta can often be determined. A large pulsating mass necessitates prompt referral to a vascular surgeon.

Radiographs should be examined for signs of aortic aneurysm in addition to abdominal palpation (Fig. 4.5) (42). Radiographic evidence of the abdominal aortic aneurysm is visualized anterior to the lumbar spine on the lateral lumbar view (Fig. 4.6). Winterstein (42) found an incidence of 35 abdominal aortic aneurysms on retrospective analysis of 2000 consecutive x-ray reports, representing 1.75% of the total group. Since not all abdominal aortas contain visible calcific plaque, the incidence is probably greater than this study reports. Of these patients, 26 were males, with an average age of 74.19 years. Of the 9 females, the average age was 70.44 years. The typical patient with an abdominal aortic aneurysm is in the sixth or seventh decade and presents with a deep boring pain in the midlumbar region (43).

Radiographic evidence of an aortic aneurysm shows a calcific streak outlining the anterior margin of the aorta just anterior to L4 and L5, the region in which the aorta normally bifurcates into the common iliac vessels. This calcific outline does not appear to be parallel to the spine but deviates at its upper portion toward the anterior abdomen (42). Suspected cases of aortic aneurysm should be promptly referred to a vascular surgeon for evaluation and treatment.

TUMORS

The possibility of pathological fracture of bone weakened by a primary or secondary tumor is the obvious omnipresent risk of manipulation of patients suffering from these conditions. Even lightly applied mobilization may be too much for patients with bone weakened by neoplastic growth. Fortunately, tumors producing lytic bone lesions are rare and usually visualized on x-ray. The importance of obtaining clear diagnostic radiographs of the area of complaint must be stressed (44).

Fisk (44) estimated that there is an incidence of less than four per 100,000 with primary or secondary bone tumors and of these, only one in 20 occurs in the spine, making the incidence of spinal tumors one per 500,000. Most of these bone tumors are secondary to primary sites in the prostate, breasts, lungs, thyroid gland, kidney, gastrointestinal tract, uterus, and bladder. Infrequently, multiple myeloma may be found. According to Fisk (44) it is usual for the primary growth to be detected before secondary spread has occurred. Where the secondary site is identified first, the patient generally does not look well, has lost weight, and may complain of a boring bone pain that is most noticeable at night. A marked local tenderness of the affected region of the spine can usually be elicited by palpation. X-ray findings suggestive of bone tumors include loss of substance where bone resorption (osteolysis) has occurred or areas of increased density due to bone deposition (osteosclerosis).

Chest x-rays often reveal a primary site in cases of suspected metastasis to bone. Laboratory investigation of patients suspected of having a malignant tumor should include a complete blood count and serum calcium, inorganic phosphate, alkaline phosphatase, acid phosphatase, and serum protein levels (45). The malignant tumor usually has an insidious onset with relentless progress and may be initially mistaken for a simple back strain. Its eventual recognition is inevitable, but early detection and referral is obviously of the essence. For this reason, poorly responding symptomatology should be reviewed with the consideration of further tests for possible organic and/or malignant causation.

BONE INFECTIONS

Bone infections are rare and usually exhibit readily identifiable patterns. The patient generally appears to have a systemic illness and has a history of febrile symptoms. Most chronic infections of bone occur in the young and are rare since the advent of antibiotic drugs. A primary site such as the lungs, urinary tract, or gastrointestinal tract is typically found with tuberculosis of bone, and a staphylococcal furuncle or carbuncle often precedes osteomyelitis.

Tuberculosis of the spine (Pott's disease) accounts for more than half of all bone and joint tuberculosis (45). It is most common during early childhood. Systemic manifestations include chronic ill health, which accompanies the primary infection of the pulmonary, urinary, or gastrointestinal tracts. Laboratory analysis shows an elevated sedimentation rate and positive tuberculin skin tests. In the early stages of tuberculosis an osteolytic lesion in the anterior part of the vertebral body may be visualized on x-ray, with a regional osteoporosis and narrowing of the adjacent intervertebral disc. In the advanced stage there may be evidence of extensive destruction and collapse of the anterior vertebral body, with spread to adjacent vertebrae and a paravertebral abscess.

Osteomyelitis of the spine is usually hematogenous from a distant primary site. The earliest clinical symptoms are pain and rigidity from protective muscle spasm (43). These precede the roentgenographic findings. After a few days, evidence of soft tissue swelling may be present and should indicate the need for laboratory procedures such as a white blood cell count, a differential count, and a sedimentation rate determination. After the first week to ten days there is evidence of destruction of bone. As with bone tumors, the primary concern with bone infection is pathological fracture, and manipulation of the affected area is absolutely contraindicated (46, 47). Radiographic examination is an essential preliminary procedure prior to treatment. When coupled with appropriate tests, it can detect suspected bone infection. Thus the harmful effects of

manipulation and a dangerous delay of treatment can be avoided.

TRAUMATIC INJURIES

Traumatic injuries to osseous and soft tissue structures can preclude forceful spinal manipulation. It is generally agreed that unstable fractures of the spine contraindicate manipulation of that area (2, 47). Stress radiographs (48–51) may prove useful in the determination of instability. Soft tissue, nonforce manipulation or mobilization procedures may still be possible under certain circumstances. Gentle manipulation of other areas of the spine for relief of muscle spasm may be indicated. Useful conservative techniques include physical therapy modalities, deep tissue massage, passive stretching, and trigger point therapy.

Articular trauma, including dislocation and severe ligamentous strain indicated by pain on motion and stress x-rays are also contraindications to the dynamic thrust of the area. In the case of "whiplash" injury, it is important that only those specific areas of joint fixation be manipulated, while sprained and strained tissue is immobilized with supports. It is necessary to differentiate these areas of hypermobility by the use of motion palpation and stress x-rays (Chapter 6) (48–51).

Spondylolisthesis does not contraindicate spinal manipulation (Chapter 8). Maitland (52) cautions against strong manipulation of patients with spondylolisthesis while Stoddard (46) recommends that manipulation is contraindicated in unstable cases. He cautions also that forced torsional adjustments are contraindicated at any stage of spondylolisthesis.

Cassidy and Potter (53) have found manipulation to be beneficial in over 80% of cases of back pain associated with spondylolisthesis. They stress, however, that such treatment does not claim to influence the spondylolisthesis itself, with treatment directed to the posterior joints above and below the level of slippage (Chapter 8). It is their observation that spondylolisthesis is an incidental finding in these patients and not a contraindication to manipulative therapy.

A progressive slip or instability of the motion segment, while rare, is a poor prognostic sign for conservative treatment (53). Spondylolisthesis or anterior slippage of the vertebral body can be best visualized on lateral radiographs. Flexion and extension views are used to evaluate stability (Chapter 6).

Among the more serious conditions requiring modification of treatment are spinal hematomas in patients on anticoagulant therapy (54). Forceful manipulation of the spine may cause intraspinal bleeding, with subsequent development of sensory and motor deficits that can progress to paraplegia, quadriplegia, or even death. An adequate medical history of the patient is essential, with a complete systems review and notation of any medication that the patient is taking. Inspection may reveal a tendency toward excessive bruising, which may indicate a platelet deficiency such as thrombocytopenia purpura. Soft tissue therapy and gentle mobilization procedures may prove useful, with avoidance of forceful manipulations.

Iatrogenic trauma can be induced by manipulation of the spine under general anaesthesia. A comparatively large amount of stress can be applied to deep structures when the protection of the reflex spasm of the erector spinae muscles is abolished by the anesthesia. Thus, already traumatized muscle fibers may be further damaged, and laxity of ligaments increased.

ARTHRITIDES

The most serious complication from the systemic arthritides (ankylosing spondylitis, rheumatoid arthritis, psoriatic arthritis, and Reiter's syndrome) is inflammatory rupture of the transverse ligament with dislocation of the atlas (55). Diagnosis of this rupture requires flexion stress x-rays of the cervical spine to accentuate any increase in the atlantoodontoid interspace. Measurements in excess of 5 mm in children or 3 mm in adults are indicative of anterior slippage of the atlas on the axis. This should preclude spinal manipulative therapy, since the possibility of total luxation with central cord compression exists. Manipulation is absolutely contraindicated for these patients.

Ankylosing spondylitis typically occurs in patients between 15 and 35 years of age and is much more common in males than females (43–44). The common presenting complaint is low back pain following a nontraumatic and insidious onset. The sacroiliac joints are generally the first sites of involvement, evidenced radiographically by ill-defined joint margins with lateral reactive sclerosis appearing on both sides of the articulations. As the disease progresses, the spine slowly fuses, with a caudal to cephalic progression. Accompanying back stiffness is the prominent characteristic (43). The most helpful laboratory finding is the presence of HLA-B27, found in the serum of greater than 80% of patients with ankylosing spondylitis (56). Mild anemia and an elevated ESR are usually present, but these tests are nonspecific.

Most authors agree that manipulation is contraindicated in the inflammatory stage of ankylosing spondylitis (2, 44, 52, 55). Stoddard (46) recommends that manipulation of the spine and exercise to maintain mobility are not contraindicated following the acute phase, but feels there is a limit to what can be achieved by manipulative techniques. Excessive use of force is never recommended. Gentle manipulation of the costovertebral joints is thought to be of benefit when the disease is quiescent, because maintenance of near normal respiratory movements will have a beneficial effect on the general health of the patient.

Rheumatoid arthritis predominantly affects the cervical region of the spine. It is a systemic disorder, characterized by destruction of synovial tissue and ultimately the joint surfaces, with subsequent development of ligamentous laxity. As the disease progresses, osteoporosis affects the osseous structures in the cervical spine. Ligamentous laxity occurs at the lower cervical spine as well as the previously discussed atlantoaxial region. Dislocation of the cervical spine in rheumatoid patients may be totally asymptomatic (43). Forward subluxation of 4 to 5 mm of the lower vertebral bodies is considered significant instability. Dynamic flexion/extension views of the cervical spine may be necessary for accurate diagnosis (48–51), and the consensus is that forceful manipulation of the patient is contraindicated (47, 55). Maitland (52) states, however, that while forceful manipulation must never be used in these cases, it is wrong to preclude palliation by gentle mobilization.

Psoriatic arthritis is roentgenographically indistinguishable from Reiter's syndrome of the spine, and there may be a sacroiliitis similar to that of ankylosing spondylitis. Paraspinal ossifications may span vertebral bodies in both conditions. They tend to develop asymmetrically (43). Reiter's syndrome, characterized by urethritis, conjunctivitis, and arthritis, generally occurs in young males but may be seen in women and children. Spinal involvement probably occurs in 20–30% of patients with psoriatic arthritis. The HLA-B27 antigen is found in 80% of patients with Reiter's syndrome and in 50% of those with spinal involvement in psoriatic arthritis (56). As with other forms of inflammatory arthritides discussed, spinal manipulation is definitely contraindicated in the active stage (47, 55). Patients with such disorders as rheumatoid arthritis, ankylosing spondylitis, psoriatic arthritis, or Reiter's disease should be carefully evaluated for any sign of acute inflammation of spinal joints before manipulation is attempted.

Osteoarthritis or degenerative joint disease of the posterior facet joints is characterized roentgenographically by hypertrophy of bone at the articular margins (Fig. 4.6). As the cartilage degenerates, the joint space narrows, and there may be erosion of articular bone with alteration of the joint surfaces, which can best be visualized on oblique projections. The most signficant symptom is backache increased by exertion and relieved by rest. The patient may also complain of stiffness after prolonged inactivity, particularly upon arising in the morning. Factors implicated in the etiology of osteoarthritis include aging, abnormal stress, trauma, obesity, diet, and an element of inherited propensity (43). Laboratory findings in these patients are normal.

Maigne (2) feels that manipulation should be avoided during the acute inflammatory phase of osteoarthritis and adjusting should only be in the direction of no pain and free movement (the acute in-

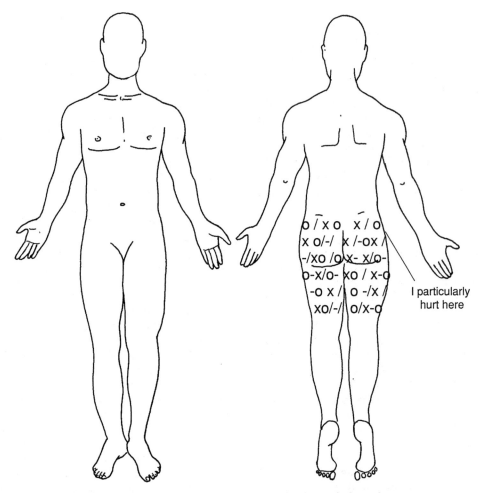

Figure 4.7. Patients magnifying their symptoms of malingering often demonstrate pain in nonanatomical patterns, utilizing multiple symbols in the same region. Symbols: numbness (−), pins and needles (o), burning (×), stabbing (/).

flammatory phase produces pain in all directions). Maitland (52) recommends gentle mobilization in the treatment of osteoarthritis, followed by more vigorous manipulation, but not in the presence of a very painful joint. Stoddard (46) recommends improving circulation in the treatment of osteoarthritis of spinal joints by articular manipulation. Mennell (57) believes that if rest increases joint stiffness or pain in a joint, some inflammatory disease process should be suspected. Further evaluation is indicated, and manipulation is contraindicated until these conditions are either ruled out or eradicated.

Pathological fracture can result from forceful manipulation applied to patients with osteoporosis and osteomalacia (46, 52). The use of soft tissue and mobilizing techniques may prove beneficial for patients with these conditions. The spine is particularly vulnerable to osteoporotic fracture. Those with a history of long-term steroid therapy and postmenopausal females are most susceptible. Osteoporosis is the most common metabolic bone disease in adults, with 70% of all fractures occurring in the elderly as the result of osteoporosis. Even minor trauma to the

spine, such as the stress caused by a cough or sneeze, may result in the collapse of weakened vertebrae (58).

The pathological process that leads to osteoporosis is usually operative for some time before diagnosis can be confirmed by radiographs. Approximately 30% or more of bone substance must be lost before there is radiographic evidence. The "codfish" vertebrae, vertebral body collapse, and rarefaction are characteristic. The horizontal trabeculae or striations are lost, but the vertical ones remain. The endplates remain well defined. Finding loss of trabeculation of the femoral heads has proven helpful in the diagnosis of osteoporosis.

Laboratory investigation should include serum calcium and phosphorous and alkaline phosphatase determinations. These values are normal in the osteoporotic patient but changed in osteomalacia. A slight increase in alkaline phosphatase level may be present if recent fractures are due to osteoporosis. Parathyroid hormone and T4 levels will also aid in the differential diagnosis. ESR, serum protein electrophoresis, CBC, and SMA-12 are helpful when it is

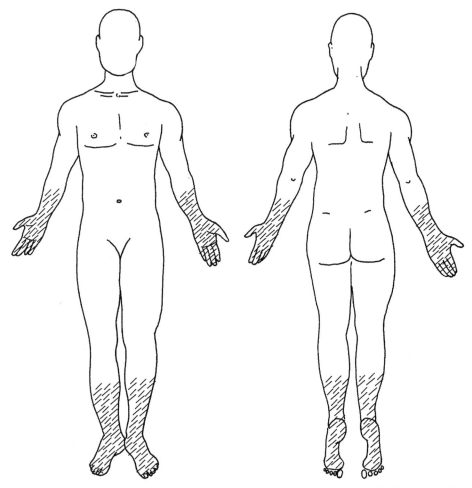

Figure 4.8. The classic stocking or glove anesthesia pattern outlined on the pain diagram should alert the chiropractor to the possibility of a psychological problem. Peripheral neuropathy should also be ruled out. Symbol: numbness (−).

suspected that the osteoporosis is secondary to malignancy (58).

PSYCHOLOGICAL CONSIDERATIONS

The term psychosomatic medicine epitomizes the dual nature of the mind and body concept, and it is not an easy task to differentiate psychogenic from organic complaints (58). A number of psychological conditions must be considered in dealing with the chiropractic patient. These include malingering, hysteria, hypochondriasis, pain tolerance, and the dependent personality. Each condition poses a diagnostic challenge and requires a modification of patient management.

Malingering

By definition the malingerer is motivated by some form of secondary gain. This is not necessarily financial, although we generally associate this problem with one who pretends slow recuperation from a disorder in order to continue to receive sickness or compensation benefits (59). Some malingerers, however, feign illness to obtain less hazardous or less physically demanding work, or they may be using a pretended illness to avoid a situation where there is a conflict with fellow workers. Occasionally a patient is seeking attention from indifferent family members, and these may benefit from family counseling (28).

Malingering can be divided into three major categories.

1. Pure malingering, in which there is a deliberate deception by the description and/or the production of nonexistent symptoms and signs;
2. Partial malingering, which involves the conscious and voluntary exaggeration of symptoms of a real disease;
3. Deliberate attribution of an actual disability to an injury or accident that did not cause it (60).

Magnifying symptoms and attributing disability to an incident that did not cause it are more common than pure malingering. The important aspect of malingering by definition rests upon the motivation of the involved individual. Malingering is found in those situations that offer benefits from the presence

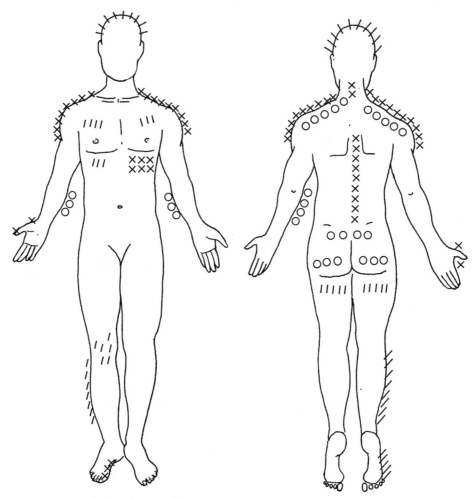

Figure 4.9. Hypochondriacs exhibit multiple complaints in multiple areas, often demonstrating total body pain and pain outside the body. Symbols: pins & needles (o), burning (×), stabbing (/).

of disease and should be suspected if the patient lacks sincerity or demonstrates incongruity or a lack of completeness of symptoms. Exaggerated symptoms and pain response may also be suspicious signs. Malingerers are often uncooperative, and defensive and angry with examinations. They can be careless about their symptoms and may readily give them up when they think no one is watching (61).

A number of tests may be used to identify the malingerer, including the pain drawing (62) (Fig. 4.7) and the Burns' bench test (63). Malingerers usually exhibit inconsistencies in pain patterns and physical findings, and they often overreact to examination procedures. Testing the same function directly and indirectly is a commonly applied method of diagnosing malingering (64, 65). The supine straight leg raise and the sitting straight leg raise (Bechterew's or Flip test) for sciatic nerve traction are examples of direct and indirect testing for the same function.

The diagnosis of malingering should be avoided, since the term is a medicolegal designation and constitutes an accusation (66). In reporting such cases,

it is better to report multiple inconsistencies between direct and indirect testing, with no objective findings to substantiate the patient's subjective complaints. Prolonged treatment of the malingerer can prove expensive and does little to enhance the credibility of chiropractors in the eyes of the third party payers, not to mention the time taken away from the patients with legitimate complaints.

Hysteria (Conversion Reactions)

The hysterical patient differs from the malingerer by unknowingly presenting nonorganic complaints. The malingerer suffering from conversion phenomena exhibits symbolic representations of physical conflict in terms of motor or sensory manifestations (67). Hysterical patients do not have conscious control over the symptoms, which differ from psychophysiologic reactions in that there is no demonstrable anatomic or pathophysiologic abnormality except in extreme cases, where there is a secondary response such as disuse atrophy. Patients with conversion disorder are frequently described as immature or dependent.

Like malingerers, hysterical patients may present with numerous symptoms and display inconsistent and exaggerated responses to examination. They often complain of abnormal neurological functions manifested by total or partial paralysis (68). The classic stocking or glove anesthesia should alert the chiropractor to suspect the possibility of a psychological problem once peripheral neuropathy such as occurs with diabetes or alcholism has been ruled out (Fig. 4.8).

Prompt referral of the hysterical patient is necessary to avoid delay in appropriate treatment. These patients have very real psychotic problems that need to be dealt with by professionals trained in the treatment of psychological or psychiatric disorders.

Hypochondriasis

Hypochondriasis is characterized by multiple somatic complaints and a preoccupation with one's physical health. The incidence increases with age. Hypochondriacs differ from malingerers, who tend to emphasize symptoms related to the injured area. The hypochondriac, on the other hand, often complains of symptoms involving different anatomical systems (Fig. 4.9). Most frequently these are symptoms referrable to the musculoskeletal system, particularly the head and neck (69–70).

Hypochondriacs exhibit few objective findings, and the results of previous tests and studies are inconclusive and nonrevealing. Invasive diagnostic or therapeutic procedures should be undertaken only on the basis of objective findings, not on the basis of subjective complaints. The hypochondriacal patient who formerly had no disease can develop genuine and incapacitating symptoms due to iatrogenically induced conditions such as those seen in some cases of failed back surgery.

Hypochondriasis may be a sign that the patient is experiencing external stress or an internal conflict. Transient syndromes can become long-standing problems if there is sufficient reinforcement (see "Dependent Personality"), which can come from the unwitting chiropractor as well as any other health care professional.

Hypochondriacs may use the sick role to avoid certain social responsibilities or to explain failure. In addition to serving as a mechanism to protect self-esteem, hypochondriasis can be used in interpersonal relationships to get attention and sympathy from others. Hypochondriacal patients have usually seen a number of physicians in the past and tend to be critical of their previous care. They are often tense individuals who seek relief from high-pressure work through psychosomatic complaints. The MMPI (Minnesota Multiphasic Personality Inventory) is useful in diagnosing these patients, and prompt referral for psychometric evaluation and appropriate treatment is in the patient's best interest.

Pain Tolerance

Pain tolerance depends on a variety of factors. Anxiety, emotional distress, and ethnocultural factors can influence pain behavior and pain tolerance, with individual differences in experience (71–74).

Italians (74), Jews (75–76), and Mexican-Americans (77) have been shown to be more demonstrative in their response to pain. They may be less tolerant of painful procedures, and as with any patient exhibiting a low pain tolerance, these patients require reassurance and gentle maneuvers. Careful monitoring of pain response will indicate when treatment modification is necessary.

Dependent Personality and Disability Syndromes

The dependent personality can become tiresome to the busy practitioner. These patients tend to not accept their responsibility in the healing process and become dependent on chiropractic care for their sense of well-being. They often refuse to follow prescribed dietary or exercise programs and expect the chiropractor to compensate for poor living habits. Reassurance and patient education are necessary when dealing with the dependent personality.

The chiropractic physician should never attempt to capitalize on the dependent personality for personal gain. To encourage such patients in their sick roles for the purpose of financial gain or ego enhancement is highly unethical. Over-emphasizing the seriousness of a condition to keep a patient returning for unnecessary treatment has become the practice of some overutilizers and is a discredit to the chiropractic profession.

Authorizing prolonged time loss to emphasize the seriousness of the patient's condition does the patient a great disservice. While the patient should not be returned to work prematurely, prolonged inactivity creates a downward spiral of disability and frequently results in weight gain and deconditioning, making it increasingly difficult to return the patient to productivity. The patient who appears to be reluctant to return to work is commonly laid off at the first opportunity by the disgruntled employer. Any financial reward gained by the patient in such cases is minimal compared to the future loss of earning power when the patient becomes unemployed and labeled a "back cripple."

The chiropractor should not play patient advocate in an effort to gain a large settlement for an accident victim. It is the chiropractic physician's responsibility to reduce human suffering and, through appropriate rehabilitation, return the injured person to productivity as expediently as possible. Objective reporting of the patient's condition allows the patient to receive just compensation when true disability exists. Authorization of excessive time loss, which leads to loss of the patient's self-esteem in addition to increased costs to employers, insurance companies, and the government, should not be encouraged by members of the chiropractic profession.

Disability syndromes can be frustrating to the physician when a patient presents the outward appearance of seeking medical care in order to get well, with a covert intention of remaining in the sick role. Although these patients may be successful in obtaining benefits, the quality of their lives is actually poor, and the trade-off of symptoms for benefits appears to be an unsatisfactory alternative to a productive life.

Whether these patients are conscious malingerers, hysterics, hypochondriacs, or dependent personalities, they have a true disability with loss of earning capacity and disruption of family life. They should, therefore, be referred for adequate evaluation and treatment. They place a strain upon chiropractors as well as other health care providers, insurance funds, and compensation boards. Adequate psychological and psychiatric examinations should be sought for these patients, because of the deleterious effects on industry, society, and business as well as on their own personal lives.

NEUROLOGICAL COMPLICATIONS

Among the more serious complications of spinal manipulative therapy are cauda equina compression (78), myelopathy (79), and paresis (80) due to aggravated radiculopathy.

Cauda Equina Syndrome

The preexisting cauda equina syndrome with loss of bowel or bladder control, impotence, perianal anesthesia, and lower limb paresis is a definite contraindication to lumbar spine manipulation. Such symptoms require immediate referral for surgical decompression. The return of neurological function is directly proportional to the total time the symptoms (including paraparesis) have been present (80). Bilateral symptoms and signs commonly precede serious compression and may indicate its imminence (78).

Cervical Disc Lesions and Myelopathy

Cervical disc lesions (Chapter 10) can cause severe neurological complications in both the upper and lower extremities. Disc protrusion affects the upper extremities due to nerve root involvement, while symptoms in the lower extremity indicate direct cord involvement. Early recognition of these conditions and immediate referral for neurological decompression is essential to prevent permanent neurological deficits.

In addition to the neurological findings, radiographs of cervical disc lesions may demonstrate loss of the normal cervical lordosis, localized immobility, and narrowing of the intervertebral disc space. These findings are more significant to the diagnosis of a herniated cervical disc if they are localized to one interspace. When multiple interspaces are involved, findings are more likely to reflect generalized spondylosis. For a more definitive diagnosis, a CT scan or myelogram may be necessary, since these radiographic findings are also characterisic of a vertebral motion segment fixation (81).

Nerve Root Damage

There is a possibility that further nerve root damage may be caused by mechanical pressure of the herniated disc during the act of manipulation. In a series of 400 cases of herniated intervertebral discs verified by surgery, Poppen (82) noted four cases in which sudden complete paraplegia followed manipulation. Thibodeau (83) reports two similar cases and states that low back manipulation is contraindicated in the presence of disc symptoms. These cases represent a very small number compared to the many cases in which the patient with a suspected disc lesion has benefited from spinal manipulative therapy. It appears that the patients with intervertebral disc syndrome may benefit from flexion distraction more than rotational manipulation (Chapter 8). However, both methods have proven successful in reducing the symptoms in patients diagnosed as having herniated discs (84–85).

Any case in which there are advancing neurological deficits should be referred for a neurological evaluation. This includes muscle weakness such as a foot drop or a weak extensor hallucis longus, diminished or absent reflexes, and sensory loss.

CONCLUSION

Most of the complications of spinal manipulative therapy can be avoided by careful evaluation of each patient based on a good working knowledge of the relevant anatomy and physiology, and prompt referral where indicated (Table 4.2). The chiropractic physician should not use more force than is necessary, preferably using specific short-lever thrusts as opposed to high-force, long-lever rotational maneuvers. Soft tissue and mobilizing techniques may prove beneficial where more forceful manipulation is contraindicated. If prolonged therapy becomes necessary, reevaluation after 6 to 8 weeks is indicated, since laxity of ligaments may result from repeated stretching of joints (86). An absolute contraindication for manipulative therapy in one area of the spine may not apply to another area of the spine, which is unaffected by the condition. Healing may be enhanced in areas of hypermobility if normal mobility is restored and maintained in another area of the spine that exhibits hypomobility.

There are no substitutes for skill, knowledge, and finesse. In the hands of a trained chiropractor, spinal manipulation is safe and effective and as such should be included as an integral part of the health

Table 4.2   General Health Problems Which Either Contraindicate or Require Modification of Spinal Manipulation

Condition	Potential Complications of Manipulation	Method of Detection	Modification of Patient Management
Vascular complication			
1. Vertebral-basilar insufficiency	Vertebral basilar infarction	Predisposition detected by cervical extension-rotation test, Doppler angiography	Cervical manipulation contraindicated in extension and rotation, use soft tissue and mobilizing techniques, refer to vascular surgeon for evaluation
2. Atherosclerosis of major blood vessels	Blood vessel rupture (hemorrhage), dislodged thrombi	Palpation, ausculation, x-ray visualization, Doppler	Soft tissue and mobilizing techniques with light adjustments, refer to vascular surgeon
3. Aneurysm	Rupture and hemorrhage	Irregular pulse, abdominal palpation, ausculation, x-ray	Refer to vascular surgeon
Tumors			
1. Lung	Metastasis to spine, ribs	Ausculation, lab findings, x-ray, MRI	Referral
2. Thyroid	Metastasis to spine	Palpation, x-ray, and lab findings, MRI	Referral
3. Prostate	Metastasis to spine	Palpation, MRI, x-ray and lab findings, rectal exam	Referral
4. Breast	Metastasis to spine	Palpation, MRI x-ray and lab findings	Referral
5. Bone	Pathologic fractures	X-ray and lab findings	Referral
Bone infections			
1. Tuberculosis	Pathologic fracture	Biopsy X-ray and lab findings	Referral
2. Bacterial infection (osteomyelitis)	Pathologic fracture	Biopsy X-ray and lab findings	Referral
Traumatic injuries			
1. Fractures	Increased instability, delayed-healing fracture	X-ray findings including CT	Referral
2. Joint instability or hypermobility	Increased instability	Stress x-ray views, palpation, stress ROM	Manipulation of area of fixation, immobilization or avoidance of area of instability; if severe, refer for surgery
3. Severe sprains or strains	Increased instability	Stress ROM, stress x-ray views, motion palpation	If severe, refer for surgery, manipulate area of fixation
4. Unstable spondylolisthesis	Increased instability	Stress x-ray, motion palpation	Avoid areas of slippage, specific manipulation to levels above and below
Arthritis			
1. Rheumatoid arthritis	Transverse ligament rupture, increased inflammation	X-ray and lab findings	Forceful manipulation of the cervical spine contraindicated, use soft tissue and mobilizing techniques with light adjustments
2. Ankylosing spondylitis	Increased inflammation	X-ray and lab findings	In the acute stage mobilizing techniques and exercise contraindicated, bed rest; mobilizing techniques useful later
3. Psoriatic arthritis	Transverse ligament rupture	X-ray findings, skin lesions	Forceful manipulation contraindicated, use soft tissue mobilizing technique
4. Osteoarthritis (unstable stage)	Increased instability	Pain and stiffness of joint, stress x-ray findings	Immobilization of area if severe
5. Osteoarthritis (late stage)	Neurologic compromise	X-ray findings	Mobilization, gentle manipulation
6. Uncoarthrosis	Vertebral artery compromise	X-ray findings	Gentle traction, mobilizing and soft tissue techniques
Psychological consideration			
1. Malingering	Secondary gain syndrome	Exaggerated response, inconsistencies in signs and symptoms	Release of patient
2. Hysteria	Prolonged treatment	Exaggerated response, inconsistencies in signs and symptoms	Refer for psychological evaluation

Table 4.2 *(Continued)*

Condition	Potential Complications of Manipulation	Method of Detection	Modification of Patient Management
3. Hypochrondriasis (dependent personality)	Dependency on chiropractic	Delayed healing time	Reevaluate patient, wean with reassurance
4. Pain intolerance	Unnecessary pain	Patient communication, excessive tension on palpation	Gentle maneuvers and reassurance
Metabolic disorders			
1. Clotting disorders	Spinal hematoma	History of anticoagulant therapy, pulse, bruises	Forceful manipulation contraindicated
2. Osteopenia (osteoporosis, osteomalacia)	Pathological fractures	History of long-standing steroid therapy, and post menopausal female, anticonvulsive medication, and malabsorption syndrome and nutritional deficiencies, x-ray findings	Forceful manipulation contraindicated, use mobilizing technique with light adjustment
Neurologic complication			
1. Sacral nerve root involvement from medial or massive disc protrusion	Permanent neurological deficits	Neurological and orthopaedic tests, CT scan and myelography	Refer patient
2. Disc lesions (advancing neurological deficits)	Permanent neurological deficits	Neurological and orthopaedic tests, CT scan and myelography	Refer patient
3. Space-occupying lesions	Permanent neurological deficits	MRI, CT scan, myelography	Refer patient

care system (87). Like any other skilled procedure, the expected results and number of complications depends on the ability of the clinician. Lack of examining and manipulative skills should therefore be considered a contraindication to spinal manipulative therapy (47).

References

1. Ligeros K: *How Ancient Healing Governs Modern Therapeutics.* New York, GP Putnam's Sons, 1937, p 402.
2. Maigne R: *Orthopedic Medicine: A New Approach to Vertebral Manipulations.* Springfield, IL, Charles C Thomas, 1972, pp 169, 208.
3. Pratt-Thomas HR, Berger KE: Cerebellar and spinal injuries after chiropractic manipulation. *JAMA* 133:600–603, 1947.
4. Kunkle EC, Muller JC, Odom GL: Traumatic brain-stem thrombosis: report of a case and analysis of the mechanism of injury. *Ann Intern Med* 36:1329–1335, 1952.
5. Shwartz GA, Geiger JK, Spano AV: Posterior inferior cerebellar artery syndrome of Wallenberg after chiropractic manipulation. *AMA Arch Intern Med* 97:352–354, 1956.
6. Ford RF, Clark D: Thrombosis of the basilar artery with softenings in the cerebellum and brain stem due to manipulation of the neck. *Bull Johns Hopkins Hosp* 98:37–42, 1956.
7. Green D, Joynt RJ: Vascular accidents to the brain stem associated with neck manipulation. *JAMA* 170:522–524, 1959.
8. Smith RA, Estridge MN: Neurologic complications of head and neck manipulations: report of two cases. *JAMA* 182:528–531, 1962.
9. Pribeck RA: Brainstem vascular accidents following neck manipulation. *Wis Arch Phys Med Rehabil* 54:237–240, 1973.
10. Nick J, Contamin F, Nicholle MH: Neurological incidents and accidents due to cervical maniulation. *Societe Med Des Hopit De Paris* 118:435–444, 1967.
11. Kaneshepolsky J, Danielson H, Flynn RF: Vertebral artery insufficiency and cerebellar infarct due to manipulation of the neck. *Bull Los Angeles Neurol Soc* 37:62–65, 1972.
12. Nagler W: Vertebral artery obstruction by hyperextension of the neck: report of three cases. *Arch Phys Med Rehabil* 54:237–240, 1973.
13. Lyness SS, Wagman AD: Neurological deficit following cervical manipulation. *Surg Neurol* 2:121–124, 1974.
14. Mechalic T, Farhat SM: Vertebral artery injury from chiropractic manipulation of the neck. *Surg Neurol* 2:125–129, 1974.
15. Miller RG, Burton R: Stroke following chiropractic manipulation of the spine. *JAMA* 229:189–190, 1974.
16. Davidson KC, Weiford EC, Dixon GD: Traumatic vertebral artery pseudoaneurysm following chiropractic manipulation. *Neuroradiology* 115:651–652, 1975.
17. Mueller S, Sahs AL: Brain stem dysfunction related to cervical manipulation: report of three cases. *Neurology* 26:547–550, 1976.
18. Rinsky LA, Reynolds GG, Jameson RM, Hamilton RD: A cervical spinal cord injury following chiropractic manipulation. *Paraplegia* 13:223–227, 1976.
19. Easton JD, Sherman DG: Cervical manipulation and stroke. *Stroke* 8:594–597, 1977.
20. Parkin PJ, Wallis WE, Wilson JL: Vertebral artery occlusion following manipulation of the neck. *NZ Med J* 88:441–443, 1978.
21. Zimmerman AW, Kumar AJ, Gadoth N, Hodges FJ III: Traumatic vertebrobasilar occlusive disease in childhood. *Neurology* 28:185–188, 1978.
22. Nyberg-Hansen R, Loken AC, Tenstad O: Brain stem lesion with coma for five years following manipulation of the cervical spine. *J Neurol* 218:97–105, 1978.
23. Krueger BR, Okazaki H: Vertebral-basilar distribution infarction following chiropractic cervical manipulation. *Mayo Clin Proc* 55:322–332, 1980.
24. Schellhas KP, Latchaw RE, Wendling LR, Gold LHA: Vertebrobasilar injuries following cervical manipulation. *JAMA* 244:1450–1453, 1980.
25. Braun IF, Pinto RS, DeFilipp GJ, Liberman A, Pasternack P, Zimmerman RD: Brain stem infarction due to chiropractic manipulation of the cervical spine. *South Med J* 76:1199–1201, 1983.
26. Horn SW: The "locked-in" syndrome following chiropractic manipulation of the cervical spine. *Ann Emerg Med* 12:103–105, 1983.
27. Fast A, Zincola DF, Marin EL: Vertebral artery damage complicating cervical manipulation. *Spine* 12:840–841, 1987.
28. Gatterman MI: Contraindications & complications of spinal manipulative therapy. *ACA J Chiro* 18:S75-S86, 1981.

29. Jaskoviak PA: Complications arising from manipulation of the cervical spine. *J Manip Physiol Ther* 3:213–219, 1980.
30. Giles LGF: Vertebral-basilar artery insufficiency. *J Can Chiro Assoc* 21:112–117, 1977.
31. Pyo J, Lowman RM: The "ponticulus posticus" of the first cervical vertebra. *Radiology* 72:850–854, 1959.
32. Selecki BR: The effects of rotation of the atlas on the axis: experimental work. *J Can Chiro Assoc* 13(4):30–31, 1969.
33. Berlin L: Unusual foramina, pseudoformina, and developmental defects of bone. *Am J Roentgenol Rad Ther Nucl Med* 91:1089–1103, 1964.
34. Buna, M, Coghlan W, deGruchy M, Williams D, Zmigwsky O: Ponticles of the atlas: a review and clinical perspective. *J Manip Physiol Ther* 7:261–266, 1984.
35. Houle JOE: Assessing hemodynamics of the vertebrobasilar complex through angiothlipsis. *J Can Chiro Assoc* 16(2):35–36, 41, 1972.
36. George PE, Silverstein HT, Wallace H, Marshall M: Identification of the high risk pre-stroke patient. *ACA J Chiro* 18:S26-S28, 1981.
37. Fisk JW: Neck manipulation (letter). *NZ Med J* 89:61, 1978.
38. Virtama P, Kivalo E: Impression on the vertebral artery by deformation of the unco-vertebral joints. *Acta Radiol* 48:410, 1957.
39. Sheehan S, Bauer RB, Meyer JS: Vertebral artery compression in cervical spondylosis. *Neurology* 10:968–986, 1950.
40. Marinelli MR: Extracranial arterial disease: assessment of noninvasive techniques part 1. *Primary Cardiology* 7:53–66, 1980.
41. Reed CA, Toole JF: Clinical technique for identification of external carotid bruits. *Neurology* 31:744–746, 1981.
42. Winterstein JF: Abdominal aortic aneurysm. *Roentgenological Briefs: Council on Roentgenology to the American Chiropractic Association Inc.* 11:84, 1984.
43. D'Ambrosia RD: *Musculoskeletal Disorders, Regional Examination and Differential Diagnosis*, ed 2. Philadelphia, JB Lippincott, 1977, pp 251, 312, 313, 315, 343.
44. Fisk, JW: *A Practical Guide to Management of the Painful Neck and Back: Diagnosis, Manipulation, Exercises, Prevention.* Springfield, IL, Charles C Thomas, 1977, p 6.
45. Salter RB: *Textbook of Disorders and Injuries of the Musculoskeletal System.* Baltimore, Williams & Wilkins, 1970, p 311.
46. Stoddard A: *Manual of Osteopathic Practice.* London, Hutchinson, 1969, p 279.
47. Haldeman S: Spinal manipulation therapy in the management of low back pain. In Finneson BE: *Low Back Pain*, ed 2. Philadelphia, JB Lippincott, 1980 pp 250–251.
48. Hviid H: Functional radiography of the cervical spine. *Ann Swiss Chiro Assoc* 3:37–65, 1965.
49. Conley RN: Stress evaluation of cervical spinal mechanics. *J Clin Chiro* 1(3):46–62, 1974.
50. Grice A: Preliminary evaluation of 50 sagittal cervical motion radiographic examinations. *J Can Chiro Assoc* 21:33–34, 1977.
51. Henderson DJ: Significance of vertebral dyskinesia in relation to the cervical syndrome. *J Manip Physiol Ther* 2:3–15, 1979.
52. Maitland GD: *Vertebral Manipulation*, ed 4. Boston, Butterworths, 1977, pp 182–183.
53. Cassidy, JD, Potter GE, Kirkaldy-Willis WH: Manipulative management of back pain in patients with spondylolisthesis. *JCCA* 22:15–20, 1978.
54. Dabbert O, Freeman DG, Weis AJ: Spinal meningeal hematoma, warfarin therapy, and chiropractic adjustment. *JAMA* 214:2058, 1970.
55. Kleynhans AM: Complication of and contraindications to spinal manipulative therapy. In Haldeman S (ed): *Modern Developments in the Principles and Practice of Chiropractic.* East Norwalk, CT, Appleton-Century-Crofts, 1979, pp 370–379.
56. Forrester DM, Brown JC, Nesson JW: *The Radiology of Joint Disease*, ed 2. Philadelphia, WB Saunders, 1978, pp 596–597.
57. Mennell J McM: *Back Pain: Diagnosis and Treatment Using Manipulative Techniques.* Boston, Little, Brown & Co, 1960, p 113.
58. Finneson BE: *Low Back Pain.* Philadelphia, JB Lippincott, 1980, pp 179, 495, 498.
59. Tabor CW: *Tabor's Cyclopedic Medical Dictionary*, ed 11. Philadelphia, FA Davis, 1972, p 852.
60. Garner HH: Malingering. *Ill Med J* 128:318–319, 1965.
61. Ford CV: *The Somatizing Disorders: Illness as a Way of Life.* New York, Elsevier, 1983, p 128.
62. Ransford AO, Cairns D, Mooney V: The pain drawing as an aid to the psychological evaluation. *Spine* 12:127–134, 1976.
63. Evanski PM, Carver D, Nehemkis A, Waugh TR: The Burns' test in low back pain: correlation with the hysterical personality. *Clin Orthop* 140:42–44, 1979.
64. Frost HM: Diagnosing musculoskeletal disability of psychogenic origin in orthopaedic practice. *Clin Orthop* 82:108–122, 1972.
65. Wiles MR: Somatic, psychogenic and false disability. *J Manip Physiol Ther* 3:149–153, 1980.
66. Szasz TS: Malingering: diagnosis or social condemnation? *AMA Arch Neurol Psychiatry* 76:432–443, 1956.
67. Campbell RJ: *Psychiatric Dictionary*, ed 5. New York, Oxford University Press, 1981, pp 298–300.
68. Helfet AJ, Gruebel Lee DM: *Disorders Of The Lumbar Spine.* Philadelphia, JB Lippincott, 1978, p 138.
69. Kengar: Hypochondriasis: a clinical study. *Br J Psychiatry* 110:478–488, 1964.
70. Pilowsky I: Primary and secondary hypochondriasis. *Acta Psychiatr Scand* 46:273–285, 1970.
71. Engel BT: Some physiological correlates of hunger and pain. *J Exp Psychol* 57:389–396, 1959.
72. Craig KD: Emotional aspects of pain. In Wall PD, Melzak R (eds): *Textbook of Pain.* New York, Churchill Livingstone, 1984, pp 153–161.
73. Mount BM: Psychological and social aspects of cancer pain. In Wall PD, Melzak R (eds): *Textbook of Pain.* New York, Churchill Livingstone, 1984, pp 460–471.
74. Zborowski M: Cultural components in response to pain. *J Social Issues* 8:16–30, 1952.
75. Sternbach RA, Tursky B: Ethnic differences among housewives in psychophysical and skin potential responses to electrical shock. *Psychophysiology* 1:241–246, 1965.
76. Mechanic D: Religion, religiosity, and illness behavior: the special case of the Jews. *Human Organization* 22:202–208, 1963.
77. Lawlis GF, Achterberg J, Kenner L, Kopetz K: Ethnic and sex differences in response to clinical and induced pain in chronic spinal pain patients. *Spine* 9:751–754, 1984.
78. Jennett WB: A study of 25 cases of compression of the cauda equina by prolapsed intervertebral discs. Radcliffe Infirmary, Oxford, Department of Neurological Surgery, 19:109, 1956.
79. Kewalromani LS, Kewalromani DL, Krebs M, Saleem A: Myelopathy following cervical spine manipulation. *J Phys Med* 61:165–175, 1982.
80. Hooper J: Low back pain and manipulation paraparesis after treatment of low back pain by physical methods. *Med J Aust* 1:549–557, 1973.
81. Shapiro R: *Myelography*, ed 3. Chicago, Year Book, 1975, p 399.
82. Poppen JL: The herniated intervertebral disc on analysis of 400 verified cases. *N Engl J Med* 232:211–215, 1945.
83. Thibodeau AA: Backache, a therapeutic conference. New England Medical Center 11:34–42, 1949.
84. Mathews JA, Yates DAH: Reduction of lumbar disc prolapse by manipulation. *Br Med J* 3:696–697, 1969.
85. Cox JM: *Low Back Pain: Mechanism, Diagnosis and Treatment*, ed 4. Baltimore, Williams & Wilkins, 1985, pp 172–237.
86. Grieve GP: Lumbar instability. *Physiotherapy* 68:2–9, 1982.
87. *Chiropractic in New Zealand: Report of the Commission of Inquiry.* Wellington, Hasselberg PD, 1979, p 3.

CHAPTER 5

Examination

SCOTT FECHTEL, D.C., B.S.

More mistakes are made from want of proper examination than for any other reason. MacNab

The steps leading to a decision about how and what to treat are the most important part of any interaction between a doctor and a patient. If the treatment is to be appropriate and the patient is to improve, the physician must understand the patient's problem. This process is the diagnostic evaluation.

The evaluation has a number of parts. The physical examination may encompass chiropractic, orthopaedic, neurologic, and general areas of inquiry. Laboratory tests may be required. Imaging of the body may be done by x-rays, gamma rays, magnetic resonance, or ultrasound. These studies may be enhanced with contrast or by computer. The chiropractic physician should be acquainted with the indications for each of these modalities and, if they are not available in the office, should know how to get the patient to them when necessary.

The scope of this chapter is spinal evaluation. The emphasis is on "in office" diagnostic evaluation. This includes the orthopaedic, neurologic, and physical examination techniques needed for routine chiropractic care of spine-related injury and disease. The organization is regional; the cervical, thoracic, and lumbosacral areas of the spine are considered individually. Critical elements of each spinal region are presented initially. An overview of general spinal considerations precedes the regional discussion.

Orthopaedic testing involves examination of the mechanical structure of the body. The interaction of bones, muscles, ligaments, tendons, and joints is evaluated. Ranges of motion and functional challenges are the hallmarks of such tests.

Neurologic evaluation in the office checks readily accessible portions of the central and peripheral nervous systems. Sensation in its various permutations (light touch, cold, heat, position, vibration, and pain) can be examined. Trophic reactions as well as motor control can be assessed. Cord-level reflexes, both normal and pathologic, should be part of the examination routine. On occasion the chiropractic physician may need to observe cranial nerve function. Ophthalmoscopic determination of intracranial pressure is sometimes needful. The individual's reaction to pain must be understood. The "functional overlay" or "supratentorial" component of pain problems is present in any clinical practice.

The chiropractic contribution to diagnosis is the integration of the orthopaedic and neurologic evaluation of spinal function leading to appropriate physical treatment. The traditional emphasis on spinal manipulation by the profession has produced a number of evaluating systems for spinal function. Both static (x-ray, postural, moire) and dynamic (motion palpation, functional radiography, and cineroentgenography) approaches are available to clinicians. These tools have been derived from the basic and clinical sciences and, as in all areas of scientific inquiry, must stand the tests of time and new knowledge. The rapid growth of interest in biomechanics and the consequent basic and clinical research in this field is hastening the review process. As in all areas of medicine, improved patient care will follow. This is part of the excitement of chiropractic practice today.

HISTORY

No introduction to diagnosis is complete without a discussion of the patient's history. Obtaining an adequate history is not just getting a list of the patient's complaints, it also includes observation of pain behavior. An adequate history will elicit clues to the direction the remainder of the evaluation will take.

70

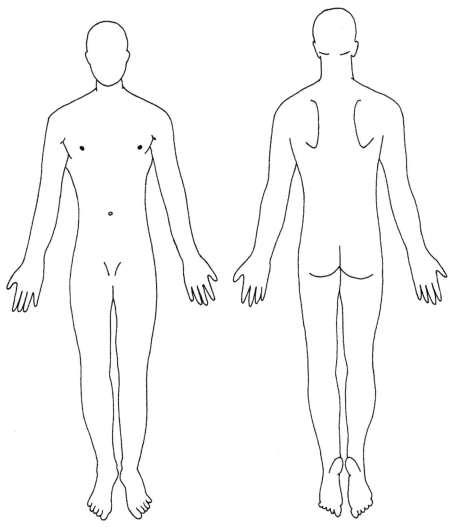

Figure 5.1. The pain drawing can indicate both physical and psychological problems. The different symbols indicate the type of pain, numbness (−), pins and needles (o), burning (×), aching (*), stabbing (/), with a scoring system for differentiation of psychological and pathological conditions (Chapter 4) (Table 5.1).

Symptomatic complaints are the beginning. Complaints should be cataloged as current or past, and the severity of this occurrence and seriousness noted. Are these problems annoying or are they disabling? Directed questioning will then fill in the details of onset, course, contributing factors, and previous treatment. It is worse than useless to repeat previously failed therapy. If, for example, your new, back pain patient just finished a series of 20 sacroiliac joint manipulations by another chiropractor without significant improvement, it is unlikely that another series of 20 manipulations to the same freely moving joint will prove beneficial. It is not efficient to evaluate body systems that are not connected to the patient's problem. With our back pain patient it would seem unreasonable to evaluate the carpal tunnels. Similarly, there is no clinical reason to evaluate the cranial nerves for a simple lumbar strain episode.

The completed history should include information in the following areas: *What?* a list of complaints arranged by system, severity, and seriousness; *When?* whether onset is insidious or sudden, traumatic or not, better or worse with specific actions, times, or motions; *Past?* contribution from previous illness or injury, previous attempts at treatment (whether at home or through consultation), previous episodes of similar problems or family involvement; and *Course?* is this episode getting better or worse? Has any past treatment been beneficial? Are the symptoms expanding in scope or intensity?

It is also helpful to discern what the patient thinks about the problem, how it started, and any underlying problems or concerns. Dealing with the patient's concerns about the illness or injury early, establishes rapport and relaxes the patient. Once patients recognize that they will be cared for as persons and that their worries or fears can be put to rest or acted upon accordingly, the remainder of the evaluation

Table 5.1 Hypothesis for Evaluating Pain Drawings[a]

A patient with poor psychometrics may show this by
1. Unreal drawings (poor anatomic localization, scores 2 unless indicated; bilateral pain not weighted unless indicated)
   a. Total leg pain
   b. Lateral whole leg pain (trochanteric area and lateral thigh allowed)
   c. Circumferential thigh pain
   d. Bilateral anterior tibial area pain (unilateral allowed)
   e. Circumferential foot pain (scores 1)
   f. Bilateral foot pain (scores 1)
   g. Use of all four modalities suggested in instructions (we feel patient is unlikely to have "burning areas," stabbing pain, pins and needles, and numbness all together; scores 1)
2. Drawings showing "expansion" or "magnification" of pain (may also represent unrelated symptomatology; bilateral pain not weighted)
   a. Back pain radiating to iliac crest, groin, or anterior perineum (each scores 1; coccygeal pain allowed)
   b. Anterior knee pain (scores 1)
   c. Anterior ankle pain (scores 1)
   d. Pain drawn outside the outline (Fig. 4.8); this is a particularly good indication of magnification (scores 1 or 2 depending on extent)
3. "I particularly hurt here" indicators (Fig. 4.6); some patients needing to make sure the physician is fully aware of the extent of symptoms may (each category scores 1; multiple use of a category is not weighted)
   a. Add explanatory notes
   b. Circle painful areas
   c. Draw lines to demarcate painful areas
   d. Use arrows
   e. Go to excessive trouble and detail in demonstrating the pain areas (using the symbols suggested)
4. "Look how bad I am" indicators (Fig. 4.8); additional painful areas in the trunk, head, neck or upper extremities drawn in. Tendency toward total body pain (scores 1 if limited to small areas, otherwise scores 2).

[a]Adapted from Ransford AO, Cairns D, Mooney U: The pain drawing as an aid to the psychologic evaluation of patients with low back pain. *Spine* 1:127–134, 1974

can be conducted in a forthright and trusting manner.

When consideration of manipulation is undertaken, it is imperative to determine if the patient is taking any anticoagulant medications. Although not firmly established, the possibility of manipulation-induced intraarticular bleeding must be seriously examined. The consequences of an intraarticular bleed or persistent hemmorrhage can be devastating, justifying the additional caution (Chapter 4).

Other symptoms that would suggest that spinal pain is referred from other body systems must be explored. Back pain coincident with claudication symptoms would indicate the need for vascular consultation. Widespread, nonradicular neurologic symptoms suggest peripheral nerve demyelinating disease, for which physical treatment would not be primary. Similarly, neurologic signs focal to one nerve would suggest the possibility of trauma or compression along the nerve and not the root. The clinician must consider symptoms and signs from the more central locations. These findings warrant referral for specialty consultation and more invasive or technological diagnostic examinations than can be conducted in the chiropractic office.

A thorough history will direct the physical examination and should provide the clinician with a suspected diagnosis. Proper attention to the history will simplify the following physical examination, saving both clinician and patient time and expense. Kern (1) reported that physicians who had completed the standard internal medicine residency training program felt that the most important clinical tools in practice (compared with the emphasis placed on

them in training) were the history and physical examination. Forewarned is forearmed!

Pain Diagram

A useful tool that gives valuable information about both physical and psychological problems is a pain drawing. The patient is given a form with outlines of the body (Fig. 5.1), which can be filled in and assessed quickly (Table 5.1). When used to differentiate psychological complaints from physical conditions the diagram is scored by anatomical consistency. The pain diagram as described by Ransford (2) had better than 80% correlation with the hysteria and hypochondriasis levels of the Minnesota Multiphasic Personality Inventory.

When the pain drawing is consistent with known anatomic referral patterns, no points are assessed, and valuable clues can be obtained for the diagnostic impression. When patients draw pain pictures that are not consistent with known referral pathways and exceed the body margins, utilize multiple pain quality descriptors (again in a nonphysiological fashion), or give verbal descriptions of symptoms not in accord with the drawing, then points are assigned for each type of variation. With a score higher than three points assigned to the pain drawing, there is less likelihood of a good outcome from treatment independent of psychologic intervention (Chapter 4).

PHYSICAL EXAMINATION

The spinal examination can be separated into orthopaedic and neurologic portions. Either orthopaedic or neurologic examination challenges

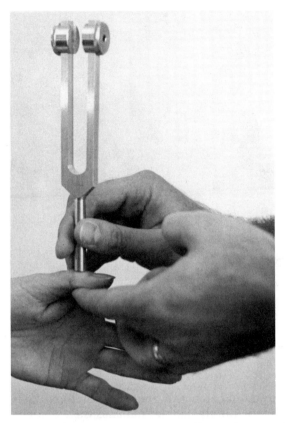

Figure 5.2. Vibratory sensation is tested by application of a vibrating tuning fork over bony prominences.

the tissue to determine its functional or pathologic state. Orthopaedic testing is more complex because there are more tissues to evaluate. Neurologic testing challenges sensory, motor, and reflex functions. Orthopaedic testing can be used to differentiate problems associated with bones, joints, ligaments, and muscles. The real world includes problems that involve all such tissues in varying degrees, as well as problems limited to a single tissue or part. The successful physician is part detective as well as an expert in application of therapies.

A note about eponyms. It is an honor to have a test named for a researcher; however, for the student and practicing physician such eponyms are of academic interest only. Being forced to memorize a vast number of names unrelated to the function of a test is cumbersome and time-consuming, and may lead to ambiguity in the reporting of clinical findings. For that reason, emphasis here will be on functional descriptions rather than eponyms.

Peripheral and central nerve testing is used to locate a lesion. The clinical tools available to the chiropractor are: sensation, reflex, and motor neural function. Sensory function can be differentiated into pain and temperature, touch, vibration, and position. Reflexes can be physiologic or pathologic. Motor function can be lost, normal, or aberrant and can be either hypo- or hypertonic. Tremors or changes in

dexterity may occur. These changes can occur in limited or widespread areas.

The initial evaluation of neural lesions determines at what level the lesion exists. A peripheral lesion manifests itself locally. The more central the lesion, the wider the area of pain, paresthesia, or motor change involved. Therefore, the physician can recognize the change of neural function involved and the extent to which it has occurred. The lesion will have altered function below and normal function above.

Vibration sensation is carried by fibers in the dorsal or posterior columns of the spinal cord. It is tested by applying a vibrating tuning fork to bony prominences from distal to proximal (Fig. 5.2). Most persons will be able to discern vibration or buzzing at the first joint of each digit. Occasionally the need to test the next proximal major joint will arise, such as going to the ankle from the great toe. Various factors such as age, previous injury, or disease may explain a deterioration of distal sensation. Symmetry between the extremities may be considered "normal" or clinically insignificant. Since fibers transmitting this sensation cross at the level of the lower medulla and not in the spinal cord, unilateral alterations of sensation point to an ipsilateral peripheral or cord lesion.

Position sense is carried by fibers in the dorsal column–medial lemniscal pathway. This sense is tested by firmly grasping a great toe or thumb and moving the digit in an up or down direction (Fig. 5.3). The patient must have closed eyes (to remove visual clues) and inform the examiner of the onset and direction of movement. Movement of between 1/16 and 1/14 inch should be distinguishable. Symmetry between the tested parts is the critical finding. Usually sensation in the hands is more sensitive than that in the feet. Because fibers cross at the level of the lower medulla, unilateral findings suggest an ipsilateral cord lesion. Bilateral losses are associated with ataxia (a loss of muscular coordination and impairment of gait).

Pain sensation is easily tested with a pin or pinwheel. By tapping the patient's skin, the clinician can determine whether a lesion involves a peripheral nerve, dermatome, myotome, the cord, or the brain. Pain and temperature information travel in the lateral spinothalamic tract. These fibers cross the cord at the level of entry; therefore a lesion in the cord will alter sensation on the contralateral side.

Pain of psychologic origin will not be confined within the above levels (Chapter 4). Stocking-glove or whole extremity distribution of pain or paresthesia are examples of such presentations. In evaluating psychogenic pain, factors such as pain behavior and secondary gain must be determined and differentiated from other pathology, such as diabetic peripheral neuropathy or stroke.

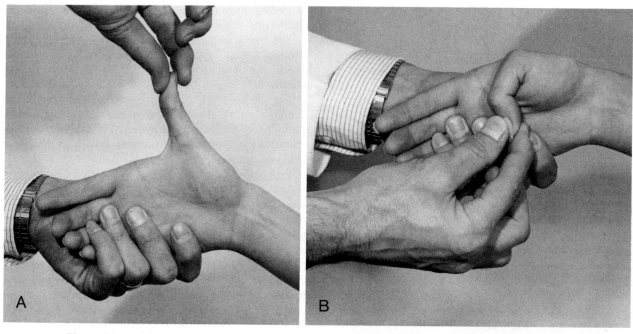

Figure 5.3. Position sensation is tested by moving the thumb in an **A** up and **B** down direction.

Table 5.2 Muscle Grading Chart[a]

Rank	Description	Grade
Normal	Complete range of motion against gravity with full resistance	5
Good	Complete range of motion against gravity with some resistance	4
Fair	Complete range of motion against gravity and only without resistance	3
Poor	Complete range of motion with gravity eliminated	2
Trace	Evidence of slight contractility, no joint motion	1
Zero	No evidence of contractility	0

[a]Adapted from Hoppenfeld S: *Physical Examination of the Spine and Extremities.* East Norwalk, CT, Appleton-Century-Crofts, 1976, p 26.

Motor losses also help define the level of the lesion. Both quality and quantity of motor change is important. Is the muscle hypo- or hypertonic? Is the muscle subject to fine control or limited to gross movement? Muscle strength can be quantified from normal to absent (Table 5.2). Strength or tone changes are limited to a discrete muscle in peripheral nerve losses, to a group of muscles (generally) in radicular damage, and to progressively greater areas as the location of the lesion ascends the neuraxis. Referral of the patient for evaluation by electromyography will provide much definitive evidence in these conditions.

Manual muscle testing requires that the clinician position the patient so that the tested muscle is isolated. Then, smooth application of force against the muscle will allow the examiner to grade the muscle strength. "Give-away" is a finding associated with pain or psychogenic problems. This occurs when the examiner smoothly increases the force against a muscle while the patient matches the examiner until a threshold is reached and the patient releases the muscle, or "lets go." This threshold is not present for neurologically impaired muscle. Rather the muscle's ability to withstand force is smoothly exceeded. Repeat testing is consistent in impaired muscle, while psychogenic losses are variable.

Deep tendon reflexes used most commonly are those associated with the biceps, triceps, and brachioradialis muscles in the upper extremities, and the patellar and achilles tendons in the lower extremities. These reflexes are associated with segmental levels of the cord and occur when the tendon stretch activates the muscle spindles, sending a phasic, synchronous discharge to the cord. Testing involves identifying the tendon and then percussing it with a rubber hammer. Before concluding that a tendon reflex is absent or impaired, the patient should be distracted or the reflex reinforced (Fig. 5.4). Distraction is often effected by diverting the patient's gaze or by having the patient grasp the hands together tightly or pull against one another. "Reinforcement" occurs as the patient increases the tone of the muscle involved in a particular reflex. This increases the amplitude of the tendon and muscle stretch.

Initial testing is done with the muscle in as relaxed a state as possible. Having the patient push with the toes against the examiner (for the patellar or achilles) or gently tense the muscle (for the biceps or triceps) will generally allow the examiner to appreciate some muscle jerk. Again the concern is with symmetry between the extremities, unless a

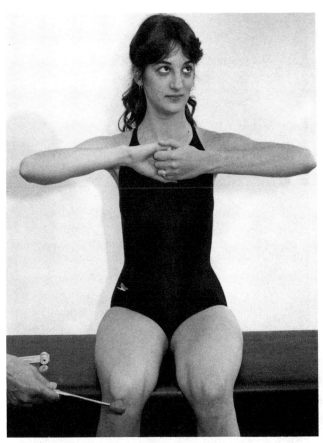

Figure 5.4. Distraction of the patient by diverting the gaze and tightly pulling against the hands may be necessary to elicit the patellar reflex.

more central lesion is suspected. Wide variations in the excursion of the "jerk" are the rule between individuals but not within the same person. It is not appropriate to label a reflex hypoactive until all available methods of reinforcement have been attempted. If the reflex cannot be elicited bilaterally and other reflexes are intact, the reduction in reflex action is clinically unimportant.

Pathological reflexes for the office-based physician are primarily the Babinski and grasp. Stroking the sole of the foot of the newborn normally produces a dorsiflexion of the big toe and fanning of the other toes. In the adult or more mature nervous system this action usually produces a plantar flexion of the toes (Fig. 5.5A), or they may be held rigid. When the pyramidal pathway of the cord is damaged, such uncomfortable stimulation of the sole of the foot results in dorsiflexion of the great toe and spreading or fanning of the other toes (Fig. 5.5B). In the normal adult this action is suppressed by the fibers of the corticospinal pathway. Infants may demonstrate these withdrawal signs up to 18 months of age. Gently stroking the palm of the hand in the newborn results in approximation of the fingers and thumb. This grasping reflex occurs in the adult with brain damage in the motor cortex area. There are a great

number of variations on these themes of pathological reflexes. These two are the most widely known. The variations are different ways of eliciting withdrawal responses from noxious stimuli.

As noted above, the musculoskeletal or orthopaedic portion of the examination involves a wider variety of tissues than the neurological. Bones, ligaments, joints, muscles, and tendons should all be evaluated, and this is made easier by noting the type of action that causes the symptoms. Pain caused by passive motion of a joint complex suggests that the bone, joint, or ligament is injured, while symptoms present with active motion alone point to the muscle or tendon. Passive motion occurs as the examiner moves the joint. Active motion occurs when the associated muscles move the joint. Similarly, by positioning the patient or requiring specific actions of the patient, a particular joint or portion of a joint complex can be challenged. This is the area with which the greatest number of eponyms have become associated. Each way of moving or stressing a joint has some researcher's name attached, and these movements are discussed at length in textbooks of neurology.

Mechanical analysis of joint function has shown that some elasticity is present in the normal ligamentous structure of each joint. Mennell (3) refers to this as "joint play." The loss of joint play is referred to as a "fixation" by Gillet (4). According to Gillet this is the entity that responds to manipulation. The analysis of joint play can be accomplished by springing each vertebra in each of its planes of motion or by monitoring the relative motion between bony landmarks. This process is described as "motion palpation" by Gillet (4) and Faye (5). The codification of this process is one of the greatest contributions of chiropractic researchers to the study of spine-related problems (Chapter 3).

Briefly, to quickly evaluate the spine for fixation, the patient is seated with the doctor behind. The doctor braces the patient with one arm across the patient's shoulders and, using the fist or back of the hand, gently pushes the spine in the anteroposterior plane (Fig. 5.6). The push should take the spine to the end of the range of physiologic motion, then test the elasticity of the ligaments with a slight springing motion. Normal motion occurs when the spine yields to the push and rebounds smoothly. The doctor should remember to keep the axis of the push parallel to that of the facets of the palpated segments.

The doctor ascends the spine one fist breadth at a time. Fixation of a segment is perceived as a failure of the spine to yield to the springing motion. As the rhythm of palpation is gained, the fixation is perceived as an abrupt stop in motion, like a pendulum hitting a wall. This routine is repeated in the lateral and oblique planes.

The cervical spine can be motion palpated in the same fashion. The occiput–cervical spine articula-

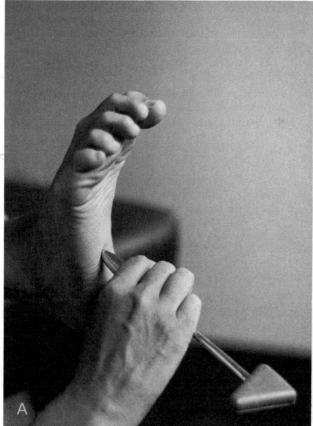 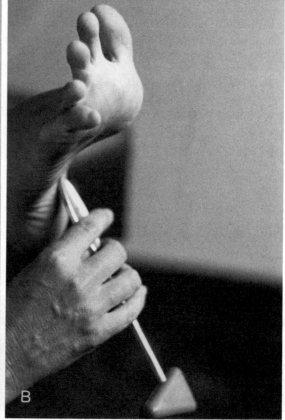

Figure 5.5. **A**, Stroking the sole of the foot produces plantar flexion of the toes in normal adults. **B**, Fanning the toes with this procedure is a pathological response indicating a pyramidal or cord lesion.

tion is palpated by grasping the transverse processes of the first cervical segment with a thumb and forefinger and directing the patient to nod the head through a full range of motion. Springing the vertebra at the end of motion will discern the elasticity of the supporting ligaments. At the second cervical segment, rotation of the head will first slide the occiput on its C1 condyles, then give rotation of C1 on the odontoid. The palpating hand again contacts the transverse processes of the second vertebra and springs at the end of the normal motion. With practice the doctor will develop a ready feel for vertebral motion and a smooth routine of palpation.

A final introductory note on physical examination is important. A well-organized pattern of examination procedures will facilitate complete examination. It should not take a prolonged time to examine each region of the spine. A ready familiarity with the anatomy and pathology of the area under consideration will direct the search. The search begins with the history, which implicates the area to begin each patient's evaluation. Recognizing the neural, vascular, musculoskeletal, and other tissues in the area leads to an organized consideration of each.

It must become habitual for each doctor to exclude those pathologic entities that carry the worst

prognosis (Chapter 4). There are many changes ongoing in the practice of all schools of health care in the United States. None of these social/societal changes remove the physician's absolute duty to guard the patient's best interest. Treating a spinal fixation through appropriate manipulation without discovering an adjacent tumor or aneurysm is not in the patient's best interest.

Cervical Spine

A regional examination of the cervical spine must consider related anatomy. Diagnostic examination of the neck must include consideration of all the anatomy that connects the structures of the head with those of the trunk. All blood supply for the brain ascends through the neck. The brain stem with its critical structures is located in the neck. The neck contains the cervical portion of the spine including discs, bones, joints, and nerve roots. The esophagus, trachea, endocrine and lymph glands, as well as the structures of the head must be considered.

The examination begins with observation. Is the head in normal anatomical position or does it list or tilt? Are there any anomalies or scars present? Does the patient appear to be in pain? Are conversational

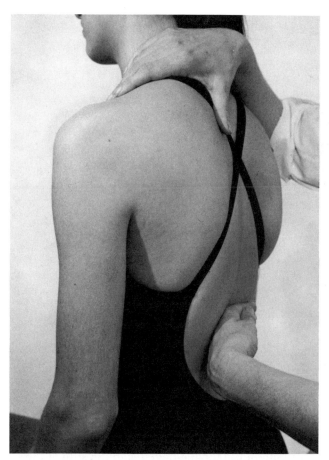

Figure 5.6. A motion palpation screen is performed with the patient stabilized while the doctor flexes and extends each vertebral motion segment.

movements fluid? Can the patient perform an active extension-rotation test without evidence of vertebral artery impairment?

To the chiropractor intending to employ manipulation, the two most critical structures in the neck, from the point of view of manipulation, are the vertebral arteries and the intervertebral discs. The most severe complications of spinal manipulation occur in these two areas. Vertebral artery stenosis caused by congenital anomaly or by arteriosclerotic disease is reported to be the predisposing element. Ponticulus posticus, the anomaly of a round spicule of bone located on the posterior arch of the atlas vertebra, encircling the vertebral artery, is now recognized as another predisposing element to this syndrome (6–10) (Chapter 4). Briefly, under these conditions, cervical manipulation may cause thrombosis with subsequent brainstem infarction.

In the literature are reports of such patients with outcomes ranging from full recovery to death. Sheehan (11) has proposed the rotation-extension test to screen for predisposition. Krueger (6) discounted the notion that preexisting vascular or bony abnormalities or both were required for the syndrome to occur, because of the absence of these findings in his series of patients. George (9) has proposed a series of screening tests including evaluating the patient's history for vascular problems, blood pressure evaluation, carotid artery palpation, and sustained cervical rotation and extension (held for 3 to 5 seconds) (Fig. 5.7).

Auscultation of the carotid arteries is more revealing than palpation. A family or personal history of vascular problems including stroke, transient ischemic attacks, hypertension, or bruit should excite suspicion in the examining doctor. Current hypertensive disease must increase the index of suspicion. Reports of dizziness, nausea, faintness, diplopia, fuzzy vision, vertigo, or nystagmus during or after the extension and rotation test should lead to very careful evaluation before attempting spinal manipulation. For patients with positive findings, consultation with a vascular surgeon should be obtained prior to cervical spine manipulation or before any form of therapy is applied to this area. It must be noted that these measures will not uncover congenital anomalies of the vertebral arteries; however, this anatomical variation is infrequent. Under such circumstances the screening tests can cause the syndrome, therefore extreme caution should be employed by the clinician in performing them. The examiner should be prepared for that eventuality with a plan of action to transport the patient to an appropriate facility in the least possible time.

The range of motion in each plane is determined next. This includes rotation (Y-axis rotation), left and right lateral bending (Z-axis rotation), and flexion and extension (X-axis rotation) (Chapter 2). Although intersegmental motion depends on the local joint anatomy, global ranges of motion are approximately (12): left and right rotation, 80°; left and right lateral bending, 45° each; flexion, 45° (depending on the amount of submandibular soft tissue), and extension, 45° (Fig. 5.8). It is important to note that there are individual variations. These depend on sex, age, anatomical variations, past injury, and degenerative disease. Briefly, neither the 80-year-old spine with its concomitant degenerative joint disease or the spine with a congenital fusion can be expected to demonstrate the ranges of motion of the unimpaired, youthful spine.

While the need to evaluate the cranial nerves is not common in chiropractic practice, everyone will see an occasional patient with symptoms of cranial nerve dysfunction. The chiropractor should be able to recognize the symptoms, to screen the patient, and to recognize the need for a more thorough diagnostic evaluation. Loss of the sense of smell without a history of skull fracture or local trauma is usually apparent to the patient and will be revealed by a simple question or two during history taking. Similarly, visual impairment such as loss of part or all of a visual field will probably be spontaneously reported.

Figure 5.7. Extension and rotation of the cervical spine held for 3 to 5 seconds can be used as a screening test to evaluate vascular flow through the vertebral arteries.

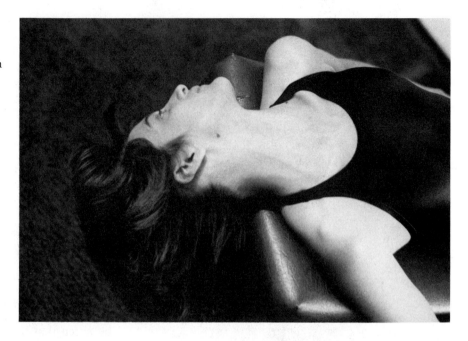

Nerves III, IV, and VI are tested by observing the motion of the eyes. The patient is directed to turn the eyes first to one side, then to the other. While the eyes are directed to one side, the patient is asked to look up and down. Weakness of the ocular muscles or subjective diplopia are positive signs. Nystagmus can be tested by having the patient track the examiner's finger in the horizontal and vertical planes. Sustained jerks in the tracking eyes is abnormal, a few low-amplitude jerks at the extremes of lateral gaze are normal. Pupillary size, shape, and reflexes can be rapidly noted.

Sensory function of nerve V can be tested with a cotton wisp applied to the facial skin served by this nerve. Motor function of the jaw is tested by directing the patient to open the mouth wide. Weakness is demonstrated by deviation of the jaw to the weak side. Nerve VII is tested by having the patient frown or smile, closing the eyes tightly, and having the examiner attempt to open them. The thoughtful observer will have noted weakness of these muscles during conversational expression and movements of the patient's face. The corneal reflex is tested with a cotton wisp applied to the cornea away from the patient's diverted gaze. A swift bilateral blink is the normal response. The corneal reflex includes fibers of both nerves V and VII.

Testing bone and air conduction of hearing (the tests of Weber and Rinne) and ascertaining the acuity of normal hearing with a watch tick will give a good idea of the status of nerve VIII.

Problems in talking or swallowing associated with nasal escape of air during talking and a soft, breathy voice suggest lesions of nerves IX and X. Asking the patient to open the mouth and say "ah" will demonstrate weakness of the palate musculature by a deviation of the uvula to the intact side. Checking the gag reflex by touching the back of the throat with a tongue blade will test the sensory function of these two nerves.

Nerve XI can be evaluated by testing the sternocleidomastoideus and trapezius muscles. Having the patient stick the tongue out in the midline will uncover nerve XII dysfunction. With a unilateral nerve impairment the tongue deviates to the side of the lesion and demonstrates ipsilateral atrophy and fasciculations. Side-to-side movement of the tongue will differentiate between upper motor neuron lesions and cranial nerve faults. A decrease in the rate of side-to-side movement occurs with higher lesions.

To evaluate the integrity of the spinal joints, traction and compression are applied. Traction is gently administered, with one hand cupping the chin and the doctor's other hand supporting the occiput. Injury to the joints will be aggravated by traction, while pain due to fixation, muscle spasm, or disc injury will be alleviated (Fig. 5.9). Compression will aggravate pain due to swelling and spasm of joint fixation, disc injury, or sprains. Compression should be applied gently, in the neutral position, with the neck rotated and extended both right and left (Fig. 5.10). Foraminal compression occurs with rotation and extension, which focuses the stress to the ipsilateral facets. A positive foraminal compression test occurs when radicular signs such as dermatomal pain, paresthesia, or motor loss are demonstrated with the maneuver, not simply when facet pain is present.

Percussion can be applied to the vertex of the head in the neutral position (Spurling's maneuver). Again, reproduction of radicular signs or symptoms are the positive result. Motion palpation is performed on the craniocervical and lower cervical sec-

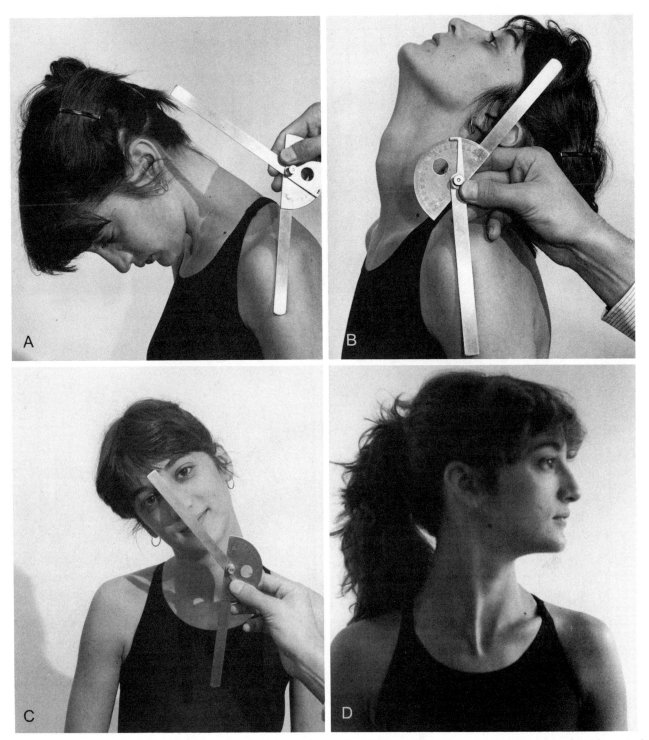

Figure 5.8. **A**, Normal cervical spine range of motion includes 45° of flexion. **B**, Normal cervical spine range of motion includes 45° of extension. **C**, Normal cervical spine range of motion includes 45° of lateral bending. **D**, Normal cervical spine range of motion includes 80° of rotation.

tions to determine endplay motion. Fixation of an apophyseal joint is a positive indication for manipulation at that level. This indication is interpreted by the clinician in light of the other findings of examination.

Intervertebral disc injuries carry less catastrophic consequences than strokes with brainstem injury, but pose a significant problem. Preexisting disc injury can usually be identified by the history of injury, physical examination findings suggestive of

Figure 5.9. Gentle traction of the cervical spine relieves pain due to muscle spasm, joint fixation, and disc injury.

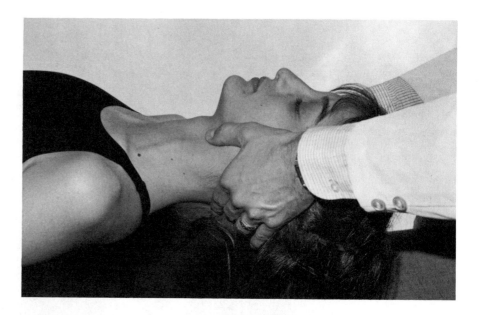

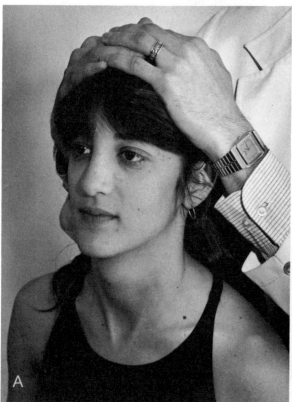

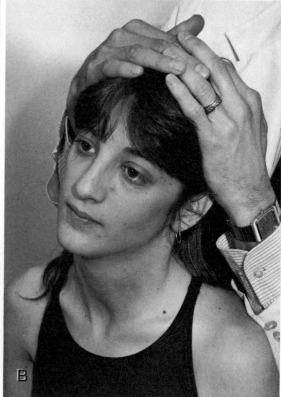

Figure 5.10. **A**, Axial compression aggravates pain from the swelling and spasm of joint fixation, disc injury, or sprains.

B, Compression of the head, with the neck in oblique extension, compresses the ipsilateral facet joints.

nerve-root irritation, and severe guarding muscle spasm. Spinal manipulation is not advisable without adequate prior evaluation because of the possibility of further disc damage (Chapter 4). Harsh or forceful spinal manipulation has been identified as a cause of disc injuries. Residual problems after disc injury range from full recovery of transient paresthe-

sia to motor and sensory loss from spinal root damage. All patients must be apprised of the relative risk of this therapy prior to its application.

A more common disorder is the myofascial pain syndrome. This disorder is characterized by acute muscle pain with accompanying "trigger points." There may be other symptoms and signs associated

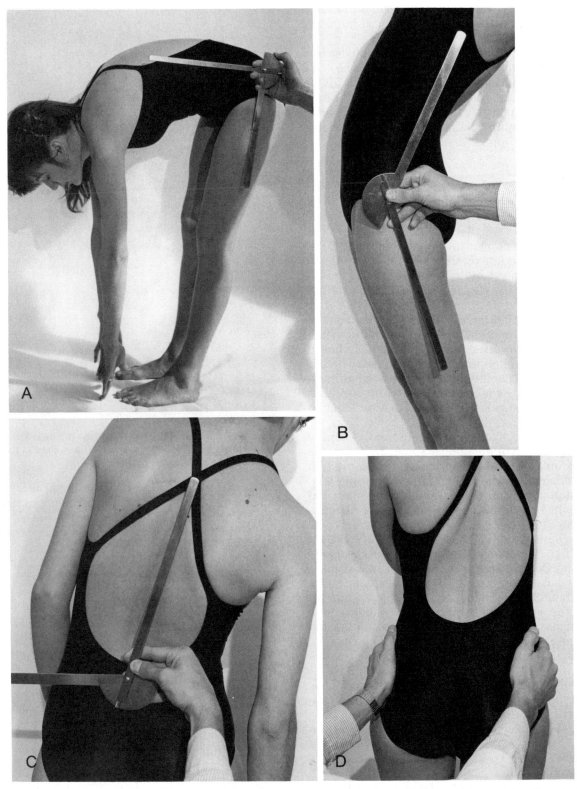

Figure 5.11. **A,** Normal thoracolumbar range of motion includes 90° of flexion. **B,** Normal thoracolumbar range of motion includes 30° of extension. **C,** Normal thoracolumbar range of motion includes 30° of lateral bending. **D,** Normal thoracolumbar range of motion includes 30° of rotation.

with myofascial disorders. Trigger points and accompanying muscle pain usually abate with chiro-

practic pressure techniques. In some cases they recur quickly, and concurrent treatment with other medical specialists for the other aspects of the disease process may be necessary for satisfactory management (Chapter 12).

Disorders of the thyroid, trachea, lymph nodes, and other prevertebral soft tissues must also be considered. Palpation and auscultation are helpful in raising the index of suspicion about these. Further evaluation by a physician specializing in this area will minimize "indirect" injuries of patients seeking relief through chiropractic services.

Thoracic Spine

The anatomy of the thoracic spine includes the ribs, which poses a variation to the anatomy of the cervical and lumbar regions. The ribs protect the organs of the chest and alter the biomechanics of the thoracic spine. Coupled to the sternum anteriorly, the ribs limit motion in all planes of the thoracic spine, thus adding stability to this region. This fundamental difference affects not only diagnosis but also treatment and prognosis of injuries to this area.

As in the examination of other spinal regions, observation plays the initial role. Subtle findings such as a high shoulder or a protruding scapula should excite suspicion of an underlying scoliosis. The clinician will occasionally uncover gross abnormalities of the chest, such as pigeonbreast, duplicate sternum, or Sprengel's deformity with or without an omohyoid bone.

Ranges of thoracic spine motion are generally tested with those of the lumbar spine. They include (12) flexion to at least 90°, extension to 30°, rotation to 30° bilaterally, and lateral bending to 30° (Fig. 5.11). Motion palpation for end-play determines fixation of the individual apophyseal joints or rib articulations.

The scapular motion should be free and without crepitation. Palpation of the scapular muscles is appropriate. Occasionally compression of the scapula will enhance the symptoms of a subscapular bursitis. In trauma cases, radiography of the scapula for fracture is appropriate. Having the patient do a "wall push-up" will determine the status of the serratus anterior muscle and hence the long thoracic nerve. Failure of this muscle to stabilize the scapula results in the "winged" scapula.

In the thoracic spine the intervertebral disc presents particular problems. Protrusion of a soft tissue mass into the narrow thoracic canal causes cord injury, where such a lesion in the cervical and lumbar canal yields nerve root compression. Protruded thoracic discs can be identified by the local muscle spasm, limited focal motion, radiation of pain and sensory loss about the chest paralleling the ribs, and cord signs such as spastic paralysis or paresis of the lower extremity, increased deep tendon reflexes, and extension of toes with foot plantar stimulation (Babinski sign), with or without other cauda equina signs (sphincter loss, sexual function loss, saddle anaesthesia). Motor innervation from the thoracic

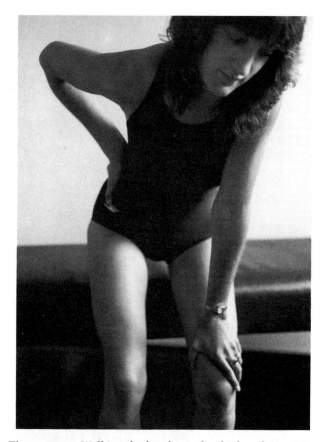

Figure 5.12. Walking the hands up the thighs when arising from a sitting position is known as Minor's sign.

spine includes the abdominal muscles. These can be tested with a bent knee sit-up. Movement of the umbilicus during sit-up (Beevor's sign) indicates weakness of the anterior abdominals in the opposite direction of umbilical travel.

Dysfunction of the organs of the chest and abdomen can cause thoracic spine pain. Pain of cardiac origin can appear in this area. Parenthetically, Brodsky (13) reminds us that cervical spine disorders can cause cardiac area pain identical to that of ischemic disease. Lung malignancies can intrude upon thoracic structures. Metastatic disease from breast cancer is well known. Mediastinal disease can also cause symptoms usually related to thoracic musculoskeletal dysfunction. Once suspected, these entities should be aggressively evaluated by laboratory, radiologic, and consultative means.

Lumbar Spine

Examination of the lumbar spine proceeds in the same fashion as before. Observation begins the cycle. Standing posture can procide important clues to the etiology of the patient's pain. A fixed forward flexion can be caused by psoas muscle spasm. Patients with posteriorly protruded or herniated discs cannot extend the spine and so find a position of relative comfort in the forward flexed position when standing. Forward list may be great, as much as 45°, or slight, as little as 10°. Often there is an element of lateral list. A common presentation of the acute disc is the anterolateral list.

The list can give a clue to the position of a fragment when herniation has occurred. If the fragment is medial to the nerve root, the list will be toward the fragment, thereby reducing the tension of the root against the fragment. If the root is lateral to the fragment, the list will be away from the fragment. The goal is still the same: to reduce the root tension against the offending fragment.

Maintaining flexion of the knee during weight-bearing on a leg with radicular irritation is common. The reason is the same, the extended knee will increase the root tension, increasing pain. Changing position from sitting to standing or the reverse will cause pain with some back injuries.

The effect on a patient's pain of remaining in one position for some time is also of diagnostic importance. With sprain and strain injuries, staying in one position will allow an increase in swelling. Depending on the nature of the injury, the swelling will be either intra- or extraarticular, or both. This patient can move fairly easily but stiffens up after remaining in one position for 10 minutes or more. When arising from a sitting position the acute back patient exhibits a characteristic "hand-walking-up-the-thighs" maneuver (Minor's sign) (Fig. 5.12). This is caused by the combination of painful extension and swelling limiting back motion. As the patient moves, greater extension becomes possible and allows a more erect posture. Usually, maximum extension will have been obtained within two to three steps.

Having observed the patient, the clinican is now prepared to continue the examination. With the patient in the standing posture, range-of-motion testing can occur. The patient is asked to attempt full movement in each of the six planes of motion: flexion, extension, lateral bending (right and left), and rotation (right and left) (Fig. 5.11).

Forcing a patient through motion testing can result in greater injury, therefore, the patient should be asked to go only as far as pain will allow. The physician should ask why the patient stopped at the chosen limit and observe the ease of motion. Inferences can be drawn about limits from the pain of stretching injured muscles or limits imposed by joint locking. The more serious the injury, the greater the limitation imposed on motion. As an example, a modest strain of the erector muscle group may impose pain only at the extreme of flexion. On the other hand, a disc herniation mandates a fixed forward-flexion posture with limits of less than half the normal allowances in all planes of motion.

Range-of-motion testing for the dorsolumbar spine is accomplished by asking the patient to lean forward to touch the toes with the outstretched fingers while maintaining the knees in an extended position. Flexion should be accomplished to 90°. Gym-

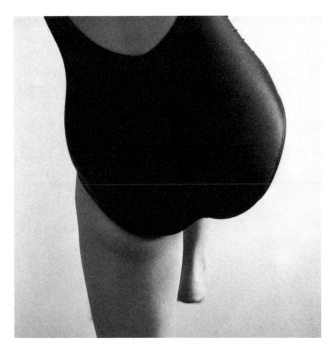

Figure 5.13. When the patient flexes one knee toward the chest (Trendelenburg's test), the pelvis should remain fixed in the horizontal plane by the gluteal muscles.

nasts and other athletes will be able to exceed this. The examiner should gently support the patient at the waist when requesting extension. The patient should bend backward from the waist 30°. Lateral bending should be at least 30°. The patient should be instructed to slide the hand toward the knee along the thigh. Rotation is also 30°. Here the examiner must stabilize the pelvis so that the patient does not rotate at the knee or ankles.

With the patient standing, the integrity and motion of the sacroiliac joints and action of the gluteal muscles can be evaluated. As the patient stands on one foot and flexes the other knee toward the chest (Trendelenburg's test) (Fig. 5.13), the pelvis should be fixed in the horizontal plane by the gluteal muscles. If the hemipelvis lowers on the side of knee flexion, the gluteal muscles are not acting appropriately. If knee flexion and elevation is stopped by a sudden sharp pain in the sacroiliac region, injury to the joint must be considered. This can be more specifically evaluated by motion palpation (Chapter 7).

The next portion of the examination of the standing patient has the patient walk on the toes and heels (Fig. 5.14). This action tests the integrity of the ankle flexor and extensor muscles. If a patient is unable to stand with the heel elevated, weakness of the myotome of the S1 nerve root must be suspected (peroneus longus and brevis, gluteus maximus, and gastrocnemius-soleus). This test must be conducted in a thoughtful fashion, since many patients with an acute back injury will report increased back pain with this maneuver. The increase in pain occurs as the patient assumes the heel-elevated posture, with

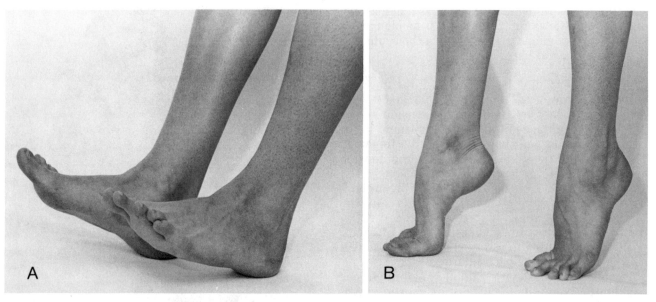

Figure 5.14.   **A,** Walking on the heels tests the neural control of the ankle dorsiflexors. **B,** Walking on the toes tests for neural control of the ankle plantar flexors.

a shift in the center of gravity of the body and consequent change in the postural muscle tension. In equivocal tests, reinforcement is possible by asking the patient to bounce up and down on the balls of the feet—forcing elevation of the heels several times. If there is impingement of the nerve root, that muscle will exhaust more rapidly than the one in the other leg.

Similarly, having the patient heel stand, elevating the toes, tests the L5 muscles. The ankle extensor (foot dorsiflexor) muscles, tibialis anterior, extensor digitorum longus, and extensor hallucis longus, must function normally to allow heel walking. (Realizing that the tibialis anterior is innervated by fibers from the L4 root, the L4, L5, and S1 roots can be differentiated with manual muscle testing while the patient is not weightbearing.)

A sitting straight-leg raise (Bechterew's test) adds valuable information when compared to the supine version indirectly testing the same function (Fig. 15.15A). The examiner may raise the heel upward, extending the leg to 180°. If the patient complains of pain, the level at which pain occurs should be determined. The quality and distribution of the pain should also be determined. Central low back pain suggests mechanical joint problems. Sciatic or femoral distribution pain suggests nerve root impingement. The patient can also be requested to attempt touching the toes while both knees are extended (Fig. 5.15B). Comparison to the earlier standing effort should shed some light on the consistency of the patient's complaints (since the biomechanical effect, discounting the direction of gravity, is the same).

In the prone position the back can be palpated. Muscle and skin tone must be evaluated. Is there

spasm of the muscles? If so, which muscles are involved? Is the patient guarding the area? Guarding is differentiated from spasm by the amount of muscle involved. If a discreet area of paravertebral muscle is hard or nodular, then it is probably spasm. If the entire muscle is tight and firm, it is probably guarding the spine. Conscious and unconscious guarding must be differentiated. If there is sufficient tissue damage to warrant gross motion guarding (and you have seen this with other tests), then guarding is appropriate. If the examination has appeared normal until now, and you are confronted with massive guarding "spasm," then it is unlikely that there is a physiological explanation for the "spasm."

"Springing" the spinous process discerns the status of the facet joints. The examiner places a thumb on the spinous process tip and pushes, varying the force. If there is no pain response to gentle pressure, the examiner might bounce the joint with a little more vigor. The spine should not be extended with this maneuver. Springing the spinous processes can be done either in the prone position or seated as part of the motion palpation screen. Capsular ligament damage, articular cartilage damage, or cortex damage will cause pain when the facet surfaces are approximated during this maneuver. A similar effect occurs when percussing the spinous tip with the pleximeter. Usually pain with gentle percussion suggests fracture or tumor destruction of the involved vertebra (Fig. 5.16).

With the patient in the prone position, one can palpate the sciatic nerve in the sciatic notch, trochanteric area, and posterior knee. Simple digital prodding of these specific areas will elicit a pain response when the nerve is inflamed. Reports of pain with digital palpation of the nerve should be dis-

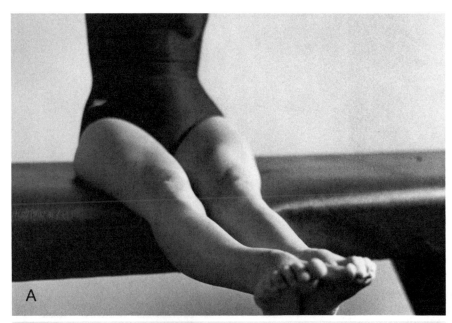

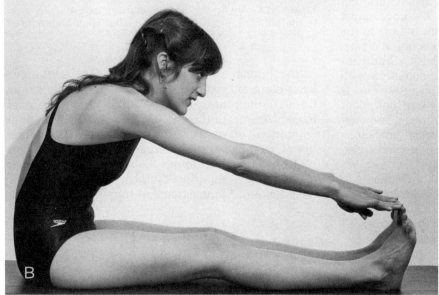

Figure 5.15. **A,** A sitting straight-leg raise (Bechterew's test) is an indirect test for sciatic nerve stretch. **B,** By having the patient touch the toes while sitting with both knees extended, forward bending is indirectly tested.

criminated from general gluteal muscle tenderness. Palpating the bodies of the muscles will provide evidence for the source of the pain complaints.

With the patient supine, palpation of the abdomen can be undertaken. Pain possibly referred from abdominal organs necessitates consideration of this procedure. Any abnormal masses must be located. The quality of internal organ tone should be assessed. For instance, is the colon soft or rigid, are the abdominal muscles pliant or guarding? Auscultation of the abdomen will provide information about the normal function of the colon and the abdominal aorta. Aneurysms of this vital vessel will require referral to a vascular surgeon prior to performing spinal manipulation in the back. Malignant disease of the uterus, ovaries, testicles, or prostate

can metastasize to the lumbar spine. If the chiropractor is uncomfortable with genitourinary tract examination, appropriate referral must be obtained. This area must be considered as a possible pain referral source.

Dermatomal sensation can be evaluated with the pinwheel or pin and cotton wisp (Fig. 5.17). Pain sensation will be elicited with the pin or other sharp object, while soft touch is elicited by the cotton. The examiner should compare dermatomal regions, either with two instruments or serially.

An early or subtle sign of nerve-root irritation reported by Gunn (14) is trophedema. Trophedema is a change in tissue texture caused by partial denervation. It consists of boggy, inelastic subcutaneous tissue (determined by rolling between thumb and fore-

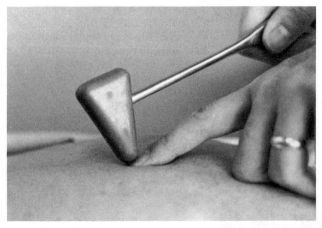

Figure 5.16. Percussion of the spinous processes can be used to help differentiate vertebral fractures or pathology.

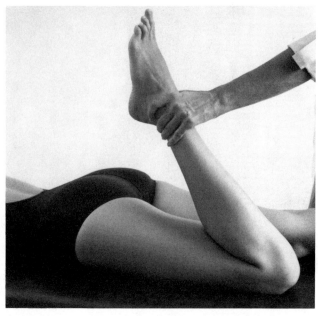

Figure 5.18. By flexing the knee and approximating the heel to the buttocks, extension of the lumbar spine is produced beyond 90° of knee flexion.

finger). This is a gradual fibrosis of the subcutaneous tissue, and the overlying skin tends to be fissured and prone to heavy folds. This alteration of the skin quality produces a *peau d'orange* effect similar to that described for malignant tumors in the breast. The matchstick test provides a quick screen for this condition. Firm palpation with a blunt instrument (matchstick) produces an indentation with sharp edges that persists for several minutes. This is similar to pitting edema, but pitting will not occur with larger instruments, such as the finger. Indentations may not be confined to a dermatomal area. They may be widespread or (in less severe cases) limited to the area of a trigger point.

Flexing the knees by approximating the heels to the buttocks (bilateral Ely's) produces an extension

of the lumbar spine (Fig. 5.18). If the facets have been damaged, pain will occur as the heels swing through their arc. More swelling causes pain at lower portions of the arc (30–45°), while the normal amount of elasticity allows complete approximation. Obese patients with enlarged thighs and calves will not be able to touch their buttocks with their heels. There is significant lumbar extension at 90° of knee flexion. Spine extension tractions the anterior

Figure 5.17. Dermatomal sensation can be evaluated with a pinwheel.

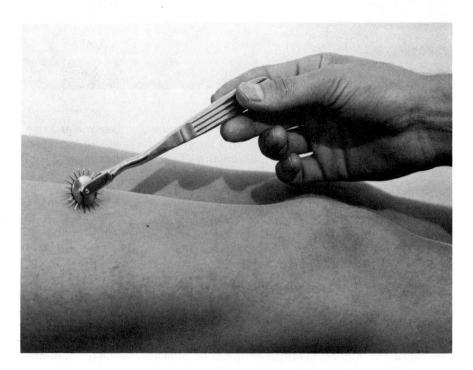

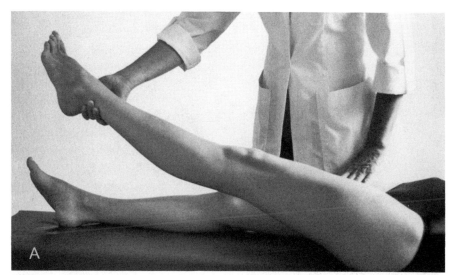

Figure 5.19. **A,** Raising the straight leg with the patient supine differentiates hamstring tightness, sacroiliac dysfunction, and sciatic nerve stretch (Chapters 7 & 8). **B,** Lowering the leg 10–15° and dorsiflexing the foot will produce radicular pain with an inflammed or irritated nerve root (Braggard's reinforcement).

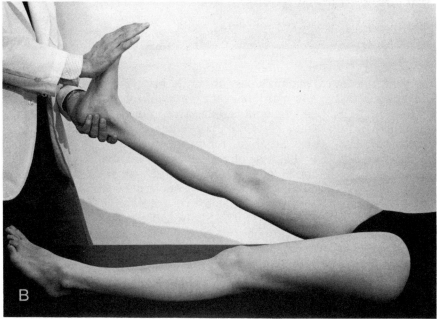

portion of the vertebrae, causing pain from traumatized discs and ligaments. A space-occupying mass in the lumbar canal will increase pressure on the cord or nerve root at that level. Extension also approximates the facets.

With the patient supine, the straight-leg raise (SLR) (Fig. 5.19A) can be accomplished. This test can have a variety of interpretations and can be either very informative or clinically valueless, depending on its interpretation. The classic test is for stretch of the sciatic nerve against the intervertebral foramen as the thigh is flexed on the hip with the knee extended. This maneuver can be augmented by lowering the leg 10–15° below the level at which the patient has reported radicular pain and dorsiflexing the foot. This will return the radicular pain with an inflamed or irritated nerve foot (Braggard's reinforcement) (Fig. 5.19B).

Muscular pain when raising the leg is caused by pull against damaged muscle, tendon, ligament, or articulations (including the disc). This is not an indication of nerve-root pressure. Therefore it should be reported as back or muscular pain caused by the straight-leg raise, not a positive SLR.

The figure-of-four test (Patrick's FABERE) (Fig. 5.20) is designed to test the integrity of the acetabulofemoral articulation. It carries the hip through a complete range of motion. The movements are: flexion, abduction, external rotation, and extension. Pain elicited by this test must be differentiated between muscular, nerve, or articular tissues.

While the patient remains supine, the femoral, dorsalis pedis, and posterior tibial pulses can be sought. These are sufficiently superficial that they can be found easily along their anatomical course. Loss of the skin appendages at the toes, such as loss

Figure 5.20. The figure-of-four test (Patrick's FABERE) differentiates hip from sacroiliac dysfunction (Chapters 7 & 8).

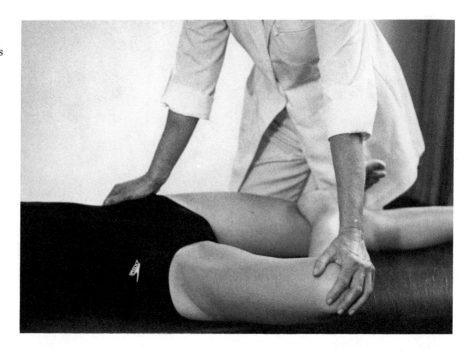

of hair from the dorsal surface of the great toes or thickened, discolored toenails would suggest that distal circulation may be impaired. These findings coupled with an inability to locate one or both of the peripheral pulses should suggest vascular consultation. It is also possible to auscultate these vessels, when in doubt.

RECORD KEEPING

An examination is performed on a given patient in order to elicit enough clinical information to reach a diagnosis. This is a decision-making process combining the anatomical, biomechanical, and pathological training the clinician has received and the information obtained from the patient through history, physical examination, radiologic examination, and laboratory examination. The process does not end until all of this information is recorded. The purpose of the record is to preserve this information.

The "SOAP" or chart-note method is useful for record keeping. The acronym SOAP stands for subjective, objective, analysis, and plan. The chart record is assembled into paragraphs for each part. The subjective paragraph contains the history and complaints recounted by the patient. The objective paragraph contains the examination evidence. The analysis is the diagnosis. And the plan is just that—the therapeutic program designed to deal with the patient's diagnosis.

Subjective information includes the patient's historical information. The history includes not just information regarding the current problem but also relevant previous medical problems. How the current problem began, what has been done for it, and the reponse to each therapy is important. Previous similar episodes and predisposing elements in the

patient's past or family history must be uncovered. As many relevant pieces of information as possible are recounted. Objective information should be specific. It is not appropriate to record just "positive" or "negative" for orthopedic tests.

Because of the wealth of information that can be obtained from a thoughtful evaluation of the patient, a simple check-off form for examination is rarely useful or reliable. An example is the straight-leg-raising test. The SLR was designed as a test of sciatic nerve root stretch. A positive SLR means that pain from the lumbosacral spine radiates in the trajectory of the sciatic nerve as the leg of the supine patient is flexed at the hip with the knee extended. If the patient reports increased pain in the low back, the information is clinically useful, but it is not a positive SLR test! Secondly, the level at which the radicular pain occurred is important, as is the distribution of the pain. So an SLR evaluation of a given patient might be recorded as: SLR yielded radicular pain to the ankle at 45° on the left, or SLR caused no radicular pain but did elicit central low back pain increase at 90°. Both notations present clinically useful information without the ambiguity of SLR+ or SLR−.

The diagnosis recounted in the analysis paragraph is a statement of the patient's problem(s). This is what will be treated. Alternatively, the diagnosis might present recognized problems for which treatment is deferred or referred to another practioner. The diagnosis is a correlative statement. That is to say, a diagnosis ties the findings of the examination to a treatable condition. For instance, a lumbosacral sprain implies that muscle spasm, edema, pain, and altered biomechanical function are present. These separate elements need not be written out. Since injuries or diseases all occur at varying levels of severity, grading the severity is appropriate. Generally accepted grading systems use numeric or narrative modifiers: Sprain grade: 1, 2, or 3 (with severity increasing up the scale) or mild, moderate, or severe sprain. When the prognosis or urgency of treatment is altered by additional information, then it should be included. A diagnosis of mild lumbosacral sprain is expected to require less treatment than severe lumbosacral sprain with left sciatic motor and sensory radiculopathy.

The plan must be specific. Another physician or therapist must be able to follow the plan in the absence of the original clinician. Such statements as "the patient will be treated with chiropractic until he is normal" do not provide that safety. A plan such as: "Complete bed rest, with bathroom and dining room privilege, with daily spinal manipulation and adjunctive ultrasound and sine wave in combination. Attempt ambulation on the fourth day. Failing ambulation, add static pelvic traction. If one week of traction, manipulation, and physical therapy fails to resolve muscle spasm and radicular symptoms, and allow ambulation, then surgical consult will be obtained" provides any person providing therapy to treat and evelute the progress of the patient. Including decision points in the plan is a reminder not to persist with ineffectual therapy. A treatment plan includes the necessary evidence that the clinician has met the standards of practice in the community.

References

1. Kern DC, Parrino TA, Korst DR: The lasting value of clinical skills. *JAMA* 254:70–76, 1985.
2. Ransford AO, Cairns D, Mooney V: The pain drawing as an aid to the psychologic evaluation of patients with low back pain. *Spine* 1:127–134, 1976.
3. Zohn DA, Mennell JM: *Musculoskeletal Pain: Diagnosis and Physical Treatment*. Boston, Little, Brown & Co, 1976, p 48.
4. Liekens ME, Gillet H: *Belgian Chiropractic Research Notes*, ed 10. Brussels, Belgium, 1973, pp 39–58.
5. Faye JL: *Motion Palpation of the Spine*. Huntington Beach, Motion Palpation Institute, 1980.
6. Krueger BR, Okazaki H: Vertebral-basilar distribution infarction following chiropractic cervical manipulation. *Mayo Clin Proc* 55:322–332, 1980.
7. Kaneshepolsky J, Danielson H, Flynn RE: Vertebral artery insufficiency and cerebellar infarct due to manipulation of the neck. *Bull Los Angeles Neurol Soc* 37:62–65, 1972.
8. Schellhas KP, Latchaw RE, Wendling LR, Gold LHA: Vertebrobasilar injuries following cervical manipulation. *JAMA* 244:1450–1453, 1980.
9. George PE, Silverstein HT, Wallace H, Marshall M: Identification of the high risk pre-stroke patient. *ACA J Chiro* 18:S26-S28, 1981.
10. Livingston MCP: Spinal manipulation causing injury: a three year study. *Clin Orthop* 81:82–86, 1971.
11. Sheehan S, Bauer RB, Meyer JS: Vertebral artery compression in cervical spondylosis. *Neurology* 10:968–986, 1960.
12. *Guides to the Evaluation of Permanent Impairment*, ed 2. Chicago, AMA, 1984, pp 47–59.
13. Brodsky AE: Cervical angina: a correlative study with emphasis on the use of coronary arteriography. *Spine* 10:699–709, 1985.
14. Gunn CC, Milbrandt WE: Early and subtle signs in low back sprain. *Spine* 3:267–281, 1978.

CHAPTER 6

Chiropractic Radiography

CYNTHIA PETERSON, R.N., D.C., D.A.C.B.R.
MERIDEL I. GATTERMAN, M.A., D.C.
TYRONE WEI, D.C., D.A.C.B.R.

The chiropractic profession has traditionally used radiography not only to locate pathology, but to analyze the structure and biomechanics of the spinal column (1).

The purpose of this chapter is to emphasize the unique contributions made by the chiropractic profession in the use of radiography for the management of spine-related disorders. Numerous excellent textbooks have been written on the subject of radiographic diagnosis. This chapter is not intended to duplicate or summarize these texts.

It must be stressed that radiographs cannot be used solely for biomechanical analysis. An x-ray examination is performed primarily for pathological screening. A number of conditions exist in which manipulation is contraindicated (2). Spinal manipulative therapy involves the application of force to the vertebrae; therefore, those pathological processes that may weaken bony architecture, or require referral for a different form of therapy (3), must be ruled out prior to manipulation (see Chapter 4). Biomechanical analysis of radiographs is important to the chiropractic profession, but is done only after pathology is excluded. Optimal radiographic quality is most essential to these diagnostic processes. It must be further emphasized that the x-ray examination in no way substitutes for a thorough patient history and physical examination; it should follow these procedures with the appropriate views (4).

HISTORY

From the early days of chiropractic, radiography and radiology have been taught in chiropractic colleges and advocated by many of the chiropractic educators and leaders (1). Wilhelm Conrad Roentgen discovered x-rays in 1895, the same year that D. D. Palmer developed his initial theories on chiropractic (5). As early as 1910, the Palmer School of Chiropractic utilized x-rays as an integral component of the chiropractic examination. These practitioners introduced the spinograph (x-ray of the spine) as a method of evaluating spinal misalignments (6–10). Chiropractors have developed spinographic analytical techniques through the years, resulting in extensive use of x-ray examinations (7–9). Most chiropractic systems of postural x-ray analysis have stressed the importance of placing the patient in the upright (weightbearing) position, so that postural relationships can be determined (6).

The erect spinograph was introduced in August 1924 at the Universal Chiropractic College in Pittsburgh, Pennsylvania (7, 8). Warren L. Sauser, a New York chiropractor, described full-spine radiography in the articles entitled "New Spinography Technique," published in 1933, and in "Entire Body X-ray Technique Perfected," published in 1935 (9). Sauser discussed the use of aluminum wedge filters for the anteroposterior and lateral views, to balance the radiographic densities over the entire spine (7). He was the first to advocate full-body AP and lateral radiographs in the upright position.

The chiropractic profession has contributed significantly to the improvement of x-ray equipment and supplies, specifically in the development of the 14-by-36-inch film, cassettes, intensifying screens, and grids (8, 9). The chiropractic profession also pioneered and has remained in the forefront in the use of filters in diagnostic x-ray (8–16). These filters were originally used to improve the quality of the diagnostic image by placing the thicker part of the

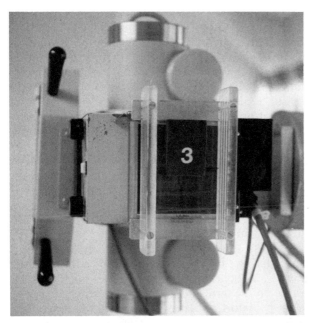

Figure 6.1. Single compensating filter placed in front of the x-ray tube (3). This reduces exposure to the filtered area and improves image quality.

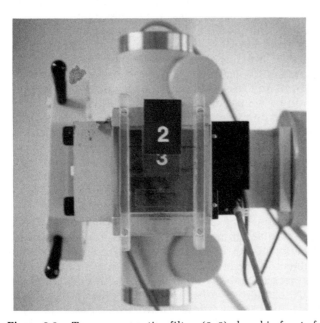

Figure 6.2. Two compensating filters (2, 3) placed in front of the x-ray tube accommodate for greater disparity in patient thickness.

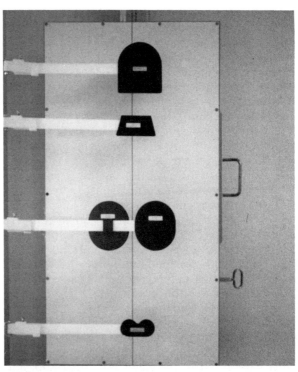

Figure 6.3. Example of eye, thyroid, breast, and gonadal shields used with an upright bucky.

filter over the less dense areas of the patient's body. More recently, emphasis has shifted from image consistency to patient safety, by offering increased protection to radiosensitive areas of the body (11, 13, 14, 16). Using such compensating filters significantly reduces exposure of the filtered areas when compared to variable-speed (graded) intensifying screens (14) (Figs. 6.1 & 6.2).

RADIATION DOSE CONSIDERATION

The radiation dosage incurred by the patient is always a consideration in radiography, as there is no "safe" level of exposure (11). This is even more important in younger patients and in those who will receive serial examinations, because radiation is cumulative (16).

While the role of compensating filters in the reduction of radiation dosage has already been discussed, additional methods of protecting the patient are available and must be used. Every effort must be made to minimize the patient's exposure, as the exposure field for spine radiography includes many radiosensitive organs such as the thyroid, lungs, spleen, ovaries, and breasts. Gonadal shielding for males must be a routine procedure (Fig. 6.3). Unfortunately, the position of the ovaries within the female pelvis may be quite variable, and small, round shields may not protect the patient. In women of small-to-moderate body type, the PA (posterioroanterior) view offers significantly less radiation dosage to both breast and ovarian tissue, with minimal reduction in osseous detail. This PA technique is particularly valuable in patients undergoing frequent examinations for the evaluation of scoliosis (14, 16).

The role of collimation in reducing exposure to nonessential areas of the body is too often overlooked. Radiation to breast tissue can and should be minimized by collimation of rays out of the field in both full-spine and thoracic spine radiographs. By reducing the size of the field, the amount of scatter radiation is reduced, and the detail of the resultant radiograph is improved (13).

The use of "split screens" in chiropractic radiography is not only antiquated but reveals a lack of concern on the part of the doctor for the safety of the patient. Split screens are intensifying screens of differing speeds that result in a more even exposure to the radiograph at the expense of the patient's safety. Rather than filter the radiation before it enters the patient, split screens affect the exposure to the radiograph after the radiation has passed through the patient. The same radiographic effect can be achieved with the use of compensating filters. Split screens should not be used under any circumstances.

The lateral full-spine radiograph has traditionally been the view that employed split screens. Lateral full-spine films require exceedingly high radiation doses and show exceedingly poor radiographic detail. The marked variability in patient thickness, combined with major divergence of the x-ray beam at the upper and lower ends of the film, make good quality, lateral, full-spine views virtually impossible to take (17). Sectional views should be substituted.

FULL SPINE RADIOGRAPHY

A major concern of a number of members of the chiropractic profession including the American Chiropractic College of Radiology is the routine use of the AP full-spine radiograph for the detection of subluxation (vertebral misalignment) (1, 6, 8, 10, 15, 16, 18). Attempting to use static x-ray findings as criteria for manipulation can be extremely harmful to the patient. Repeated manipulation to reposition a vertebra that appears "out of place" due to structural asymmetry is not only futile but also may actually create a hypermobility that perpetuates the patient's complaints. It is not possible to determine joint fixation using static radiographs and, as stated in Chapter 3, the rationale for manipulation is the restoration of joint mobility in hypomobile and fixated joints.

Other significant limitations of the full-spine radiograph include difficulty in obtaining adequate quality (as a result of marked differences in patient density), unnecessary radiation, and increased distortion (13, 16). Practitioners often take the AP full-spine view with the patient's mouth open, thus obscuring the detail of the midcervical spine. The resultant radiograph is nondiagnostic in this area, due to the superimposed mandible. Since its introduction in 1933 (7), the chiropractic full-spine postural radiograph taken on a 14-by-36-inch film has continued to evoke considerable controversy (1, 6, 11–20).

Quality control of the full-spine radiograph requires optimal equipment, a good working knowledge of the technicalities, and strict attention to related details (9, 13, 16). Clinical justification for the full-spine radiograph must insure that the benefit to the patient is greater than the radiation hazard (8, 19). If the patient's treatment regime will not be modified following review of the radiograph, then there is no clinical justification for exposing the patient to ionizing radiation. The determination of "subluxations" alone is not sufficient clinical justification to warrant this radiograph. The films must be of such quality that the presence or absence of pathology can be determined. Exactness of patient positioning for comparison to the postural norm, and adequate distance and alignment of spinographic equipment to effect known distortion parameters are prime considerations in the use of the full spine radiograph (8).

Howe (6), in 1972, defended the full spine radiograph, stating "its use is preferred to sectional studies where clinical examination shows need for radiography of several spinal sections, where a severe postural distortion is evident, where a scoliosis needs evaluation, or where a mechanical problem in one spinal area adversely affects other spinal regions." He goes on to say that "it should be equally obvious that proper visualization of a specific spinal area, structure, lesion, etc. would necessitate proper, adequate, and enough different projections of that structure on the smallest films practical."

Sectional radiographs of the area of complaint are preferred for those patients not meeting the specific criteria for full-spine radiography mentioned by Howe (6). Sectional views deliver less radiation overall and less of the often overlooked scatter radiation to the patient, with the added benefit of better radiographic detail (6, 12–14). No matter which views are selected, proper filtration, collimation, and shielding are essential for every radiograph on every patient (Fig. 6.4).

SPINOGRAPHY AS A BASIS FOR MANIPULATIVE THERAPY

The marking of spinal radiographs for malpositions, misalignments, and various angles and lines (roentgenometrics), has always been a controversial subject in the chiropractic profession because of the number of systems of adjustive techniques that base most of their premise upon small variations in radiographic mensuration. Howe (6) states that "any method of spinographic interpretation which utilizes millimetric measurements from any set of preselected points is very likely to be faulty." He continues that "if measurements are made from spinous process to edge of vertebral body—what is the conclusion if the laminae are not the same length?" Structural asymmetry is universal in the spine. The routine use of marking systems on static radiographs as the sole criterion for determining the purpose of the manipulative thrust is certainly not justified, as it has been found that the inter- and intraexaminer reliability in x-ray marking is extremely poor (18,

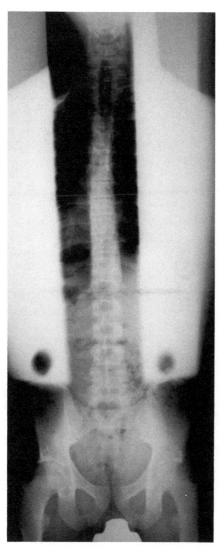

Figure 6.4. AP full-spine radiograph demonstrating a "T" shield placed in front of the x-ray tube. This acts as a collimating device for the cervical and thoracic spine, thus improving image quality. Note also the male gonad shield.

20–22). Additionally, there is a fundamental fallacy in attempting to evaluate biomechanical function on static radiographs (23–34).

The following is a list of the common causes of error in radiographic mensuration:

Image unsharpness
Projectional geometric distortion
Patient positioning
Anatomic variation
Locating standard and reference points
Observer error

Occasionally radiographic measurement of the spine offers useful information. Spinographic analysis should be handled as are other radiographic findings. Any variations from normal must be clinically correlated. As with other roentgen signs, a finding

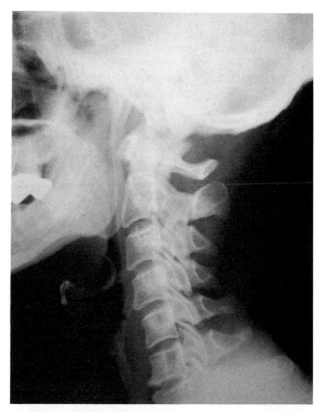

Figure 6.5. Lateral cervical-spine view taken as part of the routine x-ray series for many upper-cervical practitioners.

may or may not be significant, depending upon the clinical assessment and symptomatology. Used in this way, roentgenometrics can be clinically useful, without being the sole criterion for manipulation.

Unfortunately, chiropractic "technique" has become more of a dogma than a science or an art for some practitioners. These people are no longer unbiased and able to correctly evaluate the theory upon which they base their technique. They rationalize that their "results" should speak for themselves. The fact that patients respond favorably to a particular treatment in no way proves that the "theory" behind that treatment is sound. Every technique must be studied with good scientific methodology (21). This is the essence of our very survival as a profession. Egos must be set aside, and those theories that are proven to be unfounded must be abandoned (22, 23).

Some chiropractic techniques utilize radiographic views that do not constitute a complete diagnostic series. A classical example of this occurs with the upper cervical practitioner (23). These doctors take a series of radiographs to visualize the upper cervical vertebrae (particularly the atlas) and to make precise measurements that ultimately determine the specific treatment. The particular views taken are the lateral, nasium, vertex, and the posttreatment nasium and vertex (24) (Figs. 6.5, 6.6, & 6.7). These practitioners claim that this series offers less radia-

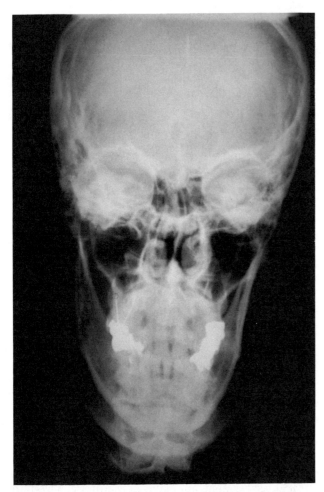

Figure 6.6. Nasium view taken by upper-cervical practitioners to visualize the atlas. Note the radiation of virtually the entire skull, and the lack of eye shields. The mandible and maxilla obscure adequate visualization of C2 through C7.

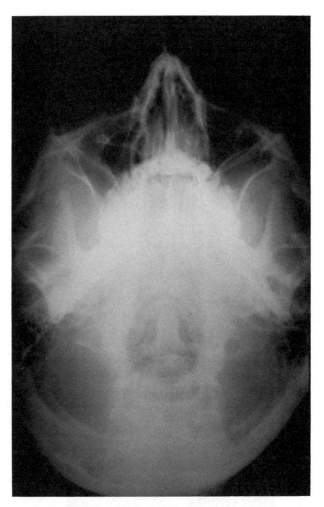

Figure 6.7. Vertex view taken by upper-cervical practitioners to visualize the upper-cervical complex. Note the radiation exposure to the orbits.

tion to the patient than a standard cervical series (24).

What these practitioners fail to recognize is that legally there are only two reasons to expose a patient to ionizing radiation. The first is for radiation therapy in the treatment of cancer and certain other diseases. Radiation therapy is beyond the scope of chiropractic practice. The second reason for exposing a patient to ionizing radiation is to diagnose pathology. As previously stated in this chapter, every radiograph must be of sufficient quality that the presence or absence of pathology can be ascertained. Additionally, a complete series of radiographs must be obtained for the area of the body being examined.

Textbooks on radiographic technique define a minimal diagnostic series for each part of the body. The views listed above do not constitute a complete diagnostic series, and the location of a "subluxation" in and of itself is not sufficient justification for taking these views. Therefore, the amount of radiation that the patient receives from these radiographs

cannot be justified. If the practitioner includes a complete cervical series in addition to the nasium and vertex views, pathology can be excluded. This is not only in the best interest of the patient but also of the treating physician. Physicians taking upper cervical radiographs must shield the radiosensitive orbits and thyroid on every view. Failure to protect the patient cannot be condoned.

UPRIGHT VERSUS RECUMBENT RADIOGRAPHY

Upright radiographs can detect some biomechanical aberrations. In the erect position, the loading of the spine will exaggerate any translatory segmental instability (25). However, diagnostic quality for bony detail cannot be sacrificed for a postural study (1). Diagnostic-quality radiographs of obese patients cannot be obtained in the upright position. These patients should always be radiographed in the recumbent position. Howe points out that "while the weight bearing relationships are seen in upright radiographs, so are antalgic and compensatory mechanisms. These may hide the true problems. Re-

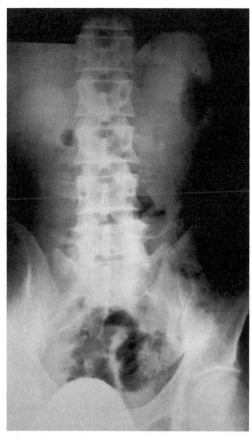

Figure 6.8. Upright AP lumbar-spine view. Note the relative lack of clarity of the osseous structures.

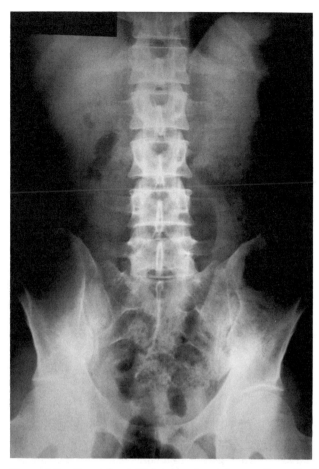

Figure 6.9. Recumbent AP lumbar view taken on the patient in Figure 6.8. The osseous detail is significantly improved. Additionally, calcifications can be noted in the spleen which were not visible on the upright radiograph.

cumbent films show non-stressed vertebral relationships and a disrelationship seen recumbent is probably more significant than one seen upright" (6) (Figs. 6.8 & 6.9).

RADIOGRAPHIC ASSESSMENT OF SPINAL SEGMENTAL MOTION

Understanding the kinetic behavior of vertebral motion segments is necessary to determine the laws of application of spinal manipulation (26). Radiographic evaluation of spinal motion obviously cannot occur using static neutral radiographs. Clinically, motion palpation assesses vertebral function using refined palpatory skills. The two radiographic techniques available to evaluate global and intersegmental vertebral motion are cineradiography and "functional" end range-of-motion radiographs (i.e., flexion, extension, lateral bending, etc.).

Cineradiography is the permanent dynamic registration of x-ray images on motion picture film (27, 28). This procedure utilizes fluoroscopy, which is routinely employed to evaluate gastrointestinal and angiographic function. Cineradiography applied to the spine allows the practitioner to review a motion repeatedly or watch it in reverse. This greatly adds to the understanding and evaluation of spinal movement (28). Members of the chiropractic profession

credited with enhancing our knowledge of spinal biomechanics through the use of cineradiography include Rich, Goodrich, and Howe in America, Illi (29) in Switzerland, and Bosman (6) in England. Unfortunately cineradiography has not proven practical for routine clinical use.

Video fluoroscopic studies have become a popular tool for assessing spinal motion. While they offer less radiation than cineradiography, only those properly qualified and trained in radiology should be using this equipment.

FUNCTIONAL X-RAY STUDIES

Of a more practical nature are the functional radiographs that employ an overlay technique to template intersegmental motion. These radiographs are taken at the end of the range of motion, then compared with the neutral radiograph (28–34) (Figs. 6.10–6.15). Based on the work of Davis in 1945, whose cervical series has become a necessary study when cervical trauma is involved, this technique discerns normal motion as well as hypomobility and hypermobility. Described by Hviid (29) in 1963, cer-

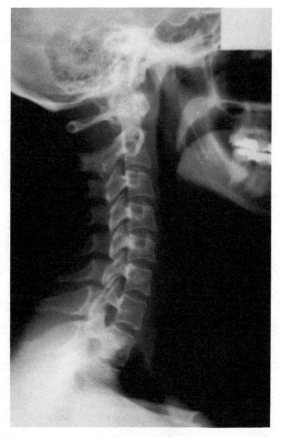

Figure 6.10. Neutral lateral-cervical radiograph. A true neutral lateral will demonstrate a horizontal Chamberlain's line.

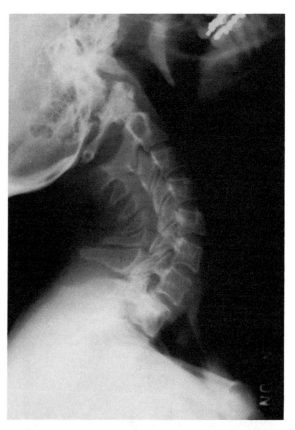

Figure 6.12. Extension lateral-cervical radiograph.

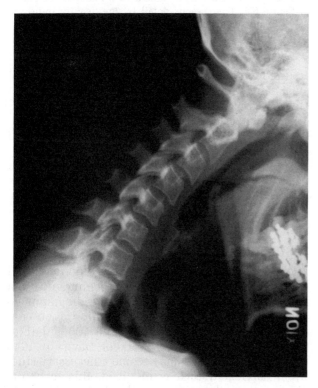

Figure 6.11. Flexion lateral-cervical radiograph. The patient's chin is fully retracted prior to flexion in order to demonstrate accurate motion of the upper cervical region.

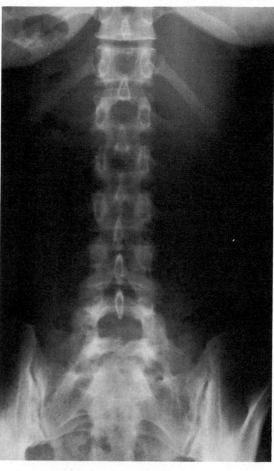

Figure 6.13. Neutral PA lumbar radiograph taken in the up-

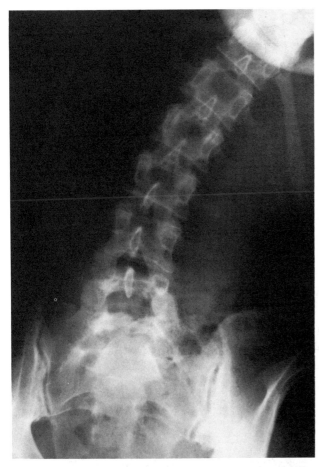

Figure 6.14. Right lateral-bending PA lumbar radiograph. Care is taken to avoid pelvic rotation. Note that the spinous processes do not rotate into the concavity as is expected.

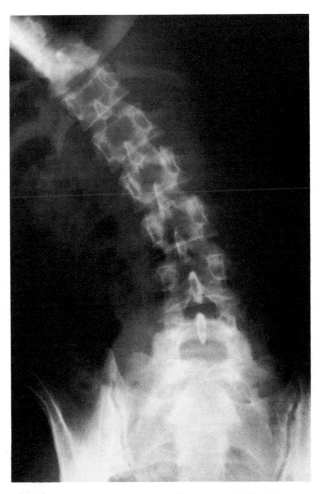

Figure 6.15. Left lateral-bending PA lumbar radiograph. The spinous processes rotate into the concavity.

vical-templating techniques have been further developed by Sandoz (30), Conley (31), Grice (33), and Henderson (26). A recent study by Friberg (25), involving the lumbar spine, found that traction-compression radiography revealed instability more reliably than functional radiographs.

The key to accurately evaluating motion on functional spinal radiographs is precise standards of patient positioning. Meticulous attention to the details of positioning cannot be overemphasized if the information obtained from the resultant radiographs is to be considered a reliable assessment of that particular patient's function. (See "Lateral Bending Study of the Lumbar Spine.")

RADIOLOGIC MANIFESTATIONS OF SPINAL SUBLUXATIONS

In 1972 the Congress of the United States passed legislation (Title 19) that enabled payment of some chiropractic services for medicare beneficiaries. The language of the legislation bound chiropractic to the concept of subluxation demonstrable by x-ray, and limited reimbursement for chiropractic services to manual manipulation for the correction of these radiographic entities.

In November 1972, in conjunction with the annual workshop of the American Chiropractic College of Roentgenology at Houston, Texas, representatives of the specialty societies and political organizations of the profession met and formulated statements of the definition, manifestations, and significance of subluxation. This classification of subluxations was designed so that medicare reporting would be uniform.

This classification of the radiological manifestations of the subluxation is based on the concept of the vertebral motion segment (intervertebral motor unit) (see Chapter 1). The vertebral motion segment was defined as two vertebrae and their contiguous structures, forming a complete set of articulations at one intervertebral level (Fig. 6.16A & B). Subluxation was defined as the alteration of the normal dynamics, anatomical or physiological relationships of contiguous articular structures. The manifestations of the complex phenomenon of subluxation were described as biomechanical, pathophysiological, clinical, and radiographic (Chapter 3). The clinical significance of subluxations was examined and discussed as they are affected by or evoke abnormal physiological responses in neuromusculoskeletal structures and/or other body systems.

In considering the possible radiological manifestations of subluxations, it was emphasized that clinical judgment must determine the advisability of

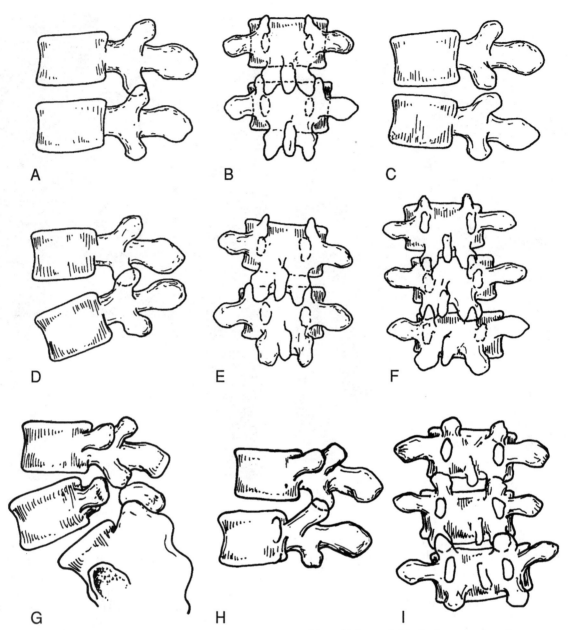

Figure 6.16. **A**, Normal vertebral motion segment positions. **B**, Normal vertebral motion segment positions. **C**, Flexion malposition. **D**, Extension malposition. **E**, Lateral flexion mal-position (right or left). **F**, Rotational malposition (right or left). **G**, Anterolisthesis (spondylolisthesis). **H**, Retrolisthesis. **I**, Laterolisthesis. **J**, Altered interosseous spacing (decreased

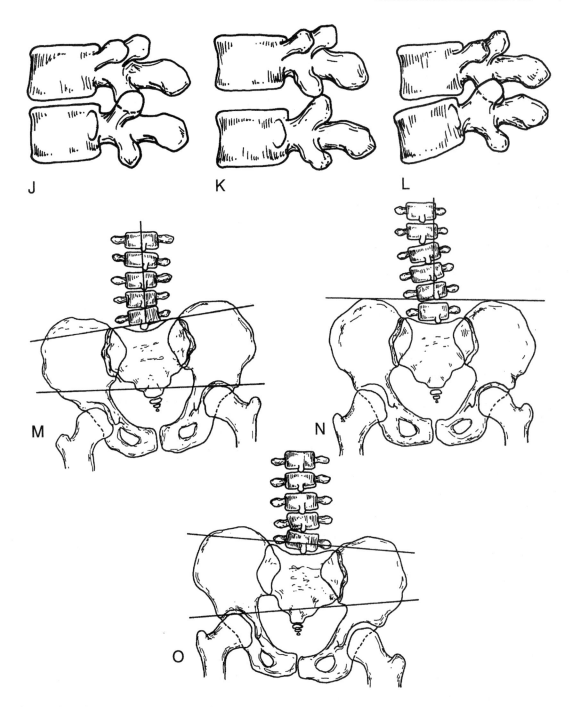

or increased). **K**, Altered interosseous spacing (decreased or increased). **L**, Osseous foraminal encroachments. **M**, Scoliosis and/or alteration of curves secondary to musculature. **N**, Sco-liosis and/or alteration of curves secondary to musculature. **O**, Decompensation of adaptational curvatures.

exposing a patient to the potential hazards of ionizing radiation. It was also noted that an important part of exposure, besides the evaluation of subluxations, is the determination of the evidence for other pathologies, and that radiographic procedures necessary to determine possible fractures, malignancies, etc., might not be the specific views needed to evaluate the possible radiological manifestations of subluxation. It was stressed that when subluxation can be evaluated by other means, it may be prudent to avoid radiation exposure. The following classification of radiologic manifestations of subluxation illustrates the consensus statement formulated by the Houston Conference of November 1972.

A. Static intersegmental subluxations
  1. Flexion malposition (Fig. 6.16C)
  2. Extension malposition (Fig. 6.16D)
  3. Lateral flexion malposition (right or left) (Fig. 6.16E)
  4. Rotational malposition (right or left) (Fig. 6.16F)
  5. Anterolisthesis (spondylolisthesis) (Fig. 6.16G)
  6. Retrolisthesis (Fig. 6.16H)
  7. Laterolisthesis (Fig. 6.16I)
  8. Altered interosseous spacing (decreased or increased) (Fig. 6.16J & K)
  9. Osseous foraminal encroachments (Fig. 6.16L)
B. Kinetic intersegmental subluxations
  1. Hypomobility (fixation subluxation)
  2. Hypermobility (loosened vertebral motion segment)
  3. Aberrant motion
C. Sectional subluxations
  1. Scoliosis and/or alteration of curves secondary to musculature imbalance (Fig. 6.16M & N)
  2. Scoliosis and/or alteration of curves secondary to structural asymmetries
  3. Decompensation of adaptational curvatures (Fig. 6.16O)
  4. Abnormalities of motion (Figs. 6.13, 6.14, 6.15)
D. Paravertebral subluxations
  1. Costovertebral and costotransverse disrelationships
  2. Sacroiliac subluxations

The above classification of radiographic manifestations of subluxation has been included to provide historical perspective regarding the development of this classification. It is important to understand that this classification was developed for political expediency. It was not designed to be used as absolute criteria on which to base manipulative therapy. While the categories indicate various components of the subluxation complex (Chapter 3), rational chiropractic therapy cannot be based solely on radiographic findings. Radiography offers a well-accepted mechanism for visualizing body structures and to some degree functional assessment, but it must be placed in proper perspective (35).

ROENTGENOMETRICS

Measurement for Basilar Impression and Basilar Invagination

The generally accepted mensurations of the base of the skull in the lateral view are Chamberlain's line and McGregor's line. The source-image distance for Chamberlain's line is 36 inches, and for McGregor's line is 72 inches (36). Since most lateral cervical-spine views are taken at a 72-inch source-image distance, McGregor's line will be the mensuration described in this text for basilar impression and basilar invagination.

MCGREGOR'S LINE

This line is constructed by connecting the posterosuperior margin of the hard palate and the most inferior surface of the occipital bone (37, 38) (Fig. 6.17). The apex of the odontoid process should be within -7.4 to $+8.0$ mm in males and -2.4 to $+9.7$ mm in females. This is the 90% tolerance range for normal, according to Lusted and Keats (37). Basilar impression or invagination is suspected if the odontoid process projects beyond the acceptable limits.

Common causes of an abnormal McGregor's line include congenital and developmental dysplasias such as hypoplastic occipital condyles, atlantooccipital assimilation, Klippel-Feil deformity, stenosis of the foramen magnum, and osteogenesis imperfecta. Acquired pathological alteration is often a complication secondary to osteomalacia, rickets, Paget's disease, and fibrous dysplasia. Although trauma is not a common cause, it should also be considered (39, 40).

ATLANTODENTAL INTERSPACE

This measurement is between the posteroinferior margin of the anterior tubercle of C1 and the anterior margin of the odontoid process (37). The space demarcates the median atlantoaxial joint (Fig. 6.18). This measurement is most useful in the evaluation of atlantoaxial subluxation (38). The distance varies with age, with the upper limits between 2.5 and 3.0 mm in adults and 3.5 and 4.5 mm in children. Since this is a synovial joint that pivots upon motion (41), the dimension also varies with flexion and extension (42).

Atlantoaxial subluxation with an increased atlantodental interspace (ADI) is most commonly associated with transverse ligament abnormality related to an inflammatory arthropathy, congenital anomaly, or Down's syndrome. Rheumatoid arthritis and ankylosing spondylitis are the most common causes within the inflammatory arthropathy category; however, psoriatic and Reiter's syndrome may also increase the ADI. According to Resnick, trau-

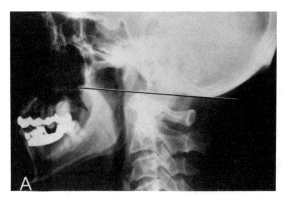

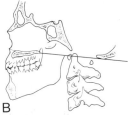

B

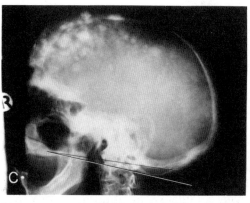

Figure 6.17. **A** & **B** McGregor's line. **C,** Abnormal McGregor's line. Note the tip of the odontoid (retouched) is well above the line due to basilar invagination from Paget's disease. (From Yochum TR, Rowe LJ: *Essentials of Skeletal Radiology.* Baltimore, Williams & Wilkins, vol 1, 1987.)

matic subluxation of the atlas and the axis is almost always accompanied by a fracture of the odontoid process (42). However, traumatically induced subluxation without fracture can be predisposed by abnormalities of the bone or ligament.

GRAVITATIONAL LINE OF THE CERVICAL SPINE

In the lateral cervical view, a plumb line is dropped perpendicular to the bottom edge of the film, from the apex of the odontoid process. This line normally falls through the anterior superior margin of the C7 vertebral body (43) (Fig. 6.19). The line is directly related to the position of the head and upper cervical spine. A flexed position of the head or a kyphotic cervical curve results in an anterior gravitation. An increased kyphosis of the upper thoracic spine may also cause this finding. A posterior gravitation is most often visualized with exten-

sion of the head or hyperlordosis of the cervical curve. This line gives a gross assessment of the gravitational stresses at the cervicothoracic junction (43).

CERVICAL STRESS LINES

These lines are constructed in the flexion lateral and extension lateral views. The superior line is drawn tangent to the posterior surface of the C2 body, and the inferior line is drawn tangent to the posterior surface of the C7 body.

In the hyperflexed position, these lines normally intersect in the C5–6 interspace. In the hyperextended position, these lines intersect at the C4–5 interspace (44). The point of intersection indicates the point of maximum stress in that position (Fig. 6.20).

ANGLE OF CERVICAL CURVATURE

This angle is taken from the neutral lateral-cervical view for evaluation of the cervical lordosis. A line is drawn through the anterior and posterior tubercles of C1. A second line is drawn tangent to the inferior endplate of C7. Perpendicular lines are constructed and the angle is measured at the intersection. Normal range is 30–45° (43).

A reduction of the lordosis may suggest muscular spasm, degenerative disc disease (45), anomalous vertical hyperplasia of the articular pillars (46), or the patient being placed in a slightly flexed position (47) (Fig. 6.21).

GEORGE'S LINE

A continuous line is drawn along the posterior vertebral bodies of the cervical spine (48, 49). In the neutral position, a break in this line is usually indicative of a segment displaced anteriorly or posteriorly in relation to the adjacent levels. This could represent sequelae secondary to trauma, degenerative disease of the disc or posterior joints, or ligamentous laxity. However, it is not an indication of instability unless confirmed by motion study such as flexion and/or extension views. Simulated disruption of George's line may be created by rotation of the spine. This line can also be used for similar interpretation of the thoracic and lumbar spine when extended inferiorly through the proximal sacrum (Fig. 6.22).

SCOLIOSIS

The Cobb method of scoliosis mensuration is currently the most accepted method of scoliosis evaluation and is standardized by the Scoliosis Research Society (50). The Cobb method is more accurately reproducible by different observers and gives larger angles. Correction can be more easily compared during the course of treatment.

The Cobb method is the mensuration method described in this text. The upper and lower end vertebrae, known as *the maximally tilted vertebrae,* are

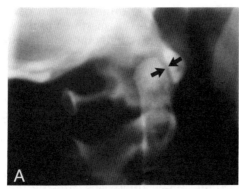 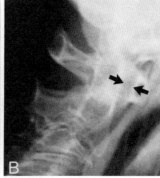 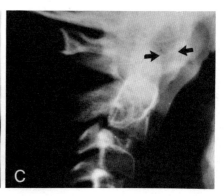

Figure 6.18. Atlantodental interspace (ADI). **A,** Adult atlantodental interspace (less than 3 mm) (*arrows*). **B,** Abnormal atlantodental interspace in a patient with rheumatoid arthritis (5 mm) (*arrows*). **C,** Childhood atlantodental interspace (less than 5 mm) (**arrows**). (From Yochum TR, Rowe LJ: *Essentials of Skeletal Radiology.* Baltimore, Williams & Wilkins, vol 1, 1987.)

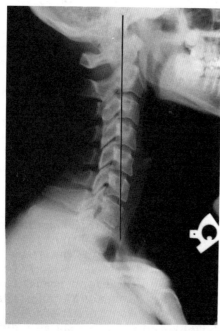

Figure 6.19. Cervical gravity line. (From Yochum TR, Rowe LJ: *Essentials of Skeletal Radiology.* Baltimore, Williams & Wilkins, vol 1, 1987.)

those that tilt most acutely towards the concavity of the curvature. A horizontal line is drawn along the superior endplate of the superior end vertebra. A similar horizontal line is drawn at the inferior endplate of the inferior end vertebra. Perpendicular lines are drawn from each horizontal line, and the intersecting angle is measured. On severe curvatures, the horizontal lines may intersect each other, eliminating the necessity of drawing perpendicular lines (51) (Fig. 6.23).

Curve classification using the Cobb method standardized by the Scoliosis Research Society is as follows (51):

Group I	00–20°
Group II	21–30°
Group III	31–50°
Group IV	51–75°
Group V	76–100°
Group VI	101–125°
Group VII	120° and above

LUMBAR SPINE

The lumbosacral angle (sacral base angle), lumbosacral disc angle, gravitational line of L3, MacNab's line, George's line, and Hadley's curve are the more commonly used mensuration procedures to evaluate biomechanical relationships of the lumbar spine and lumbosacral junction. Each measurement is an analysis of a certain part of this entire motion complex. However, complete evaluation requires a combination of these above-mentioned methods of mensuration. A single line or angle may reveal a certain interpretation but be contradicted by another. Consistency must be achieved for accuracy. Examples of true facetal imbrication usually reveal an increased sacral base and lumbosacral disc angle. Gravitation of L3 is generally posterior with a positive MacNab's line and a break in Hadley's "S" curve. However, a posterior gravitational line associated with a decreased sacral base and lumbosacral base angle is not consistent with facetal imbrication but rather with findings of hypolordosis.

LUMBOSACRAL ANGLE

In the lateral lumbosacral view, the lumbosacral angle (sacral-base angle) is constructed by intersecting the plane of the superior sacral surface (sacral base) and the horizontal (52). This is usually the bottom edge of the film (Fig. 6.6). The mean angle is 41.1° in the erect position (37, 43). This angle is increased when the sacrum is in an extended position, and decreased in a flexed position. The normal range (±2 standard deviation units) is 26–57° (37) (Fig. 6.24).

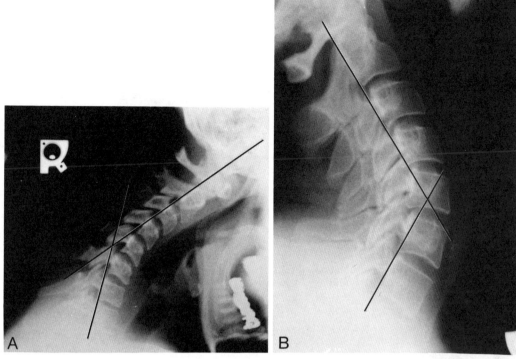

Figure 6.20. Stress lines of the cervical spine. **A,** Flexion. **B,** Extension. (From Yochum TR, Rowe LJ: *Essentials of Skeletal Radiology.* Baltimore, Williams & Wilkins, vol 1, 1987.)

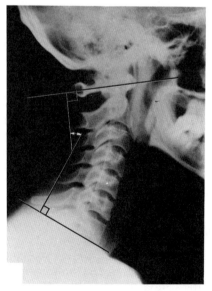

Figure 6.21. Angle of cervical curve.

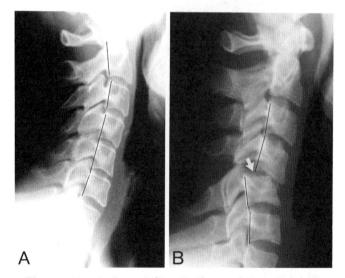

Figure 6.22. **A,** George's line. **B,** Abnormal George's line due to traumatic bilateral facet dislocation (*arrow*). (From Yochum TR, Rowe LJ: *Essentials of Skeletal Radiology.* Baltimore, Williams & Wilkins, vol 1, 1987.)

LUMBOSACRAL DISC ANGLE

Lines tangent to the inferior vertebral body surface of L5 and the superior sacral surface converge and intersect posteriorly to form the lumbosacral disc angle (Fig. 6.25). The normal range is 10–15° (43). An increased angle results in an imbrication of the zygapophyseal joints. Parallel lines are sometimes associated with a posterior disc protrusion (43).

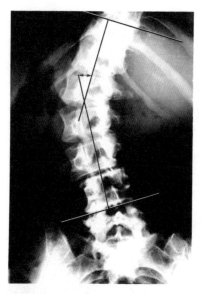

Figure 6.23. Cobb method of scoliosis evaluation. (From Yochum TR, Rowe LJ: *Essentials of Skeletal Radiology.* Baltimore, Williams & Wilkins, vol 1, 1987.)

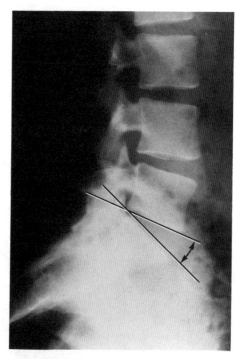

Figure 6.25. Lumbosacral-disc angle. (From Yochum TR, Rowe LJ: *Essentials of Skeletal Radiology.* Baltimore, Williams & Wilkins, vol 1, 1987.)

of the zygapophyseal joints and narrowing of the intervertebral disc spacing. The reliability of this line has not been documented, and the original description was based on recumbent radiographs (24) (Fig. 6.26).

HADLEY'S "S" CURVE

On the AP or oblique radiograph, a line is drawn along the inferior aspect of the transverse process, extending down the lateral margin of the lamina and inferior articular process. This line is continued across the zygapophyseal joint to the opposing superior articular process of the immediate caudad segment (53, 54). This line should form a smooth "S" configuration. (Fig. 6.27) A break in this "S" is indicative of telescoping or imbrication of the facet joints.

GRAVITATIONAL LINE OF L3

In the lateral lumbosacral view, a plumb line is dropped perpendicular to the bottom edge of the film, from the center of the L3 vertebral body. This line normally falls through the anterior third of the sacral base (42) (Fig. 6.28). If this line falls anterior to the sacrum, it is indicative of either an extended sacrum or a flexed lumbar spine. A flexed sacrum or hyperextended lumbar spine would allow this gravitational line to drop posterior to the anterior third of the sacral base. The significance of this should be related to the sacral-base angle and the lumbosacral-disc angle.

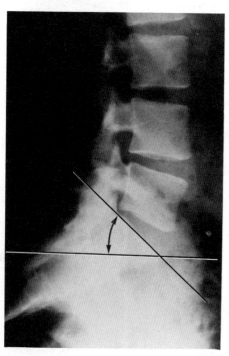

Figure 6.24. Lumbosacral angle. (From Yochum TR, Rowe LJ: *Essentials of Skeletal Radiology.* Baltimore, Williams & Wilkins, vol 1, 1987.)

MACNAB'S LINE

A line drawn across the inferior body surface of any lumbar vertebra should not intersect the superior articular process of the immediate caudad segment (43). This finding is positive with imbrication

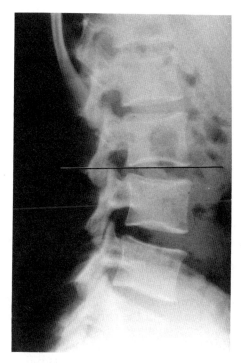

Figure 6.26. MacNab's line. (From Yochum TR, Rowe LJ: *Essentials of Skeletal Radiology.* Baltimore, Williams & Wilkins, vol 1, 1987.)

MEYERDING'S CLASSIFICATION FOR SPONDYLOLISTHESIS

This classification is used to determine the degree of anterior displacement in a spondylolisthesis (anterolisthesis). In a lateral view of the lumbosacral junction, the superior surface of the sacral base is divided into four equal quadrants, with the most posterior quadrant listed as the first division. The position of the posterior inferior corner of L5 is determined relative to the adjacent quadrant. The anterolisthesis is classified as grade I if the posterior L5 body is aligned to the first quadrant. A grade II anterolisthesis is listed if the posterior L5 body is aligned to the second quadrant and so forth (55) (Fig. 6.29). This same classification can be used for evaluating any vertebral body level other than C1. A more accurate method for evaluating the severity of anterolisthesis involves determining the *percentage* of displacement.

SPINAL CANAL STENOSIS

Spinal canal stenosis can be secondary to a developmental variant or degenerative or pathological processes. Developmental stenosis is most frequently due to hyperplastic laminae and/or shortened pedicles. Degenerative stenosis can be due to posteriorly directed spondylophytosis, zygapophyseal joint proliferative degeneration, or ligamentum flavum hypertrophy. Plain-film examination is not always conclusive; however, the lateral view does offer some value.

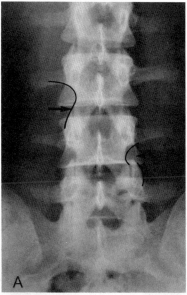
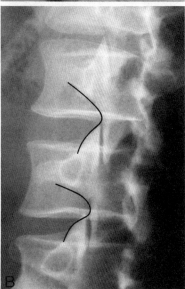

Figure 6.27. Hadley's "S" curve. **A,** Anteroposterior normal (*arrow*), anteroposterior abnormal (*arrowhead*). **B,** Oblique normal. (From Yochum TR, Rowe LJ: *Essentials of Skeletal Radiology.* Baltimore, Williams & Wilkins, vol 1, 1987.)

In the cervical spine, the sagittal spinal-canal diameter is determined by the distance between the posterior vertebral body and the spinolaminar line. At the level of C4 to C7, cord compression is suspected if the measurement is under 10 mm. Cord compression is unlikely if the diameter is 13 mm or more (45).

In the lumbar spine, the lower limit of normal for the transverse diameter of the spinal canal is 20 mm. This is determined by measuring the distance between the inner aspect of the pedicles (45). The sagittal spinal-canal diameter is determined by measuring the distance between the upper posterior vertebral body and the line created by connecting the

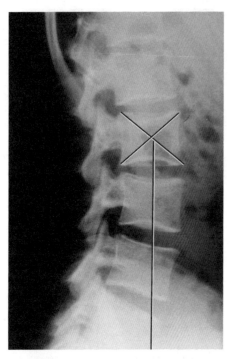

Figure 6.28. Lumbar gravity line. (From Yochum TR, Rowe LJ: *Essentials of Skeletal Radiology*. Baltimore, Williams & Wilkins, vol 1, 1987.)

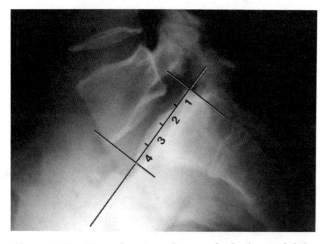

Figure 6.29. Meyerdings' grading method of spondylolisthesis. Meyerding classification of spondylolisthesis. (From Yochum TR, Rowe LJ: *Essentials of Skeletal Radiology*. Baltimore, Williams & Wilkins, vol 1, 1987.)

apex of the superior and inferior articular process (56). The lower limit of normal is 15 mm according to most investigators; a diameter of 12 mm is unequivocally pathological (45).

CHAMBERLAIN METHOD TO DEMONSTRATE ABNORMAL SACROILIAC MOTION

Instability or loosening of the sacroiliac joint and/or symphysis pubis is best demonstrated with this method. The reinforcing ligaments of these structures may be hyperextended, torn, or ruptured due to acute or chronic trauma.

The method of examination includes an erect study of the pubic bones. Two posteroanterior projections of this area are taken with weightbearing on alternate legs. The patient stands on two blocks, approximately 6 inches from the floor. The blocks are removed alternately to allow one leg to hang free (57).

In addition, a neutral view of this area and inclusion of the sacroiliac joints in all views is recommended, as any separation or disease can be observed. A loosening of the pelvic articulations is confirmed by separation of the symphysis pubis in the vertical plane (58) (Figs. 6.30, 6.31, & 6.32).

FLEXION AND EXTENSION STUDY OF THE CERVICAL SPINE

This study employs the neutral, flexion and extension lateral views of the cervical spine. There are many methods of analysis described in the literature. The following method of mensuration was pioneered by Appa Anderson, D.C., D.A.C.B.R., Professor of Radiology at Western States Chiropractic College.

The neutral lateral view is taken in the same manner as a routine erect lateral view of the cervical spine at a 72-inch source-image distance. The mandible is retracted in the nod position prior to full flexion (59, 60). On full extension, the subject is told to focus the eyes on the ceiling without extending the mid or lower back (Figs. 6.10, 6.11, & 6.12).

Analysis of these radiographs is twofold. First, the cervical spine is templated by tracing the inferior surface of the occiput behind the foramen magnum, anterior and posterior tubercles of C1, vertebral bodies, and spinolaminar junction of C2 through C7. Next, the template of neutral C7 is superimposed upon C7 in flexion. The posterior aspect of the vertebral body of C6 is traced. The template of neutral C6 is then superimposed upon C6 in flexion. The posterior aspect of the vertebral body of C5 is traced. This sequence is followed through the occiput and treated similarly for the extension view (60).

Often, when the cervical spine is in a straight or kyphotic position, there is little or no motion in flexion but extreme movement upon extension. Interpretation of the intersegmental motion of the cervical spine should consider the range from maximum flexion to maximum extension at each level. According to Henderson and Dorman, a total excursion of less than 25% of the sagittal body diameter represents articular fixation, and values exceeding 75% suggest radiographic instability.

The second point of this analysis should be to determine whether there are any anterolistheses or retrolistheses in these extreme states of bending. Pseudosubluxation of the cervical spine in adolescents should also be considered. Anterior step-off of

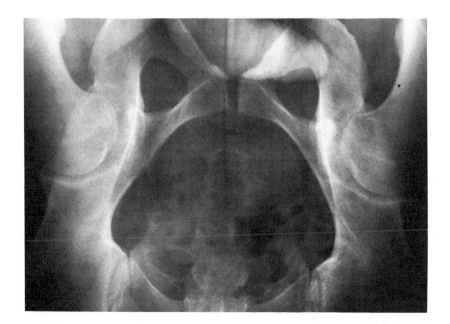

Figure 6.30. Standing neutral PA view of symphysis pubis and sacroiliac joints.

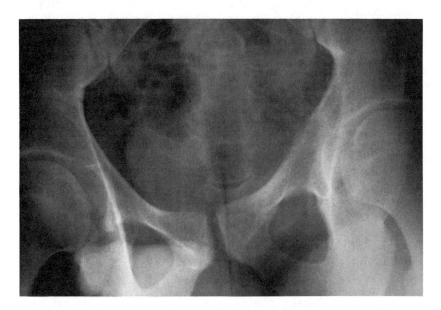

Figure 6.31. Patient is standing on the left leg while the right leg hangs free. Note the superior shear of the left pubic bone.

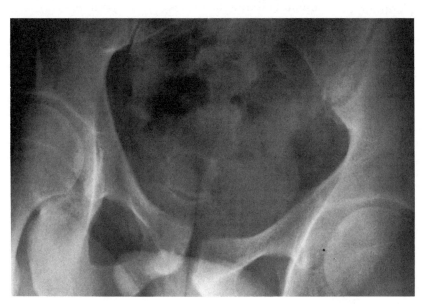

Figure 6.32. Patient is standing on the right leg while the left leg hangs free. The pubic bones are now aligned.

2 to 4 mm of C2 and C3 in flexion is considered normal with correction in neutral or extension (60 & 61).

Marked anterior displacement of C2, resembling subluxation, was noted in 19% of the children between 1 and 7 years of age by Cattell and Fitzer (62). They report a similar finding, although less frequently, between C3 and C4. An excess of this 2 to 4 mm in children is considered hypermobility or instability. An anterior subluxation, as described by Harris (63), demonstrates a straight or kyphotic cervical curve with the involved segment at the apex. The interspinous space is abnormally wide, and the intervertebral disc–spacing is narrowed anteriorly. There is a distraction of the facet joints. All findings are accentuated upon flexion and reduced in extension.

A segment that exhibits significant anterolisthesis or retrolisthesis upon bending in the sagittal plane may demonstrate reduced motion between maximum flexion and extension upon templating. This pivoting motion is replaced by abnormal gliding or translation from ligamentous instability.

An accurate interpretation of cervical intersegmental motion should include a combination of these two methods of analysis.

FLEXION AND EXTENSION STUDY OF THE LUMBAR SPINE

Stability of the lumbar spine is best studied by placing the part in hyperflexion and hyperextension. A disruption of George's line (48) upon motion could indicate a loss of the integrity of the zygapophyseal joints, intervertebral disc, and/or supporting soft tissue structures.

This study is important in evaluating the degree of stability of a spondylolisthesis. According to Yochum (24) an anterolisthesis or retrolisthesis of 4 mm or greater displacement in either direction indicates radiographic instability. Surgical fixation should be entertained if the clinical symptoms of the patient correlate. Evaluation of the stability of a previously surgically fused segment prior to manipulation is critical.

LATERAL-BENDING STUDY OF THE LUMBAR SPINE

Many articles have been written describing the normal or ideal lumbar spine motion (33, 34, 64). Understanding ideal motion is a prerequisite of identifying pathological motion (34, 67). Research is continuing in an attempt to confirm the patterns attributed to normal motion and the clinical significance of the varieties of abnormal motion in the lumbar spine.

Lateral bending of the lumbar spine requires a complex muscular and ligamentous coordination that results not only in intersegmental lateral tilt but also in a coupled rotation at each vertebral level (34, 67). It is beyond the scope of this chapter to discuss the functions of each muscle group in this complex

motion. Early recognition of abnormal lumbar spinal motion may lead to specific manipulative and soft tissue treatment programs to restore normal mobility (67) (Figs. 6.13, 6.14, & 6.15). The significance of long-term aberrant motion is still being investigated. However, acute low-back injury, especially disc herniation, has been shown to result in specific types of abnormal motion upon lateral bending, which may help in diagnosing the specific level of disc herniation (64).

A lateral-bending study is a relatively simple procedure. This examination includes an AP or PA neutral, left and right lateral-bending view in either the standing or seated position. In the thin-to-moderately-built patient the PA lumbar projection is recommended. In this position the divergence of the x-ray beam is along the plane of the disc spaces. It is important that the knees be locked in all three positions if the patient is standing. Bending should occur at the waist without lifting the heel off the ground. Pelvic shift must be avoided, and stabilization bands may be necessary.

Normal motion of the vertebral motion segments includes wedging of the disc on the ipsilateral side of bending and contralateral vertebral body rotation (6, 33, 34). Lateral flexion at the L3–4 and L4–5 motion segments is approximately 7–8°, and at the L5–S1 level approximately 1–2° (64).

Abnormal motion includes a lack of adequate lateral flexion, contralateral vertebral body rotation, or both. Lateral disc protrusion causes a lack of lateral flexion on the ipsilateral side of involvement, whereas a medial disc protrusion causes a lack of lateral flexion to the contralateral side (64).

Weitz (64) noted that a normal lateral-bending study does not rule out midline disc protrusions or spinal stenosis. Multilevel disc protrusions also may not be enhanced by lateral-bending studies. Occasionally contralateral flexion of the vertebral body upon bending is observed. Bilateral contralateral movement of L5 is believed to be of no clinical significance.

Inadequate contralateral vertebral-body rotation upon lateral bending is often attributed to unilateral paravertebral muscular hypertonicity. The axis of rotation is then shifted toward the side of hypertonicity, resulting in unilateral facet-joint fixation (34). Cassidy (34) also suggests that the contralateral facet and corresponding posterolateral annulus fibrosis are subjected to increased motion, predisposing them to strain and degenerative change.

References

1. Howe JW: Some considerations in spinal x-ray interpretations. *J Clin Chiro Archives*, Spring, 75–95, 1971.
2. Gatterman MI: Contraindications and complications of spinal manipulative therapy. *ACA J Chiro* 15:75–86, 1981.
3. Phillips RB: The use of x-rays in spinal manipulative therapy. In Haldeman S: *Modern Development in the Principles*

and *Practice of Chiropractic*. East Norwalk, CT, Appleton-Century-Crofts, 1980, pp 189–208.

4. Wyatt LH, Schultz GD: The diagnostic efficacy of lumbar spine radiography: a review of the literature. From the proceedings of the 4th Annual Current Topics in Chiropratic: Reviews of the Literature. Palmer Research Consortium, February 1987.

5. Coelho LR: Spinal radiographic techniques, quality, assurance and radiation safety. In Haldeman S: *Modern Development in the Principles and Practice of Chiropractic*. East Norwalk, CT, Appleton-Century-Crofts, 1980, pp 209–229.

6. Howe JW: Facts and fallacies, myths and misconceptions in spinography. *J Clin Chiro Archives*, ed 2. winter, 34–35, 1972.

7. Poehner WG: First erect spinograph. *Natl Chiro J* 11:18, 1942.

8. Hildebrandt RW: Chiropractic spinography and postural roentgenology: Part I history of development. *JMPT* 3:87–92, 1980.

9. Sausser WI: Entire body x-ray techniques perfected. *Natl Chiro J*, Feb, 17-18, 1935.

10. Hildebrandt RW: *Chiropractic Spinography: A Manual of Technique and Interpretation*, ed 2. Baltimore, Williams & Wilkins, 1977, pp 6–9.

11. Levine JI, Howe JW, Rolofson JW: Radiation exposure to a phantom patient during simulated chiropractic spinal radiography. *J CCA*, May, 21–26, 1973.

12. Hardman LA, Henderson DJ: Comparative dosimetric evaluation of current techniques in chiropractic full spine and sectional radiography. *J CCA* 25:141–145, 1981.

13. Field TJ, Buehler MT: Improvements in chiropractic full spine radiography. *JMPT* 4:21–25, 1981.

14. Merkin JJ, Sportelli L: The effects of two new compensating filters on patient exposure in chiropractic full spine radiography. *JMPT* 5:25–29, 1982.

15. Gatterman BG: Filtration in chiropractic. *ICA International Review of Chiro*, winter, 62–64, 1985.

16. Gray JE, Hoffman AD, Peterson HA: Reduction of radiation exposure during radiography of scoliosis. *J Bone Joint Surg* 5:5–11, 1983.

17. Thurlow R: Comparative radiation dose from spinal radiography. *J CCA*, Oct, 99–100, 1978.

18. Phillips RB: An evaluation of the graphic analysis of the pelvic or the AP full spine radiograph. *ACA J Chiro* IX:139–148, 1975.

19. Fickel T: An analysis of the carcinogenicity of full spine radiography. *J Am Chiro Asso* 20:61–66, 1986.

20. Hildebrandt RW: Full spine radiography: a matter of justification. *J Am Chiro Asso* 20:61–66, 1986.

21. Keating JC: Traditional barriers to standards of knowledge produced in chiropractic, *Proceedings: Concensus Conference on the Validation of Chiropractic Methods*. Seattle Wash. Mar. 2 1990, Williams & Wilkins (Forthcoming)

22. Anderson RT: A radiographic test of upper cervical chiropractic theory. *JMPT* 4:129–133, 1981.

23. Sigler DC, Howe JW: Inter and intra-examiner reliability of the upper cervical x-ray marking system. *JMPT* 8:75–80, 1985.

24. Yochum TR, Rowe LJ: *Essentials of Skeletal Radiology*. Baltimore, Williams & Wilkins, vol 1, 1987, pp 169, 191, 268.

25. Friberg O: Lumbar instability: a dynamic approach by traction-compression radiography. *Spine* 12(2):119–129, 1987.

26. Henderson DJ, Dorman TM: Functional roentgenometric evaluation of the cervical spine in the sagittal plane. *JMPT* 8:219–227, 1985.

27. Fielding JW: Cineroentgenography of the normal cervical spine. *J Bone Joint Surg* 39a:1280–1288, 1957.

28. Howe JW: Cineradiography evaluation of normal and abnormal cervical spinal function. *J Clin Chiro* 76–88, 1972.

29. Hviid H: Functional radiography of the cervical spine. *Ann Swiss Chiro Assoc* 3:37–65, 1963.

30. Sandoz R: Newer trends in the pathogenesis of spinal disorders. *Ann Swiss Chiro Assoc* 5:112, 1971.

31. Conley RW: Stress evaluation of cervical mechanics *J Clin Chiro* 3:46–62, 1974.

32. Grice AS: Preliminary evaluation of fifty sagittal cervical motion radiographic examinations. *J CCA* 21(1):33–34, 1977.

33. Grice AS: Harmony of joint and muscle function in the prevention of lower back syndromes *J CCA*, July 7–10, 1976.

34. Cassidy JD: Roentgenological examination of the functional mechanics of the lumbar spine in lateral flexion. *J CCA*, July:13–16, 1976.

35. Howe JW: Radiologic investigation of spinal biomechanics *J CCA*, Dec., 16–21, 1976.

36. Schafer RC: *Chiropractic Physical and Spinal Diagnosis* ed 1. Oklahoma City, Associated Chiropractic Academic Press, 1980, IV/39-IV/47, p 48.

37. Lusted LB, Keats TE: *Atlas of Roentgenographic Measurement*, ed 4. Chicago, Year Book, 1978, pp 48–50, 113, 141.

38. McGregor M: The significance of certain measurements of the skull in the diagnosis of basilar impression. *Br J Radiol* 21:171, 1948.

39. Epstein B: *The Spine, A Radiological Text and Atlas*, ed 4. Philadelphia, Lea & Febiger, 1976, pp 161–162.

40. Reeder MM, Felson B: *Gamuts in Radiology Comprehensive Lists of Roentgen Differential Diagnosis*, Cincinnati, Audiovisual Radiology of Cincinnati, 1975, pp A7, 4–7.

41. Warwick R, Williams P: *Gray's Anatomy*, Br ed 35. Philadelphia, WB Saunders, 1973, p 416.

42. Resnick D, Niwayama G: *Diagnosis of Bone and Joint Disorders*. Philadelphia, WB Saunders, 1981, vol 3, pp 19, 26, 49, 52, 53, 94–95, 2295.

43. MacRae JE: *Roentgenometrics in Chiropractic*, Toronto, Canadian Memorial Chiropractic College, 1974, p 19.

44. Jackson R: *The Cervical Syndrome*, ed 4. Springfield, IL, Charles C Thomas, 1977.

45. Resnick D, Niwayama G: *Diagnosis of Bone and Joint Disorders*. Philadelphia, WB Saunders, 1981, vol 1, pp 1380, 1408, 1411.

46. Peterson CK, Wei T: Vertical hyperplasia of the cervical articular pillars. *ACA J Chiro* 21:78–79, 1987.

47. Keats TE: *An Atlas of Normal Roentgen Variants*, ed 2. Chicago, Year Book, 1979.

48. George AW: A method for more accurate study of injuries to the atlas and axis. *Boston Med Surg J* 181:13, 1919.

49. Litterer WE: A history of George's line. *ACA J Chiro* 24:39–40, 1983.

50. Cailliet R: *Scoliosis, Diagnosis and Management*. Philadelphia, FA Davis, 1978, p 28.

51. Keim HA: *Scoliosis, Cibia Clinical Symposia* 30 (1):18–19, 1978.

52. Cox JM: *Low Back Pain: Mechanism, Diagnosis and Treatment*, ed 4. Baltimore, Williams & Wilkins, 1985.

53. Hadley LA: *Anatomico-Roentgenographic Studies of the Spine*. ed 4. Springfield, IL, Charles C Thomas, 1979, p 174.

54. Hadley LA: Intervertebral joint subluxation, bony impingement and foraminal encroachment, with nerve root changes. *Am J Roentgenol* 65:377, 1951.

55. Meyerding HW: Spondylolisthesis. *Surg Gynecol Obstet* 54:371, 1932.

56. Eisenstein S: The morphometry and pathological anatomy of the lumbar spine in South Africans, negroes and caucasoids with specific reference to spinal stenosis. *J Bone Joint Surg* 59B:173, 1977.

57. Ballinger PN: *Merrill's Atlas of Radiographic Positions and Radiologic Procedures*, ed 5. St. Louis, C V Mosby, vol 1, p 247.

58. Dihlmann W: *Diagnostic Radiology of the Sacroiliac Joints*. Chicago, Year Book, 1980, pp 12–16.

59. Henderson DJ, Dorman TM: Functional roentgenometric evaluation of the cervical spine in the sagittal plane. *JMPT* 8(4):219, 1985.

60. Anderson AL: Lecture notes, Western States Chiropractic College, 1975.

61. Fechtel SG: Pseudosubluxation of the cervical spine in adolescents: A case report. *JMPT* 6(2):81, 1983.

62. Cattell HS, Fitzer DL: Pseudosubluxation and other normal variations in the cervical spine in children. *J Bone Joint Surg* 47A(7):1295, 1965.
63. Harris JH: *The Radiology of Acute Cervical Spine Trauma.* Baltimore, Williams & Wilkins, 1978, pp 49–52.
64. Weitz EM: The lateral bending sign. *Spine* 6(4):388–397, 1981.
65. Tanz S: Motion of the lumbar spine: a roentgenologic study. *Am J Roent* 69(3):399–412, 1953.
66. Miles M, Sullivan WE: Lateral bending at the lumbar and lumbosacral joints. *Anat Rec* 139:387–398, 1958.
67. Grice, AS: Radiographic, biomechanical and clinical factors in lumbar lateral flexion: part I. *J Manip Physiol Ther* 2(1):26–34, 1977.

68. Allbrook D: Movements of the lumbar spinal column. *J Bone Joint Surg* 39B(2):339–345, 1957.
69. Pearcy MJ, Tebreual SB: Axial rotation and lateral bending in the normal lumbar spine measured by three dimensional radiography. *Spine* 9(6):582–587, 1984.
70. Simnet J, Fischer LP, Gonon G, Carret JP: Radiographic studies of lateral flexion in the lumbar spine. *J Biomech* 11:143–150, 1978.
71. Schalintzek M: Functional roentgen examination of degenerated and normal intervertebral discs of the lumbar spine. *Acta Radiol* [Suppl](Stockh) II:300–306, 1954.

CHAPTER 7

Disorders of the Pelvic Ring

As the subject of perennial academic debate, the sacro-iliac joint seems born to trouble as the sparks fly upward.

This statement (1) by Grieve summarizes the controversial nature of the function of the sacroiliac articulations with respect to the pelvic ring. An understanding of this function is necessary if one is to comprehend pelvic biomechanics, since the sacrum through its articular surfaces forms the keystone in the pelvic ring (2) (Fig. 7.1). In addition to the paired

sacroiliac joints, three other articulations contribute to pelvic motion, the pubic symphysis, and the two coxofemoral articulations.

The closed-kinetic-chain model (Chapter 3) is useful in the understanding of the interdependence of these joints, with each articulation having determinate relations with each of the other joints in the ring (3). The sacroiliac joints posteriorly and pubic symphysis anteriorly comprise the joints of the pelvic ring and form a mechanism that functions similarly to the three-joint complex of the typical vertebral motion segment (4) (Fig. 7.2). The paired

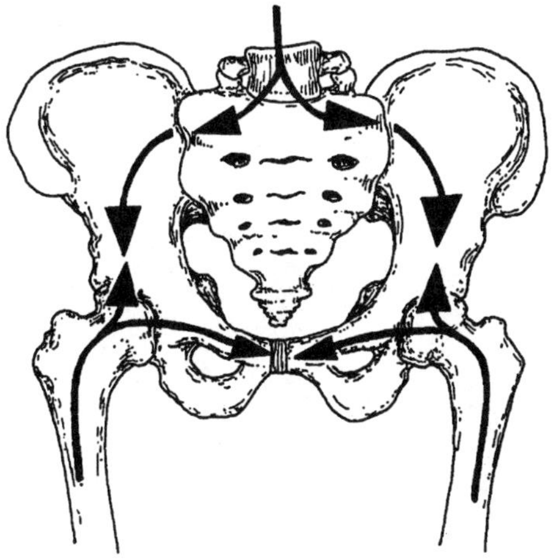

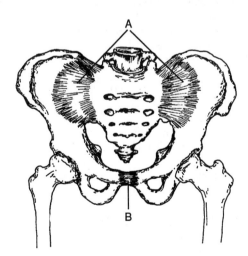

Figure 7.1. The sacrum, through its articular surfaces, forms a keystone in the pelvic ring. It is tightly held in the ring by strong ligaments, and because it is wider above than below, the heavier the weight placed on it, the more the sacrum becomes locked in place as the downward forces are dispersed anteriorly in the pelvic ring. (After Kapandji) Kapandji IA: *The Physiology of the Joints: The Trunk and Vertebral Column,* vol 3. New York, Churchill Livingstone, 1974, p 59.)

Figure 7.2. The pelvic ring forms a mechanism that functions similarly to the three-joint complex of the typical vertebral motion segment. The paired sacroiliac joints (A) guide and restrict motion in the manner of the posterior facet joints, while the elastic and compressable symphysis pubis (B) functions like the intervertebral disc, allowing six degrees of freedom of motion, similar to the small amount of movement allowed in the vertebral motion segment. Motion of the coxa femoral joints (C) contributes to pelvic ring motion during walking.

sacroiliac joints guide and restrict motion in the same manner as the posterior facet joints of the typical vertebral motion segment, while the elastic and compressible amphiarthrodial disc at the symphysis pubis allows for six degrees of freedom, similar to the action of the intervertebral discs. An additional element in this closed kinetic chain, is introduced during the bipedal gait, with motion of the coxofemoral joints contributing to pelvic ring motion during walking (5).

Disorders involving any one of these joints will affect each of the other joints in the closed kinetic chain. For example, fixation of one sacroiliac joint often causes hypermobility and subsequent pain of the contralateral sacroiliac joint, while hip-joint fixation often leads to hypermobility and pain in the ipsilateral sacroiliac joint (6). It is essential that the reciprocal relationships between joint fixation and hypermobility be considered whenever examination and manipulation are performed.

ANATOMY OF THE SACROILIAC JOINTS

The paired sacroiliac joints lie within the pelvic ring, at an oblique angle to the sagittal plane. Ligamentous support of the joints consists of the thicker and stronger posterior sacroiliac ligament, and the less dense anterior capsules supporting the front of the joints (7). The interosseous sacroiliac ligaments are massive and form the chief bond between the sacrum and the ilia. They fill the irregular space above and behind the joint and are covered by the posterior sacroiliac ligament. The sacroiliac joint has an auricular or "C" shape, with a convexity that faces anteriorly and inferiorly. The relative length of the cephalic and caudal extensions is variable. The joints appear in a multitude of forms, with not only individual differences but also considerable contralateral variations in the same individual.

Morphologically and functionally, the sacroiliac joint is recognized as a true diarthrodial joint with a joint cavity containing synovial fluid, articular cartilage, and a joint capsule lined with synovial membrane. The joint capsule is reinforced by ligamentous connections allowing movement between the contiguous bony surfaces. Microscopic examination of the joint surfaces reveals a bluish fibrocartilage that covers the iliac side, while the sacral surface shows a thicker, whiter hyaline cartilage (7, 8).

By puberty, irregularities develop in the form of elevations and depressions on the sacroiliac joint surfaces. The iliac side develops a convexity, while a corresponding concavity forms on the sacral side (8) (Fig. 7.3). The contours of the joint surfaces continue to change with age and, by the third decade, there is an increase in the number and size of the elevations and depressions, which interlock to limit mobility. After the third decade, the articular cartilage becomes roughened, fused, and frayed. In the elderly, degeneration leads to fibrous or fibrocartilaginous adhesions and occasionally, ankylosis (8).

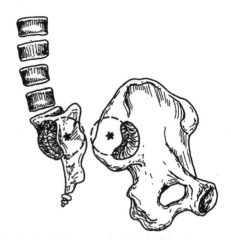

Figure 7.3. Motion at the sacroiliac joint primarily occurs in the oblique sagittal plane, with the axis of rotation centered around the iliac tubercle (*). The joint surfaces appear to move along the tram rail, the convex ridge of the iliac surface gliding in the sacral grooves. (After Kapandji IA: *The Physiology of the Joints: The Trunk and Vertebral Column*, vol 3. New York, Churchill Livingstone, 1974, p 59.)

Accessory articular facets, ranging in size from 2–10 mm in diameter, have been observed posterior to the articular surface between rudimentary transverse processes of the second sacral vertebrae and the ilium (9) (Fig. 7.4). These accessory sacroiliac joints may be unilateral or bilateral. Trotter (10) observed them in approximately one out of every three persons. Degenerative changes in accessory sacroiliac joints lead to a narrowing of the joint spaces and to marginal osteophytes. A synostosis occasionally develops between the opposing joint surfaces (11).

The sacrum, sacroiliac, and lumbosacral regions are common sites of congenital and developmental anomalies and deficiencies. More severe are agenesis, dysgenesis, and dysplasia. Minor asymmetries or variations are of clinical significance because

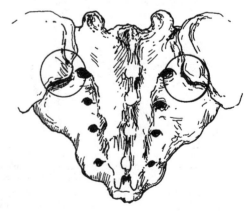

Figure 7.4. Accessory articular facets between rudimentary transverse processes of the second sacral vertebrae and the ilium form a diarthrodial joint subject to degenerative changes.

they may produce functional imbalances and result in spinal instability and altered biomechanics. It may be concluded that asymmetry and maldevelopment of the sacrum and its articulations represent a predisposing etiologic factor in low back pain syndromes.

ANATOMY OF THE PUBIC SYMPHYSIS

The pubic bones are joined in the median plane by the cartilaginous pubic symphysis, which functions in a manner similar to that of the intervertebral disc. This fibrocartilaginous connection is reinforced from above by the superior pubic ligament, from below by the arcuate pubic ligament, and from the front by a layer of oblique fibers that serve to prevent loss of disc integrity due to torsional forces. The intertwining of these semielastic fibers permits movement through transient compression and sustains joint integrity during the strong shearing forces that occur during walking (7).

MOTION AT THE SACROILIAC JOINT

While sacroiliac motion is commonly considered to be very slight (3–5°), it has been demonstrated in both anatomical specimens and the living subject (12–14). Sacroiliac motion is affected by a number of factors, including age and sex of the individual and configuration of the joint surface. Motion at this joint decreases gradually with age, more rapidly in the male than in the female (7). The joint in the female tends to be more excavated, with a wider retroarticular space and longer interosseous ligaments, all promoting greater mobility. Hormonal influences of pregnancy and, to some extent, the menstrual cycle participate in a reversible laxity process (15, 16).

Motion of the sacroiliac articulations occurs primarily in the oblique sagittal plane, with the axis of rotation centered around the iliac tubercle, located immediately posterior to the sacroiliac joint (Fig. 7.3). Bowen and Cassidy (8) suggest that opposing joint surfaces probably move along, and are directed by, the convex ridge of the iliac surface gliding in the concave sacral depression (17) (Fig. 7.3). While this track-bound motion is the easiest to verify, it appears that there is sufficient separation of the joint surfaces to allow for some translation to occur as well (18).

Gillet and Liekens (19) have described the sacrum as floating within the pelvic ring. While this concept appears paradoxical to the notion of the sacrum as a keystone, this floating or gliding motion is consistent with the idea that the sacroiliac joint functions as a shock-absorbing structure that cushions the slight amount of physiological movement observed (14). For translational movement also to occur, the articular surfaces must separate a sufficient distance to allow them to move upon one another. The energy involved in separating the two articular surfaces is absorbed by the ligamentous tissue, giving the joint its shock-absorbing ability (18). This separation of articular surfaces is enough to allow the small amount of movement noted in the frontal and horizontal planes, produced in the process of sitting and during walking. Rotary motion of the sacroiliac joints in the sagittal plane, combined with translatory motion, produces a coupled motion and results in a change in the axis of rotation. This changing axis of rotation (referred to as the instantaneous axis of rotation (2)) may account for the controversy that surrounds the location of the axis of rotation of the sacroiliac joint (13, 14, 17, 18, 20, 21).

Mennell (22) has observed clinically that the change in distance between the posterior superior iliac spines with the patient seated and prone, can be measured as a means of monitoring sacroiliac motion (Fig. 7.5). He found that normally this distance decreases by 1/4 to 3/4 inch when changing from a sitting to a lying position. This coronal-plane movement is accompanied upon sitting by nutation of the sacrum, in which the sacral promontory moves inferiorly and anteriorly as the apex of the sacrum and tip of the coccyx move posteriorly in the sagittal plane. This movement is checked by both the sacrotuberous and the sacrospinous ligaments (Fig. 7.6). As the iliac crests approximate, the ischial tuberosities move apart, widening the base of support when assuming a seated position (17). In addition to this paired-joint motion in which both ilia move symmetrically, paired reciprocal motion occurs at the sacroiliac joints during walking (see Chapter 13).

Pitkin and Pheasant (23) have discussed the paired motions as flexion and extension, in which the sacrum is the moving member and the ilia are fixed. They describe the reciprocal motion as lateral bending and rotation of the sacrum, in which the ilia are the moving members and the sacrum follows passively. As with typical vertebral motion segments of the spine, it appears that lateral bending and rotation of the sacrum do not occur separately, but rather are coupled movements (23). Grice and Fligg (24) have discussed this mechanism as a coupled motion, which was first described by Illi as a gyroscopic action producing a figure-of-eight movement of the sacrum between the ilia. This action was seen by Illi (25) to be translatory motion, and certainly some degree of translation must occur (18) if this composite theory of sacroiliac motion is correct (14).

The biomechanics of the pelvis during walking were aptly described by Grice in 1972 (5). On heel strike, the ipsilateral innominate moves posteriorly into flexion as the same side of the sacrum moves anteriorly and inferiorly. This creates a cushioning effect on the forces transmitted from the ground up the shaft of the femur. Conversely, the contralateral ilium is extended forward in the toe-off phase as the sacrum moves posteriorly and superiorly on the same side. Through the action of the iliolumbar liga-

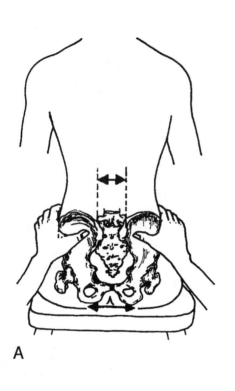
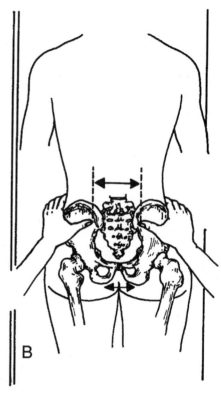
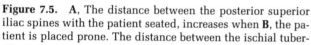

Figure 7.5. **A,** The distance between the posterior superior iliac spines with the patient seated, increases when **B**, the patient is placed prone. The distance between the ischial tuber- osities is greater in the sitting position, widening the base of support.

ment, the motion of L5, and therefore the whole spine, is dampened (5).

THE SACROILIAC SYNDROME

The sacroiliac syndrome (26) is composed of a number of factors that should be considered when dealing with pelvic ring disorders. Like typical vertebral-motion-segment lesions, sacroiliac dysfunction may take the form of simple joint locking, or joint locking with compensatory hypermobility in adjacent articulations. Occasionally, there is a sacroiliac sprain with unilateral or bilateral hypermobility without joint locking (14). It must be stressed that repeated manipulation of a joint that is moving normally is not only futile but also contraindicated because of the danger of creating and/or perpetuating a hypermobile state (27). Acuteness of pain in a sacroiliac joint is not always indicative of the site of causation. A locked sacroiliac joint may result in increased motion demands on the opposite side, in turn causing pain and inflammation of that joint (28). The most acute tenderness is frequently found in the sacroiliac joint contralateral to the one that is jammed or locked.

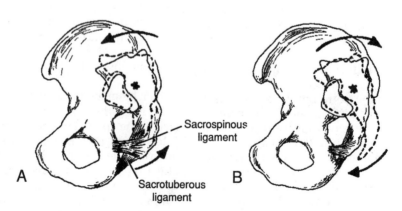

Figure 7.6. Movement of the sacrum in the sagittal plane is known as **A**, nutation and **B**, counternutation. Nutation is checked by the sacrotuberous and sacrospinous ligaments.

The site of joint locking is important in determining patient positioning and the subsequent direction of the manipulative thrust. In order that a minimum of force may be employed, causing the least amount of trauma to the patient, it should be determined whether the joint locking has occurred at the superior or inferior joint surfaces or if the sacrum is locked in the horizontal plane.

CLINICAL CONSIDERATIONS

History and Etiology

The etiology of sacroiliac dysfunction can usually be determined through the patient's history. Frequently, the patient describes a fall or lifting injury that involved torsional stress. Stepping off a curb or twisting in bed have been implicated in sacroiliac joint locking. The mechanism is thought to be a jamming of the joint at the extreme of normal motion in either the sagittal or horizontal plane. Turek (29) describes this as occurring when an irregular prominence of one articular surface becomes wedged upon a prominence of the apposed articular surface. Concomitantly the ligaments are taut, reflex muscle spasm is intense and severe, and continuous pain occurs until reduction is effected. He states, "The sacroiliac joint appears anatomically susceptible to jamming because of the surface irregularities which must work in synergy with the opposing articular surface."

Ligamentous laxity, both during and following pregnancy, predisposes to the sacroiliac syndrome (15, 16). Sacroiliac fixation is a common finding in postpartum back pain, and it responds with rapid resolution of symptoms following appropriate spinal manipulative therapy (30). Similarly, ligamentous loosening due to hormonal influence prior to the onset of menstruation enhances the vulnerability of sacroiliac joint slipping with subsequent fixation. Stabilization during this period may be maintained by the use of a trochanteric belt (Fig. 7.7).

Signs and Symptoms

Pain accompanying the sacroiliac syndrome is typically unilateral, dull in character, and located over the buttocks. It may radiate posteriorly down the thigh (high sciatia) or to the groin and anterior thigh (Fig. 7.8). Occasionally it may extend down the lateral or posterior calf to ankle, foot, and toes (26). Sensory changes are rare.

Referred pain from the sacroiliac joints is experienced in the posterior dermatomal areas of L5, S1, and S2; over the sacrum; or in the buttocks. Pain produced by pathologic changes of the anterior sacroiliac ligaments radiates into anterior dermatomal areas of L2 and L3, particularly into the thigh region immediately below the groin. Referred pain may be produced some distance away from the joint in sacroiliac disease, if the pathologic process involves the nerves that run close to these joints. These nerves include the lumbosacral trunk, the obturator nerve, and the anterior branch of the first sacral nerve. If the pathological process in the sacroiliac joints spreads to these nerves, pain and motor deficits in the lower extremities may occur. Pain from a hypermobile sacroiliac joint may be experienced in the ipsilateral hip, due to contraction of the piriformis muscle, which originates at the sacrum and at the ilium. When this muscle contracts, it tends to press the sacrum and ilium together in an attempt to stabilize the joint.

Erhardt (31) has noted that "eight different segments of the spinal cord are involved in the sensory supply of the sacroiliac joints. Pain may be referred throughout the distribution of the broad sensory supply." He further notes that this broad sensory supply is the reason why low back, buttock, and thigh pain originating in the sacroiliac joints may be easily and erroneously attributed to the lumbar spine or to hip disease (31).

The sensory supply of the sacroiliac ligaments, as established by Pitkin and Pheasant (23), is described as follows:

> The anterior sacroiliac ligaments contain fibers from the anterior branches of L2 and L3; the interosseous sacroiliac ligaments, from the posterior branches of L5, S1 and S2; the dorsal ligaments, from the anterior branches of L5, S1 and S2, as well as the posterior branches of L1 to L5 and S1 to S3.

Radiographically, the joint is difficult to visualize and is best viewed with the beam passing posteriorly to anteriorly. Pelvic instability can be demonstrated by radiokinetic tests that stress the joint (Chapter 6).

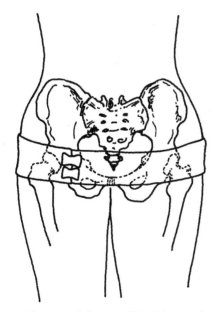

Figure 7.7. A hypermobile sacroiliac joint can be stabilized with a tight, encircling, elastic trochanteric bandage. The sacroiliac joint generally stabilizes within 3 to 6 weeks of continous immobilization.

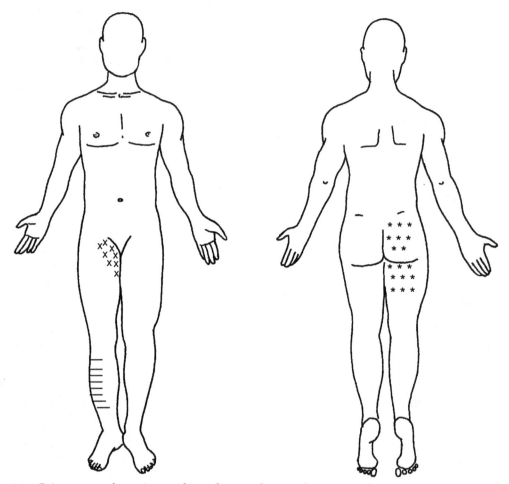

Figure 7.8. Pain pattern of a patient with a right sacroiliac syndrome. (*, aching; ×, burning; −, numbness.)

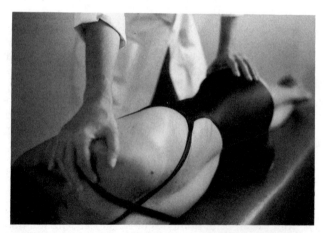

Figure 7.9. With the patient lying on the side, firm compression over the iliac crest may produce sacroiliac pain in the involved joint.

Examination

As with most other areas of the spine, biomechanical lesions of the pelvis are most effectively demonstrated by motion palpation. Manipulation specifically

directed to restore the small, normal range of motion is also a helpful retrospective diagnostic aid when it results in restoration of movement and relief of pain.

Orthopaedic Tests for Pelvic Ring Dysfunction

A number of orthopaedic tests are useful in determining sacroiliac involvement, but they give no indications as to whether or not manipulation is indicated.

Pelvic Compression

Pelvic compression places strain on the sacroiliac joints and elicits pain if inflammation is present (33). With the patient in side posture, firm compression over the up-side iliac crest may produce posterior sacroiliac joint pain (Fig. 7.9). With the patient supine on a firm surface, posterior joint pain can also be elicited when the anterior superior iliac spines are pressed toward each other (Fig. 7.10A). Also, with the patient supine, if the examiner exerts pressure on both anterior inferior and superior iliac spines bilaterally, anterior sacroiliac joint pain can be produced by forcing the ilia laterally (Fig. 7.10B). A stretching force is placed upon the anterior sacroiliac ligament, which results in pain in the affected sacroiliac joint.

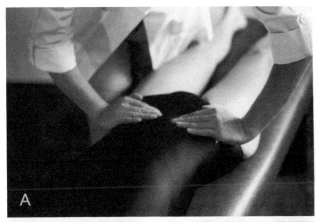

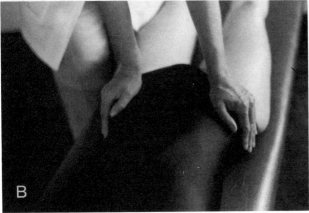

Figure 7.10. If pain results in the sacroiliac joints when the iliac bones are **A**, pressed together or **B**, forced apart, then a sacroiliac dysfunction is suspected.

Pain provoked in the sacroiliac regions indicates a positive test on any of these maneuvers, but it does not differentiate the exact nature of the sacroiliac problem or give an indication of the appropriate treatment.

FABERE Test (Figure-of-Four Test)

FABERE (33) stands for flexion, abduction, external rotation, and extension. Also known as the figure-of-four test, this maneuver places strain on the ipsilateral hip joint and sacroiliac joint. With the patient supine, the examiner grasps the ankle and the flexed knee. The thigh is flexed (F), abducted (AB), and externally rotated (ER), and extended (E). Pain or loss of joint play at the hip indicates a hip lesion, as opposed to sacroiliac involvement, which is indicated by pain localized usually to the ipsilateral sacroiliac joint.

Joint play at the hip can be tested by moving the knee through an arc, beginning with the knee and thigh flexed and internally rotated and ending with the thigh flexed, abducted, and externally rotated (Fig. 7.11A & B). In the absence of hip pathology, restriction of motion in the FABERE position indicates hip-joint fixation, and therapy should be di-

rected to the hip rather than the sacroiliac joint. Sacroiliac joint pain may be produced on the FABERE test by articular fixation at the site of pain or by compensatory hypermobility of that joint, produced by fixation of the ipsilateral hip or contralateral sacroiliac joint (Fig. 11C). This test does not differentiate between these possibilities.

Straight-Leg Raise (Lasegues' Sign)

The straight-leg raise, which produces pain by stretching the sciatic nerve, is often slightly restricted with sacroiliac lesions. A herniated disc usually produces pain and restricted motion at 45° or less, while the sacroiliac lesion does not usually restrict the straight-leg raise until 70–90° (34).

The test is performed with the patient lying supine while the leg is elevated with the knee extended. The normal person can tolerate the leg being raised to 90° without discomfort. When pain is felt on the posterior aspect of the thigh as a result of stretching the hamstrings in people with diminished flexibility, the test may give a false positive result.

With a herniated disc, the patient experiences a burning pain down the distribution of the sciatic nerve, which is accentuated by dorsiflexion of the foot (Braggard's reinforcement). A sacroiliac lesion is characterized by pain in the ipsilateral sacroiliac joint as the straight leg is raised (34) (Fig. 7.12). Manual stabilization of the contralateral ilium will increase the range of motion in the straight-leg raise and decrease the pain with sacroiliac dysfunction.

Thigh Hyperextension (Yeomann's Test)

Pain localized to the sacroiliac joints on hyperextension of the ipsilateral thigh in the prone, supine, or lateral position provides useful information for the differential diagnosis (Fig. 7.13). Pain with this maneuver indicates the site of involvement but not the nature of the problem. With a sacroiliac lesion, the prone patient is often able to extend the leg much higher on the side that is less involved.

INDICATIONS AND CONTRAINDICATIONS FOR MANIPULATION OF THE SACROILIAC JOINT

Sacroiliac dysfunction can be identified by palpating for joint play with the patient seated. This method (discussed in Chapter 5) gives a general impression of joint fixation. To determine the site and plane-of-motion restriction, the sacroiliac joint is palpated with the doctor seated and the patient standing in front of and facing away from the doctor. As the patient raises one leg, relative motion between the ilium and sacrum can be monitored (26, 35). The superior sacroiliac joint tends to become locked in flexion with restriction of extension movement in the sagittal plane.

By far the most common site of sacroiliac fixation, this lesion is characterized by a number of clinical findings. Asymmetry of the positions of the posterior superior iliac spines (PSIS) is frequently noted,

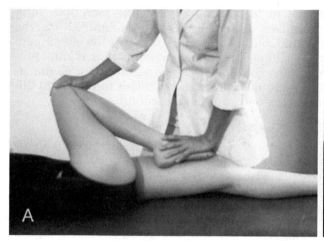

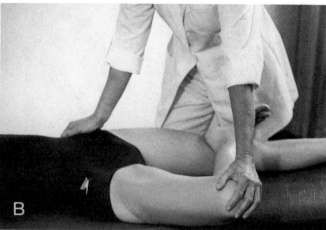

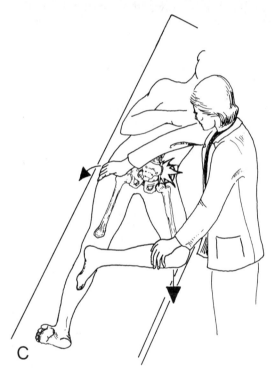

Figure 7.11.   A, Joint play at the hip can be tested by moving the knee through an arc beginning with the knee and thigh flexed, adducted and internally rotated and ending **B,** with the thigh flexed, abducted, and externally rotated. **C,** Pain in the sacroiliac joint can be differentiated from hip pain by the Patrick FABERE test.

with the PSIS on the side of superior joint-locking appearing inferior when the patient is examined in the upright position. The ipsilateral leg may also appear shorter on recumbent examination and in upright radiographs. An effective manipulation of the sacroiliac joint can be made with the patient in a side posture position, using a specific, short-lever, high-velocity thrust.

PALPATION FOR SUPERIOR JOINT FIXATION (FLEXION FIXATION)

When the sacroiliac joint is fixed in flexion, motion in the upper joint is restricted around the X-axis in the sagittal plane. The line of drive of the manipulative thrust is in the sagittal plane, to restore motion. With the patient standing, one thumb is placed over the second sacral tubercle and the other over one PSIS (Fig. 7.14A). The patient then flexes the ipsilateral thigh and knee and lifts the leg as high as possible. With normal motion, the thumb over the ipsilateral PSIS moves downward 1 to 2 centimeters (Fig. 7.14B). In a fixed joint, the thumb over the PSIS does not move downward (Fig. 7.14C). The patient will consequently rotate the entire buttock downward and forward, and with the superior portion of the joint fixed in flexion, the PSIS does not move posteriorly and inferiorly as it should (26, 35).

MANIPULATION FOR A SUPERIOR JOINT FIXATION (FLEXION FIXATION)

Manipulation of the upper sacroiliac joint is achieved with the patient positioned in side pos-

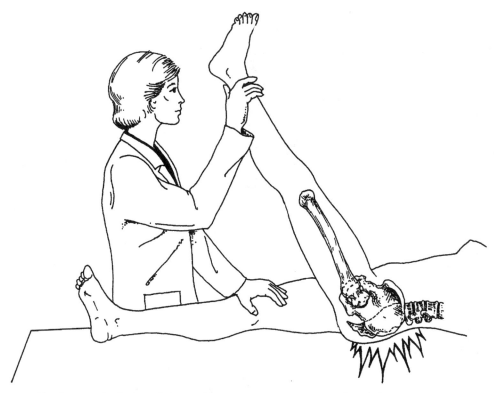

Figure 7.12. Normally the straight leg can be raised to 90° without discomfort. Pain at 45° or, less particularly, of the electric type that radiates into the feet, the back, or the opposite side indicates nonspecific irritation of the sciatic nerve or root. Pain produced from 70 to 90° and localized to the sacroiliac joint (illustrated above) is more indicative of a sacroiliac lesion.

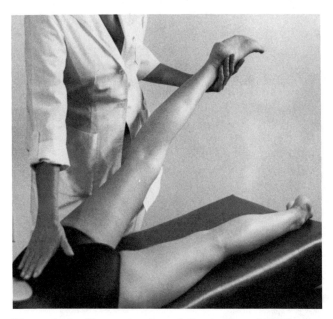

Figure 7.13. Hyperextension of the ipsilateral thigh produces pain, with lesions of the sacroiliac joint.

ture, with the side of joint fixation placed up. The inferior leg is held straight, the superior leg is flexed, and the shoulders and hips are brought into vertical alignment. The inferior arm is tractioned gently toward the head, then flexed and placed above the chest. The clinician's hand is placed on the patient's upper shoulder with moderate pressure executed toward the head, locking the patient's spine against rotation (36). The clinician's lower hand then contacts the upper posterior superior iliac spine, and traction is exerted to the point of tension. The patient's superior leg is tractioned with the clinician's inferior thigh (Fig. 7.15).

As the patient relaxes, usually following a deep breath, a high-velocity, low-amplitude thrust is delivered through the clinician's inferior arm and through the thigh down the long axis of the patient's flexed leg. The clinician's superior arm must maintain tension to stabilize the trunk and spine through the delivery of the thrust. The directional thrust of the inferior hand is anterior and slightly toward the patient's inferior shoulder. Care must be taken not to thrust with the superior hand, since this torsional movement may further compromise an injured disc.

The position of the doctor may be varied depending on the amount of leverage desired. The most common position is with the doctor's inferior thigh in contact with the patient's upper thigh. A body drop can then be initiated to employ the leverage of the femur. A longer lever arm may be employed by hooking the doctor's inferior knee in the patient's flexed upper knee using a downward thrust. Repalpation should confirm normal motion, with the PSIS mov-

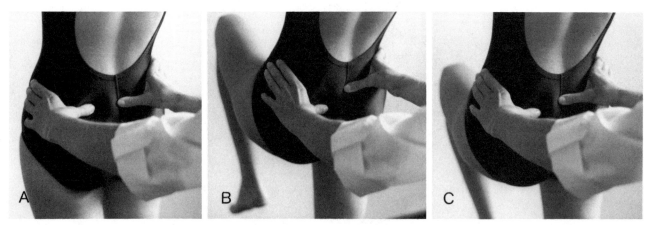

Figure 7.14. **A**, Relative motion of the left sacroiliac joint is palpated with the thumb placed over the second sacral tubercle and the other over the PSIS. **B**, With normal motion, the PSIS moves downward 1–2 cm as the leg is raised. **C**, If the joint is fixed the PSIS does not move downward.

Figure 7.15. The side posture technique for manipulation of a right superior sacroiliac joint fixation has the doctor's stabilizing hand tractioning the patient's superior shoulder while the thrusting hand contacts the affected ilium. The manipulative thrust is directed through the ilium, down the thigh and the long axis of the patient's flexed leg. The patient's superior leg is tractioned with the doctor's inferior thigh, and a body drop is simultaneously instituted as the thrust is delivered.

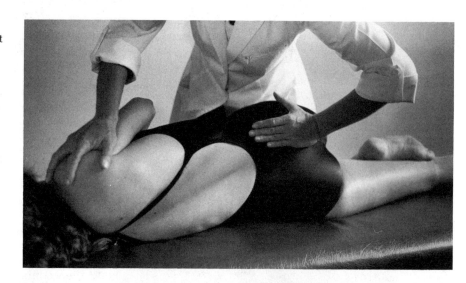

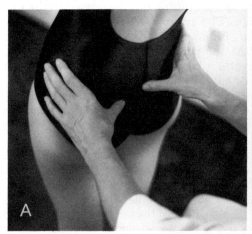
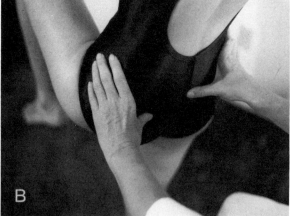

Figure 7.16. **A**, Inferior sacroiliac joint motion is monitored with one thumb placed on the sacral apex and the other over the ipsilateral ischial tuberosity. **B**, As the patient flexes the ipsilateral thigh and knee, the thumbs should move apart 1–2 cm.

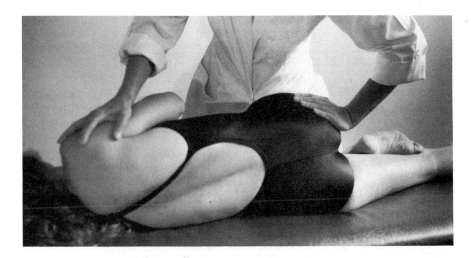

Figure 7.17. Manipulation of the patient with an inferior joint fixation is performed with the patient positioned in side posture with the upper leg flexed past 90°. The thrust is delivered anteriorly and inferiorly, with a scooping cephalad motion toward the patient's lower shoulder.

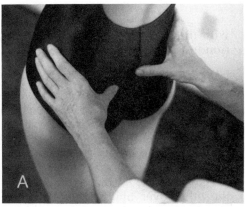

Figure 7.18. **A**, To test sacral rotation, one of the examiner's thumbs is placed over the second sacral spinous process and the other over one PSIS. **B**, When the contralateral leg is raised, the thumbs should come together 1–2 cm. Absence of this motion indicates a sacral rotational fixation.

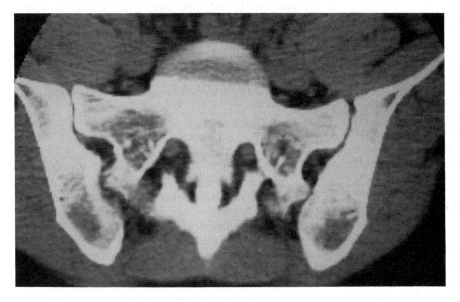

Figure 7.19. CT scan of sacral rotation. Sacral rotation indicating a possible sacral fixation is visualized on this CT scan. This patient had been subjected to a bone scan, myelogram and MRI in addition to the CT scan, all of which were read as negative. Following this the patient responded favorably to chiropractic manipulation of the sacroiliac joint. (Courtesy of Jasmar Reddin, D.C.)

Figure 7.20. The patient with a sacral rotational fixation is positioned in side posture, with the side of fixation involvement placed down. The hand contacts the upper portion of the sacrum, and with a scooping motion the thrust is delivered anteriorly away from the locked joint.

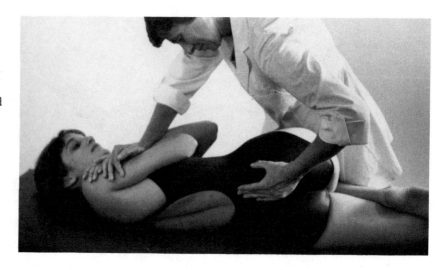

ing downward in relation to the second sacral tubercle.

PALPATION FOR INFERIOR JOINT FIXATION (EXTENSION FIXATION)

When the sacroiliac joint is fixed in extension, motion in the lower joint is restricted around the X-axis in the sagittal plane. To detect inferior joint locking (extension fixation) one thumb is placed on the sacral apex and the other over the ipsilateral ischial tuberosity. As the patient flexes the ipsilateral thigh and knee, lifting the leg as high as possible, the ischial tuberosity normally moves laterally 1–2 cm (Fig. 7.16). With joint fixation, there is no lateral movement of the tuberosity, and the joint is locked in extension.

MANIPULATION FOR INFERIOR JOINT LOCKING (EXTENSION FIXATION)

Fixation of the sacroiliac joint in extension restricts motion in the sagittal plane. Palpation of the joint reveals restricted motion in the lower portion of the joint. Occasionally, an extension fixation in one sacroiliac joint is accompanied by a flexion fixation in the contralateral joint, producing a pelvic distortion or "tortipelvis" (Chapter 11).

Manipulation of the patient with an extension fixation of the sacroiliac joint is performed with the patient positioned in side posture (as for a flexion fixation) with the side of fixation placed up and the upper thigh flexed past 90° (36).

The clinician's inferior hand contacts the ischial tuberosity, and following a deep breath and relaxation by the patient, a high-velocity, low-amplitude thrust is delivered anteriorly and inferiorly with a scooping cephalad motion toward the patient's lower shoulder (Fig. 7.17). The clinician's upper arm maintains tension on the patient's upper shoulder, to stabilize the trunk and spine. Following the thrust, repalpation should confirm normal motion,

with the ischial tuberosity moving laterally in relation to the sacral apex.

PALPATION FOR SACRAL ROTATIONAL FIXATION

When the sacrum is fixed in rotation, sacral motion is restricted around the Y-axis in the horizontal plane. While rare, this fixation may be released with the least amount of force by contacting the sacrum, rather than the ilium or ischium.

To test for sacral rotation, the examiner places one thumb over the second sacral spinous process and the other over one PSIS. The patient is then instructed to raise the contralateral leg as high as possible. With normal motion the sacrum moves 1–2 cm laterally, approximating the PSIS (Fig. 7.18). With this lesion it is common to find hypertonic adductors on the affected side and hypertonic tensor facial latae on the contralateral side. Sacral rotation may be visualized on a CT scan (Fig. 7.19); however, routine scanning for this lesion is not recommended.

MANIPULATION FOR A SACRAL ROTATION FIXATION

The patient with a sacral rotational fixation is positioned in side posture, with the side of fixation placed down. The fingertips of the adjusting hand contact the second sacral tubercle above and below for a pull maneuver, assisted by knee-to-knee kick start, while stabilizing the contralateral shoulder in extension. If the sacrum is wide enough, a knife-edge contact can be made on the second sacral tubercle, and the adjustment made with a scooping, rotational, anterior thrust. This manipulation requires minimal force with proper contact and positioning. This maneuver is effective when the superior ilium is rotated and flexed internally onto the sacrum (Fig. 7.20).

Alternatively, when the superior ilium is rotated and flexed externally with respect to the sacrum, the side of the sacroiliac fixation is placed up, and the

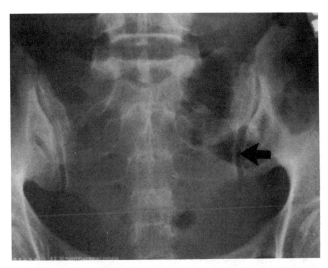

Figure 7.21. Sacroiliac instability following trauma can be demonstrated in this case by the widening of the left inferior sacroiliac joint (*arrow*).

clinician's superior hand contacts the sacrum, thrusting toward the external fixation with the same scooping motion described above. Repalpation following manipulation should verify the establishment of normal motion with the sacrum, approximating the posterior superior iliac spine.

The prognosis is good for a simple sacroiliac syndrome involving only joint fixation. This condition commonly resolves with one to six treatments over a 2-week period. A 6-year study, in which 283 patients with low back pain were treated with manipulation, showed the best results in patients with a posterior joint or sacroiliac syndrome (37). More than 90% of patients with a diagnosis of sacroiliac syndrome were either symptom-free, with no re-

striction for work or other activities, or they suffered only mild constant or intermittent pain and had no restriction for work or other activities following a course of spinal manipulative therapy. It is notable that these patients had not previously responded to simple conservative care, had suffered from low back pain for many years, and were disabled by pain at the start of the treatment.

DIFFERENTIAL DIAGNOSIS OF SACROILIAC JOINT LESIONS

Sacroiliac Sprain

Pain in a hypermobile sacroiliac joint is usually due to a ligamentous sprain. Instability following trauma is indicated by widening of joint space (Fig. 7.21). Excessive ligamentous laxity inevitably leads to traumatic degenerative arthrosis of the sacroiliac joints, with symptoms of morning stiffness, limited forward bending, and pain when rising from a seated position (10, 27). The characteristic signs of sacroiliac degeneration seen on radiographs are joint erosion and condensation in the form of subchondral sclerosis (38) (Fig. 7.22). If motion palpation of the sacroiliac joints reveals excess motion unilaterally, a sacroiliac sprain should be suspected.

Manipulation of a hypermobile joint is contraindicated, and treatment should be directed toward restriction of abnormal motion by an encircling trochanteric bandage. It is important that the slight amount of normal motion not be restricted, and for this reason an elastic tensor bandage (such as used to wrap a sprained extremity joint) is recommended, rather than a more restrictive belt or support (Fig. 7.7) (39). This bandage should be worn at all times, for a period of 3 to 6 weeks. Healing of this joint rarely takes longer in healthy individuals. It is imperative that manipulation not be introduced into

Figure 7.22. Bilateral degenerative sacroiliac arthrosis.

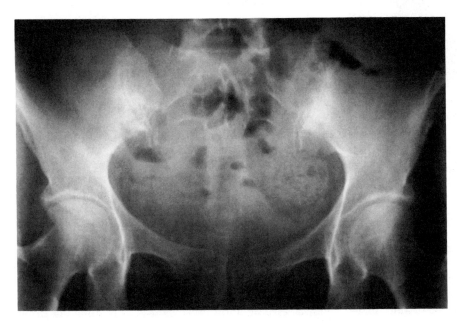

Figure 7.23. Microtrauma and repeated pregnancies can lead to degenerative changes seen on radiographs as sclerosis in the iliac bones, known as hyperostosis triangularis.

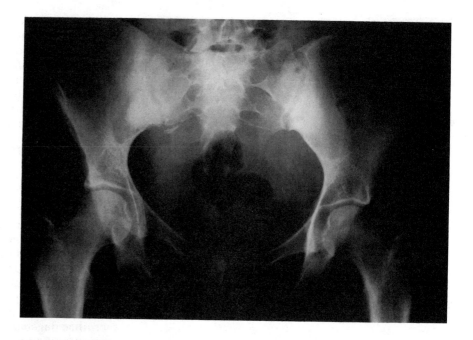

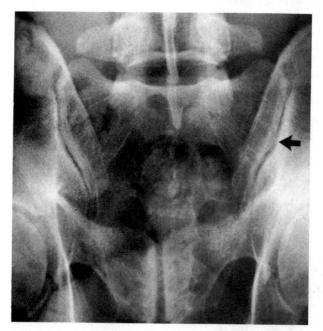

Figure 7.24. Early degenerative changes of the right sacroiliac joint are noted in this avid golfer (*arrow*).

such hypermobile joints, since repetitive stretching of lax ligaments can perpetuate the patient's problem (40).

Pregnancy and Postpartum Instability

Pelvic instability beginning as early as the end of the first trimester of pregnancy is due to ligamentous relaxation resulting from the effect of the ovarian hormone relaxin (11, 15, 16). Microtrauma and repeated pregnancies with resulting sacroiliac insta-

bility can lead to the initiation of degenerative changes, some of which may be seen on radiographs as sclerosis in the iliac bones, known as hyperostosis triangularis ilii (11) (Fig. 7.23).

Instability In Athletes

Trauma (Fig. 7.24) or vigorous physical activity, which places repeated strain on athletes such as long-distance runners, hurdlers, jumpers, football and soccer players, ballet dancers, golfers, and bowlers, can lead to sacroiliac strain (34). The onset of such sprains may be gradual, with symptoms ranging from a painful irritation to hypermobility of one or both sacroiliac joints. Some degree of pelvic torsional stress may occur when the repeated stress is unilateral (Chapter 13).

Sacroiliac Sprain with Attendant Muscle Strain

A longer course of treatment with adjunctive physiotherapy may be necessary when muscle strains or their residuals occur along with the articular fixation (Chapter 12).

Mild injury resulting from minor trauma generally resolves within one week, with 4 to 6 treatments. Maximum treatment in these cases is 30 days.

Complicated strains result when tissues are physiologically deficient at the time of injury, which can prolong the inflammatory response and delay healing. Such cases can require 1 to 3 months of care and up to 24 visits. When patients fail to show progress at any time, they should be referred for evaluation and a second opinion.

SACROILIAC DYSFUNCTION

The sacroiliac articulations are moving, weightbearing synovial joints exhibiting the same characteristic joint dysfunction that plagues other

Table 7.1 Differential Diagnosis of Common Pelvic-Ring Disorders

Condition	History & Symptoms	Diagnostic Indicators & Procedures	Therapy
Biomechanical disorders			
Traumatic & movement syndromes			
Sacroiliac joint fixation	Sacroiliac joint pain/ tenderness, pain radiating into the buttocks	Motion palpation reveals restricted SI joint motion	Manipulation (see text)
Sacroiliac sprains (hypermobile joints)	History of trauma or stress of SI joint; unilateral pain in hip, buttock & upper posterior thigh	Pain on compression of the SI joints & over the symphysis pubes; motion palpation may reveal one joint hypermobile compared to other	Immobilize with trochanteric belt
Coccygeal subluxation & dislocation	Coccygeal pain usually post-traumatic from fall on the buttocks or obstetrical delivery; rectal complaints	Radiographic examination demonstrates coccygeal displacement	Sacrotuberous ligament pressure, manipulate
Pubic instability	Pubic & inguinal pain aggravated by movement	Radiokinetic views show pubic assymetry	Immobilize with trochanteric belt
Postural syndromes			
Obesity	Low back & buttock pain due to increased anterior pelvic tilt	Excess weight for height & body type, positive skin-fold test, radiographs show increased sacral base angle & increased lumbar lordosis	Reduce weight, exercise to decrease anterior pelvic tilt
Pregnancy	Low back & buttock pain due to increased anterior pelvic tilt & ligamentous softening	A reverse Patrick's FABERE test (figure-of-four test), with internal rotation, produces pain on distraction of the SI joints, increased lumbar lordosis	Support with a trochanteric belt; manipulate where indicated by motion palpation; decrease activity; weight control
Dysmenorrhea	Painful menstruation	Gynecological examination	Exercise; decrease pelvic tilt with traction
Muscle Syndromes			
Piriformis syndrome	Pain in the buttock extending down the course of the sciatic nerve, trigger points at the origin & insertion of the muscle	Palpable muscle spasm & trigger points in the piriformis muscle; pain on internal rotation of the hip with the knees in flexion	Apply deep pressure to the trigger points in the belly of muscle & at the insertion on the capsule
Psoas spasm	Low back pain, occasional inguinal pain & increased lumbar lordosis	+ Thomas test; discrepancy in arm length with arms extended over head	Stretching exercises; avoid sit-ups; manipulate
Tensor fascia lata syndrome	Pain between iliac crest & greater trochanter	Palpable muscle spasm; pain on internal hip rotation; check for contralateral sacral rotation	Deep pressure therapy; manipulate; exercise
Gluteus medius spasm	Buttocks pain	Palpable trigger points in the gluteus medius muscle	Apply deep pressure to the trigger points
Stress disorders			
Hyperostosis triangularsis illii (osteitis condensans illii)	Low back pain radiating into the buttock, symptoms aggravated by activity; occurs primarily in females of child-bearing age, proportion female to male 9:1	Muscle spasm & increased lumbar lordosis common; radiographs demonstrate condensation of bone of the articular portion of the ilium; does not involve the joint space	Decrease lumbosacral angle by decreasing anterior pelvic tilt; immobilize with a lumbosacral corset
Sacroiliac osteoarthritis	Morning stiffness & low back pain	Radiographic examination reveals narrowed joint space, subchondral sclerosis, subchondral cysts, & marginal osteophytes	Mobilization, swimming & exercise
Fractures	History of trauma or pathology, back pain exaggerated by weight-bearing, neurological deficits	Radiographic examination most commonly reveals disrupted sacral foramen	Immobilization & stabilization for 6 to 8 weeks

Table 7.1 *(Continued)*

Condition	History & Symptoms	Diagnostic Indicators & Procedures	Therapy
Pathological Lesions			
Infectious disorders			
Ankylosing spondylitis	More common in males (5:1), buttock pain, aching & stiffness after inactivity; bilateral involvement of the sacroiliac articulations	Restriction of chest expansion, pain on SI joint compression, elevated sedimentation rate, positive HLA B27 predisposition; radiographs of SI joints show bilateral marginal erosion & irregularities, sclerosis with bony ankylosis in the late stages	Heat, mild exercise; manipulation when acute phase has passed; refer for pain & anti-inflammatory medication when severe
Pyogenic sacroiliitis	Fever, localized pain & tenderness radiating to the buttock in a sciatic distribution; child or history of drug abuse common	Positive radioisotope scan & thermogram; radiographs demonstrate marginal erosion, blurred joint contours, & early joint narrowing	Refer for antibiotic medicine
Tuberculosis sacroiliitis	Affects young adults; SI joint pain commonly referred to the groin & less commonly along the sciatic distribution; rarely bilateral	Pain on SI joint compression, positive tuberculin test & increased ESR; radiographs demonstrate blurred joint contours & pseudowidening; late stages show bony ankylosis	Immobilize & refer for medication
Reiter's syndrome	Preceded by diarrhea or sexual contact; history of urethritis, conjunctivitis, & inflammatory nonsuppurative arthritis; skin lesions not uncommon, more frequent in men	Serological evidence of infection; radiographic evidence of sacroiliitis	Refer for medication
Inflammatory bowel disease (Crohn's disease)	History of chronic bowel disorders, acute onset of peripheral arthritis	Radiographic evidence of sacroiliitis R/O systemic candidiasis	Refer for medication or dietary management
Metabolic disorders			
Paget's disease (osteitis deformans)	Over 55 affected, aching pain in buttocks unrelieved by rest, bones are often enlarged	Radiographs demonstrate exaggerated bizzare bony trabeculation; bone expansion common; heat-labile alkaline phosphatase is high	Refer for medication
Gout	Sacrogluteal pain	Elevated serum uric acid level; radiographic examination reveals erosion of joint borders, sclerosis of joint margins, cyst-like areas	Diet, refer for medication (colchicine)
Space-occupying lesions			
Tumor	Pain increased on rest	Radiographs demonstrate osteolytic or osteoblastic lesions, positive bone scan	Refer for biopsy
Aneurysms	Low back pain	Radiographs may demonstrate ballooning of involved artery	Refer for surgery

diarthrodial joints (14). They are subject to reversible joint fixation within their limited range of motion, frequently at the extreme of the possible range of movement. They become irritated and have a tendency to hypermobility when motion at adjacent or contralateral articulations is restricted. They may exhibit instability due to ligamentous insufficiency and are prone to develop degenerative disease, as do other synovial joints.

Because the sacroiliac joint is a diarthrodial joint characterized by movement in addition to weightbearing, it is crucial that normal movement, however small the range, be maintained. It is of fundamental importance that motion at this joint is sometimes a synchronous, paired, symmetrical motion (as in sitting), while at other times, it is an unpaired reciprocal motion (as in walking). Postural asymmetry and pelvic distortion involving pelvic torsion are discussed in Chapter 11.

COCCYGODYNIA

Many cases of coccygodynia are considered psychogenic (41, 42), and often only severe cases receive serious consideration. The treatment of such cases is often surgical excision of the offending segment.

The most common causes of coccygodynia are flexion injury or direct contusion of the coccyx, which results from a fall in the sitting position. When sitting upright on a hard surface, the weight of the body is born by the two ischial tuberosities, the coccyx lying approximately 2 cm above this level. When a fall occurs, however, with the body tilted backward to an angle of 45°, the coccyx can become contused and anteriorly displaced in flexion. The coccyx can also receive the impact if a fall occurs on an uneven surface or on a projection smaller in width than the distance between the ischia (approximately 13 cm). Occasionally childbirth causes an extension sprain of the coccyx (4, 42).

Both flexion and extension displacements can be identified by lateral radiographs. Rectal examination of the coccyx facilitates palpation. Normally only flexion and extension (23) are possible at the sacrococcygeal joint. External palpation can reveal the site of tenderness, with lateral, forward, or backward displacement detectable.

Coccygodynia can sometimes be treated with the patient prone while cephalad pressure is applied to the sacrotuberous ligament. The patient is placed prone, with the hips slightly elevated. The point of contact is midway between the ischial tuberosity and the apex of the sacrum. Pressure is applied, lifting slightly headward, with the thumb medial to the ischial tuberosity and deep toward the coccyx. The direction of contact can be varied, moving a slight amount at a time, until relief of pain has been achieved. Contact is usually maintained for several minutes, promoting patient relaxation (43).

Manipulation of the coccyx should be done with caution and only after biomechanical analysis, with appropriate regard for the radiographic and static palpatory findings. Manipulation of a displaced coccyx without symptoms is not advised, since this may induce pain and distress for the patient. When manipulation is indicated, the anteriorly displaced coccyx can be manipulated through the rectum (43).

DIFFERENTIAL DIAGNOSIS OF PELVIC-RING DISORDERS

Differential diagnosis of pelvic-ring disorders is not limited to biomechanical dysfunction (Table 7.1). Like other joints, the sacroiliac articulations can be affected by inflammatory diseases including pyogenic and granulomatous infections as well as ankylosing spondylitis. Metabolic disorders such as osteitis deformans and gout can also be manifested in the pelvis, and as with other areas of the spine, one must always be mindful of space-occupying lesions when differentiating the patient's problem (11).

Among the most common disorders to affect the pelvic ring are muscle syndromes and postural asymmetries. These subjects are discussed in depth elsewhere (Chapters 11 and 12).

The variety of sacroiliac problems makes diagnostic differentiation difficult at best, when one considers that the sacroilac joints are more than passive transmitters of body weight to the femoral heads. The biomechanics of these articulations must be fully considered when diagnosing disorders of the pelvic ring. While the precise mechanical nature of sacroiliac joint dysfunction may seem difficult to determine, motion palpation and analysis of the corresponding pelvic function makes the choice of treatment more than arbitrary manipulation of these joints based on theoretical concepts.

References

1. Grieve GP: The sacro-iliac joint. *Physiotherapy* 62:384–400, 1976.
2. White AA, Panjabi MM: *Clinical Biomechanics of the Spine.* Philadelphia, JB Lippincott, 1978, p 265.
3. Brunstrom S: *Clinical Kinesiology*, ed 3. Philadelphia, FA Davis, 1979, p 11.
4. Sandoz RW: Structural and functional pathologies of the pelvic ring. *Ann Swiss Assoc* 8:106, 1981.
5. Grice A: Mechanics of walking, development and clinical significance. *JCCA* 16:15–23, 1972.
6. Gatterman MI: Indications for spinal manipulation in the treatment of back pain. *ACA J Chiro*, 19:51–66, 1982.
7. Warwick R, William R: *Gray's Anatomy*, ed 35 British. Philadelphia, WB Saunders, 1973, p 444.
8. Bowen V, Cassidy JD: Macroscopic and microscopic anatomy of the sacro-iliac joint from embryonic life until the eighth decade. *Spine* 6:620–628, 1981.
9. Schunke GB: The anatomy and development of the sacroiliac joint in man. *Anat Rec* 72:313–331, 1972.
10. Trotter M: A common anatomical variation in the sacroiliac region. *J Bone Joint Surg* 22A:293–299, 1940.
11. Dihlmann W: *Diagnostic Radiology of the Sacro-iliac Joints.* Translated by Michaelis L.S. Chicago, Year Book, 1980, p 5.
12. Weisl H: The movement of the sacro-iliac joint. *Acta Anat* 23:80–89, 1955.
13. Colachis SC Jr., Warden SC, Bechtal CO, Strohm BR: Movement of the sacroiliac joint in the adult male: a preliminary report. *Arch Phys Med Rehabil* 44:490–498, 1963.
14. Frigerio NA, Stowe RR, Howe JW: Movement of the sacroiliac joint. *Clin Orthop* 100:370–377, 1974.
15. Goldthwait SE, Osgood RB: A consideration of the pelvic articulations from an anatomical, pathological and clinical standpoint. *Boston Med Surg J* 152:593–634, 1905.
16. Ohlsen, H: Moulding of the pelvis during labor. *Acta Radiol Diagn* 14:417, 1973.
17. Kapandji IA: *The Physiology of Joints: The Trunk and Vertebral Column.* New York, Churchill Livingstone, 1974, vol 3. p 64.
18. Wilder DG, Pope MG, Frymoyer JW: The functional topography of the sacroiliac joint. *Spine* 5:575–579, 1980.

19. Gillet H, Liekens M: *Belgian Chiropractic Research Notes*. ed 4. Motion Palpation Institute Huntington Beach, CA 1981, p 9.

20. Illi WH: Sacro-iliac mechanism keystone of spinal balance and body locomotion. *National College Journal of Chiropractic*, 12:3–23, 1940.

21. Weisl H: The articular surfaces of the sacro-iliac joint and their relation to the movement of the sacrum. *Acta Anat* 22:1–14, 1954.

22. Mennell JM: *Back Pain: Diagnosis and Treatment Using Manipulative Technique*. Boston, Little, Brown & Co, 1960, p 62.

23. Pitkin JC, Pheasant JC: Sacrothrogentic telalgia: A Study of Sacral Mobility. *J Bone Joint Surg*, 18:365–374, 1936.

24. Grice AS, Fligg DB: Biomechanics of the pelvis. Denver conference monograph. ACA Council of Technic, Des Moines, p 103, 1980.

25. Illi F: The Vertebral Column: Life line of the body. *National College Journal of Chiropractic*, 23:8–11, 1951.

26. Kirkaldy-Willis WH: *Managing Low Back Pain*, ed 2. New York, Churchill Livingstone, 1988, pp 135–137.

27. Gatterman MI, Contraindications and complications of spinal manipulative therapy. *ACA J Chiro* 15:S-75, 1981.

28. Beal MC: The Sacro-iliac problem: review of anatomy, mechanics and diagnosis. *J Am Osteopath Assoc* 81:667–679, 1982.

29. Turek SL: *Orthopaedics Principles and their Application*, ed 3. Philadelphia, JB Lippincott, 1977, p 1469.

30. Potter GE, Cassidy JD: Diagnosis and manipulative management of post-partum back pain: a case study. *JMPT* 12:99–102, 1979.

31. Erhardt R: The often forgotten sacroiliac joint. Proceedings, 5th Annual Dr. Donald B Tomkins Lecture, American Chiropractic College of Roentgenology Annual Workshop, Denver, 1985, p4.

32. Chamberlain WE: The symphysis pubis in the roentgen examination of the sacroiliac joint. *Am J Roentgenol* 24:621–625, 1930.

33. D'Ambrosia RD: *Musculoskeletal Disorders Regional Examination and Differential Diagnosis*. Philadelphia, JB Lippincott, 1977, p 259.

34. Grieve GP: *Common Vertebral Joint Problems*. New York, Churchill Livingstone, 1981, p 281.

35. Grecco MA: *Chiropractic Technique Illustrated*. New York, Jarl Publishing, 1953, pp 48–57.

36. Haldeman S: Spinal Manipulative Therapy in the Management of Low Back Pain. In Finneson BE (ed): *Low Back Pain*. Philadelphia, JB Lippincott, 1980, p 263.

37. Kirkaldy-Willis, WH: *Managing Low Back Pain*. New York, Churchill Livingstone, 1983, pp 175–183.

38. Cohen AS, McNeil JM, et al.: The "normal" sacroiliac joint. *Am J Roentgenol Rad Ther & Nuc Med* 100:559–563, 1967.

39. Macnab I: *Backache*. Baltimore, William & Wilkins, 1977, p 68.

40. Stoddard A: *Manual of Osteopathic Technique*, ed 3. London, Hutchinson, 1980, p 217.

41. Richard HJ: Causes of coccydynia. *J Bone Joint Surg* 36B:142, 1954.

42. Cyriax J: *Textbook of Orthopaedic Medicine, Vol 1 Diagnosis of Soft Tissue Lesions*, ed 6. London, Bailliere & Tindall, 1975, p 439.

43. Reinert OC: *Chiropractic Procedure and Practice*, ed 4. Floriasont, MI, Marian Press, 1976, p 156.

CHAPTER 8

Disorders of the Lumbar Spine

MERIDEL I. GATTERMAN, M.A., D.C.
DAVID PANZER, D.C.

Mechanical low back pain results from the inherent susceptibility of the lumbar spine to static loads due to muscle and gravity forces and to kinetic deviations from normal function. While no one therapeutic procedure is a panacea for all etiological factors producing low back pain, a large percentage of disorders of the lumbar spine due to biomechanical dysfunction respond favorably to chiropractic management.

The inherent susceptibility of the lumbar spine to biomechanical disorders can be attributed to various factors. Developmental anomalies and variations occur with such frequency at the lumbosacral junction that Schmorl and Junghanns refer to this area as an ontogenetically unstable region (1). The "developmental unrest" present in this area creates a predisposition for serious disease processes resulting from mechanical low back dysfunction (1).

Anomalous transitional segments, especially those involving accessory joints and asymmetrical joint facings (tropism), are common causes of biomechanical dysfunction (1–3). Restriction of motion due to anatomical variations may contribute to stresses, with the burden of motion transmitted to other segments of the spine. This produces abnormal strain on the soft tissues that must check the tendency toward hypermobility in the adjacent segments (4). Abnormal static loading may occur in the lumbar spine from postural faults, such as anterior pelvic tilt, or may be due to spondylolisthesis (see Chapter 11). Tropism and degenerative changes in the three-joint complex predispose to kinetic deviations from normal function with resulting hyper- and hypomobility. Cassidy, Kirkaldy-Willis and Mc-

Gregor (5) have studied the response of five differentiated lumbar spine conditions to spinal manipulation. These conditions responded to varying degrees, which supports the contention that biomechanical dysfunction of the lumbar spine responds favorably to chiropractic management.

ANATOMY

Anatomically, the five lumbar vertebrae are distinguished by their greater weight. The kidney-shaped body is large and wider from side to side. Because of the relatively large size of the vertebrae, the lumbar spine comprises approximately 25% of the spine's total length (6).

The vertebral foramina that form the spinal canal are triangular, and the pedicles are short. The spinous processes are almost horizontal, quadrangular, and thickened along the posterior inferior borders (7). The superior articular facets are slightly concave and face dorsally and medially, while the inferior facets are slightly convex and face ventrally and laterally. The posterior border of the superior articular process bears a rough elevation known as the mamillary process, the site of attachment of the multifidus and medial intertransverse muscles. The transverse processes are long and thin. The posterior inferior aspect of the root of each transverse process bears a small, rough accessory process (Fig. 8.1) (7). The fifth lumbar spinous process is frequently smaller, with more massive transverse processes connected to the whole of the lateral surface of the pedicles, encroaching on the side of the body. The fifth lumbar body is usually the largest of the lumbar vertebrae and has a greater anterior vertical dimension, which increases the lumbar lordosis.

Posterior Facet Joints

The paired posterior facet articulations (zygapophyseal joints) are classified as diarthrodial plane

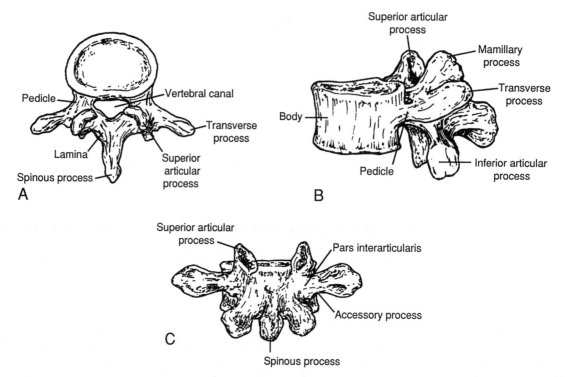

Figure 8.1. **A,** The typical lumbar vertebra exhibits short pedicles and a triangular spinal canal. **B,** The posterior border of the *superior articular process* bears a rough elevation known as the *mamillary process.* **C,** The *transverse processes* are long and thin with a rough *accessory process* in the posterior inferior aspect.

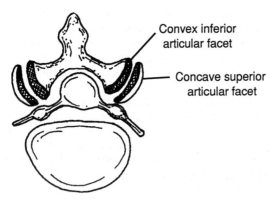

Figure 8.2. The medial-facing concave facets of the superior articular processes clasp from below the convex lateral-facing facets of the vertebra above. Shown in cross section.

joints designed to restrict and guide spinal motion. Unlike the intervertebral disc, these freely movable joints are not designed to bear weight. King, Prasad, and Ewing (8) have concluded that, depending on spine posture, the facet joints share up to 33% of the axial load (see Chapter 11). Adams and Hutton (9) found that the lumbar apophyseal joints resist about 16% of the intervertebral compressive forces in the erect standing posture, whereas in the erect sitting posture they resist none. Although such contact relieves the intervertebral disc of compressive force, it might be a cause of low backache. Degenerative changes in the disc also affect the posterior joints by increasing the axial load on the posterior joints. As the disc thins, the interaction of changes in the component parts of the three-joint complex produces vertebral motion segment dysfunction.

The plane of the facet joints is vertical in the lumbar region of the spine. The medial-facing concave facets of the superior articular processes clasp from below the convex lateral-facing facets of the vertebra above (Fig 8.2). The orientation of the facet articulations most commonly changes from a sagittal facing in the upper lumbar region to a more coronal facing in the lower joints (2, 3). The loose fibroelastic capsule is rendered even more lax than that of most diarthrodial joints by the elastic ligamentum flavum, which is blended with the medial capsular ligament (10).

The presence of meniscoids in the posterior facet joints and their clinical significance is controversial. It has been suggested that entrapment of meniscus-like bodies is an etiological factor in facet-joint locking (1, 11–17) (see Chapter 3). These meniscoids have been described as fibrous tissue that has developed secondarily in synovial fat pads as a result of mechanical stress. They are composed of a connective tissue rim extending along the dorsal and ventral margin of the joint, with an adipose base extending into the joint. They are located at the superior and inferior poles of the articular facets (Fig. 8.3). Other adipose tissue pads occur superoventrally and infradorsally.

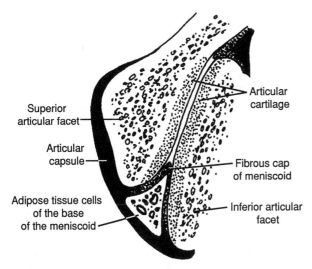

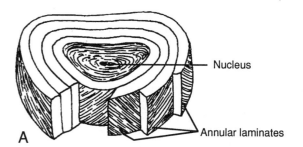

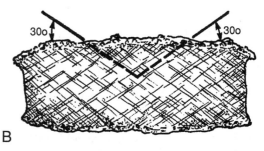

Figure 8.3. Fibroadipose meniscoids of a facet joint. (Modified from Engel R, Bogduk N: The menisci of the lumbar zygapophyseal joints. *J Anat* 135:795, 1982 and Bogduk N, Engel R: The menisci of the lumbar zygapophyseal joints: a review of their antatomy and clinical significance. *Spine* 9:454–460, 1980.)

Figure 8.4. Intervertebral disc. **A,** The annular fibers form a restraining outer ligament that contains the inner nucleus pulposus arranged in concentric lamelle. **B,** The reinforcing fibers are oriented in opposite directions at about 30°. (Modified from White AA, Panjabi MM: *Clinical Biomechanics of the Spine.* Philadelphia, JB Lippincott, 1978, p 18.)

Functionally, they act as "space fillers," providing greater stability and helping distribute the load on the joint over a greater area (17). Lewit (13) describes these meniscoids as having a soft base and a hard edge that cannot be compressed. He postulates that constant pressure from the meniscoids produces a cavity in the cartilage in which it is trapped. Bogduk and Engle (17), however, consider the theory of meniscoid entrapment to have been overstated, suggesting that future studies consider other causes of "acute locked back" outside the lumbar zygapophyseal joints, specifically abnormalities in the lumbar intervertebral disc. They state that the connective tissue rim is too short to become trapped, and the tension of the ligamentum flavum (ventrally) and multifidus muscles (dorsally) protect against them being drawn into the cavity of the joint. They point out that adipose tissue parts are too soft and pliable to create a recess and get trapped. While this may be true of smooth, symmetrical planar facets, it would seem that surface irregularities (3) coupled with translatory motion would increase the probability of entrapment.

Intervertebral Discs

Endplates

The intervertebral discs are separated from the adjacent spongiosa and cancellous bone of the vertebral bodies above and below by a plate of hyaline cartilage. The circumference of the endplate is bound by margins of cortical bone of the vertebral body, which forms a bony ring. This bony ring is created through ossification of the epiphyseal plate, which is the growth zone of the immature vertebral

bodies. It is thicker in front and sides than in back (18) and helps to anchor the disc to the vertebral body. The endplates provide a permeable barrier between the nucleus pulposus and the spongiosa of the vertebral bodies, allowing the transfer of the tissue fluid that meets the nutritional demands of the disc.

The intervertebral discs are interposed between adjacent surfaces of the vertebral bodies, serving to unite the vertebrae as well as separate them. They are thicker in front than behind in the lumbar region and contribute to the anterior convexity of the lumbar spine (7). They are thick enough to be an important factor in controlling movement at the intervertebral joint (18) and are securely anchored to the vertebral endplates, thus making the popular concept of a "slipped disc" impossible.

Annulus Fibrosus

The annular fibers form a restraining outer ligament that contains the inner nucleus pulposus (Fig 8.4A). The outer annular fibers are more elastic peripherally and are gathered in concentric lamellae, with successive layers overlapping in alternating oblique directions (Fig. 8.4B). The outermost fibers are much more numerous anteriorly and are attached to the periosteum and vertebral body just beyond the epiphyseal ring of cortical bone.

The posterior part of the annulus, especially the posterolateral part, is a site of potential weakness because of the thinning and bifurcation of annular fibers posteriorly and the eccentric position of the nucleus pulposus, which lies closer to the posterior aspect of the disc. There is also less reinforcement from the posterior longitudinal ligament, which is attenuated and thin, narrowing caudally from L1. By the time it reaches L5, it is less than half of the posterior disc margin. At the S1 interspace, it is half of the width above L1. This deficiency at L5-S1 contributes to the inherent structural weakness at this level, where the greatest static stress and spinal movement produce the greatest kinetic strain (19).

Nucleus Pulposus

The nucleus pulposus is a semifluid gel that makes up 40% of the intervertebral disc. It is composed of stellate cells sparsely scattered throughout a matrix of fine, interlacing collagen fibers and mucopolysaccharides. The mucopolysaccharides (proteoglycans) are large, strongly hydrophilic molecules. This protein-polysaccharide gel exerts an imbibition pressure, which binds over eight times its volume of water and is responsible for the high water content of the nucleus, which decreases steadily with age. The hydrophilic properties of the nucleus pulposus depend on the proteoglycans' ion exchange capacity and its charge density, rather than its molecular weight.

Because the hydrophilic attraction of the proteoglycans is not a biochemical bonding, significant amounts of water can be expressed from the nucleus by continued mechanical pressure, which explains the diurnal variation in body height. Upright posture during the day creates mechanical pressure, with a decrease in the disc height. On recumbancy, the disc imbibes water through the endplates, resulting in an increase in disc height (20). The average person is 1% shorter at the end of the day than in the morning. When relieved of mechanical stresses in space, the astronauts' discs imbibed water to such an extent that they returned to earth two inches taller than when they left. Adams, Polan, and Hutton (21) have shown that diurnal variations in the stresses on the lumbar spine were greater in the morning, with a 5° increase in range of motion during the day. They concluded that lumbar discs and ligaments are at greater risk of injury in the early morning, due to the increased hydrostatic pressure in the nucleus pulposus. The turgor of the nucleus pulposus creates a dynamic hydraulic suspension system that adds to the mobility of the spine through an even distribution of compression forces, which are redistributed evenly in all directions (22).

Ligaments of the Lumbar Spine

For the most part, the spinal ligaments are stronger and denser in the lumbar region than in other regions of the spine, with the exception of the posterior longitudinal ligament (19). The ligamentum flavum is thickest in the lumbar region (7), contributing to the intrinsic stability of the spine and protecting the nerve root from mechanical impingement, while prestressing the disc. The elasticity of the disc is balanced by the elasticity of the medial anterior capsule of the posterior joints, formed by the lateral extension of the ligamentum flavum (10).

The supraspinous ligament is thicker and broader in the lumbar region, connecting the apices of the spinous processes. The interspinous ligaments are broad, thick, and quadralateral in the lumbar region. The posterior longitudinal ligament generally narrows between the first lumbar vertebra and the sacrum, where it is merely a narrow strip of fibrous tissue blending with the fibers of the posterior annulus. This inadequacy of the posterior longitudinal ligament in the lower lumbar segments decreases the protection against intervertebral disc herniation, increasing the risk of lateral disc bulge into the spinal canal (19).

The anterior longitudinal ligament extends down the anterior surface of the intervertebral bodies as far as the upper part of the anterior sacrum. It is firmly fixed to the margins of the vertebral bodies and anterior intervertebral discs. Traction at the attachment points may produce the "anterior lipping" of the vertebrae seen clinically (23).

The fifth lumbar vertebra (and occasionally the fourth) is also stabilized by the iliolumbar ligaments. These ligaments attach to the lower anterior borders and tips of the transverse processes, radiating in two main bands to the pelvis. The lower band attaches to the anterior part of the upper surface of the ipsilateral sacrum, blending with the ventral sacroiliac ligament. The upper part attaches to the crest of the ilium and gives partial origin to the quadratus lumborum. It is continuous above with the thoracolumbar fascia (7).

Inconstant transforaminal ligaments appear with relative frequency in the lumbar spine (24) (Fig. 8.5). Discussed by a number of authors (18, 24–27), these ligaments have been shown to traverse the intervertebral foramen, diminishing the space available for the emerging nerve root. Bachop and Stern (27) compare these ligament-like thickenings to "bars over a window or cage. Anything entering or leaving has to squeeze by them on one side or the other."

While the precise nature and origin of these ligaments has not been determined, they appear to be condensations in the fascia overlying the foraminal exit, which are distinct and discrete structures. It has been theorized that they are homologous with the radiate ligaments of the thoracic region. They insert anterior to the base of the transverse processes and expand in a fan-like manner by fine but very resistant fibers. Panzer and Peterson have demonstrated that a strong tug with a probe is not sufficient to tear these ligamentous fibers (personal communication).

Golub and Silverman (24) have shown that these tough fibrous bands are able to stretch, deform, or

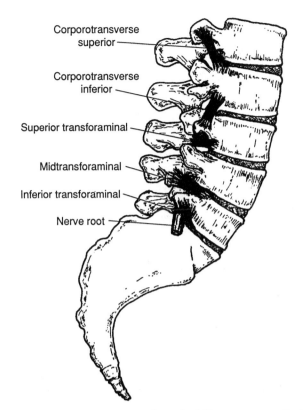

Corporotransverse superior

Corporotransverse inferior

Superior transforaminal

Midtransforaminal

Inferior transforaminal

Nerve root

Figure 8.5. Inconstant transforaminal ligaments can diminish the space available for emerging nerve roots. The *corporotransverse superior* ligament runs from the accessory process of the transverse process obliquely, anteriorly, and inferiorly to insert into the posterolateral aspect of the vertebral body or the adjacent annulus or both. The *corporotransverse inferior* ligament runs from the superior surface of the transverse process obliquely, superiorly, and anteriorly to insert into the vertebral body or adjacent annulus, or both. The *superior transforaminal* ligament extends from the posterior to the anterior aspect of the inferior vertebral notch. The *midtransforaminal* ligament extends from the articular capsule and ligamentum flavum across the midforamen to the annulus. The *inferior transforaminal* ligament extends from the superior facet across the superior vertebral notch to the junction of the annulus and vertebral body. (Modified from Golub BS, Silverman B: Transforaminal ligaments of the lumbar spine. *J Bone Joint Surg* 51A:947–956, 1969.)

abrade the spinal nerve during its back-and-forth excursions when straight-leg raising and lowering. The signs elicited can easily mislead the diagnostician into misdiagnosing a disc herniation. MacNab (25) refers to corporotransverse entrapment against the alae of the sacrum as a rare source of nerve root pressure. Bachop (27) contends that since the blood vessel is generally superior to the ligament and the nerve root inferior to it, a superiorly placed ligament would place the blood vessel at risk, while an inferiorly placed ligament would endanger the nerve. He concludes that a positive straight-leg raise can be the result of a "guillotine effect" on the nerve, as described by MacNab (25).

Five major types of transforaminal ligaments were noted by Golub and Silverman (24) (Fig. 8.5), who designated them (a) corporotransverse superior, (b) corporotransverse inferior, (c) superior transforaminal, (d) mid-transforaminal, and (e) inferior transforaminal. Because some transforaminal ligaments were hidden, Bachop and Stern (27) suggest that these be referred to as intraforaminal ligaments.

Muscles and Fascia of the Lumbar Spine

Lumbodorsal Fascia

The lumbodorsal fascia covers the deep muscles of the back (Fig 8.6). In the lumbar region it is in three layers. The superficial layer attaches to the spinous processes of the lumbar vertebrae, the sacrum, and the supraspinous ligaments. The middle layer attaches medially to the tips of the transverse processes of the lumbar vertebrae and the intertransverse ligaments, caudally to the iliac crest, and cephalad to the lower border of the twelfth rib and the lumbocostal ligament. The ventral layer covers the quadratus lumborum and is attached medially to the anterior surfaces of the transverse processes of the lumbar vertebrae, anterior to the lateral part of the psoas major. Caudally, it attaches to the iliolumbar ligaments and the adjacent iliac crests (7). Cephalad, it attaches to the front of the transverse processes of the first lumbar vertebra and to the lower margin of the twelfth rib (7).

Sacrospinalis (Erector Spinae)

The sacrospinalis are attached to the median sacral crest, the spinous processes and, the supraspinous ligaments of the lumbar vertebrae, the eleventh and twelfth thoracic vertebrae, and the medial dorsal aspect of the iliac crests by a broad thick tendon. Some of its fibers form a large fleshy mass that splits in the upper lumbar region into three columns. Laterally it becomes the iliocostalis, intermediately the longissimus, and medially the spinalis (Fig. 8.7).

The iliocostalis lumborum attaches by flattened tendons to the inferior borders of the angles of the lower ribs. The longissimus lumborum attaches to the posterior surfaces of the transverse processes and the accessory processes of the lumbar vertebrae. The spinalis lumborum attaches to the first and second lumbar vertebrae, uniting to form a small muscle that attaches to the spines of the upper thoracic vertebrae. The erector spinae are extensors of the spinal column. The iliocostalis and longissimus muscles, in addition to extending the spine, also assist in lateral flexion of the trunk.

Transversospinalis and Intrasegmental Muscles

The multifidus muscles attach in the lumbar region from all of the mamillary processes, passing upward and attaching to the vertebrae above. The more superficial fibers pass from one vertebra to the third or fourth vertebra above, while the intermediate fibers span from one vertebra to the second or

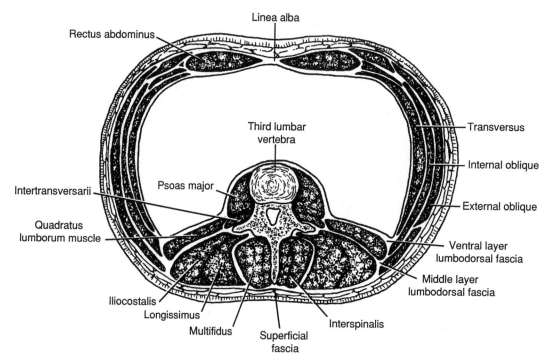

Figure 8.6. Transverse section through the abdominal wall showing the lumbodorsal fascia and muscles at the level of the *third lumbar vertebra*. This musculature and fascia acts as a girdle to support the abdominal viscera and add support to the lumbar spine. (Modified from Finneson BE: *Low Back Pain*, ed 2. Philadelphia, JB Lippincott, 1980, pp 6–7.)

third vertebra above, and the deepest fibers connect contiguous vertebrae. The rotatores muscles run deep to the multifidus and are not well developed in the lumbar region of the spine. They are represented by irregular and variable bundles that extend from the transverse processes of one vertebra to the lower border of the lamina of the next vertebra above.

The interspinalis muscles are short, paired muscles running between the spines of contiguous vertebrae, one on each side of the interspinous ligaments. The intertransversarii are small muscles spanning the transverse processes of the vertebrae. In the lumbar region they consist of two sets of muscles. The intertransversarii medius connects the accessory processes of one vertebra with the mamillary processes of the next vertebra. The intertransversarii lateralis run between the transverse processes and attach dorsally to the accessory processes, as well as ventrally to the transverse process. The transversospinalis and intrasegmental muscles are thought to act as postural stabilizers, steadying vertebral motion segments during motion of the vertebral column as a whole and insuring the efficient action of the long spinal muscles (7) (See Chapter 1).

Deep Lateral Muscles

The two pair of deep lateral muscles, the quadratus lumborum and psoas major muscles, attach to the transverse processes of the lumbar vertebrae. The quadratus lumborum attaches to the last rib, the transverse process of the lumbar vertebrae, and the iliac crest. It is irregularly quadrilateral and broader caudally. It assists in inspiration by fixing the last rib, and if the pelvis is fixed, it flexes the trunk to the same side. When both muscles act together, they assist in extension of the lumbar portion of the spinal column.

The psoas muscles arise from the bodies and transverse processes of the lumbar vertebrae and the interposed discs, attaching to the lesser trochanter of the femur. Acting conjointly with the iliacus, the psoas flexes the thigh upon the pelvis. During a full sit-up from the supine position, it increases the lumbar lordosis (see Chapter 13).

Diaphragm

In addition to the spinal attachment of the quadratus lumborum and the psoas muscles, the diaphragm attaches to the vertebral column by the crura. These tendinous attachments blend with the anterior longitudinal ligament (Fig. 8.7). The right crus is broader and longer than the left, arising from the anterolateral surface of the bodies and intervertebral discs of the upper three lumbar vertebrae. The left crus arises from the corresponding part of the upper two. These central tendons anchor the diaphragm as it contracts, pulling down the dome during inspiration. Chronic stress in the diaphragm can thus lead to low back pain through unreleased tension in the upper lumbar vertebrae.

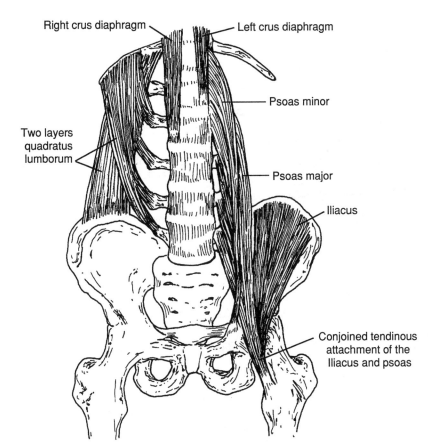

Right crus diaphragm

Left crus diaphragm

Psoas minor

Two layers
quadratus
lumborum

Psoas major

Iliacus

Conjoined tendinous
attachment of the
Iliacus and psoas

Figure 8.7. Deep muscles of the lumbar spine. Two pair of deep lateral muscles attach to the transverse processes of the lumbar spine. The diaphragm attaches to the anterior bodies of the lumbar region with the tendinous fibers blending into the anterior longitudinal ligament. Tension in any of these three muscles can produce low back pain. (Modified from Kirkaldy-Willis WH: *Managing Low Back Pain*, ed 2. New York, Churchill Livingstone, 1988, pp 117–131.)

Lumbar Innervation

The structures of the lumbar spine can be divided into ventral and dorsal compartments by a coronal plane passing through the intervertebral foramen, according to the innervation (28). The components of the ventral compartment are innervated by branches from the lumbar ventral rami and the lumbar plexus. These structures include the psoas, quadratus lumborum, and intertransversarii muscles, and the anterior longitudinal ligament, annulus fibrosus and dura. In addition, the sinuvertebral (recurrent meningeal) nerve supplies the skeletal elements of the ventral compartment (Fig. 8.8). Passing back into the intervertebral foramen, this nerve divides into transverse and descending branches and a major ascending branch. The transverse and descending branches supply the posterior longitudinal ligament and the intervertebral disc at the level of entry of the nerve, while the ascending branch passes to the next higher level, overlapping with the supradjacent nerve.

The posterior compartment is innervated by branches from the lumbar dorsal rami. The posterior primary rami pass back medially to the medial intertransverse muscle and divide into medial intermediate and lateral branches (28). The medial branch descends at the back of the transverse processes and superior articular processes, lying in a groove formed by these structures. It supplies the structures that lie medial to the line of the posterior vertebral joints. This strip increases from 2 cm at the first lumbar level to 3 cm on either side of the midline at the fifth lumbar level. The structures innervated by the medial branch include the multifidus and interspinalis muscles, the ligaments, articular capsules, ligamenta flava, and the interspinous and supraspinous ligaments. The posterior vertebral joint receives innervation from two segmental levels. At each level the ramus sends branches to that level and to the superior capsule of the joint at the level below. Free and complex, unencapsulated nerve endings are found in the capsule and are thought to mediate pain and proprioception (29). The intermediate branches of the lumbar dorsal rami supply the longissimus muscles, while the iliocostalis muscles are innervated by the lateral branches of the rami.

ANOMALIES OF THE LUMBAR SPINE

Variations of the lumbar spine, while common, are not always clinically significant (30). Tropism or asymmetry of the posterior lumbar joints occurs in approximately one-quarter of human spines (19) and predisposes the individual to facet-joint locking (3).

Transitional lumbosacral vertebrae are often symptomatic when accompanied by accessory joints, which are subject to degenerative change like any synovial joint. When this malformation is uni-

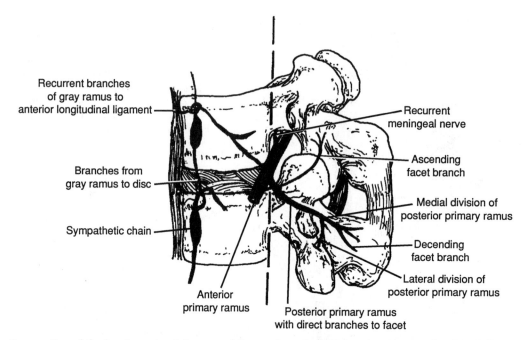

Figure 8.8. Innervation of the lumbar spine is by way of the lumbar spinal nerves that divide into the ventral and dorsal *primary rami.* (Modified from Kirkaldy-Willis WH: *Managing* *Low Back Pain*, ed 2. New York, Churchill Livingstone, 1988 pp 117–131.

lateral, it creates asymmetrical motion that can lead to biomechanical dysfunction. Congenital absence of pedicles, dysplasia, or absence of spinous processes and clefts in pedicles have all been reported (1). A greatly enlarged spinous process at L5 may accompany a spina bifida of S1. Since soft-tissue anomalies such as transforaminal ligaments (Fig. 8.4) escape radiological detection, the frequency of anomalous development in the lumbar spine may be higher than estimated.

MOVEMENT OF THE LUMBAR SPINE

Movement of the lumbar spine is dependent on the interaction of the three-joint complex composed of the intervertebral disc and two posterior facet joints. Lumbar motion is controlled by many combinations of articular curvature, ligamentous arrangement, and muscle forces. Motion is restricted by the discs, articular facets, and numerous ligaments. Muscle force facilitates and resists active motion.

Mechanics of the Intervertebral Disc

Normal vertebral-motion-segment movement is contingent upon a healthy intervertebral disc. The disc height controls spinal movement (18), with the amount of motion dependent upon the ratio of disc height to vertebral body height. In the lumbar spine this 1:3 ratio is made possible by the approximately 9 mm of average disc thickness (31). The healthy intervertebral disc is noncompressible, due to the turgor of the nucleus, which stiffens the annulus and thus supports shear and compression loads. This ac-

tion is similar to a ball-bearing mechanism (31) with the spherical nucleus placed between adjacent vertebral bodies.

The hydrophilic properties of the nucleus pulposus creates a preloaded state in which the pressure in the center is never zero, even when the disc is unloaded. The pressure in the center of the nucleus is confined within the relatively inextensible casing formed by the annular fibers, which separate adjacent vertebral bodies and give the disc a greater resistance to compressive forces (31). The nucleus pulposus distributes stresses uniformly to the annulus fibrosus and cartilaginous endplates.

When an asymmetrical load is applied axially to a disc, the upper vertebra tilts toward the overloaded side. The displaced disc material produces a bulge of the "criss-crossed" annular fibers. Contrary to Cailliet (19) and Kapandji (31), who have theorized that the disc is displaced toward the side of convexity, Farfan (18), White and Panjabi (23), and Brown, Hansen, and Yorra (32) have demonstrated that the disc is displaced toward the side of concavity. Mechanical tests performed on fresh autopsy specimens of the lumbar spine showed that the disc expanded on the concave side and contracted on the convex side of the curve, while at points 90° to the plane of motion, little or no expansion or contraction occurred (32). Krag et al. (33), using metal markers in vitro, demonstrated that during flexion the annulus expanded anteriorly and retracted posteriorly, and the nucleus shifted posteriorly.

Disc Loads

Nachemson (34), utilizing a pressure transducer attached to the tip of a needle inserted into the disc, has demonstrated in vivo that the disc nucleus behaves hydrostatically. This method of evaluation demonstrated that disc loads vary with posture. For example, the pressure in the L3 disc is about 40% higher when sitting unsupported than when standing. Disc pressure at this level has also been found to increase more than 100% during bending forward or carrying loads. The greatest increase in disc pressure appears to be during forward flexion and rotation, which increases the load by 400%. Reclining reduces the pressure on the disc by 50 to 80% (34).

Planes of Movement in the Lumbar Spine

The shape and orientation of the articular facets and the ligaments and muscles guide movement to provide restraint against excessive motion. In the lumbar spine, the large range of motion is proportionate to the thickness of the intervertebral discs, so that with disc degeneration a significant amount of lumbar motion may be lost.

Flexion - Extension

Flexion and extension in the sagittal plane in the lumbar spine occurs concurrently with anterior and posterior pelvic tilt (see Chapter 11). There is a gradual decrease in flexion and extension ranges from the lower to the upper segments (35). Sagittal-plane movement involves both rotation and translation, with the superior vertebra sliding forward as well as rotating around the X (coronal) axis, which is located in the posterior annulus of the intervening disc.

Flexion and extension are restricted more by the apposition of the facet-joint surfaces than by tension in the posterior ligaments (36). The facet joints guide the rotation of both flexion and extension and resist translation (Fig. 8.2).

The capsular ligaments and the intervertebral disc play the next most important role in resisting flexion, with the supraspinous and interspinous ligaments making a lesser contribution. The ligamentum flava also offer some restraint (35). They offer elastic resistance to flexion because they are placed behind the axis of sagittal movement of the vertebral segments.

Lateral Bending and Rotation

Lateral bending and rotation were identified as coupled movements as early as 1905 by Lovett (37). While Tanz (38) reported in 1953 that lateral bending was frequently not associated with rotation, subsequent studies support the early work of Lovett (23, 34, 37, 39). This coupled motion results in a shift in the axis of rotation (see "Instantaneous Axis of Rotation" in Chapter 2), which is generally located in the posterior part of the disc. Farfan (18) reported a relationship between the location of the center of rotation and the direction of rotation. He found that the center of rotation appeared to move toward the side to which rotation was found.

This coupled motion in the lumbar spine results in the spinous processes moving toward the concavity of the curve during lateral bending. Pearcy and Tibrewal (39) demonstrated that there was no simple mechanical coupling of rotation in the lumbar spine. They found approximately 2° of axial rotation at each intervertebral joint, with L3–4 and L4–5 being slightly more mobile. Ten degrees of lateral bending was reported in the upper three levels, with 6° at L4–5 and 3° at L5-S1. Lateral bending and rotation are restricted by the antagonistic muscles and surrounding ligaments.

BIOMECHANICAL DISORDERS OF THE LUMBAR SPINE

Nachemson (34) has stated that "mechanical factors are the greatest importance in the development of low back pain." Farfan (40) agrees that the etiological factor in backache is mechanical, stating that when the mechanical problem is neutralized or removed, the patient is cured. While many of the doctors treating low back pain hold this view, the differentiation of biomechanical disorders of the spine is complex.

An accurate and complete diagnosis depends on an understanding of the pathology and pathogenesis of low back pain as well as the biomechanical factors involved. Central to this understanding is the concept of the three-joint complex formed by the intervertebral disc and two posterior facet joints (Chapters 1 and 2). Changes affecting the posterior joints also affect the disc, and vice versa.

Compressive forces and rotational strains have been identified as the two major factors involved in the mechanism of injury (41). Compressive forces commonly result from falls onto the buttocks, and while they tend to cause pathological changes in the disc, they may first result in facet-joint locking at the time of injury. Degeneration of the posterior joints follows at a later stage.

Rotational stresses lead to pathological changes in both the disc and posterior joints (41) (Fig. 8.9). Rotational forces may also cause facet-joint locking when unguarded movement forces the posterior joints to the extreme range of normal motion (Fig. 8.10). This is especially common where facet tropism is present (18). Three phases have been identified in the degenerative process: dysfunction, instability, and stabilization (42).

A definitive diagnosis by the chiropractor involves two parts, (a) the pathological diagnosis, which reflects the tissue damage incurred and allows an accurate prognosis, and (b) the biomechanical diagnosis, which allows formulation of the type of manipulation to be employed. An appropriate treatment plan requires both.

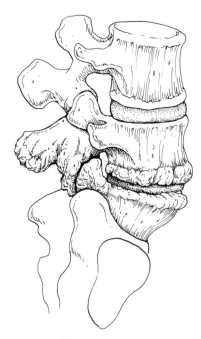

Figure 8.9. Rotational stresses lead to pathological changes in both the disc and posterior joints. (Modified from Cox JM: *Low Back Pain: Mechanism, Diagnosis and Treatment*, ed 4. Baltimore, Williams & Wilkins, 1985, pp 18, 36.)

Clinical Considerations

A carefully elicited history of the onset of low back pain not only determines the etiology of biomechanical disorders of the lumbar spine, but also gives the chiropractor an understanding of the location of the problem as well as the structures damaged by the injury. Disorders of the pelvic ring (see Chapter 7) must also be considered, because many of the conditions that affect the lumbar spine produce findings similar to those affecting the pelvis.

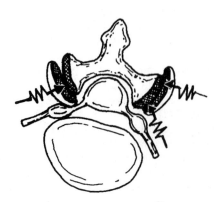

Figure 8.10. Rotational forces may cause facet-joint locking when unguarded movement forces the posterior joints to the extreme range of normal joint motion where they become jammed.

History and Etiology

Patients with an acute locked low back frequently complain of a sudden sharp pain following which they are unable to straighten up (42). Facet-joint locking in the lumbar spine occurs with a sudden, unguarded movement, frequently in a position of flexion and rotation. Patients complain of a "catch in the back" or say that "something slipped out of place." They may have heard a "pop" or a "snap" at the time of joint locking.

In the absence of any direct trauma (such as incurred by a blow, or lifting or lowering a heavy weight), simple joint locking is not likely to cause major soft-tissue damage. Leading questions about discomfort following long automobile trips, heavy lifting, or extended periods of stooping may elicit a history of previous low-back dysfunction (6). Although the onset of pain may be attributable to trauma, the symptoms may be caused by unsuspected underlying pathology, such as metastatic neoplasm (6).

It is important to determine which mechanical factors make the pain worse and what relieves the pain. Pain that is worse on sitting is commonly due to sacroiliac dysfunction, while increased pain with prolonged standing, especially with the arms outstretched in front, is more apt to originate in the lower lumbar facet joints. Back pain or sciatic pain increased by forward bending may be indicative of a herniated disc however less than 10% of low back pain is due to herniation of the intervertebral disc (43). Pain that is eased by bed rest is generally mechanical, while pain that is worse at night while lying in bed is characteristic of many tumors. Perianal or genital pain with numbness and/or paresthesia, disturbances of sphincter function, or impotency, require immediate referral for neurological evaluation (Chapter 4). Disorders of the pelvic ring (Chapter 7) must not be overlooked, because sacroiliac syndromes produce findings similar to those in conditions involving acute locking of the lumbar spine.

Signs and Symptoms

The patient with an acute locked low back complains of pain in the lumbar region (11), restricted motion (42), and an inability to straighten. Observation reveals antalgia (11) with slow, guarded movements. The pain is generally unilateral and paravertebral (19). Extension and lateral bending, away from the side of the pain, frequently hurt the patient most. Flexion is cautious and limited (19) but can be achieved, producing the inability to straighten and a typical grabbing of the back followed by walking the hands up the thighs in slow increments to prevent further spasm in the paraspinal muscles. Similarly, on rising from the sitting position, the patient may place one hand on the back while the other presses on the thigh (Minor's sign, Fig. 8.11). This sign is often seen with

Orthopaedic Tests of Lumbar Spine Dysfunction

Straight-Leg Raising

Passive straight-leg raising affects numerous tissues and should be conducted following a standard protocol (Chapter 5). Recording the results of a straight-leg raising test as either positive or negative (19) gives little guidance to the clinician. In addition to neuromeningeal tension, passive straight-leg raising stretches the hamstring muscles, the tissues of the buttock, and the posterior facet joints as well as stressing the sacroiliac joints (19).

Pain arising from the nerve root can be confirmed by qualifying or adjunctive tests. When pain is felt, the range of motion (in degrees) and the site of pain should be recorded. Straight-leg raising in the presence of sciatica caused by nerve-root pressure produces severe pain in the back, in the sciatic distribution of the affected leg, or in both (Fig. 8.12A). To confirm that the nerve root is the source of the pain, the involved leg is raised to the point of pain and then lowered a few degrees. Nerve-root stretch is then produced by forced dorsiflexion of the ankle (25, 44) (Braggard's test, Fig. 8.12B) or by firm pressure applied to the popliteal fossa over the posterior tibial nerve. If the pain is reproduced by either of these tests, altered root tension is indicated.

If the sciatic pain is reproduced on internal rotation of the femur after the straight leg is lowered a few degrees, it is indicative of irritation of the sciatic nerve by the piriformis muscle, not a sign of nerve-root tension, and is known as a positive piriformis sign (see Piriformis Syndrome, Chapter 12).

Non-neurogenic pain may be elicited in patients with tight hamstrings and is felt as tightness or a muscle pull behind the knee (6). Pain in the sacroiliac joints is usually elicited on straight-leg raising past 70° in patients with a sacroiliac syndrome (Chapter 7). When pain is elicited in the affected extremity by straight-leg raising of the opposite leg (Fajersztajns sign or the well-leg-raising test, Fig. 8.12C), it is strongly suggestive of a disc herniation, usually lying medial to the root within the "axilla" between the dura and the exiting root sleeve (6). Pain that occurs with less than 30° of straight-leg raising is strongly indicative of disc herniation.

Sitting Straight-Leg Raising (Bechterew's Test, Sitting Root Test)

In a sitting position, the patient extends each leg, then both legs together. The results should be consistent with straight-leg raising in the supine position. The patient may lean backward in order to avoid radiating pain from disc lesions. Extending both legs will usually increase the back and sciatic discomfort (45) (see Chapter 5). To obviate malingering, the doctor may elevate each lower extremity individually while feigning the purpose of checking the dorsalis pedis pulse, thus putting the potential

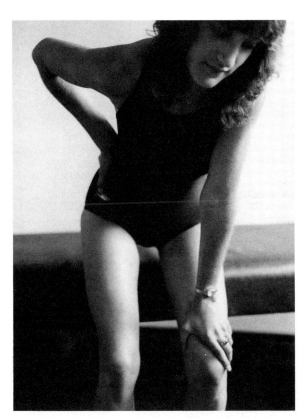

Figure 8.11. Minor's sign. The patient with acute low back pain straightens from the seated or flexed position by grabbing the back, followed by walking the hands up the thighs in slow increments, to prevent further spasm of the paraspinal muscle.

sacroiliac lesion; lumbosacral strains, sprains, and fractures; and radiculitis due to intervertebral disc syndrome.

Lumbar Spine Examination

Motion palpation to determine posterior joint locking is the most definitive indicator of lumbar facet-joint fixation. AP radiographs of lateral bending (see Chapter 6) are useful in the determination of the level of blocked movement, but give no indication as to whether the blockage is due to posterior joint dysfunction or an intervertebral disc lesion.

Orthopaedic tests are useful in making a differential diagnosis, but subjective response to treatment is often the most definitive indication of appropriate treatment. Manipulation of an acute locked low back brings prompt relief of symptoms, and most residual pain subsides in two to three days. Symptomatology that lasts longer indicates more substantial soft-tissue damage and should be evaluated accordingly to rule out complicating factors. The muscle spasm that accompanies simple articular blockage is commonly due to protective muscle splinting, which reflexly protects joints adjacent to the locked joints when they are required to provide compensatory mobility for the blocked articulation.

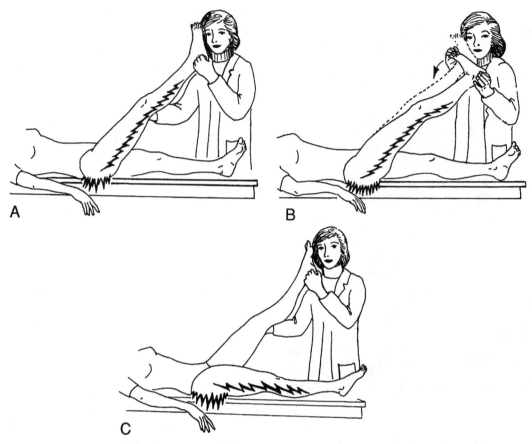

Figure 8.12. **A,** A severe pain in the back and in the sciatic distribution is described as a positive straight-leg-raising test (SLR). **B,** To confirm that the nerve root is the source of pain, the involved leg is raised to the point of pain, then lowered a few degrees. In this position, dorsiflexion of the foot repro-duces sciatic pain (dorsiflexion reinforcement). **C,** Pain elic-ited in the affected extremity by straight-leg raising of the op-posite leg is strongly suggestive of a disc herniation medial to the nerve root (Well leg raising).

malingerer off guard. No backward leaning and no radiation on elevating the leg suggests no pathology.

Femoral Nerve Traction Tests

To traction the femoral nerve, the patient lies on the unaffected side with the unaffected limb flexed slightly at the hip and the knee (Fig. 8.13). The patient's back is kept straight (not hyperextended), and the neck is slightly flexed. The doctor grasps the patient's affected (painful) limb and extends the knee while gently extending the hip to approximately 15°. The knee is then flexed, which further stretches the femoral nerve.

Pain radiating to the anterior thigh is a positive result. Pain in the groin and hip, radiating along the anterior medial thigh, is indicative of an L3 nerve root lesion, while pain extending to the midtibia indicates an L4 nerve root problem (46).

Heel Walk

The patient is asked to heel walk toward the examiner to determine foot extensor weakness (46). Walking on the heels tests the strength of the tibialis anterior, extensor digitorum longus, and the hallucis longus muscles. Weakness of this muscle group is consistent with L5 nerve-root compression (Fig 8.14).

Toe Walk

The patient is asked to toe walk away from the examiner to determine plantar flexor weakness. If one heel drops closer to the floor, weakness of the gastrocnemius, soleus, and plantaris muscles is indicated. Weakness of this muscle group is consistent with S1 nerve root compression (Fig 8.15).

Squatting

Full squatting evaluates muscular strength and hip and knee function. If dysfunction is present, this movement usually produces pain at the site of pathology (6).

Hip Flexion (Thomas Test)

With the patient supine, one knee is flexed to the chest, while the other leg remains extended. Initially as the hip flexes, the lumbar spine is flattened and the pelvis is stabilized. Further flexion can then originate only in the hip joint. With a fixed flexion

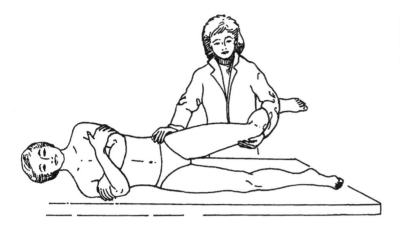

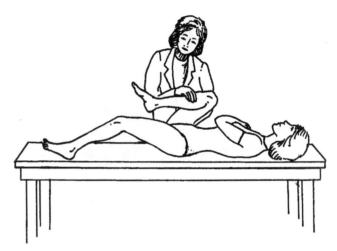

Figure 8.13. Femoral nerve traction test. The femoral nerve can be tractioned by first extending the hip and knee, followed by knee flexion while maintaining hip extension at approximately 15°.

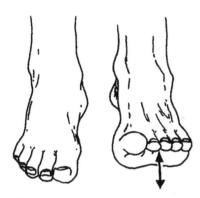

Figure 8.14. Heel walk. Weakness of the tibialis anterior, extensor digitorum longus, and extensor hallucis longus muscles can be observed as the patient walks on the heels toward the examiner.

Figure 8.16. Hip flexion (Thomas test). A spasm of the psoas muscle will cause the extended (neutral) leg on the affected side to rise off the table when the contralateral leg is maximally flexed.

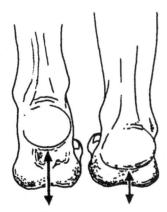

Figure 8.15. Toe walk. Plantar flexion weakness can be observed as the patient walks on the toes away from the examiner. If one heel drops closer to the floor, weakness of the gastrocnemius, soleus, and plantaris muscles is indicated.

Axial Compression (Kemp's Test)

Axial compression of the trunk is performed with the patient sitting. The examiner reaches around the patient's shoulders from behind and rotates and extends the patient. Axial compression is then applied with the patient maximally extended and rotated right and then left. This procedure stresses both the ipsilateral sacroiliac and the lumbar facet joints. Pain in either region differentiates lumbar from sacroiliac dysfunction.

The patient is then rotated and flexed, with axial compression of the trunk applied at the end point of motion on both sides. This produces a stress on the contralateral paravertebral musculature and suggests a muscle strain if pain is produced in the stretched muscle. Radicular pain should be noted and suggests nerve-root compression from a herniated disc. This must be differentiated from referred pain, which is common in lumbar facet and sacroiliac lesions (44) (see Chapter 7).

contracture or tight psoas muscle, the thigh of the extended leg will raise off the table. The extent of a flexion contracture can be determined by estimating the angle between the table and the patient's leg (Fig. 8.16) (48).

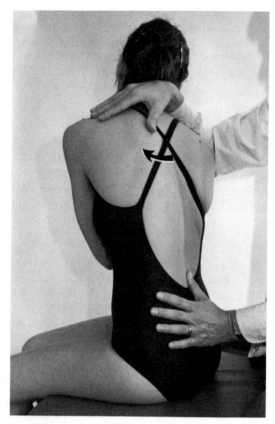

Figure 8.17. Palpation of lumbar vertebrae fixed in rotation. The doctor's stabilizing arm is positioned as for lateral bending for efficiency of examination (see Fig. 8.18).

MANIPULATION OF THE LUMBAR SPINE

Manipulation of the lumbar spine can be successfully performed with the patient in a prone, side-lying, sitting, or sometimes supine position. When motion palpation reveals restricted movement, a specific manipulation is chosen to restore motion. A key goal in lumbar manipulation, as in manipulation of other areas, is to restore specific desired movement at a chosen motion segment, with minimal force and minimal involvement of adjacent segments. This goal is aided by proper patient positioning, doctor positioning, generation of joint tension, a proper vector of manipulative thrust, and application of a controlled high-velocity thrust. This specific approach is distinct from more general mobilization techniques with the goal of mobilizing many joints.

Contraindications to Lumbar Manipulation

General contraindications to manipulation have been discussed elsewhere (Chapter 4). The major contraindication in the lumbar spine is disc herniation with increasing neurological deficit (43), which is generally considered a contraindication to rotational manipulation, especially with the patient in the side-lying position. Some investigators have re-

ported positive results, which are apparently due to more favorable positioning of the nuclear fragment and/or nerve root rather than an actual reduction of the herniation (11, 48–50). This must be considered a very risky endeavor at best. Since long-lever rotational manipulation may increase already existing torsional damage to posterior annular fibers (51–54), worsening of a disc herniation is a potential outcome, and such cases have indeed been reported (53–57).

Palpation of Lumbar Vertebrae Fixed in Rotation and Lateral Flexion

As in the thoracic spine, lumbar rotation and lateral flexion are coupled movements (Chapter 2), and manipulation of the lumbar spine is generally designed to release movement restriction in both the coronal and horizontal planes around the Z and Y axes. Either of these motions can be emphasized in the manipulative vector, depending upon the relative predominance of fixation noted in motion palpation.

The procedure for palpating lumbar rotation is essentially the same as that for the lower thoracic spine. With the patient seated and facing away from the doctor, the palpating thumb is placed against the side of the spinous process, and the patient is rotated to the extreme range-of-motion toward the ipsilateral side (Fig. 8.17). Segmental motion should be felt as well as a springy joint play while springing the spinous process further into rotation. Loss of either of these indicates restricted motion in the horizontal plane around the Y axis (i.e., rotation). This palpation is often facilitated by spanning two spinous processes with thumb contact to give a reference point immediately below the segment being tested.

Palpation of lumbar lateral flexion is also the same as that for the lower thoracic spine. With the patient seated facing away from the doctor, the palpating thumb is placed against the side of the spinous process, and the patient is laterally flexed ipsilaterally (Fig. 8.18). The spinous process should move slightly toward the thumb, and as the contralateral facets separate, the normal articulation exhibits the springiness of joint play. When the vertebra is fixed in lateral flexion, the springiness of joint play is absent. If the lumbar spine is positioned in flexion as this test is performed, the physiological coupling of movement changes, and the spinous process will fall away from the thumb (i.e., toward the convex side of the curve). A distinctly springy joint play should still occur (58–60).

Manipulation of Lumbar Vertebrae Fixed in Lateral Flexion and Rotation

Patient Prone (61–63)

With the patient in a prone position, the doctor faces the patient, using a broad stance on the side of spinous process rotation. The doctor takes a rein-

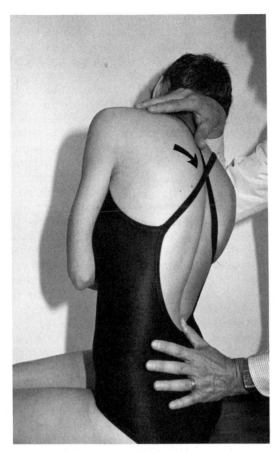

Figure 8.18. Palpation of lumbar vertebrae fixed in lateral flexion.

forced pisiform contact on the spinous process and uses a lateral-to-medial and slightly caudad tissue pull to take out slack (Fig. 8.19). The fingers should point approximately 45° to the spine and, after tension is produced in the joint by taking out tissue slack, a short-amplitude, high-velocity thrust is de-

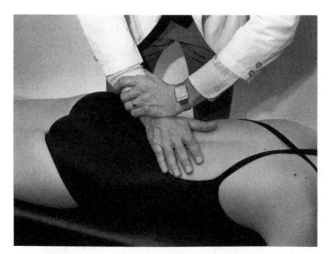

Figure 8.19. Prone pisiform-spinous manipulation for lumbar vertebrae fixed in rotation and/or lateral bending.

livered at the end of exhalation. The vector is lateral-to-medial, posterior-to-anterior, with a slight caudad torque to help facilitate ipsilateral lateral flexion.

An alternative vertebral contact point is the lumbar mamillary process (61, 63–65). The doctor stands on the side of the more posteriorly rotated mamillary process and takes a pisiform contact with a medial-to-lateral tissue pull, while reinforcing the contact hand with the other hand (Fig. 8.20). A high-velocity, short-amplitude thrust is delivered in a posterior-to-anterior direction toward the end of exhalation. A cephalad, caudad, or torquing vector may be added to increase lateral flexion as needed.

Patient Sitting (49, 50, 61, 65)

Manipulation to restore lateral flexion and/or rotation can be performed with the doctor sitting behind the seated patient. A pisiform contact is taken over the mamillary process, while the doctor's other hand grasps the crossed arms of the patient. This arm contact allows the doctor to control rotational movement of the torso, as the mamillary contact isolates this gross movement at a particular vertebral level, producing rotation away from the side of contact. A short-amplitude dynamic thrust is usually necessary to complete this procedure. Lateral flexion may be added by bending the patient's torso.

An alternate vertebral contact point is the spinous process, which can be used instead of the mamillary process in the above maneuver, allowing the introduction of more lateral flexion. The doctor uses pisiform, thenar, or thumb contact on the side of the spinous process and grasps the patient's arms as above, or drapes the forearm across the patient's shoulders, grasping one shoulder with the hand and the other with the bend of the elbow. This position allows more control over lateral flexion, and the patient's torso can be positioned to control the degree of rotation, lateral flexion, and even flexion or extension to be introduced by the manipulation. A virtually pure lateral flexion movement can be induced by bending the patient to one side and thrusting laterally to medially against the spinous process in the opposite direction.

Patient Side-lying

Mamillary Push (61, 62, 64, 66). A variety of side-lying manipulations are possible to restore lateral flexion and/or rotation. A few examples are given below.

With the patient lying on one side, the doctor positions the patient's spine slightly into flexion, lateral flexion, and rotation by pulling on the arm nearest the table. The patient's superior leg is flexed at the knee and hip and rests on the straightened inferior leg, with the foot in the popliteal space. The doctor faces the patient. Either the patient's knee is between the doctor's or the doctor's more caudad thigh contacts the patient's thigh. The patient's arms are

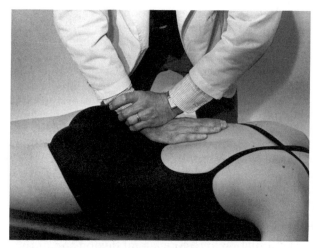

Figure 8.20. Prone pisiform-mamillary manipulation for lumbar vertebrae fixed in rotation and/or lateral bending.

folded, and care is taken not to introduce excess thoracolumbar torsion by allowing the superior shoulder to fall posteriorly. The doctor's cephalad hand contacts this shoulder, and the other hand takes a pisiform contact on the mamillary process further from the table (Fig. 8.21). Tension is created at the joint by pushing anteriorly with the contact hand, tractioning the patient's shoulder cephalad, and rolling the patient's pelvis anteriorly as the doctor holds it against the table. When tension is achieved, a sudden body drop occurs by the doctor, and a high-velocity impulse is made in a posterior-to-anterior direction, causing rotation and a small amount of lateral flexion of the segment contacted.

Spinous Push (50, 59, 62–63). An alternative vertebral contact point is the spinous process. With the patient and doctor positioned as above, the doctor takes a pisiform contact on the spinous process of the vertebra to be adjusted. As the doctor performs a body drop and high-velocity impulse with

the contact hand, the vector of thrust is lateral to medial (i.e., toward the table) and posterior to anterior. Thus, if the patient is lying on the right side, left rotation and left lateral flexion are produced at the segment being contacted.

Spinous Pull (61, 63–65). The spinous process can also be utilized by grasping it with the second and third fingers and pulling upward (i.e., away from the table) (Fig. 8.22). The patient is positioned as in the previous two adjustments, and the superior hip and knee are flexed and rotated until tension is developed between the leg and contact point. The doctor, standing on the superior leg, which rests against the table, controls the patient's bent leg by grasping it at the knee, using the instep of the doctor's inferior foot. At tension, a quick, short, pulling impulse is delivered by the contact hand simultaneous with a short thrust of the foot. The vector is lateral to medial and slightly posterior to anterior, which would cause right rotation and slight right lateral flexion at the motion segment being adjusted if the patient were placed on the right side.

Increased counterrotation of the patient's shoulders can be utilized to manipulate the joints immediately above the doctor's contact. (59).

Patient Supine

The upper lumbar segments can also be manipulated with the patient in the supine position.

Palpation of Lumbar Vertebrae Fixed in Flexion (58–59)

When a lumbar vertebra is fixed in flexion, motion is restricted in a sagittal plane around the X-axis. With the patient seated in front of and facing away from the doctor, the palpating thumb or finger is placed between the spinous processes. When the patient is passively extended, the spinous processes should approximate (Fig. 8.23). At the extreme of extension, a posterior-to-anterior push with the fin-

Figure 8.21. Pisiform-mamillary push manipulation for lumbar vertebrae fixed in rotation and/or lateral bending.

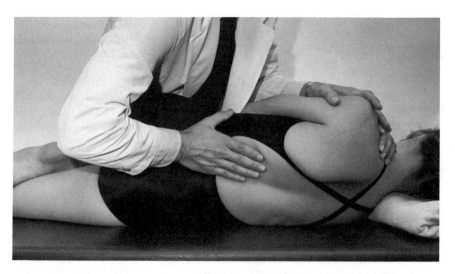

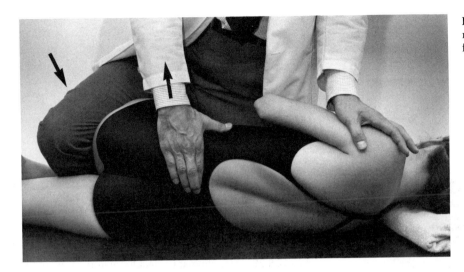

Figure 8.22. Spinous pull maniplation for lumbar vertebrae fixed in rotation.

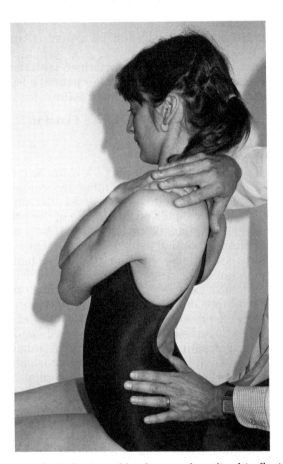

Figure 8.23. Palpation of lumbar vertebrae fixed in flexion.

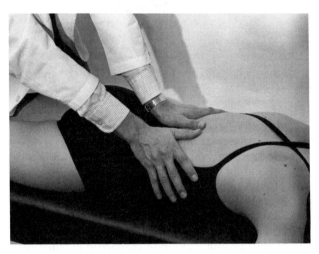

Figure 8.24. Bilateral thenar contact for manipulation of lumbar vertebrae fixed in flexion, with patient prone.

Manipulation of Lumbar Vertebrae Fixed in Flexion

Patient Prone

With the patient prone, a bilateral thenar contact may be taken over the mamillary processes of the fixed segment. The doctor stands alongside the table in a low fencer stance, facing the patient's head (Fig. 8.24). Joint tension is produced by pressing posterior to anterior and cephalad, producing extension and slight axial distracton of the joint (61).

This same procedure can be done with the patient kneeling on a knee-chest table. Rotational movement can be added by altering the contact and vector appropriately. Extension is facilitated in this position because the abdomen hangs freely (63–64).

Patient Side-Lying (63–65)

With the patient in a side-lying position, the superior knee and hip are flexed, and the superior foot

gers or back of the hand should produce a distinct springy joint play. When a vertebra is fixed in flexion, the spinous processes do not approximate and joint play is diminished. An alternative contact can be made with the thumbs over the facet joints. This may show greater fixation of the left or right posterior joint of a given motion segment.

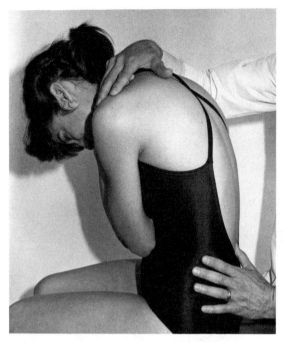

Figure 8.25. Palpation of lumbar vertebrae fixed in extension.

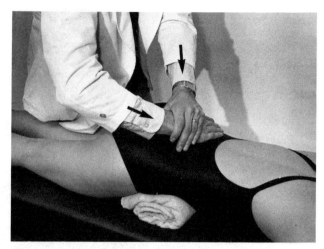

Figure 8.26. Hypothenar contact for manipulation of lumbar vertebrae fixed in extension, with patient prone.

placed in the popliteal fossa of the inferior leg. The hip is not flexed far enough to flex the vertebra to be contacted, since the purpose of this adjustment is to produce extension. Contact is taken with the pisiform over the up-side facet joint, which is restricted, and a thrust is delivered in a posterior-to-anterior direction, with a body drop as needed.

Alternatively, the spinous process may be used as a contact to produce bilateral extension of the joints. Again the vector is posterior to anterior to produce extension, but either of these techniques lend themselves to the introduction of rotation and/or lateral flexion along with extension by simply altering the corrective vector.

Patient Supine

The upper lumbar segments can be manipulated with the patient in the supine position to produce extension. The procedure is essentially the same as that for the thoracic spine (Chapter 9).

Palpation of Lumbar Vertebrae Fixed in Extension (59)

When a lumbar vertebra is fixed in extension, motion is restricted in a sagittal plane around the X-axis. With the patient seated in front of and facing away from the doctor, the palpating thumb or finger is placed between the spinous processes (Fig. 8.25). When the patient is passively flexed, the spinous processes should separate, and if lifted superiorly they should exhibit the springiness of normal joint play. When a vertebra is fixed in extension, the spinous

processes do not separate and joint play is diminished.

This palpation can also be performed with the patient lying on the side, utilizing the patient's legs as levers to assist in the flexion motion (59).

Manipulation of Lumbar Vertebrae Fixed in Extension

Patient Prone

With the patient prone and a pillow under the abdomen to induce flexion, a knife-edge contact is taken between the spinous processes that do not open. The doctor stands on either side of the patient in a low fencing stance facing the patient's head. Skin traction is applied cephalad prior to contact to take out tissue slack, and the stabilizing hand is placed on top of the contact hand, with the pisiform of the stabilizing hand placed in the anatomical snuffbox of the contact hand for reinforcement. The contact hand presses cephalad to the point of tension as the doctor's body weight is shifted cephalad (Fig 8.26). The patient is then instructed to inhale, at the end of which the manipulative thrust is applied in a posterior-to-anterior and strongly cephalad direction, to release the fixation and allow the spinous processes to open. A body drop is used to provide additional force as needed to release the fixation.

An alternative method with the patient prone involves a hinged table and slow flexion-distraction rather than a high-velocity manipulative thrust. This technique has been described by Cox (67–69) and is described more completely later in this chapter, as a procedure for lumbar disc protrusion.

Patient Side-Lying

With the patient lying on the side and the lumbar spine in a flexed position, the hip and knee of the patient's superior leg are flexed until the segment to be adjusted receives maximum tension. At the same time, the heel of the doctor's hand is softly cupped

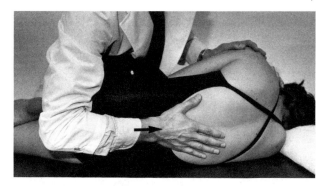

Figure 8.27. Pisiform-spinous push manipulation for lumbar vertebrae fixed in extension.

around the inferior portion of the spinous process that exhibits lack of flexion (Fig 8.27). With the patient's hip held in flexion by the doctor's leg and a cephalad tissue pull applied, a quick manipulative thrust and body drop are delivered, with a cephalad and posterior-to-anterior vector to restore flexion.

Patient Supine (61)

A supine manipulation can be achieved in the upper lumbar segments with the patient's arms crossed or the patient grasping the back of the neck with interlaced fingers and elbows together. The patient is held by the doctor in a flexed position, with the apex of flexion at the involved segment. The palmar contact hand is placed over the segment just inferior to the one to be flexed, with the fingers curled to form a flat fist. With the patient in adequate flexion, the doctor utilizes a body drop through the patient's arms and chest in an anterior-to-posterior direction with a cephalad vector, to isolate flexion at the segment desired. The approximated spinous processes will fall between the curled fingers and thenar pad, while the hand serves as a fulcrum on which flexion will occur.

Manipulation of the Lumbar Disc Lesion

Special considerations are necessary when applying manipulative therapy to a prolapsed or herniated disc. Once this diagnosis has been reached through clinical and/or radiographic examination (Chapters 5 and 6) care must be taken not to further injure already damaged annular fibers. Farfan and coworkers (51–53) have described the role of rotational forces in the injury of annular fibers and, in general, rotational manipulation is considered to be contraindicated in cases of lumbar disc herniation. However, many authors have described success with rotational manipulation, particularly in cases of relatively minor herniation. Even when successful, this technique does not seem to actually replace a displaced nucleus to its normal position but apparently moves it away from the neighboring nerve root, and hence relieves radicular symptoms. This procedure carries a definite risk of worsening a disc herniation, which has also been reported (54–56) (Chapter 4).

A safer approach to manipulative management of the disc lesion involves movements other than rotation. This approach emphasizes the movements of flexion, extension, or lateral bending depending on the tolerance of the patient.

Flexion Technique

Passive intersegmental flexion-distraction has been described in the osteopathic literature (50) and more recently by Cox (67–69), who believes it provides the following:

1. Decompression of the neural structures and enlargement of the IVF;
2. Centripetal force from posterior annular fibers and the posterior longitudinal ligament to push the nucleus anteriorly;
3. Enhancement of disc nutrition through imbibition;
4. Suction and traction.

Finneson (6) has also compared the effects of flexion and extension of the lumbar spine, emphasizing that flexion increases the size of the spinal canal. Studies using CT scanning and myelography have demonstrated greater nerve root and dural sac pressure in extension than in flexion in cases with facet hypertrophy (70).

Clearly, benefits from flexion will be more likely in less severe herniations, where the integrity of the posterior annular fibers and posterior longitudinal ligament have been preserved. In more severe cases, flexion may allow further posterior migration of nuclear material, with worsening of symptoms. Patient response must be carefully monitored to establish whether this form of therapy is appropriate. Long-term management emphasizing flexion techniques will often include pelvic tilt (Chapter 11) and William's flexion exercises.

Treatment consists of strapping the ankles of the prone patient to the caudad end of a table that is hinged to flex in the middle. Axial traction of the caudad half of the table is also utilized. With the patient positioned so that maximum flexion occurs at the involved segment, the doctor uses a thenar contact on the spinous process, pushing cephalad in a pumping motion while the other hand flexes and pumps the caudad end of the table. Motorized tables may also be utilized. Care must be taken to monitor patient tolerance and to avoid excessive flexion, which may cause injury. Two inches of movement is commonly recommended (67). The distal half of the table is also hinged to allow lateral flexion and/or rotational movements if necessary. Ancillary physiotherapy may be added as needed (Chapter 13). This type of flexion manipulation also has value in such non-disc conditions as facet syndromes, tropism, spinal stenosis, and spondylolisthesis (68, 69, 71, 72), which have been implicated as factors causing sciatica and back pain (73–75).

In apparent contrast to the preceding technique is treatment emphasizing extension. The rationale of this approach is that a disc injury almost invariably occurs during a flexed position, allowing the nucleus to migrate posteriorly due to annular damage (76). Extension of the joint reverses this process, decompresses the disc, and may help shift the nucleus more anteriorly (77, 78). Again, patient tolerance becomes an obvious factor, since many patients are unable to extend during an acute phase of a disc injury. Quite commonly, however, a disc lesion is associated with a vertebra fixed in a flexed position, and extension treatment may be the most appropriate and best tolerated by the patient.

Boumphrey (72), using MRI, showed that McKenzie extension exercises increased the disc height in normal and degenerated discs but did not have an effect on the position of the nucleus pulposus of normal, degenerated, or herniated discs. Passive extension, as it increases facetal weightbearing, apparently distracts the vertebral bodies enough to enhance intradiscal imbibition.

Aside from passive McKenzie-type exercises, the principle of extension can be applied with segmental manipulation in a prone, side-lying, supine, or knee-chest position. Even patients who are unable to extend actively when weightbearing, may often quite easily be placed in this position passively when on their side and not weightbearing. Again, patient tolerance is an important guide, and previously described techniques to produce extension may be appropriate.

DIFFERENTIAL DIAGNOSIS OF LUMBAR SPINE DISORDERS (Table 8.1)

A number of conditions coexist with the articular dysfunction due to simple joint locking. This complicates diagnosis and treatment because of the indistinguishable symptoms in the early stages of these disorders. Congenital and developmental anomalies such as tropism, transitional segments, and spondylolisthesis may create biomechanical stresses that predispose the patient to vertebral joint locking. Others, such as muscle strain, may prolong healing time and necessitate adjunctive procedures. In many cases, recurrent episodes of acute pain may necessitate periodic intensive care to promote healing, in addition to manipulation to relieve the loss of joint motion. Such passive care should not become a compensation for unhealthy living habits. Substitution of passive patient care for active participation in exercise programs, weight control, and good spinal hygiene should not be encouraged.

Pathological degenerative changes in the three-joint complex must be understood, with disc degeneration, posterior joint syndrome, disk herniation, and stenosis all etiological conditions to be differentiated. The spontaneous onset of low back pain due to neoplasm, although not common, can be misleading and is a crucial factor to be considered. A history

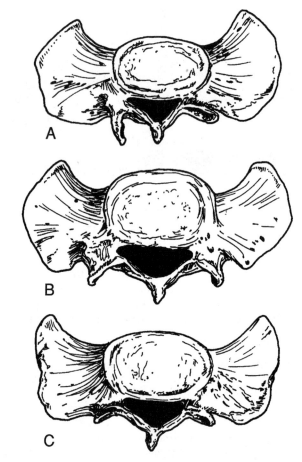

Figure 8.28. Facet tropism. **A,** Asymmetrical facet facings (tropism). **B,** Sagittal-facing facets. **C,** Coronal-facing facets.

of injury or trauma must be kept in proper perspective, since patients with metastatic neoplasm may give a history of trauma coincidental with the onset of low back pain that is perpetuated by the malignancy (6). Muscle spasm is a protective mechanism accompanying spinal fractures, and these must be ruled out, particularly with trauma to the elderly and the postmenopausal female.

Tropism

Tropism is asymmetrical articular facings (Fig 8.28A). It is derived from the Greek word *trope,* meaning turning (6). Putti (73), in 1927, described the biomechanical instability produced by asymmetrical facets. Badgeley (75) pointed out that asymmetrically formed articular processes strongly suggest mechanical instability and susceptibility to ligamentous injury. Sagittal facet facings are normal for the upper lumbar spine (Fig. 8.28B), with coronal facet facings normal in the lower lumbar spine (2, 4) (Fig. 8.28C).

Cyron and Hutton (76) have found that articular tropism (in which one facet faces coronally while the other faces more sagittally) can lead to lumbar

Table 8.1 Differential Diagnosis of Common Disorders of the Lumbar Spine

Condition	History & Symptoms	Diagnostic Indicators & Procedures	Therapy
Biomechanical disorders			
Facet-joint fixation	History of unguarded movement, increased pain on extension, focal tenderness over affected facet joint, faulty posture, low back pain, radiation into groin, hip, buttock, and/or thigh	Motion palpation reveals restricted facet joint motion; radiographs may reveal increased sacral base angle with sclerosed and overriding facets; stress radiographs reveal abnormal movement; tropism may accompany	Manipulation (see text), pelvic tilt exercises
Facet-joint sprain	History of trauma, increased pain on extension, focal tenderness over affected facet joint, low back pain radiating into groin, hip, buttock, and/or thigh	Motion palpation reveals absence of fixation at site of pain; stress radiographs reveal abnormal movement	Treat reflex muscle spasm directly (Ch 12), manipulation is contraindicated in absence of joint fixation
Intervertebral disc herniation	Patient usually 30–50 years of age with episodes of low back pain, leg pain, or both	CT and MRI reveal disc herniation; pain may increase on flexion and straight-leg raise (30° or less), muscle weakness, absent reflex, and sensory deficits may be present	Mild to moderate cases may respond to manipulation (see text) and a few days of bed rest followed by an elastic support and exercise program; severe cases with advancing neurological deficit, bladder or bowel symptoms require prompt referral for neurological evaluation
Traumatic disorders			
Transverse process facture	History of trauma, pain lateral to spine	Spasm of quadratus, radiographs reveal displaced transverse processes, usually unilateral	Immobilize and stabilize with lumbar support 4–8 weeks, restricted activities for 12 weeks; urinalysis to rule out urinary tract injury
Vertebral compression fracture	History of trauma or pathology, back pain	Paraspinal spasm, bone scan, radiographs reveal vertebral wedging	Immobilize with bed rest for 12 weeks, body cast if severe
Spinous process fracture	History of trauma, back pain and pain on forward bending	Focal tenderness over fracture site, bone scan, radiographs reveal displaced spinous process	Immobilize with lumbar support for 4 weeks
Unstable fractures	History of trauma, back pain, neurological deficits	Radiographs reveal radiolucent areas, soft tissue swelling, possible dislocations or evidence of ligamentous injury	Refer for neurological evaluation
Spondylolisthesis	Childhood history of trauma or repeated infant falls; hyperextension injuries have been implicated	Oblique radiographs reveal separation of pars interarticularis, degree of slipping determined by lateral view, instability determined by flexion-extension lateral radiographs	Manipulation directed to dysfunctional joints above and below; refer for surgical evaluation if unstable
Muscle syndromes			
Acute paraspinal muscle strain	History of trauma, repetitive bending (overuse), immediate transitory pain followed by pain free interval and subsequent stiffness, limited mobility and muscle spasm	Pain radiates upward to thoracic region and down into buttocks. List or functional scoliosis due to muscle spasm; bending away from side of spasm increases pain; palpation reveals muscle spasm & tenderness. Radiographs reveal flattening of lumbar curve	Short-lever manipulation when indicated, ice and ultrasound initially, bed rest in severe cases for 2–3 days, lumbar support belt for several weeks followed by exercise and spinal hygiene instruction

Table 8.1 *(Continued)*

Condition	History & Symptoms	Diagnostic Indicators & Procedures	Therapy
Chronic recurrent lumbar strain	History of repeated episodes of low back pain with complaints of a mild persistent ache between episodes of disabling pain	Increased lumbar lordosis, persistent mild muscle spasm, and/or trigger points in lumbar musculature	Short lever manipulation when indicated, avoid repeated, long-lever nonspecific manipulation; ultrasound and deep tissue massage at times of exacerbation; stretching exercises and postural retraining, lumbar support for aggravating activities
Paraspinal myofascial pain	History of trauma or overuse with muscle strain	Chronic stiffness, trigger points in involved muscles	Short-lever manipulation when indicated, avoid repeated long-lever nonspecific manipulation; trigger point therapy, massage, ultrasound, passive mobilization followed by active stretching and postural retraining
Quadratus lumborum	Pain between the 12th rib and iliac crest lateral to the sacrospinalis	Tenderness to palpation of affected muscle, pain increased with bending to contralateral side, rule out fracture of transverse process	Passive stretching of muscle followed by active stretching exercises; manipulation when indicated
Psoas	Low back pain, occasional pain and increased lumbar lordosis	Positive Thomas test, discrepancy in arm length with arms extend-overhead	Passive & active stretch-exercises, full sit-ups contraindicated, manipulation and trigger point therapy when indicated
Piriformis	Pain in buttock extending down the course of the sciatic nerve, trigger points in belly and insertion of the muscle of the involved hip	Palpable muscle spasm & trigger points in piriformis muscle with pain on internal rotation of the hip with the knee flexed	Trigger point pressure therapy, passive and active stretching of the piriformis muscle, sacroiliac manipulation where indicated
Gluteus medius	Posterior & lateral thigh and calf pain	Palpable muscle spasm in the gluteus medius muscles, weakness on Trendelenburg's test	Trigger point pressure therapy, passive and active stretching of the piriformis muscle, sacroiliac manipulation where indicated
Gluteus maximus	Pain in the buttock and posterior thigh	Palpable muscle spasm, trigger points in gluteus maximus muscle	Trigger point pressure therapy, passive & active stretching of piriformis muscle, sacroiliac manipulation where indicated
Tensor fascia latae	Lateral thigh & leg pain	Palpable muscle spasm & trigger points in tensor fascia latae; positive Ober's test	Trigger point pressure therapy, passive and active stretching of the tensor fascia latae
Hamstring	Pain and tenderness over the hamstring origin from the ischial tuberosity; knee pain.	Palpable muscle spasm & trigger points in hamstring muscles	Trigger point pressure therapy, passive and active stretching of the hamstring
Anomalous development Tropism	Related episodes of facet-joint locking	AP radiographs reveal facet asymmetry; simulated when segmental rotation is present	Manipulation when indicated
Transitional vertebrae	Delayed healing following trauma	Radiographs reveal transitional segment; frequently rudimentary or accessory articular processes	Manipulation when indicated, avoidance of excess rotation; support belt; surgical evaluation if signs of nerve entrapment

Table 8.1 *(Continued)*

Condition	History & Symptoms	Diagnostic Indicators & Procedures	Therapy
Spinal canal stenosis	Bizzare complaints in both legs; neurogenic claudication, night pain relieved by walking	Lateral radiographs suggest small canal, confirmed by CT or MRI scan; flexion of the lumbar spine may reduce symptoms	Trial of manipulation, exercise to reduce lumbar lordosis, avoidance of extension & back support; if symptoms persist, refer for surgical evaluation
Iatrogenic disorders			
Dependency syndrome	History of ongoing passive therapy (drugs, manipulation, physical therapy)	Absence of objective findings; psychometric testing	Patient education, exercise, psychological counseling if severe
Joint hypermobility	History of trauma, nonspecific manipulation, recurring muscle spasm	Stress radiographs reveal hypermobile segments; motion palpation may reveal excess joint play with typical "boggy" sensation	Therapy directed toward reduction of muscle spasm (trigger point therapy, ultrasound, massage, and stretching exercises)
Failed surgery syndrome	Chronic unrelenting pain & functional incapacitation as a consequence of having undergone back surgery	MRI and CT scanning may reveal postfusion stenosis; psychometric testing, spinal nerve block	Manipulation when indicated, postural education, exercise; reparative surgery only after careful screening
Arachnoiditis	History of surgical myelographic or spinal anesthetic procedures; symptoms include leg pain, low back pain, or occasional loss of sphincter control, impotency in males & other symptoms of cauda equina syndrome; symptoms markedly increased with activity	MRI is preferable to enhanced CT or myelography; follow-up myelography shows nonfilling of the root sleeves, nonvisualization of the nerves within the cul-de-sac & deformity/narrowing of cul-de-sac; CT scan may show calcium deposit suggesting arachnoid ossification	Refer for surgical evaluation; epidural steroid injection or caudal block may be beneficial
Pathological conditions			
Degenerative disc disease	Commonly may not have symptomatic back pain	Radiographs reveal decreased disc height with listheses in unstable phase; MRI and CT for further evaluation	Manipulation if indicated and exercise
Degenerative joint disease	Morning stiffness & back pain; commonly not be symptomatic	Radiographs reveal narrowed joint space, subchondral sclerosis and marginal osteophytes, MRI & CT for further evaluation	Manipulation if indicated and traction, exercises
Lateral stenosis (lateral recess entrapment)	Buttock and lower extremity pain, unilateral exertional claudication, back pain less common	Rotational and hyperextension stress radiographs may reveal osteophytic overgrowth and subluxation of the posterior joint; MRI or CT confirms	Manipulation if indicated and exercises & instruction in back care; avoid excess rotation
Osteoporosis	Postmenopausal females & over 65 affected; back pain	Radiographs reveal thinning of the cortex and trabeculae of the vertebral body, concave endplates, "codfish" vertebrae	Nutritional supplements & increased activity, refer for hormone therapy if severe
Viscerosomatic	Back pain with concurrent visceral complaints	Radiographs & laboratory findings support visceral pathology	Refer to appropriate specialist for concomitant care

instability manifesting itself as joint rotation (Fig. 8.29A). This rotation occurs toward the side of the more oblique (coronally) facing facet, which can place additional stress on the annulus fibrosus of the intervertebral disc and the capsular ligaments of the apophyseal joints. Cox (2) notes that patients with anomalous facet facings are at high risk for de-veloping a disc lesion on rotation. Steindler (4) noted that the asymmetry results in the sagittal artic-ulations mutually locking each other, restricting both lateral and rotatory motion (Fig. 8.29B). Farfan and Sullivan (77) describe this locking as the "cam" effect of the facet, when one facet is rotated against its "fellow" (Fig. 8.30).

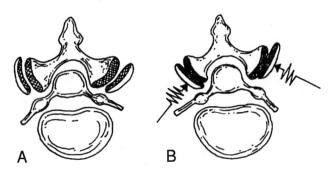

Figure 8.29. A&B Facet tropism permits greater rotation on the side of the more coronal facing facet, which increases the likelihood of facet-joint locking.

The predisposition to facet-joint locking in patients with articular tropism makes the biomechanical effects of this specific congenital anomaly especially amenable to spinal manipulation. Cyron and Hutton (76) report that if sliding is prevented by the locking of the facets, there will be a high compressive force generated in the oblique-facing facet. The unlocked joint will then manifest stress concentration with the ligaments put under extra tensile strain. The persistent extra strain on the highly innervated synovial joints can undoubtedly cause pain. With prolonged strain, compensatory hypermobility may be produced in the oblique unlocked joint.

This supports Farfan and Sullivan's contention (77) that the more oblique-facing facet fails to resist torsion as sheer force, with strains of higher magnitude than usual falling directly on the disc. This is supported by the high correlation between asymmetrical orientation of the facet joints and the level

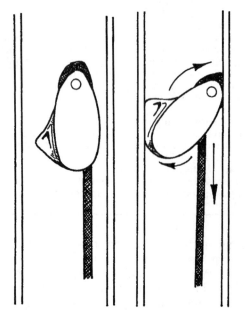

Figure 8.30. Cam effect. A cam effect occurs when an eccentric or off-center object locks on rotation.

of disc pathology, with the side of disc prolapse corresponding to the more oblique-facing facet. Like any synovial joint, degenerative changes can occur, with stress concentrations and cartilage breakdown predisposing to osteoarthritis in the posterior spinal articulations (4).

Normal lumbar spine facet joints are visible on anterior, posterior, or PA linear projections of the lumbar spine, as a radiolucent region between each superior and inferior articular process. Tropism at any level will manifest as an absence of the joint space on one side and a clear delineation on the opposite side (Fig. 8.31). This presumes that the patient is properly positioned for the radiograph, since a false appearance of tropism may result from patient rotation.

While jamming of asymmetrical facet joints has a tendency to recur, response to manipulation is rapid (3) (see "Acute Locked Back"). Repeated manipulation of joints manifesting tropism is not recommended in the absence of joint locking, but prompt manipulative therapy when joint fixation does occur prevents the development of the pain-spasm-pain cycle seen in chronic low back pain patients, quickly resolving the recurring symptoms.

Transitional Lumbosacral Vertebrae (Lumbarization, Sacralization)

The term transitional lumbosacral vertebrae encompasses both lumbarization and sacralization. Lumbarization means that the first sacral segment has the characteristics of a lumbar vertebra (44). The vertebral body of S1 assumes the form of the last presacral segment, with lack of formation of the lateral masses (1). Sacralization means that the fifth lumbar vertebra has the characteristics of the first sacral segment (44), with the last vertebral body incorporated into the sacrum, and the vertebral arches and transverse processes adapted to the lateral masses of the sacrum (1). The term transitional segment is less descriptive than classifying this anomaly as either lumbarization or sacralization, but because of the difficulty of distinguishing between lumbarization and sacralization, lumbosacral transitional vertebra is the preferred term (1). The name is considerably less important than the biomechanical or clinical significance (78).

A transitional vertebra itself does not cause pain (1). When bilaterally symmetrical, the lumbarized S1 segment and sacralized L5 segment create little additional biomechanical stress at the lumbosacral junction. In the case of sacralization, the burden of motion is transmitted to other levels of the lumbar spine (4), with movement that is normal to 5 vertebral motion segments demanded in 4 segments. In the case of lumbarization, the strain falls primarily on the soft-tissue structures of the lumbosacral and sacroiliac regions, which must maintain stability.

If lumbarization or sacralization is unilateral, there is greater potential for mechanical strains and

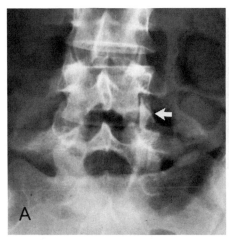
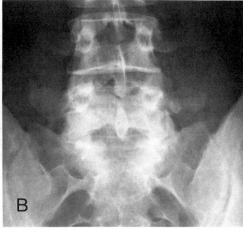
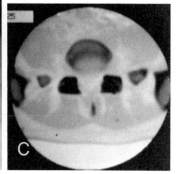

Figure 8.31. **A,** Tropism is seen on x-rays as an absence of the joint space on one side while clearly delineated on the other side, illustrated here at L4. Tropism at L5 is evident on the AP radiograph (**B**) and on the CT scan (**C**) of this patient.

the production of back pain caused by the transitional segment. If a joint is established between the transverse process and the sacrum (transverse-sacral articulation) on one side (Fig. 8.32), lateral bending to the opposite side causes tensile stress on the contralateral posterior articulation and iliolumbar ligaments. Bending to the same side as the extra articulation causes compression stress on that joint. Rotation and flexion-extension stresses tend to be referred to the vertebral motion segment above a unilateral transitional segment.

The asymmetrical torque movement that occurs with unilateral sacralization or lumbarization predisposes to disc stress, often causing herniation of the disc one level above the transitional segment (Bertolotti's syndrome) (79). This is probably due to the reduced capacity for movement of the four-joint complex at the transitional segment (41) transmitting the biomechanical stress to the segment above.

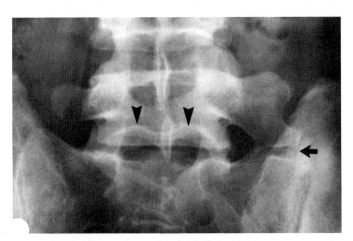

Figure 8.32. Transitional segment with accessory articulation. (From Yochum TR, Rowe LJ: *Essentials of Skeletal Radiology.* Baltimore, Williams & Wilkins, 1986, p. 122.)

Unilateral asymmetrical transitional vertebrae may be associated with varying degrees of scoliosis, showing a rotation and torsion of the vertebral bodies (1). Usually the unsacralized side is lower. The variation of the lumbosacral transition not only involves changes in the transverse processes and vertebral bodies but commonly includes anomalous changes in the apophyseal joints. Frequently, transitional segments have only rudimentary articular processes. The intervertebral disc beneath the transitional vertebra usually shows a considerable decrease in height (1).

In addition to radiographic visualization of the lumbosacral transitional segment on AP or PA lumbar views, oblique projections are necessary to evaluate the condition of the apophyseal joints. The behavior of the disc spaces and degree of inclination in relation to the sacrum are best seen on lateral weightbearing radiographs (1).

Treatment of patients exhibiting a lumbosacral transitional segment is first directed toward removing any joint fixations determined by motion palpation. Herniation of the disc above the transitional segment, producing symptoms of nerve-root entrapment, has been diagnosed with increasing frequency in recent years (79). Cox (68) recommends flexion-distraction manipulation in cases of disc herniation accompanying a transitional segment, utilizing the same therapy applied to other patients with disc herniation. He recommends elimination of rotatory movements of the lumbar spine and pelvis and prescribes a 10-inch-wide lumbosacral support belt. The patient is instructed to avoid activities in which twisting is involved. Heel lifts and muscular strengthening exercises may also prove beneficial (1).

In a study of 576 patients with back pain, Cox and Shreiner (80) reported that it was more difficult to relieve pain caused by transitional segments than that caused by any other condition studied. Patients

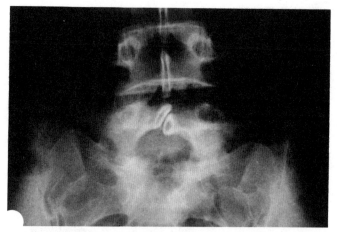

Figure 8.33. Spina bifida occulta at the lumbosacral junction. (From Yochum TR, Rowe LJ: *Essentials of Skeletal Radiology.* Baltimore, Williams & Wilkins, 1986, p 120.)

with a transitional segment had a 21% favorable response in 10 days, while those with tropism showed a 45% favorable response in the same period. Should surgical intervention be necessary to relieve the effects of nerve entrapment, spinal fusion of the transitional vertebrae has been recommended to eliminate further torque stresses (79).

Spina Bifida Occulta

Minor degrees of absence of the neural arch are referred to as spina bifida occulta. The cleft that results from the absence of the spinous process is easily identified on AP or PA radiographs of the lumbar spine (Fig. 8.33). Spina bifida is seen so frequently in the general population that it is considered to be an anatomic variant of normal that rarely causes a serious pain problem in adult life (6, 79). There may be some loss of stability normally furnished by the muscle and tendinous attachments to missing posterior elements (6). Whether or not this predisposes to instability and/or articular locking has not been established.

Spondyolisthesis

Spondylolisthesis is derived from the Greek roots *spondylos* meaning vertebra and *olisthesis* referring to slippage (81). Literally translated, it means slipping of the vertebra, but traditionally spondylolisthesis is defined as an anterior slippage of a vertebral body on the vertebra below. Commonly the result of a spondylolysis or interruption of the pars interarticularis, spondylolisthesis can also be the result of dysplasia of the neural arch or degenerative and pathological changes. The pars separation may be unilateral or bilateral. The unilateral separation causes an asymmetrical stress pattern often seen on radiographs as unilateral sclerotic pedicle (82). The most widely accepted classification of spondylolisthesis is based on the work of Wiltse and coworkers (83) (Table 8.2).

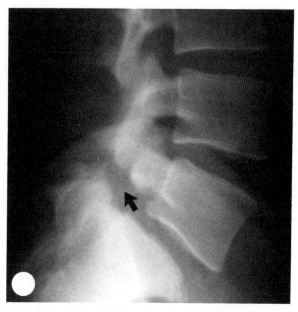

Figure 8.34. Spondylolisthesis due to pars interarticularis separation at L5 (*arrow*) and anterolisthesis of the L5 body. (From Yochum TR, Rowe LJ: *Essentials of Skeletal Radiology.* Baltimore, Williams & Wilkins, 1986, p 244.)

Isthmic Spondylolisthesis

Incidence. The most common form of spondylolisthesis is isthmic spondylolisthesis with separation of the pars interarticularis. The incidence of this type of spondylolisthesis varies with sex and racial background. In the Caucasian population the incidence has a 5–7% frequency of pars defect (84). Stewart (85) reported a higher incidence of spondylolisthesis with neural arch defects in the Northern Eskimo. A lower incidence of spondylolisthesis has been noted in the Black and South African populations (86). Frederickson et al. (87) found a male to female ratio of 2:1. An increased prevalence of spondylolisthesis has been noted in Olympic athletes (16–17%) (88), with the highest incidence found in divers and gymnasts. There appears to be a hereditary predisposition to the defect and a strong association with spina bifida occulta (87, 89).

Etiology. There has been considerable controversy over the etiology of the pars interarticularis defect. For many years the defect was considered a congenital anomaly (1). Cadaver studies of newborns by Batts in 1939 (90) and Rowe and Rocke in 1953 failed to demonstrate this lesion. Troup, in 1977, (91) concluded that spondylolysis is an acquired fracture. More recent studies continue to support the theory that spondylolysis is acquired, probably as the result of fatigue fractures (91, 92).

Rosenberg, Berger, and Friedman (93) reported that no cases of spondylolysis or spondylolisthesis were detected in a 1981 radiographic examination of 143 patients who had never walked, which supports

Table 8.2 Classification of Spondylolisthesis[a]

Type	Defect	Characteristics
Dysplastic	Anterior displacement due to congential abnormality of the upper sacrum or the neural arch of L5	Frequently accompanied by a wide spina bifida occulta involving the sacrum and L5 vertebra, which progresses to more severe grade of displacement
Isthmic	Defect in the pars interarticularis due to:	Four times more common than dysplastic
	1) Lytic or stress (fatigue) fracture	1) Caused by biomechanical stress (fatigue fracture) not noted in the newborn, most common type found in persons under age 50
	2) Elongated but intact pars	2) Secondary to repeated minor trabecular stress fractures of the pars which heal with an elongated pars as the body of L5 is displaced anteriorly
	3) Acute fracture of the pars	3) Rare, result from acute pars fractures following severe trauma, usually involving hyperextension of the lower lumbar spine, displacement rare
Degenerative (pseudospondylolisthesis)	Secondary to long-standing degenerative arthrosis of the zygapophyseal joints and discovertebral articulations without pars separation	Ten times more common at L4 than L3 or L5, six times more common in females over 60 than males, three times more common in blacks than whites, four times more likely to be found in association with sacralization of L5
Traumatic	Secondary to fracture of part of the neural arch other than pars interarticularis	Results from severe injury in which the neural arch is fractured, tends to heal with immobilization
Pathological	Localized bone disease, Paget's disease, metastatic bone disease, osteoporosis	Pathological bone disorders affecting the neural arch result in spondylolysis

[a]Modified from Wiltse LL, Newman MD, MacNab I: Classification of spondylolysis and spondylolisthesis. *Clin Orthop* 117:23–29, 1976.

the theory that spondylolysis and isthmic spondylolisthesis result from fatigue fractures from activities associated with ambulation.

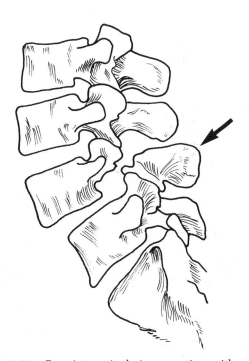

Figure 8.35. Pars interarticularis separation with anterior slippage of the body of L4 is palpable as a depression above the L4 spinous process. (From Yochum TR, Rowe LJ: *Essentials of Skeletal Radiology*. Baltimore, Williams & Wilkins, 1986, p 254.)

While spondylolysis in children can occur shortly after walking begins, clinical and radiographic evidence suggests that the most frequent age of onset is after the age of 5 years. A prospective radiographic study of 500 unselected first grade children from 1955 through 1957 (87) showed that the incidence at age 6 years was 4.4%, which increased to 6% in adulthood. This study concluded that slipping usually is demonstrable at about the same time that the pars interarticularis defect is first detected, and slipping may increase up to the age of 16 years but rarely does so. Progression of a slip was never symptomatic in the population studied.

The mechanism of fracture has been variously attributed to flexion (94) and the combination of extension and rotational stresses. The development of lumbar lordosis and repeated infant falls, particularly if premature walking occurs, have also been implicated (95). The higher incidence in sports producing hyperextension (88) (i.e., diving and gymnastics) suggests that mechanical stress plays a part in the etiology of spondylolysis. The higher incidence in males might also be due to their activity level rather than to a sex-linked predisposition (96).

Clinical Findings. Spondylolisthesis due to pars interarticularis defect is seen most commonly at the L5 vertebral motion segment, with the body of the 5th lumbar vertebra slipping anteriorly on the sacrum (83) (Fig. 8.34). The posterior part of the separated vertebra retains the normal position relative to the sacrum, with the inferior articular process and the posterior arch attached to the spinous process.

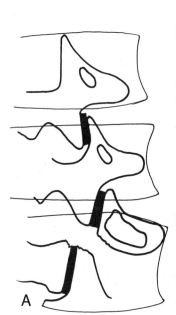

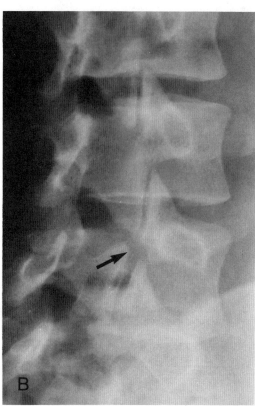

Figure 8.36. Classic signs of spondylolisthesis. **A,** The outline of a Scottie dog can be visualized on posterior oblique views of the lumbar spine. The superior facet corresponds to the ear, the pedicle to the eye, the transverse process to the nose, and the inferior articular process to the foreleg. The alignment of the facet joints changes abruptly at the level of slippage known as the stepladder sign. **B,** A lucent collar appears on the Scottie dog produced by the pars defect. (From Yochum TR, Rowe LJ: *Essentials of Skeletal Radiology.* Baltimore, Williams & Wilkins, 1986, p 261.)

The anterior portion of the segment slips forward, along with the pedicle, superior articular processes, and transverse processes (4).

Approximately half of the patients with radiographic evidence of spondylolisthesis do not develop symptoms (97–99). This suggests that the presence of a spondylolysis and spondylolisthesis are often incidental findings not necessarily related to the patient's symptomatology (96). Frederickson et al. (87) found that the development of spondylolysis with or without spondylolisthesis does not cause pain in most patients. If slippage has reached an advanced stage, a depression may be palpable above the spinous process of the separated vertebra when the displacement of the body allows the segments above to move forward, producing a step along the row of spinous processes (4) (Fig. 8.35).

Radiographic Findings. Radiological evaluation is the definitive method of confirming spondylolysis and spondylolisthesis (Chapter 6). The most diagnostic radiograph for determining separation of the pars interarticularis is the oblique view (78). The appearance of the neural arch and its processes seen on the oblique film has been likened to a Scottie dog (Fig. 8.36A). A pars defect will appear as a linear radiolucency that simulates a collar or broken neck of the dog (Fig. 8.36B). Misalignment of the zygapophyseal joints at the involved level (referred to as the "stepladder sign") may also be seen on the oblique view (Fig. 8.36A).

If there is significant anterior displacement, the superimposition of the L5 body over the sacrum creates the appearance of the inverted "Napolean hat" sign (Fig. 8.37). The lateral view is used to determine the degree of slippage (Meyerding method) (Chapter 6). Flexion and extension lateral radiographs are useful in evaluating intersegmental stability (see Chapter 6).

Chiropractic Management of Spondylolisthesis. Spinal manipulation offers rapid symtomatic relief to many patients with back pain associated with spondylolisthesis. Cassidy, Potter, and Kirkaldy-Willis (81) stress that treatment is not directed at the level of slippage nor at influencing the slippage. Rather, specific manipulation directed at the dysfunctional joints above and/or below the defect can reduce the pain and disability in chronic low back pain patients with spondylolisthesis (96). There is no evidence that a slip can be reduced by manipulation, and even if this were possible, the normal holding elements of the vertebral motion segment would not be able to maintain the reduction (96).

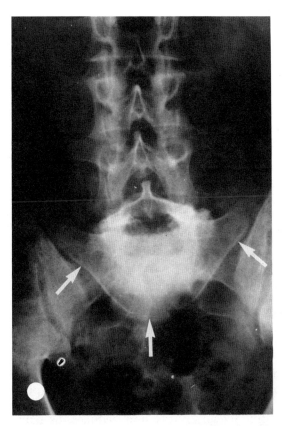

Figure 8.37. "Napoleon hat" sign. Anterior slippage producing the superimposition of the L5 body over the sacrum creates the appearance of the inverted Napolean hat visualized on the AP view. (From Yochum TR, Rowe LJ: *Essentials of Skeletal Radiology.* Baltimore, Williams & Wilkins, 1986, p 256.)

The treatment of choice is specific high-velocity, low-amplitude manipulation to the dysfunctional joints above and below the defect with the patient in side posture (96). Prone lumbar manipulation is not recommended.

The treatment outcome is not significantly different between patients with chronic low back pain exhibiting spondylolisthesis and those without spondylolisthesis. In most cases spondylolisthesis is considered an incidental finding and no contraindication to manipulative therapy (81). A small number of patients with unstable spondylolisthesis (4 mm or more of segmental movement evaluated on flexion/extension lateral radiographs) fail to respond to conservative care. Individuals with progressive biomechanical instability and/or advancing neurological deficits may be surgical candidates. Arthrodesis with vertebral body or bilateral transverse process fusion may be necessary to achieve stability (23, 78). Instability and progressive slip are signs of poor prognosis with conservative treatment (81). Instability is not common in vertebral motion segments exhibiting spondylolisthesis and is unlikely to progress past adolescence (86).

Disability due to Spondylolisthesis. The degree of disability attributed to spondylolisthesis is controversial (1, 78, 100, 101). If one considers that spondylolisthesis predisposes a worker to back injury or prolongs healing time after injury, then preemployment screening perhaps unfairly eliminates those patients with spondylolisthesis as high risks in occupations involving heavy labor. High disability awards to patients with persistent back pain that is coincidentally associated with spondylolisthesis, will also limit opportunities for the worker with spondylolisthesis if employers fear high insurance premiums to cover the high awards. Frederickson et al. (86) have concluded that "a child with spondylolysis or spondylolisthesis can be permitted to enjoy a normal childhood and adolescence without restriction of activities and without fear of progressive listhesis or disabling pain." The same consideration should be given to the adult.

Acute Lumbar Strain

The most common diagnosis given for sudden low back pain is lumbar strain (102). This is easily understood when one considers that the paraspinal muscles serve as the first line of defense in the prevention of spinal injury. While this condition may be the most frequent cause of acute low back pain, the diagnosis of lumbar strain should not be made indiscriminately before more complex syndromes have been considered.

Lumbar strains involve stretching or tearing of spinal muscles and their attachments. This results from muscle contraction associated with uncontrolled movement, or direct trauma to the back (contusion). A fall in which the low back musculature is stretched can also produce a lumbar strain. Minor muscle strain can occur with overuse following unaccustomed repetitive tasks. This results in low back pain and stiffness through the increased demands of muscle activity. In these cases, the complaints tend to be of short duration (2–3 days) and are relieved by a period of rest followed by a graduated return to the repeated activity.

Uncontrolled movements frequently associated with lumbar strain include sudden ballistic motion, bending and twisting concomitantly, and the lowering of a heavy weight. During the latter, the overall muscle is lengthening while the muscle contracts (eccentric contraction). The force of gravity pulling on the weight overrides the stretch reflex that normally protects the muscle from overstretching.

Acute strains from a single act are frequently characterized by an immediate transitory pain followed by a pain-free interval, after which the patient develops stiffness, limited mobility, and muscle spasm. Patients often report that they experienced a sudden pain of short duration at the time of the precipitating injury (4, 102). Since the pain subsides, it is not disabling, and the patient may complete the task with only minor discomfort. Several hours later (of-

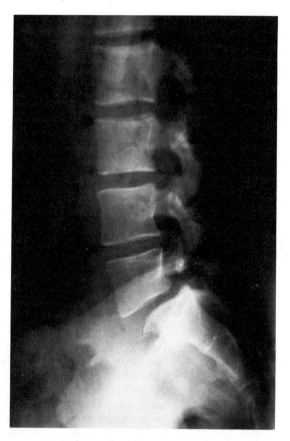

Figure 8.38. Radiographs of a patient with a lumbar strain reveal flattening of the lumbar curve on the lateral view. Incidently noted is the spondylolisthesis at L5.

ten after a rest break) or the following morning, the patient is unable to arise due to intense pain produced by muscle spasm. If unaccompanied by joint fixation or more extensive soft tissue damage, the episode subsides in a few days with a gradual resumption of normal activities. If the injury results in more serious damage to the spine, involving ligaments or joints, then by definition it is not a simple lumbar strain. Factors that interfere with physiological relaxation of the muscle will produce a vicious cycle of spasm, pain, spasm, producing further impairment of relaxation, which can lead to chronic pain syndrome. Reassurance about the nondisabling nature of lumbar strain can help to prevent this cycle. The severity of the clinical features of acute lumbar strain depends directly upon the degree of paravertebral muscle spasm present.

Clinical Features of Acute Lumbar Strain

The patient's gait is slow and guarded with painful movement of the spine. The back may be flexed slightly or listing to one side. Patients often complain that they cannot stand up straight. Spinal movements are limited in direct proportion to the amount of spasm present (102). The pain in the low back may radiate upward into the thoracic spine and

into the buttocks. Forward bending causes increased discomfort, and if the paraspinal muscle spasm is unilateral, a functional scoliosis that is reduced on forward bending (Adams' test) may be present. Lateral bending of the body away from the side of spasm produces pain, while the same movement toward the muscle spasm is less uncomfortable and may relieve the pain.

Palpation will reveal diffuse tenderness along the paravertebral muscle mass. Motion palpation will determine if joint fixation is present indicating the need for manipulation. Coughing, straining, and turning on the table aggravate the low back pain. Supine and sitting straight-leg raising may elicit complaints of back pain without sciatic radiation. Axial compression (Kemp's test) does not cause severe discomfort, and differential tests for pelvic dysfunction are negative (Chapter 7). Radiographs of the spine are negative except for a flattening of the lumbar curve on the lateral view, indicating paravertebral muscle spasm (Fig. 8.38).

Management

The purpose of treatment is removing the stimulus for muscle spasm. The patient should be first palpated for facet-joint locking, and manipulation should be appropriately applied. Physical therapy, including ice and ultrasound, reduces the pain and muscle spasm. Bed rest may be necessary for several days if the pain is severe but should not be prolonged beyond 2 weeks with few exceptions (103). The patient may be referred for analgesic, antiinflammatory, or myorelaxant medication in severe cases. A lumbar support belt offers protection during convalescence but should not be encouraged for a prolonged period of time. Management should include teaching spinal hygiene to prevent reinjury (Chapters 13 and 14). The recumbent 90/90 position and stretching the paraspinal muscles by bringing the knees close to the chest can be introduced before the patient is ambulatory. If satisfactory recovery is not complete by the end of 3 weeks, the patient should be reevaluted to rule out complicating factors.

Chronic Recurrent Lumbar Strain

Acute lumbar strain progresses to chronicity with repeated episodes of partial tears of spinal muscles and their attachments. In addition to the precipitating factors causing acute lumbar strain, faulty posture and inadequate musculature have been implicated as causes of chronic lumbosacral strain (6). With time, the pathological changes of degenerative joint disease begin to complicate the low back dysfunction.

Clinical Features

The signs and symptoms of chronic lumbar strain vary greatly in both intensity and periodicity (6). Prolonged intervals of mild discomfort may be interrupted by a severe exacerbation of pain. A mild, persistent ache may remain largely in the background and is ignored by the patient who considers this state normal. The patient remains mindful of the latent nature of the back pain and models physical activities defensively, in an attempt to avoid provocative activities that cause incapacitating flare-ups of severe body pain. This pattern of presentation is referred to as chronic recurrent lumbar strain. Chronicity indicates a prolonged history of recurrences, rather than the duration of each specific attack (6).

The primary ongoing complaint is diffuse aching in the lumbosacral region. It often covers a wide area and is described as mild or annoying. In addition to the constant aching sensation, the patient often complains of fatigue or a tired feeling in the back. Although patients may give a history of a fall or injury, they have often had low back discomfort prior to the trauma (6). Finneson (6) reports that almost any activity can aggravate the pain and that posture and general carriage are usually poor. The patient is often overweight, with atonic and flabby musculature. Whether these associated findings are a significant cause of the syndrome or the effect of longstanding inactivity due to low back dysfunction has not been established. In either case, treatment must be directed at changing the patient's mode of living and aimed at increasing the overall level of physical fitness.

Examination may reveal an increase in lumbar lordosis, which is aggravated by obesity, pregnancy, and the routine wearing of high heels (Chapter 13). Certain developmental anomalies such as vertebral epiphysitis (adolescent kyphosis) result in malposture, which may produce lumbosacral strain (4). Palpation may reveal some mild paraspinal muscle spasm in the lumbar area (7) with tender nodules (4, 25, 48, 103) characteristic of myofascial pain syndrome (Chapter 12).

A careful evaluation to rule out occult conditions is essential. Just because the patient has had a similar exacerbation of the symptoms in previous acute episodes, the diagnostician cannot assume that the patient's symptoms are due to a recurrence of muscle strain, without first ruling out other underlying causes of back pain. Because the symptoms are indistinguishable in the early stages from those produced by other low back disorders, lumbar strain has been considered a "wastebasket" diagnosis. Chronic lumbar strain is probably the most frequently employed diagnosis of low back dysfunction. Despite this fact, considerably less is known about lumbosacral strain than about many of the less frequently encountered conditions that cause low back pain. Although lumbar strain is most readily identifiable, factual knowledge of this clinical entity is wanting. Thus, the diagnosis becomes one of exclusion, with careful, painstaking evaluation. Routine laboratory studies and enhanced imaging may

be necessary in addition to radiographic evaluation and orthopedic and neurological tests before a diagnosis can be made.

Management. Treatment of chronic lumbar strain must be directed to the involved muscles. Manipulation of locked joints should not be used routinely to reduce reflex muscle spasm. Repeated long-lever, nonspecific manipulation offers only brief relief and directs treatment away from the involved muscles, which respond to ultrasound (44), deep tissue massage (104), and exercise (6, 101). (Chapter 13). Hypertonic muscles characterized by muscle spasm and tender nodules respond favorably to stretching exercises, while electrical stimulation tends to perpetuate the increased motoricity (Chapter 12). Nutritional deficiencies resulting from electrolytic imbalance must be addressed (44). Changes in muscle metabolism with resulting cramps can perpetuate back pain due to muscle spasm.

A detailed explanation of basic spinal biomechanics enhances patient participation in exercise and postural retraining programs. Adequate rest is enhanced by appropriately firm mattresses and chairs that provide proper lumbar support. All activities of daily living need to be reviewed to determine how to avoid excessive stress on the low back. Back schools are helpful in training patients in the body mechanics of standing, walking, sitting, lifting, and sleeping (6).

Anything that intereferes with the physiological relaxation of muscle will start a vicious cycle of spasm-pain-spasm. The flow of venous blood and lymph away from muscles depends on the pumping action of alternate relaxation and contraction of muscles. Accumulation of tissue fluids and catabolites, the waste products of metabolism, are noxious and lead to an inflammatory process with further pain and spasm. Stress reduction techniques including biofeedback may prove beneficial in chronic cases.

In the acute stage, a lumbosacral support may be necessary to support the low back and abdominal muscles, but as muscle tone and strength improve through exercise, this support should be discontinued, usually by 6 weeks (6). It must be remembered that extensive support will further weaken the back muscles if used as a substitute for a graduated exercise program. Such dependency should not be encouraged (102). Overzealous exercise in the beginning may cause exacerbation of the muscle spasm, while excessive rest may not only prolong the recovery period but also create a so-called low back neurosis, in which the patient considers himself an invalid (6). To prevent permanent disability, which may accompany chronic pain syndromes, patients should be encouraged to return to work and recreational activities as soon as safely possible. A lumbosacral support belt may be necessary for activities that require repetitive lifting and bending.

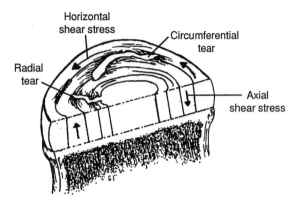

Figure 8.39. Pathological changes of the disc. Circumferential tears in the annulus fibrosus enlarge and spread with repeated torsional trauma. Radial tears allow nuclear material to stream out through the torn annulus. Torsion produces both horizontal shear stress and axial shear stress. (Modified from White AA, Panjabi MM: *Clinical Biomechanics of the Spine.* Philadelphia, JB Lippincott, 1978, p 16.)

Disc Degeneration and the Three-Joint Complex

Degenerative changes in the intervertebral disc are progressive and almost universal (105). In some, the disc retains a relatively stable appearance through many decades, showing only a gradual involution with advancing age. In others, probably some additional factors such as trauma or a pathological process precipitate degenerative changes (16). Sex, body weight, body habits, posture, nutrition, smoking, and sedentary life-styles may also play a role in disc pathology (104–106).

Radiological and postmortem studies have met with little success in correlating symptoms with degenerative changes in the spine. The peak incidence of disabling symptoms occurs between the ages of 35 and 55, which does not parallel the progression of degeneration. This suggests the premise that the degenerative process has a protective effect. The works of Kirkaldy-Willis (30, 42, 107, 108) outline stages of spinal degeneration, providing a working model for the management of low back pain. This model supports the concept that there is a natural mechanism provided by the body to compensate for the pathological changes that lead to spinal stability. Degenerative changes leading to a decrease in disc height increase the compressive force exerted on the posterior facet joints (109), while changes affecting the posterior joints also affect the disc. This interaction at the three-joint complex results in vertebral motion segment dysfunction, which in many cases is amenable to chiropractic management that significantly reduces low back pain (108).

Three Phases in the Degenerative Process

Kirkaldy-Willis (108) outlines three phases of degenerative change in the spine, each one blending into the other. The earliest phase is dysfunction characterized mainly by abnormal function. Anatomic changes at this stage are slight.

The unstable stage follows, with increased abnormal movement recognized in lateral radiographs in flexion and extension. One vertebra moves on the one below, usually backward. As instability increases, the degree of movement backward and forward becomes greater.

The third phase is restabilization, when the apophyseal joints and disc become stiff from degeneration of cartilage, loss of disc substance, fibrosis, and the formation of osteophytes around the posterior joints and disc. This process leads to stabilization of the unstable vertebral motion segment.

Sequence of Pathological Changes

The earliest change in the disc is the formation of one or more circumferential tears in the annulus fibrosus, most commonly in the outer layers and often at the posterolateral corner of the disc (Fig. 8.39). These tears can enlarge and spread with repeated torsional trauma. As the circumferential tears enlarge and spread inward toward the center of the disc, radial tears are formed.

Enlargement of radial tears continues, coalescing to one large tear from front to back and side to side within the annulus. This results in internal disruption of the disc, with progressive loss of nuclear contents. The annulus then bulges around the periphery of the disc like a half-inflated car tire, with resulting loss of stiffness and disc height. The end result of this stage is instability.

Stability eventually returns, with fibrosis of the disc and approximation of the vertebral bodies. Vertebral body bone on either side of the disc becomes dense and sclerotic. Formation of osteophytes around the periphery of the disc further stabilizes the segment-restricting movement. In extreme cases, a bar of bone connects one body with another and produces a bony ankylosis.

Concomitant pathological changes in the posterior joints accompany the degenerating intervertebral disc. The earliest change is probably synovitis due to irritation, inflammation, or nipping of a synovial tag. Fissures in the articular cartilage follow the superficial lesions, becoming ragged and thin. Later this cartilage becomes linear and may be lost in places. Formation of fibrous synovial tags may occur, starting with nipping of the synovium. This process may continue until a fibrous band is formed between the cartilage surfaces.

Succeeding rotational injuries to the three-joint complex cause small tears and capsular laxity. These tears normally heal with collagen that is not as strong as normal capsular collagen. Repeated injury increases capsule laxity, producing the phase of instability. Restabilization occurs as osteophytes are formed at the periphery of the joint when the cells of the cambial layer of the periosteum surrounding the inferior and superior articular processes proliferate.

The progression of the interacting changes between the posterior joint and disc produces abnormal movement, with restricted segmental motion sometimes seen in lateral-bending anteroposterior radiographs (Chapter 6). This is common in the dysfunctional phase and continues into the stage of instability. Manipulation of articular fixation at this point generally brings prompt relief, while frequent repeated manipulation of unstable segments protected by muscle splinting may perpetuate the pain-spasm-pain cycle.

Herniation of the nucleus pulposus can occur toward the end of the first phase of dysfunction or may take place during the unstable phase. Posterior facet syndrome with capsulitis and subluxation begins in the dysfunction phase, progressing through the stage of instability as the superior articular process slides upward and forward on the inferior process. As restabilization occurs there is a progressive loss of disc height with narrowing of the intervertebral foramen and stenosis of the lateral canal medial to it. Enlargement of the inferior articular processes causes central canal stenosis.

Lumbar spinal nerves may be entrapped at the back of the disc, laterally in the central canal, centrally in the cauda equina, more laterally in the nerve canal, and posteriorly in the zygapophyseal joints (107). Manipulation has proven beneficial to varying degrees in the treatment of nerve entrapment syndromes, but in all cases, advancing neurological deficits must be referred for further evaluation (see Chapter 4).

Posterior Facet Syndrome

The term facet syndrome pertains to posterior joint dysfunction characterized by an overriding of the facets of adjacent vertebrae, whereby the intervertebral foramina are narrowed from the superior to the inferior. For over 50 years the posterior facet joints have been considered a source of back pain, but following the work of Mixter and Barr in 1934 (110) the majority of interest by the medical profession became focused on the intervertebral disc with related irritation of the nerve roots.

Ayers, in 1929 (111) and again in 1935 (112), discussed involvement of the articular facets as well as the intervertebral disc in the production of back pain. Ghormley, in 1933 (113), introduced the term facet syndrome, pointing out that many of the aches and pains of backache represent the same type of joint pain seen in arthritis of other synovial joints. Badgeley, in 1941 (75), discussed the articular facets in relation to low back pain and sciatic radiation, indicating that 80% of cases of low back pain with sciatic radiation were based on referred pain and not direct nerve irritation. Hadley, in 1961 (114), studied spinal radiographs and found various kinds of joint destruction with imbrication, impingement, bumper formation, eburnation, and erosion in the posterior facet joints. He proposed that pinching of

soft tissues causes the "sudden catch" type of low back pain and that the degenerative changes noted probably play a part in the production of local back pain. In 1976, Mooney and Robertson (115), suggested that the structure related to the facet joint can be a persistent contributor to the chronic pain complaints of individuals with low back and leg pain. They proposed that menisci-like folds within the facet joint may account for pinching of the synovium and capsule, suggesting that perhaps this is the problem that is often successfully treated by chiropractors.

In 1985, Anderson (116) stated that the facet syndrome has been clinically overshadowed by the focus on the intervertebral disc, which has lead to a situation that may have resulted in misdiagnosis and inappropriate therapy for some patients. He concludes that the "dynasty of the disc" is gradually drawing to a close. Helbig and Casey in 1988 (117) noted that with the classic work of Mixter and Barr in 1934 (110) the role of the herniated intervertebral disc overshadowed the importance of facet-joint disorders as a source of low-back pain and sciatica.

Clinical Considerations

Etiological factors producing lumbar facet syndrome include trauma, degeneration, and faulty posture. Trauma affecting the posterior facet articulations of the low back results from hyperextension of the lumbar spine. Overthrowing the legs in diving accidents can produce this type of trauma, as can a fall to the buttocks accompanied by hyperextension of the spine. Such injury to the facet joints produces inflammation of the vertebral joint capsule, giving rise to intraarticular pressure and subsequent acute pain. This may exist without any demonstrable radiographic evidence of malalignment immediately following trauma.

Subsequent degenerative changes may occur over time if damage to the articular cartilage has occurred. Thinning of the articular disc (see Disc Degeneration) (Fig. 8.40A) permits approximation of the articulating surfaces of posterior joints, which become roughened and sclerosed (eburnation) (Fig. 8.40B). Oblique radiographs show degenerative changes with facet overriding (Fig. 8.40C).

Postural changes with an increased angulation of the sacral base and increased lumbar lordosis result in posterior displacement of the center of gravity. This allows the facet joints to become more weightbearing. Yang and King (118) found that if the facet joint was arthritic, the load could be as high as 47%. They hypothesized that excessive facet loads stretch the joint capsule and can be a cause of back pain. Overriding of the facets may also produce narrowing of the intervertebral foramina (114).

The symptoms of a classic facet syndrome are low back pain radiating into the groin, hip, buttock, and often the leg, in most cases above the knee (114, 115) (Fig. 8.41). Hyperextension movements of the back

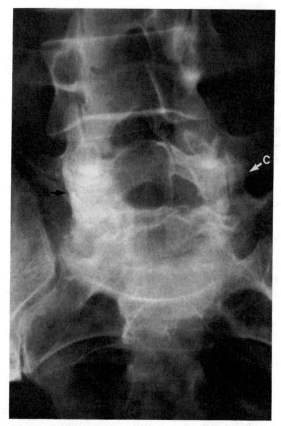

Figure 8.40. Radiographic signs of posterior facet syndrome. (A) Thinning of the articular disc with approximation of the articulating surfaces. (B) Roughened and sclerosed joint surfaces (eburnation). (C) Facet overriding.

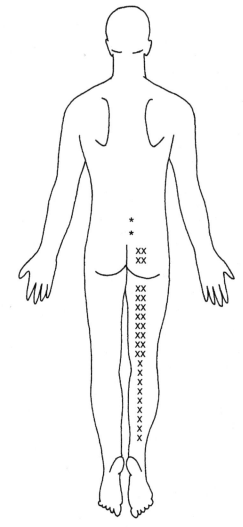

Figure 8.41. Pain diagram of a patient with chronic posterior facet syndrome. Areas of localized tenderness (*) refer pain (×) into the buttocks and down the posterior thigh and calf.

increase the pain, whereas flexion reduces it. Activities that may increase the pain include sleeping on the abdomen, sitting in an upright position, lifting a load in front of the body at or above the waistline, working with the hands and arms above the head, and arising from sitting. When the symptoms are acute, sneezing and coughing accentuate the pain, unless done with the knees and the chest approximated. Radiation of pain into the groin and anterior thigh is occasionally seen but, as with back, buttock, and thigh pain, is not related to any specific facet joint.

Minor sensory changes may be experienced by the patient, with subjective numbness accompanying the pain. These sensory changes may be a reflex phenomena that is not a true loss of sensation. Subjective muscle weakness is commonly due to pain and not a true motor deficit. Clear-cut muscle weakness, progressive sensory loss, and bladder or bowel dysfunction require prompt referral for neurological evaluation (119).

Low back stiffness, especially in the morning or with inactivity, is a common complaint. The classic signs of posterior joint syndrome are palpable muscle spasm with focal tenderness over the affected facet joint (114, 117). Pain may be relieved by hav-

ing the patient draw both knees to the chest and locking the hands around the knees, by assuming the 90/90 position, and by the Cox method of flexion and distraction (Chapter 15). Pain is increased in spine hyperextension, in upright sitting, and prone positions. Straight-leg raising may be mildly diminished due to back pain.

Radiographic findings on oblique and lateral views may show facet overriding, with change in MacNab's line and Hadley's "S" curve (Chapter 6). Subluxation of the facets may be demonstrated with posterior displacement of the segment immediately above. There is often an increase in the lumbar intervertebral disc angle (78) and increased lumbar lordosis, which shifts the weightbearing posteriorly into the posterior facet joints. Long-term compressive forces produce an increase in facet sclerosis with joint narrowing and osteophyte formation. Anomalies such as a flattened sacral kyphosis and posterior sacrum predispose to lumbar facet syndrome.

Radiographic abnormalities alone are not conclusive of a facet syndrome unless they correlate with clinical findings. The clinical findings are more diagnostic of posterior joint syndrome than are radiographic indicators. With the outline of better criteria for accurate diagnosis of the lumbar facet syndrome (7), it is expected that this frequently overlooked disorder will be more readily recognized.

Helbig and Casey (117) have formulated a scoring system with a total of 100 points. Thirty points are assigned to back pain associated with groin or thigh pain, 30 points are given for reproduction of pain with extension-rotation, and 20 points each for well-localized paraspinal tenderness and corresponding radiographic changes. Ten points are subtracted for pain below the knees. A score of 60 points or more indicates a very high probability of lumbar facet syndrome. In both acute and chronic posterior joint syndrome, articular movement, previously restricted is increased by manipulation (106).

Chiropractic management of posterior joint syndrome includes manipulation and corrective exercises. Manipulation has proven highly effective (80, 107, 120). Favorable responses to manipulation over 7–10 days may clinch the tenative diagnosis. When manipulation directed to the posterior joints at a specific level results in alleviation of the pain, it is almost certain that joints are the main site of pain (120).

Postural correction to decrease anterior pelvic tilt reduces compressive forces on the posterior joints as well as weight reduction in the obese patient. Exercises to strengthen the abdominal wall musculature helps to provide optimal postural relationships. Reclining in a 90/90 position opens the posterior joints and may be enhanced by the use of pelvic traction. Injection of anesthetic solutions into the facet joints has proven an effective medical treatment for facet syndrome (114–116, 119), but is not recommended until a less invasive trial of manipulative therapy has proven unsuccessful.

Intervertebral Disc Syndrome/Disc Herniation

With the dynasty of the disc gradually drawing to a close (115), it is imperative that biomechanical disorders of discogenic origin not be overlooked. There is ample evidence that lumbar pain and sciatica can be caused by other than lumbar disc herniation (115–117, 120). In our haste to recognize other etiological factors we must not overlook disc lesions, but it is just as important that we do not attribute the patient's complaints to the innocuous disc bulge, mindless of the paucity of substantiating clinical findings. Referred pain into the lower extremity must not be misinterpreted as a radicular pain from nerve root compromise (Table 8.3). A disc bulge visualized by enhanced imaging without

clinical findings has no more significance than freckles on the face.

An accurate differential diagnosis is nowhere more difficult than in the evaluation of low back and radiating lower extremity pain. The doctor is faced with two main problems in the diagnosis of low back pain (120). The first is the interaction of the disc and posterior joints in the three-joint complex. In practice this means that even when the main lesion is a herniation of the nucleus pulposus, the posterior joints are abnormal and are usually a source of part of the patient's symptoms. Conversely, when the posterior joints are abnormal the concomitantly degenerated disc may also be a source of pain. The second problem is that several low back syndromes produce much the same symptom complex (122).

To complicate matters, the patient may have more than one mechanical and/or degenerative problem, which throws the diagnostician off course. The piriformis syndrome (Chapter 12), for example, typically causes sciatica and is often misdiagnosed as nerve-root entrapment. This can cause prolonged, inappropriate care and in some cases needless surgery. This syndrome coupled with degenerative disc disease at corresponding lumbar levels makes a precise diagnosis even more difficult.

Degrees of Herniated Nucleus Pulposus

Three degrees of herniated nucleus pulposus are differentiated (121) (Fig. 8.42). The first is disc protrusion in which the annulus is intact. The annular fibers are thinned but not ruptured, allowing nuclear material to move posteriorly with a localized protrusion into the spinal canal. Secondly, rupture of the annular fiber allows the nucleus to extrude into the canal. With disc extrusion most of the nuclear material has not herniated beyond the annulus (41). Thirdly, with sequestration, the nucleus has herniated entirely beyond the annulus. The sequestrated nuclear material may move about, so that in some positions it is either asymptomatic or causes some combination of spine pain, referred pain, or true radiculopathy (23).

Etiological Factors in Disc Herniation

The chain of events that leads to a disc protrusion or extrusion is still unclear. It is arguable whether disc herniation is due to a traumatic event such as a single episode of mechanical overload or whether a long-term degenerative process interacts with mechanical stress to produce disc herniation.

With axial overload, it is known that the endplate fractures before the disc ruptures, even with partial separation of the annular fibers (18). The joint with a fractured endplate shows a decreased resistance to torsion and is prone to torsional stress (108). Farfan (18) proposes a mechanism of disc destruction due to an interaction of degenerative changes and mechanical influences. The most common mecha-

Table 8.3 Distinguishing Referred Pain from Radicular Pain in the Low Back[a]

	Referred Pain	Radicular Pain
Symptoms	Deep, boring, ill-defined pain, poorly localized	Sharp, well-localized electric shock-like pain
Radiation	Distant from origin in posterior joints, sacroiliac joints or muscles (i.e., gluteus medius and piriformis); pain may radiate to groin, posterolateral thigh or calf, rarely to foot	Most common presentations follow sciatic nerve root distribution from the back of the posterolateral thigh and calf to the foot or femoral nerve root distribution to the anterior thigh
Sensory alteration	Rare; occasional hyperesthesia	Frequent, follows a dermatomal distribution
Motor weakness	May have subjective weakness but objective weakness or atrophy is rare	Frequent objective weakness and atrophy with prolonged duration of symptoms
Reflex deficit	Rare, reported with posterior joint syndrome	Frequent
Nerve-root tension signs	Absent; straight-leg raising may cause increased low back pain at posterior joint or sacroiliac joint or may reveal tight hamstring muscles	Straight-leg raising produces pain in sciatic distribution, sciatic notch tenderness, popliteal and perineal nerve tenderness; hip extension with knee flexion produces pain in femoral distribution down anterior thigh

[a]Modified from Kirkaldy-Willis WH: *Managing Low Back Pain*, ed 2. New York, Churchill Livingstone, 1988, p 211.

nism of herniation is thought to be a series of rotational injuries that produce circumferential and radial tears, with one final traumatic event when the annulus yields. This produces a localized bulge with complete rupture in some cases. A severe compression injury with the spine flexed may cause a sudden rupture of the annulus (42), however this is rare.

Most disc herniation is thought to be due to torsional strain rather than to compression loads. Data suggest that men who spend 50% or more of their work time driving a motor vehicle are three times more likely to develop a herniated disc than those in other occupations. This may be due to vibration forces that are transmitted to the spine as well as the fact that sitting puts more pressure on the disc (34). The restricted position of the legs may also predispose to disc herniation. Jobs involving heavy lifting, pushing, pulling, or carrying do not seem to be significantly related to lumbar disc disease. Weight lifting and bending are not among the factors frequently associated with radiculopathy.

Clinical Considerations

History. Patients with disc herniation are usually between the ages of 30 and 50 years. They have frequently had prior episodes of low back pain. They may relate a precipitating event such as lifting, twisting, or heaving a heavy object, but may only recount a minimal provocation incident. It is not unusual to hear "I just bent down to tie my shoes" or "I

bent over to pick up the soap in the shower" from a patient with a herniated disc.

Signs and Symptoms. The patient with a herniated disc may complain of back pain, leg pain, or back and leg pain (Fig. 8.43). Often the back pain disappears with the onset of leg pain. The pain is made worse by forward bending, coughing, or sneezing and is relieved by rest in the recumbent position with the knees flexed. Placing the patient in the 90/90 position can determine this and suggests the possibility of a trial traction therapy in this position.

Commonly, numbness (hypoesthesia) can be detected over one dermatome on pinwheel testing (Fig. 8.44). Muscle weakness may be evident on heel walking or toe walking or by more direct testing of the quadriceps, dorsiflexors, and plantar flexors of

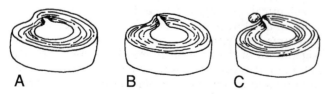

Figure 8.42. Degrees of herniated nucleus pulposus (HNP). **A**, Disc protrusion. **B**, Nuclear material protrudes into the spinal canal. **C**, Sequestration of nuclear material.

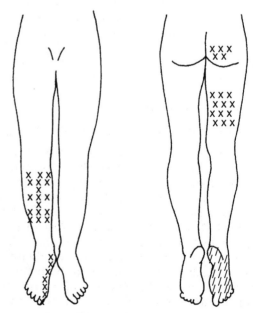

Figure 8.43. Pain diagram of a patient with a herniated L4 disc. The patient exhibited buttock and lower extremity pain but no back pain. Symbols: (×) aching, (/) stabbing pain.

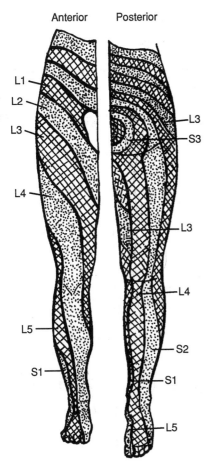

Figure 8.44. Lower extremity dermatomes.

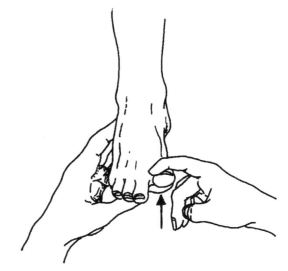

Figure 8.45. Weakness of the extensor hallucis longus is an early indicator of an L5 nerve root lesion.

the ankles (Figs. 8.14 and 8.15). Weakness of the great toe should alert the examiner to the possibility of disc herniation affecting the L5 neurological level, since this is often one of the first indicators (Fig. 8.45). The knee or ankle reflex may be markedly diminished or absent, depending on the level of herniation (Fig. 8.46).

All movements are restricted and an antalgic list is common. Straight-leg raising is frequently markedly diminished, with adjunctive tests used to further differentiate the diagnosis. Centrally located protrusions tend to produce low back pain and leg pain. Leg pain only is commonly produced by laterally located protrusions.

Radiographic findings are of limited value; however, the lateral view may demonstrate a slight reduction in disc height. AP lateral-bending views give an indication of the level of involvement, but are not definitive by themselves (see Chapter 6). The radiographic changes are characteristic of the unstable phase of disc degeneration. A small area of lucency adjacent to the upper or lower part of the vertebral body may be present (Fig. 8.47A). A minor degree of retrolisthesis may be noted in the lateral view (Fig. 8.47B).

MRI and CT scanners have replaced myelography in the diagnosis of lumbar spine lesions (107–108). Bony structures are well visualized, and with high-resolution scanning, it is now possible to demonstrate soft-tissue shadows. Magnetic resonance imaging (MRI) has proven a valuable adjunct to computed tomography, providing markedly improved soft-tissue contrast resolution of lumbar discs or neural elements (123). The more invasive myelography is commonly reserved now for verification of CT and MRI findings when the patient is deemed a surgical candidate. The water-soluble contrast medium, metrizamide, creates fewer side effects than the previously used oil-based contrast medium. Headaches, nausea, and vomiting are not as common or as persistent with metrizamide, which reduces the risk of arachnoiditis (108).

Antalgic lean is also indicative of the position of protrusion. When the disc protrudes lateral to the nerve root, the patient assumes an antalgic lean away from the side of radicular symptoms (Fig. 8.48A). When the disc protrudes medial to the nerve root (in the axilla), the patient assumes an antalgic lean into the side of radicular symptoms (Fig 8.48B). With a central disc lesion, the patient assumes a flexed posture guarding against hyperextension (68).

Chiropractic Management of Disc Herniation. A herniated disc does not preclude spinal manipulative therapy. A conservative trial of distraction manipulation or side-posture manipulation can help to reduce the symptoms of disc herniation and should be employed along with 90/90 traction in the absence of advancing neurological defects or cauda equina syndrome. Mathew and Yates (124) have demonstrated reduction in the size of the disc herniation using epidurography before and after manipulation.

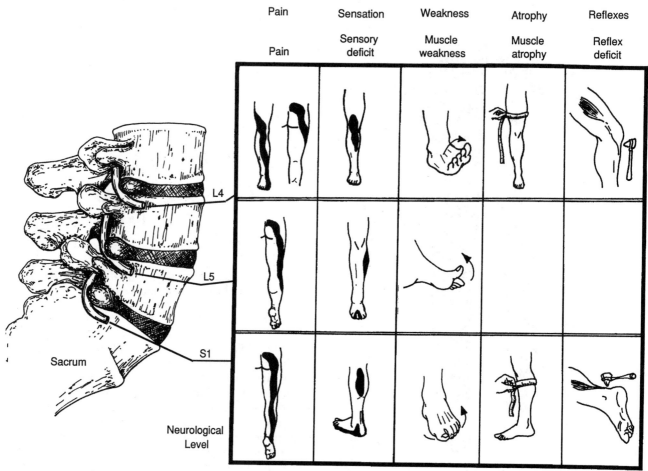

Figure 8.46. Clinical findings of herniated nucleus pulposus (HNP) by disc level.

Cox (68) recommends flexion-distraction manipulation for the treatment of lumbar disc protrusion, suggesting that this allows the intervertebral disc to resume its central position within the annulus and relieves irritation of the pain-sensitive annular fibers.

In many patients, a few days of bed rest followed by wearing an elastic support, an exercise program, and instruction in back care will result in marked relief of symptoms (122). The indications for discectomy are pain of continuing severity, increase in neurological deficit, or the onset of bladder and bowel symptoms. In such cases, prompt referral for a neurological evaluation is imperative. Removal of the disc herniation can usually be done safely and often produces a dramatic result. Fusion is rarely needed, and manipulation, exercise, and an elastic support are often effective following surgery (122).

Lateral Spinal Nerve Entrapment

Entrapment of the spinal nerve lateral to the spinal canal may occur with disc herniation, subluxation of the posterior joint, and osteophyte outgrowth (107). The lateral canal extends from the dura to the foramen. Entrapment occurs between the medial facet and the foramen (108).

When the disc degenerates, the posterior facet capsule becomes lax and permits subluxation of the facet joints. The internal disruption of the disc results in loss of disc height and stability, with annular bulging. Subluxation follows, with the superior facet joints slipping upward and forward, producing a narrowing of the lateral canal, medial to the intervertebral foramen (Fig. 8.49), and a diminution in the size of the intervertebral foramen.

Laxity of the facet capsule allows the superior facet to move backward and forward with flexion, extension, and rotation (108). Kirkaldy-Willis (108) refers to this type of lesion as a recurrent dynamic entrapment. He differentiates this from lateral entrapment with a fixed deformity, which occurs when the degenerative changes are sufficiently advanced to stabilize the affected segment. The narrowing of the canal is then fixed because of permanent deformity, with little or no movement at the affected level. Osteophytic overgrowth further narrows the lateral canal as degenerative changes advance.

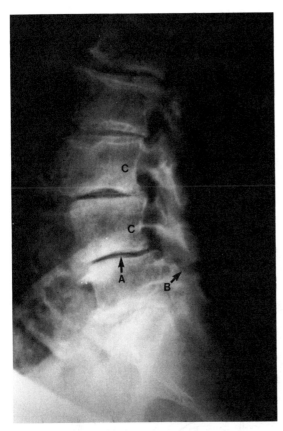

Figure 8.47. Signs of disc instability. (A) Vacuum phenomenon, (B) Retrolisthesis, (C) Anterolisthesis.

Lateral spine stenosis produces complaints of buttock and lower extremity pain. Exertional claudication involving only one extremity is common. Definitive diagnosis is dependent on enhanced imaging (108).

Computerized tomography can determine the patency of the radicular canal. MRI is a valuable adjunct to CT in the evaluation of lateral spinal stenosis. Tests for dynamic lateral entrapment include rotational and hyperextension stress of the lumbar spine (108).

Rotational stress may be applied with the patient lying on the painful side. With the doctor standing behind the patient, the shoulder is stabilized with one hand as the pelvis is rotated away from the doctor with the other hand.

Rotation may be applied with the patient standing as well. The doctor stands behind the patient and holds the pelvis firmly, while an assistant stands in front of the patient and rotates the shoulders to one side and then the other. Increased pain on rotation or hyperextension is indicative of lateral spinal nerve entrapment.

Passive hyperextension of the spine can be achieved with the patient prone. The examiner presses lightly over the lumbar spine with one hand, while the other flexes the knees and extends the hips (108). The hyperextension produced by this maneuver may result in leg pain, which occurs because the lateral canal is narrowed by forward displacement of the superior articular process. These tests are not conclusive and results are not always positive, even when dynamic lateral stenosis is present (41).

Chiropractic management of lateral spinal nerve entrapment is more effective for recurrent dynamic entrapment, but it has shown benefit in some cases with fixed deformity. Kirkaldy-Willis (41) reports that 50% of patients with lateral entrapment were markedly improved by manipulation and as a result did not require surgery. Manipulation of the spine with flexion and axial rotation in the pain-free directions opens up the lateral canal and foramen, providing relief of symptoms due to lateral spinal nerve entrapment (41). An exercise program and instruction in back care are helpful, but care should be taken not to overdo rotational exercises, as these may increase the entrapment in the lateral recess.

Wiltse et al. (125) have described entrapment of the L5 spinal nerve between the sacral ala and the transverse process. Referred to as "the far-out syndrome," this syndrome occurs in the elderly person with degenerative scoliosis and in younger adults with isthmic spondylolisthesis and at least 20% slip. The symptoms are classical for nerve root impingement, and referral for decompression should be made promptly.

Spinal Stenosis

Goldthwait (126) in 1911 was probably the first to note that cauda equina compression could be precipitated by hyperextension of the low back. Early work by Verbiest (127, 128) in the 1950s identified developmental stenosis of the lumbar spinal canal as a factor in the production of intermittent claudication. Later authors (129, 135) have delineated various other causes for spinal stenosis including degenerative arthritis (130), vertebral-body fracture (41) isthmic spondylolisthesis, fibrous tissue formation following surgery, hypertrophic bone formation following fusion (131), hypertrophy of the ligamentum flava (132), and pathological enlargement of the vertebral body (133). The sequela of spinal stenosis is compromise of the dura and cauda equina or spinal nerves.

Developmental stenosis occurs during growth years, which results in a narrowing of the spinal canal in the coronal or sagittal diameter or both. Narrowing can occur at one or more levels and can involve the entire lumbar spinal canal (131). In many cases, this anomaly does not cause symptoms but leaves less margin for safety when coupled with a small disc herniation or minor degenerative pathology. In these cases, the developmental stenosis becomes an enhancing factor that causes a minor lesion to become symptomatic (41). Collapse of a vertebral body due to compression fracture may result

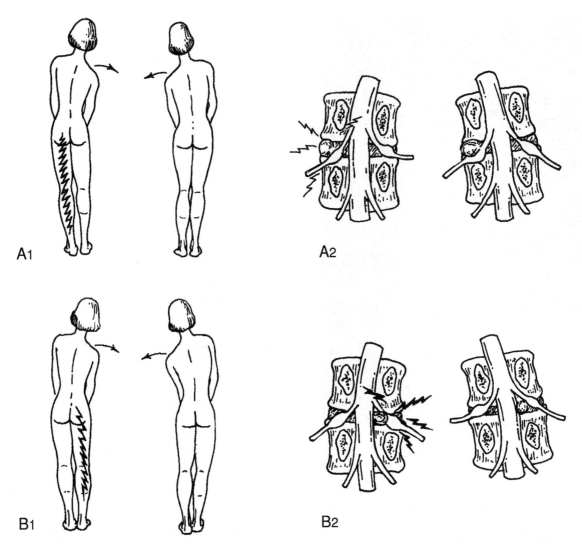

A1

A2

B1

B2

Figure 8.48. **A,** A patient with disc protrusion lateral to the nerve root exhibits an antalgic lean toward the side of radicular symptoms. **B,** Pain from a protrusion medial to the nerve root is relieved when the patient assumes an antalgic lean away from the side of radicular symptoms.

in narrowing of the bony canal (41). While not evident immediately following fracture, late changes can produce symptoms attributable to canal stenosis.

Degenerative spondylosis occurs mainly at the L4–5 level in patients over 60 years of age (131), but it may be encountered at L3–4, L5-S1, and other levels. Stenosis is produced mainly by osteophytic enlargement of the inferior facets and retrolisthesis of the upper or lower vertebra, which accompanies marked reduction of disc height due to the degenerative process. This encroachment of the central canal may begin with the unstable spine and progress during the phase of stabilization. Compromise of the cauda equina and its blood vessels may occur, and to a lesser extent the individual spinal nerves may become involved.

Isthmic spondylolisthesis can produce narrowing of the spinal canal cephalad to the pars interarticu-laris separation. At the L5-S1 level, the L5 nerve becomes entrapped by the body of L4 as the body of L5 slips anteriorly (108). Postsurgical complications can result in spinal canal stenosis by fibrosis tissue scarring following laminectomy and hypertrophic bone formation following fusion (131). Pathological enlargement of a vertebral body, due to Paget's disease (134), may cause spinal canal stenosis.

The signs and symptoms of central spinal stenosis are frequently described as bizarre (132). In addition to back pain, the patient complains of pain in one or both legs (Fig. 8.50). Neurogenic claudication occurs after walking 3–4 blocks, and the patient must stop. Night pain on recumbency is relieved by walking around the room. The patient may complain of bizarre paresthesias of the legs. Neurologic deficits are atypical and may be suggestive of malignancy. CT scanning and MRI may reveal stenosis at one or more levels. Myelography may be useful to confirm

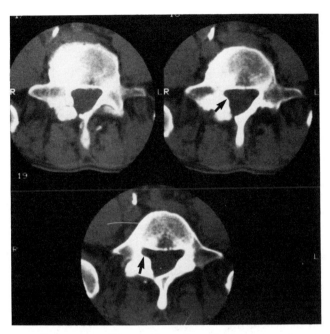

Figure 8.49. CT scan shows lateral recess stenosis.

the diagnosis (see "Lateral Spinal Nerve Entrapment").

Conservative management of central spinal stenosis includes an exercise program with instruction in back care. An elastic back support may help some patients with the syndrome. Reduction of the lumbar lordosis through pelvic tilt exercises and assumption of the 90/90 position with hips and legs flexed at 90° have proven the most beneficial. Stenosis may be reduced by flexion and accentuated by

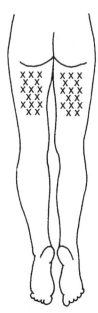

Figure 8.50. Patients with spinal stenosis complain of bizarre symptoms including bilateral leg pain. Symbol: (×) pain.

extension. Manipulation may bring dramatic relief and should not be discounted (107). Laminectomy with decompression of the cauda equina and spinal nerves may be necessary if conservative methods fail to relieve severe pain, when walking is severely restricted, or bizarre sensory changes become intolerable.

Venous Hypertension

Venous hypertension may produce pain by causing pressure on small nerves in bone, annulus fibrosus, or ligaments. It may also interfere with the circulation of the spinal nerves in the intervertebral foramen (IVF) or those of the cauda equina, producing complaints of bizarre sensations in the legs of the patient with spinal stenosis (108). Hayland, Freemont, and Jayson (136) have proposed that venous obstruction in the IVF associated with disc herniation through disc protrusion causes compression of veins and may be an important pathogenic mechanism in the development of perineural and intraneural fibrosis.

It remains to be demonstrated whether spinal manipulation increases venous drainage. It can be postulated that pain due to ischemia as a result of reduced venous outflow can be relieved by manipulation. This would account for the relief following manipulation seen in some patients with bizarre leg symptoms and in cases with disc protrusion causing compression of veins, which produces venous stasis and ischemia.

Segmental Hypermobility and Instability

Disturbances of function of the vertebral motion segments include hypermobility (hyperkinesia) as well as hypomobility (hypokinesia) and aberrant movement (dyskinesia). Obviously, manipulation is concerned with movement restriction (137), whether totally blocked segmental movement or aberrant movement due to a shifting in the axis of rotation. In general, restricted movement at one segment produces hypermobility in another (137, 138).

Segmental hypermobility is frequently a difficult problem to treat, in addition to being of considerable significance for pathogenesis (135, 139). Differentiation between segmental hypermobility and instability remains controversial. Grieve (140) contributes to the debate by describing a hypermobile joint as an overflexible link in a series of articulated bodies—a chain of joints, each with a norm of available movement. "By comparison then, there is aberrant segmental mobility, which need not be so in all its degrees of freedom." He notes that "it does not follow that the joint is therefore unstable."

Muhlemann (141) states that "hypermobile joints or segments commonly preserve their stability under normal conditions, i.e. they are functional as far as weight bearing and motion with certain limits go." Grieve (140) elaborates that "excessions of movement (repetitively imposed by gliding and twisting coupled with angular or distraction forces are greater than in adjacent segments sustaining the same stress, before deceleration effects are exerted by restraining factors e.g. disc muscles, ligaments, etc.''

Grieve (140) further notes that the stresses sustained by the restraining structures of the vertebral motion segment are likely to be greater in the loose joint, as a minutely larger momentum of movement is damped. He suggests that the inexorable accumulation of minute delayed restraints must eventually tax restraining structures in a proportion of individuals, leading to covert instability. Muhlemann (141) supports this, stating that "hypermobility can evolve into segmental instability," cautioning that "instability" should be used exclusively to refer to clear pathomorphologic derangements and changes, not for any unspecified increase in mobility.

White and Panjabi (23) define clinical instability as "the loss of the ability of the spine under physiologic loads to maintain relationships between vertebrae in such a way that there is neither damage nor subsequent irritation to the spinal cord or nerve roots and, in addition, there is no development of incapacitating deformities or pain due to structural changes."

Following these definitions, segmental hypermobility can be considered to be a reversible physiological joint dysfunction, while instability denotes a pathological process with morphological changes of the joint structures. Farfan (18) notes that sprained intervertebral joints become unstable when either the original injury was too great or the injury was repeated. In either case the increased deformability of the joint becomes permanent.

Clinically, the difference between segmental hypermobility and instability appears to be the reversibility of the articular dyskinesia. The biomechanics of functional incompetence (hypermobility and instability) of vertebral motion segments is characterized by an increase in translatory movement. Excessive intersegmental translatory movement can be determined by palpatory examination (141) and radiographic findings (135, 140, 142) (Chapter 6).

Etiology

The etiology of segmental instability appears varied and includes those situations that produce factors of overload by axial compression and axial torsion (52, 53, 107, 132, 143). Causes may be trauma, occupational stress, activities requiring excessive flexibility (e.g., gymnastics and ballet), hormonal influences (pregnancy and the effects of estrogen medication), compensation for adjacent hypomobile segments (congenital, functional, or surgical), generalized joint laxness, infections, neoplasms, and metabolic bone disease (138–140, 144).

While segmental hypermobility of the spine can occur in any individual, it is much more likely to occur if the person exhibits generalized hypermobil-

ity (constitutional hypermobility) (140, 145). Stoddard (145) suggests that the etiology of hypermobile lumbar lesions involves:

1. A severe initial sprain caused by hyperflexion injury;
2. Habitual ligamentous strain from faulty sitting posture, habitual standing on one leg, an anatomical short leg, or pregnancy;
3. Degenerative processes involving the discs and the ligaments of the vertebral complex.

Grieve (146) notes that "a degree of localized or generalized degenerative change may be hastened by repetitive and unusually vigorous manipulation—one of the most common errors in manipulative work is failure to recognize the hypermobile lumbar segment." Stoddard (145) emphasizes that "if subluxation or joint bind has occurred, the joint should be manipulated and then treated as a simple sprain. It should not be repeatedly manipulated."

Clinical Findings

The early symptoms of joint hypermobility are a mild, aching, low back pain during activities that place strain on the previously stretched ligaments. Prolonged bending or sitting in a slumped position can overstretch supraspinous and interspinous ligaments in the lumbar area. Initially, symptoms may be delayed because stretch must be sustained before the relaxed ligaments become painful. With repeated strain the ligaments become more irritable, and the length of delayed pain becomes shorter and shorter, until eventually the pain may be felt at the moment of stretch (145).

A careful history will indicate that the symptoms appear after increasingly shorter periods of the precipitating activities (145). Early complaints of stiffness and dull low back pain are followed later by symptoms of muscle tightness or spasm. The loss of ligamentous control becomes compensated for by muscles, with reflex contractions initiated by joint mechanoreceptors and muscle spindles (140).

Dynamic activities do not cause discomfort at the time of participation but are followed by increased pain, minutes to hours afterwards, depending on the severity of the condition and the activity thereafter (141). Eventually, maintaining any position causing axial pressure on the spine for more than a few minutes results in an increase in symptoms, and physical activity that exceeds the normal will cause pain upon cessation (141).

Much psychic distress is created by failure to recognize this condition. The patient is rarely comfortable, and the hypermobile state is frequently mislabeled as functional or psychogenic. Moderate to heavy physical labor is impossible for such patients because they are "punished" by pain following increased activity. Grieve notes that "this can only go on for so long before an apparently unrelated and sometimes trivial event, out of all porportion to its effects, transforms a quiescent state of affairs into a full blown, prolonged and sometimes crippling back pain episode" (140).

Examination

Postural evaluation of patients with hypermobile vertebral segments typically reveals hyperlordosis when standing and exaggerated lumbar kyphosis when sitting relaxed (135). Frequently a crease can be observed at the level of increased movement on ROM testing of extension or lateral bending. Overall, ROM is not restricted in the absence of acute muscle spasm. Motion palpation is of utmost importance, since both hypomobile and hypermobile segments can cause the same symptoms (140, 145).

Palpation of hypermobile joints reveals a boggy type of end-feel, with edematous soft tissue overlying the involved segment. The following tests for hypermobility reported by Muhlemann (141) are specifically designed to evaluate translatory segmental movement, which is indicative of hypermobility:

1. With the patient prone and the lumbar spine supported in neutral position by a cushion, the doctor moves the inferior segment with the thenar eminence of one hand while stabilizing the superior segment with the other. It is important to return to the neutral position each time the test is performed at a new segment. Translatory motion at each segment can then be evaluated.

2. With the patient in side posture, the hips flexed to 60°, and the knees at 90°, translatory motion is palpated between the spinous processes as the doctor produces anterior and posterior translation of the vertebral segments through the pelvis via the femora. Movement must be parallel to the disc plane of the segment to be evaluated, with the segment tested in neutral position. Other positions decrease translational gliding motion.

3. With the patient supine and hips and knees flexed as above, the doctor's hand palpates anterior glide of the lumbar vertebra between the spinous processes. With the doctor's hand beneath the patient and contacting the spinous processes, the patient attempts to lift the thigh by action of the psoas major muscle. Contraction of the psoas muscles will cause anterior glide of the lumbar vertebra due to its attachment to the bodies, discs, and transverse processses.

To be successful, each test depends on complete relaxation of the patient, with the segment tested in neutral position. The direction of translatory motion induced by the doctor must be parallel to the disc plane (141).

Radiographic Findings

Radiographic findings of hypermobility are indicated by excessive translation observed in lateral views of the extremes of flexion/extension and on AP views of the extremes of lateral bending (Chapter 6). The presence of gas in the disc (the Knuttson airvacuum phenomenon) is considered by some as indicative of instability (25, 141). Small traction spurs are described by MacNab as indicative of abnormal instability, while large traction spurs indicate that the segment has been unstable for some time in the past but may be stable now (25).

MacNab also describes other specific radiological changes of segmental instability such as disc narrowing, rocking or flexion/extension films, and posterior joint subluxations (147). Lumbar instability was observed by Friberg (148) by producing a physiological posterior glide on translational movement through traction compression, using a loaded backpack to pull the patients into a position of slight extension, viewed on lateral radiographs.

Chiropractic Management of Hypermobility Syndrome

Initial treatment includes manipulation of adjacent hypomobile segments by the use of specific, short-lever, segmental thrusts, avoiding undue stress on the hypermobile segment. Stretching of tight muscles (which may include the iliopsoas, rectus femoris, tensor fascia latae, hamstrings, piriformis, and quadratus lumborum) with specific trigger-point therapy, especially in the segmental muscles, is also helpful.

After 4–6 weeks, Muhlemann (141) recommends stabilization exercises utilizing isometric contraction, with short levers moving to continuously longer levers while avoiding trunk movement. He also recommends guided and optimally measurable resistance exercises after 8–12 weeks to develop static endurance through maximum strength (141).

An increase in overall fitness is strongly recommended through a graduated aerobic program. Fisk (149) considers walking the best exercise for patients with hypermobile backs. Lewit (135) recommends swimming, with the backstroke and crawl best for a hypermobile back. Breast stroke and butterfly are not recommended, because they tend to produce hyperlordosis of the lumbar spine.

NONORGANIC PHYSICAL SIGNS IN LOW BACK PAIN

Waddell et al. (150) have identified and standardized nonorganic signs in low back pain that correlate with other psychological data (Table 8.4). By helping to separate the physical from the psychological condition, they can be used as a simple clinical screen to help identify patients who require a more extensive psychological assessment. The examination technique involves five types of physical signs. A positive sign for that type of physical finding counts as one, with three or more of the five types clinically significant.

Tenderness related to physical disease is usually localized with nonorganic tenderness, either superficial or nonanatomic. Superficial tenderness is indicated if the patient is sensitive to light touch over

Table 8.4 Nonorganic Physical Signs in Low Back Pain[a]

Physical Sign[b]	Type	Example of Patient Reaction
1. Tenderness	Superficial nonanatomic	Pain response to light touch, pain over wide area
2. Simulation	Axial loading/rotation	Axial loading back pain/back pain when shoulder and pelvis are rotated in the same plane
3. Distraction	Indirect observation	Patient can cross legs to remove shoes but is unable to assume the same position on figure-of-four (Patrick's) test
	Indirect testing	90° sitting straight leg (flip test) with marked restriction of straight-leg raising while supine
4. Regional	Weakness	Partial cogwheel, "give-away" of multiple muscle groups
	Sensory	Stocking or glove distribution of sensory disturbance
5. Overreaction	Magnification of symptoms	Disproportionate verbalization, facial expression, muscle tension and tremor collapsing, or sweating

[a]Modified from Waddell G, McCulloch JA, Kummel E, Venner RM: Nonorganic physical signs in low back pain. *Spine* 5:117–123, 1980.
[b]Any individual sign counts as a positive nonorganic sign for that type, a finding of three or more of the five types is clinically significant. The examiner must avoid observer bias and rule out those conditions that can produce a patient response similar to any of the five types (see text). The nonorganic signs should be correlated with other clinical nonorganic assessment.

a wide area of lumbar skin. A localized band in a posterior primary ramus distribution may be caused by nerve irritation and should be discounted. Patients with fibromyalgia are sensitive to superficial touch over a wide area also, and differentiation of this entity must be considered (Chapter 12). Nonanatomic tenderness felt over a wide area that is not localized to one structure may be nonorganic. Nonanatomic tenderness may extend to the thoracic spine, sacrum, or pelvis, but with superficial tenderness. Muscle pain syndromes can give a false positive result (Chapter 12).

Simulation tests give the patient the impression that a particular examination is being carried out, when in fact it is not. Simulation tests are usually based on movement producing pain. If a particular movement causes the patient to report pain, that movement is then simulated without actually being performed. If pain is reported on simulation, a nonorganic influence is suggested. Axial loading produced by vertical compression over the standing patient's skull is positive for simulation if low-back pain is reported. Neck pain is commonly produced by this procedure and should be discounted. Passive rotation of the patient, with the shoulders and pelvis fixed in the same plane, is positive if the patient complains of low back pain. In the presence of root irritation, leg pain may be produced and should be discounted.

If distraction or indirect testing are inconsistent with direct testing, then this constitutes a positive nonorganic sign. A positive physical finding is demonstrated in a routine manner and then tested indirectly or with the patient's attention distracted. The distraction must be nonpainful, unemotional, and nonsurprising. Indirect observation of the patient is the simplest form of indirect testing, as the patient is unaware of being examined. Removing the shoes and stockings, with the ankle of one foot placed on the knee of the other, tests for hip function, as does the figure-of-four test. Supine straight-leg raising can be compared to the sitting straight-leg raise in this manner, as can forward bending with the legs

extended in both the standing and seated position. Any finding that is consistently present is likely to be physically based. Findings that are present in formal testing but disappear at other times may have a nonorganic component.

Regional disturbances that diverge from accepted neuroanatomy may indicate a nonorganic problem and should be noted. Stocking-and-glove paresthesias or involvement of the entire leg, a quarter, or half of the body are suspect. Patients with peripheral neuropathy or muscle pain syndromes may have physical problems exhibiting this pattern, and these conditions must be ruled out. Weakness demonstrated on formal testing by a partial cogwheel "give-way" of many muscle groups unexplained on a localized neurological basis constitutes a positive nonorganic sign, as does nondermatomal sensory change. Waddell et al. (150) warn that care must be taken, particularly in patients who have spinal stenosis or who have had repeated spinal surgery, not to mistake multiple root involvement for a regional disturbance.

Overreaction during examination may take the form of disproportionate verbalization, facial expression, muscle tension, and tremor, collapsing, or pulling away.

Three nonorganic signs out of the five categories (tenderness, simulation tests, distraction tests, regional signs, and overreaction to examination) indicate a psychological component, which should be further investigated through psychometeric testing (150).

Conclusion

Successful management of low back pain requires that the treatment be directed to the pain-producing structures. It is not possible to formulate a rational therapeutic approach without a precise diagnosis that recognizes both the biomechanical and the pathological condition of the patient. Bernard and Kirkaldy-Willis (151) reported that of 1293 cases of low back pain evaluated, 33.5% of the patients presented with combined lesions. They noted that referred pain syndromes occurred nearly twice as often as nerve-root compression syndrome, with posterior joint syndrome and sacroiliac joint syndrome the most common referred-pain syndromes. Muscle syndromes were also common but less recognized as causes of low back pain.

Spinal manipulation is one of the oldest forms of therapy for back pain. Of the over 50 clinical trials of spinal manipulation for back pain conducted since 1952, most have shown that manipulation tends to shorten the episode of pain (43). Coupled with adjunctive procedures, chiropractic manipulation provides relief for many patients suffering from disorders of the lumbar spine.

References

1. Schmorl G, Junghanns H: *The Human Spine in Health and Disease*, ed 2. New York, Grune & Stratton, 1971, pp 55, 60, 64–65, 94, 223, 377–378, 398, 415–417, 419.
2. Cox JM: Statistical data on facet facings of the lumbar spine. *ACA J Chiro* 14:S-39–S-49, 1977.
3. Helfet AJ, Gruebel Lee DM: *Disorders of the Lumbar Spine*. Philadelphia, JB Lippincott, 1978, pp 21, 28, 161.
4. Steindler A: *Kinesiology of the Human Body under Normal and Pathological Conditions*. Springfield, IL, Charles C Thomas, 1973, pp 13, 163, 165–166, 175, 376.
5. Cassidy JD, Kirkaldy-Willis WH, McGregor M: Spinal manipulation for the treatment of chronic low back and leg pain: an observational study. In Buerger AA, Greenman PE (eds.): *Empirical Approaches to the Validation of Spinal Manipulation*. Springfield, IL, Charles C Thomas, 1985, pp 119–147.
6. Finneson BE: *Low Back Pain*, ed 2. Philadelphia, JB Lippincott, 1980, pp 6–7, 45–46, 50, 54, 69, 282–285, 428–432, 541.
7. Warwick R, Williams PL: *Gray's Anatomy*, ed 35, British. Philadelphia, WB Saunders, 1973, pp 240, 282, 410, 412–414, 513, 516.
8. King AI, Prasad P, Ewing CL: Mechanism of spinal injury due to caudocephalad acceleration. *Orthop Clin North Am* 6:19, 1975.
9. Adams MA, Hutton WC: The effect of posture on the role of the apophyseal joints in resisting intervertebral compression forces. *J Bone Joint Surg* 62-B 3, pp 358–362, 1980.
10. Yong-Hing K, Reilly J, Kirkaldy-Willis WH: The ligamentum flavum. *Spine* 1:226–234, 1976.
11. Maigne R: *Orthopedic Medicine: A New Approach to Vertebral Manipulations*. Springfield, IL, Charles C Thomas, 1972, pp 9, 282, 285.
12. DeSez S: Les accidents de la deterioration structurale due disque. *Sem Hop Paris*, 6–30–55, pp 2267–2290.
13. Lewit K: The contribution of clinical observation to neurobiological mechanisms in manipulative therapy. In Korr IM (ed): *The Neurobiological Mechanisms in Manipulative Therapy*. New York, Plenum, 1978, pp 3–25.
14. Wolf J: The reversible deformation of the joint cartilage surface and its possible role in joint blockage. In Proceedings of the 4th Congress of the International Federation of Manual Medicine, Prague, *Rehabiliticia* (supp) 10–13:30, 1975.
15. Giles LGF: Lumbar apophyseal joint arthrography *JMPT* 7(1): 21–24, 1984.
16. Engel R, Bogduk N: The menisci of the lumbar zygapophyseal joints. *J Anat* 135(4):795, 1982.
17. Bogduk N, Engel R: The menisci of the lumbar zygapophyseal joints: a review of their anatomy and clinical significance. *Spine* 9:454–460, 1980.
18. Farfan HF: *Mechanical Disorders of the Low Back*. Philadelphia, Lea & Febiger, 1973, pp 17–18, 27, 33, 51, 69, 181, 204, 217.
19. Cailliet R: *Low Back Pain Syndrome*, ed 2. Philadelphia, FA Davis, 1968, pp 1, 7, 23–24, 74, 253–254, 567.
20. Tyrell AR, Reilly T, Troup JDG: Circadian variations in stature and the effects of spinal loading. *Spine* 10:2, 161–164, 1985.
21. Adams MA, Polan P, Hutton WC: Diurnal variations in the stresses in the lumbar spine, *Spine* 12:130-137, 1987.
22. Morris JM: Biomechanics of the lumbar spine. In Finneson BE: *Low Back Pain*, ed 2. Philadelphia, JB Lippincott, 1978, p 30.
23. White AA, Panjabi MM: *Clinical Biomechanics of the Spine*. Philadelphia, JB LIppincott, 1978, pp 15, 18, 79, 182, 192, 228.
24. Golub BS, Silverman B: Transforaminal ligaments of the lumbar spine. *J Bone Joint Surg (Am)* 51A:947–956, 1969.
25. MacNab I: *Backache*. Baltimore, Williams & Wilkins, 1977, pp 53, 85, 97, 125, 282.
26. Drum D: The vertebral motor unit and intervertebral foramen. In Goldstein (ed): *The Research Status of Spinal Manipulative Therapy*. Bethesda, US Department of Health, Education and Welfare, 1975, pp 67–75.
27. Bachop W, Stern H: The transforaminal ligaments in the straight leg raising test of Laseque. Twelfth Annual Biomechanics Conference on the Spine. University of Boulder, CO, Dec 1981.
28. Bogduk N: The innervation of the lumbar spine. *Spine* 8:286–293, 1983.
29. Reilly J, Yong-Hing K, MacKay RW, Kirkaldy-Willis WH: Pathological anatomy of the lumbar spine. In Helfet AJ, Gruebel Lee DM: *Disorders of the Lumbar Spine*. Philadelphia, JB Lippincott, 1978.
30. Epstein JA, et al: *The Spine: A Radiological Text and Atlas*, ed 3. Philadelphia, Lea & Febiger, 1969, p 182.
31. Kapandji IA: *The Physiology of the Joints, Vol III: The Trunk and Vertebral Column*, ed 2. Edinburgh, Churchill Livingstone, 1978, pp 30, 32, 38, 80.
32. Brown T, Hansen RJ, Yorra AJ: Some mechanical tests on the lumbosacral spine with particular reference to the intervertebral disc: a preliminary report. *J Bone Joint Surg (Am)* 39A:1135, 1957.
33. Krag MH, Serousi RE, Wilder DG, Pope M: Internal displacement distribution from in vitro loading of human spinal motion segments: experimental results and theoretical prediction. *Spine* 12(10): 1001–1007, 1987.
34. Nachemson A: The lumbar spine: an orthopedic challenge. *Spine* 1:40, 59–71, 1976.
35. Allbrook D: Movements of the lumbar spinal column. *J Bone Joint Surg (Br)* 39B:339–345, 1957.
36. Twomey LT, Taylor JR: A quantitative study of the role of the posterior vertebral elements in sagittal movements of the lumbar vertebral column. In Glasgow EF, Twomey LT, Scull AM, Kleynhams AM, Jaczak RM: *Aspects of Manipulative Therapy*, ed 2. New York, Churchill Livingstone, 1985, p 38.
37. Lovett RW: The mechanism of the normal spine and its relation to scoliosis. *Boston Med Surg J* Vol Ch III N131:349-358, 1905.
38. Tanz SS: Motion of the lumbar spine. *Am J Roentgenol* 69:399–412, 1953.
39. Pearcy MJ, Tibrewal SB: Axial rotation and lateral bending in the normal lumbar spine measured by three-dimensional radiography. *Spine* 9:582–587, 1984.
40. Farfan HF: The scientific basis of manipulative procedures. In Graham R: *Clinics in Rheumatic Disease*. Philadelphia, WB Saunders, 1980, vol 6, pp 158–177.
41. Kirkaldy-Willis: *Managing Low Back Pain*, New York, Churchill Livingstone, 1983, pp 24, 37, 94, 99, 180–181.
42. Bogduk N, Jull G: The theoretical pathology of acute locked back: a basis for manipulative therapy. *Manual Medicine* 1:23–43, 78–82, 96, 1985.
43. Kirkaldy-Willis WH, Cassidy JD: Spinal manipulation in the treatment of low back pain. *Can Fam Physician* 31:535–540, 1985.

44. Mennell JM: *Back Pain*, Boston, Little, Brown & Co, 1960, pp 67, 148, 151, 169.
45. Shaefer RC: *Basic Chiropractic Procedural Manual*, ed 2. Des Moines, Iowa, 1977, ACA II-18, II 25.
46. Magee DJ: *Orthopedic Physical Assessment*. Philadelphia, WB Saunders, 1987, p 191.
47. Hoppenfeld: *Physical Examination of the Spine and Extremities*. East Norwalk, CT, Appleton-Century-Crofts, 1976, p 156.
48. Chrisman OD, Mittnacht A, Snook G: A study of the results following rotatory manipulation in the lumbar intervertebral disc syndrome. *J Bone Joint Surg* 46A:517–524, 1964.
49. Bourdillon JF: *Spinal Manipulation*. East Norwalk, CT, Appleton-Century-Crofts, 1982, pp 128–132, 148, 181–182, 186.
50. Stoddard A: *Manual of Osteopathic Technique*. London, Hutchinson, 1980, pp 203–205, 241–246.
51. Farfan HF, Cossette JW, Robertson GH, Wells RV, Kraus H: The effects of torsion on the lumbar intervertebral joints: the role of torsion in the production of disc degeneration. *J Bone Joint Surg* 52A:468–497, 1970.
52. Farfan HF, Huberdeau RM, Dubow HI: Lumbar intervertebral disc degeneration: the influence of geometric features on the pattern of disc degeneration. *J Bone Joint Surg* 54A:492–510, 1972.
53. Farfan HF, Cossette JW, Robertson GH, Wells RV: The instantaneous center of rotation of the third lumbar intervertebral joint. *J Biomech* 4:149, 1971.
54. Farfan HF: Symptomology in terms of the pathomechanics of low back pain and sciatica.
55. Richard J: Disc rupture with cauda equina syndrome after chiropractic adjustment. *NY State J Med* 67:249, 1967.
56. Hooper J: Low back pain and manipulation, paraparesis after treatment of low back pain by physical methods. *Med J Aust* 1:549, 1973.
57. Gitelman R: A chiropractic approach to biomechanical disorders of the lumbar spine and pelvis. In Haldeman S: *Modern Developments in the Principles and Practice of Chiropractic*. East Norwalk, CT, Appleton-Century-Crofts, 1980, pp 312–319.
58. Faye LF: *Motion Palpation of the Spine* (seminar and videotape). Motion Palpation Institute, Huntington Beach, CA, 1981.
59. Peterson DH, Panzer DM, Muhlemann D: *Biomechanics-Palpation Manual*. Portland, OR, Western States Chiropractic College, 1987, pp 52–53, 125–129.
60. Cassidy DJ, Potter GE: Motion examination of the lumbar spine. *JMPT*, 2(3):151–158, 1979.
61. Peterson DH: *Adjustive Technique Manual*. Portland, OR, Western States Chiropractic College, 1988, pp 37–38, 50–51, 54–55, 60–65, 68–70.
62. Maitland GD: *Vertebral Manipulation*. Boston, MA, Butterworth, 1986, pp 46, 209–214, 284.
63. Bovee ML, Burns JR. Carrigg PM, Harmon RO, Johnson MR, Kern DP, Swearingen TL, Willhite FS: *Adjusting Technique Manual*. Davenport, Palmer Chiropractic College, 1981, pp 174–178, 182, 203, 205, 209–211.
64. Herbst RW: *Gonstead Chiropractic Science and Art* (seminar notes). Sci-Chi Publications, 1981, pp 205, 209–214, 217–223.
65. States AZ: *Spinal and Pelvic Techniques*. Lombard, IL, National College of Chiropractic, 1967, pp 73–77, 79, 82.
66. Cyriax J: *Textbook of Orthopedic Medicine*. London, Baillière-Tindall, 1980, pp 266–271.
67. Cox JM: *Low Back Pain*, ed 3. Fort Wayne, IN, JM Cox, 1980, pp 71–84.
68. Cox JM: *Low Back Pain: Mechanism, Diagnosis and Treatment*, ed 4. Baltimore, Williams & Wilkins, 1985, pp 19, 149, 186–194.
69. Cox JM: Pediogenic stenosis: its manipulative implications. *JMPT*, 2(1):35–40, 1979.
70. Penning L, Wilmink JT: Posture-dependent bilateral compression L5 or L5 nerve roots in facet hypertrophy: a dynamic CT-myelographic study. *Spine* 12:488–500, 1987.
71. Robertson JA: Intermittent lumbar flexion-distraction applied in the treatment of spondylolisthesis: a statistical analysis. *JMPT* 2(3):159–169, 1979.
72. Boumphrey F: The challege of the lumbar spine (seminar notes). San Francisco, CA, 1986.
73. Putti V. New conceptions in the pathogenisis of sciatic pain. *Lancet* 2:53-60, 1927.
74. Badgeley DE: The articular facets in relation to low back pain and sciatic radiation. *J Bone Joint Surg* 23:481–496, 1941.
75. Cyron BM, Hutton WC: Articular tropism and stability of the lumbar spine. *Spine* 5(2):168–172, 1980.
76. McKenzie RA: *The Lumbar Spine*. Waikana, New Zealand, Spinal Publications, 1981, pp 16–17.
77. Farfan HF, Sullivan JB: The relation of facet orientation to intervertebral disc failure. *Can J Surg* 10:179–185, 1967.
78. Yochum TR, Rowe LJ: *Essentials of Skeletal Radiology*. Baltimore, Williams & Wilkins, 1986, pp 123, 253.
79. Kevin HA, Kirkaldy-Willis WH: Clinical Symposia, Ciba Foundation, 32(6):8, 89, 1980.
80. Cox J, Shreiner S: Chiropractic manipulation in low back pain and sciatica: statistical data in the diagnosis, treatment and response of 576 conservative cases. *J Manip Physiol Ther* 7(1):1–11, 1984.
81. Cassidy, JD, Potter GE, Kirkaldy-Willis KW: Manipulative management of back pain in patients with spondylolisthesis. *JCCA* Mar. 15–20, 1978.
82. Albers VL, Yochum TR: Reactive sclerosis of a pedicle due to unilateral spondylolysis, a case study. *ACA J of Chiropractic*, Radiology Corner, Sept 1980.
83. Wiltse L, Wihell EH, Jackson DW: Fatigue fracture: The basic lesion in isthmic spondylolisthesis. *J Bone Joint Surg* 57-A, 17–22, 1975.
84. Taillard WF: Etiology of spondylolisthesis. *Clin Orthop* 117:30–39, 1976.
85. Stewart TD: The age incidence of neural arch defects in Alaskan natives considered from the standpoint of etiology. *J Bone Joint Surg* 35-A:937, 1953.
86. Rowe GG, Kocke MB: The etiology of separate arch. *J Bone Joint Surg* 35-A:102–110, 1953.
87. Frederickson BE, Baker D, McHolick WJ, Yuan HA, Libichy JP: The natural history of spondylolysis and spondylolisthesis. *J Bone Joint Surg* 66-A No 5, 699–707, 1984.
88. Rossi F: Spondylolysis and sports. *Sports Med* 18:317–340, 1978.
89. Wiltse LL: The etiology of spondylolisthesis. *J Bone Joint Surg* 44-A: 539–560, 1962.
90. Batts M: The etiology of spondylolisthesis. *J Bone J Surg* 21:879–884, 1989.
91. Troup JDG: The etiology of spondylolysis. *Orthop Clin North Am* 8(1):13, 57–64, 1977.
92. Wertzenberger K, Peterson HA: Acquired spondylolysis and spondylolisthesis in the young child. *Spine* 5(5):14, 437–442, 1980.
93. Rosenberg NJ, Berger WL, Friedman B: The incidence of spondylolysis and spondylolisthesis in nonambulatory patients. *Spine* 6(1):35, 1981.
94. Farfan HF, Osterra V, Lomey C: The mechanical etiology of spondylolysis and spondylolisthesis. *Clin Orthop* 117(40):40–55, 1976.
95. Newman PH, Stone KH: The etiology of spondylolisthesis. *J Bone Joint Surg* 45:39, 1963.
96. Mierau D, Cassidy JD, McGregor M, Kirkaldy-Willis WH: A comparison of the effectiveness of special manipulative therapy for low back pain patients with and without spondylolisthesis. *JMPT* IV(2):49–55, 1987.
97. Baily W: Observation on the etiology and frequency of spondylolisthesis and its precursors. *Radiology* 48:107, 1947.

98. McKee BW, Alexander WJ, Dunbar JS: Spondylolysis and spondylolisthesis in children, a review. *J Radiol* 22:100, 1971.

99. Pease CN, Nojat H: Spondylolisthesis in children. *Clin. Orthop* 52:187, 1967.

100. Pearcy M, Shepherd J: Is there instability in spondylolisthesis? *Spine* 10(3):175–177, 1985.

101. Swere JJ: The chiropractic industrial exam. *AJA J of Chiro* 16-1189:39–49, 322, 1982.

102. Gartland JJ: *Fundamental of Orthopaedics*, ed 2. Philadelphia, WB Saunders, 1974, pp 318, 323.

103. LeBlanc F: Scientific approach to the assessment and management of activity-related spinal disorders. A management for clinicians. *Report of the Quebec Task Force on Spinal Disorders* 12(7S):523, 1987.

104. Simons DG, Travell JG: Low back pain. *Postgrad Med* Part 1, 73(2):66–77, 1983.

105. Wedge JH: The natural history of spinal degeneration. In Kirkaldy-Willis WH: *Managing Low Back Pain*. New York, Churchill Livingstone, 1984, p 4.

106. Drum DC: Conservative management of lumbar disc degeneration. *J of Clin Chiro Archive* Ed 2:96–113, 209, 1972.

107. Kirkaldy-Willis WH, Wedge JH, Yong-Hing K, Reilly J: Pathology on pathogenesis of lumbar spondylosis and stenosis. *Spine* 4:291, 293–294, 319, 1978.

108. Kirkaldy-Willis WH: *Managing Low Back Pain*, ed 2. New York, Churchill Livingstone, 1988, pp 26, 61, 63, 69–70, 117–131, 147, 156, 215.

109. Brinkman P, Horst M: The influences of vertebral body fracture, intradiscal injection, and partial disectomy on the radial bulge and height of human lumbar discs. *Spine* 10(2):138, 1985.

110. Mixter WJ, Barr JS: Rupture of the intervertebral disc with involvement of the spinal cord. *N Eng J Med* 211:210–215, 1954.

111. Ayers CE: Lumbo-sacral backache. *New Eng J Med* 200:592, 1929.

112. Ayers CE: Further case studies of lumbo-sacral pathology with consideration of the involvement of the intervertebral discs and the reticular facets. *New Eng J Med* 213:716, 1935.

113. Ghormley RK: Low back pain with special reference to the articular facets with presentation of an operative procedure. *JAMA* 101:1773–1777, 1933.

114. Hadley LA: Anatomico-roentgenographic studies of the posterior spinal articulations. *Am J Roent* 86:270, 1961.

115. Mooney V, Robertson J: The facet syndrome. *Clin Orthop* 45:149–156, 1976.

116. Anderson JE: Lumbar facet arthropathy and injections: a preliminary report. *Wash Chiro Assoc Clin J* 3(1):24–27, 1985.

117. Helbig T, Casey KL: The lumbar facet syndrome. *Spine* 13(1):61–64, 1988.

118. Yang KH, King AI: Mechanism of facet load transmission as a hypothesis for low back pain. *Spine* 9(6):557–565, 1984.

119. Shealy CM: Facet denervation in management of back and sciatic pain. *Clin Orthop* 115:157–164, 1976.

120. Kirkaldy-Willis WH, Hill RJ: A more precise diagnosis for low back pain. *Spine* 4:102–109, 1979.

121. Cassidy JD: Report on the international society for the study of the lumbar spine June 1978. *J CCA* 139–141, 1978.

122. Kirkaldy-Willis WH: Five common back disorders: how to diagnoses and treat them. *Geriatrics*, Dec 1978, pp 32–41.

123. Heithoff KH: Magnetic reasonance imagery of the lumbar spine. In Kirkaldy-Willis WH: *Managing Low Back Pain*, ed 2, New York, Churchill Livingstone, 1988, p 195.

124. Mathew JA, Yates DAH: Treatment of sciatica. *Lancet*, 1:352, 1974.

125. Wiltse LL, Guyer RD, Spencer CW, Glenn WV, Porter IS: Alar transverse process impingement of the L5 spinal nerve: the far out syndrome. *Spine* 9(1):31–41, 1984.

126. Goldthwait JG: The lumbo-sacral articulation: An explanation of many cases of "lumbago," "sciatica," and "paraplegia." *Boston Med J* 164:365–372, 1911.

127. Verbiest H: A radicular syndrome for developmental narrowing of the lumbar vertebral canal. *J Bone Joint Surg* 36B:230–237, 1954.

128. Verbiest H: Further experiences on the pathological influence of a developmental narrowing of the bony lumbar vertebral canal. *J Bone Joint Surg* 37B:576–583, 1955.

129. Murro D: Lumbar and sacral compression radiculitis (herniated lumbar disc syndrome). *N Engl J Med* 254:243–252, 1956.

130. Kirkaldy-Willis WH, Paine KWE, Cauchoix J, McIvor G: Lumbar spinal stenosis. *Clin Orthop* 99:30–50, 1974.

131. Yamada H, Ohya T, Okade T, Shiozawn Z: Intermittent cauda equina compression due to narrow spinal canal. *J Neurosurg* 37:83–88, 1972.

132. Kirkaldy-Willis WH, Wedge JH, Yong-Hing K, Reilly J: Pathology and pathogenesis of lumbar spondyosis and stenosis. *Spine* 3(4):319–328, 1978.

133. Dyck P, Pheasant HC, Doyle OB, Reider JJ: Intermittent cauda equina compression syndrome. *Spine* 2(1):75–81, 1977.

134. Turek S: *Orthopaedics: Principles and Their Application*, ed 3. Philadelphia, JB Lippincott, 1977, p 1350.

135. Lewit K: *Manipulative Therapy in Rehabilitation of the Motor System*. Boston, Butterworth, 1985, pp 13, 93, 156, 347.

136. Hayland JA, Freemont AJ, Jayson MIV: Intervertebral foramen venous obstruction: a cause of periradicular fibrosis. *Spine* 14:558–568, 1989.

137. Hunter LY, Baumstein EM, Bailey RW: Radiographic changes following anterior cervical fusion. *Spine*, 399–401, 1980.

138. Casey LK, Weiss AB: Isolated congenital block vertebrae below the axis with neurological symptoms. *Spine* 6:118–124.

139. Scott D, Brid H, Wright V: Joint laxity leading to osteoarthrosis. *Rheumatol Rehabil* 18: 167–169, 1979.

140. Grieve GP: Lumbar Instability. In Grieve GP (ed): *Modern Manual Therapy and the Vertebral Column*. London, Churchill Livingstone, pp 43, 416–441.

141. Muhlemann D: Hypermobility as a common cause for chronic back pain. *Ann Swiss Chiro Assn*, in press.

142. Sandoz RW: Technique on interpretation of functional radiography of the lumbar spine. *Ann Swiss Chiro Assn* 3:66–110.

143. Kirkaldy-Willis WH, Farfan HF: Instability of the lumbar spine. *Clin Orthop* 165:110–123, 1982.

144. Posner I, White AA, Edwards WT, Wilson CH: A biomechanical analysis of the clinical stability of the lumbar and lumbosacral spine. *Spine* 7:374–389, 1982.

145. Stoddard A: *Manual of Osteopathic Practice*, ed 2. London, Hutchinson, 1983, pp 123, 127–129.

146. Grieve GP: *Lumbar Instability Physiotherapy* 68:2–8, 1982.

147. MacNab I, Forward IN, White AA, Panjabii MM: *Clinical Biomechanics of the Spine*, Philadelphia, JB Lippincott, 1978, xi.

148. Friberg O: Lumbar instability: A dynamic approach by traction compression radiography. *Spine* 12:119–129, 1987.

149. Fisk JW: *The Painful Neck and Back: Diagnosis, Manipulation, Exercises, Prevention*. Springfield, Charles C Thomas, 1977, p 189.

150. Waddell G, McCulloch JA, Kummel E, Venner RM: Nonorganic physical signs in low back pain. *Spine* 5(2):117–125, 1980.

151. Bernard TN, Kirkaldy-Willis WH: Recognizing specific characteristics of nonspecific low back pain. *Clin Orthop* 217:265–280, 1987.

CHAPTER 9

Disorders of the Thoracic Spine

MERIDEL I. GATTERMAN, M.A., D.C.
DAVID M. PANZER, D.C.

The ominous significance of thoracic pain can cause unnecessary worry when biomechanical joint dysfunction goes undiagnosed.

Biomechanical disorders of the thoracic spine differ significantly from those of the lumbar and cervical regions. This is primarily due to the persistence of the primary kyphotic curve and the stability imparted by the rib cage. Postural faults tend to increase the thoracic kyphosis, and instead of the articular facets being jammed together, they are more apt to be pulled apart. Thus, the thoracic articulations tend to separate and become locked at the extreme of their range of motion in flexion.

Increased thoracic kyphosis produces a crowding of the viscera, which interferes with normal physiologic functioning (Chapter 11). The costovertebral joints where the ribs articulate with the spinal column may also become fixed, producing sharp pain upon respiration. Strain of the postural muscles that support the upper extremities is also a common cause of thoracic pain. Among the most common sites of myofascial pain are the rhomboid and trapezius muscles. These muscles frequently exhibit trigger points that produce chronic thoracic pain (Chapter 12).

ANATOMY OF THE THORACIC VERTEBRAE AND RIBS

Thoracic vertebrae are generally classified as typical or atypical, according to their rib attachments. The typical thoracic vertebrae are the second through the eighth, with two pair of demifacets for articulation of the ribs. Each of the ribs attaching to the typical thoracic vertebra articulates with the ver-

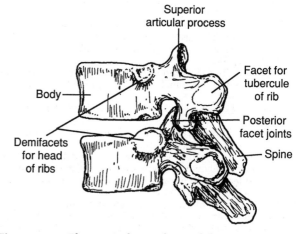

Figure 9.1. The typical vertebra exhibits two pairs of *demifacets* on the vertebral body for articulation of the rib heads, and *costal facets* on each transverse process, which articulate with the tubercle of the rib. The *spinous processes* are long and slender, their angle increasing from 35° in the upper thoracic area to 45° in the lower thoracic area.

tebrae above and below at the site of the articular facets (Fig. 9.1).

The typical thoracic vertebral body is heart-shaped when viewed from above or below (Fig. 9.2). The pedicles are short, while the laminae are only slightly longer, forming a more circular neural canal in this region. The articular facets face posteriorly and laterally, becoming more vertical as they approach the coronal plane in the lower thoracic region. The transverse processes are relatively long and angled dorsolaterally at about 45° to the midsagittal plane of the body, with costotransverse facets on their ventrolateral surfaces for articulation with the ribs (Fig. 9.2). The spinous processes are long, slender, and triangular on cross section. Their

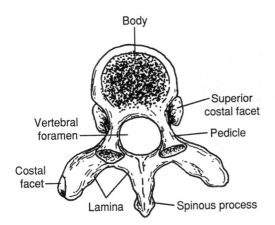

Figure 9.2. The typical thoracic vertebral body is heart-shaped when viewed from above, with a circular neural canal. The transverse processes are relatively long and angled dorsolaterally at about 45°.

angle increases from 35° in the upper thoracic area to about 45° in the lower thoracic area (Fig. 9.1).

The atypical thoracic vertebrae are the first, and the ninth through the twelfth. The first thoracic vertebral body is shaped like the lower cervical bodies, with uncinate processes on the cephalic surface. There is one full costal facet on each side of the cephalic aspect of the body for articulation with the first ribs, and one pair of demifacets on the caudal aspect for articulation with the cephalic half of the second pair of ribs (Fig. 9.3).

The body is shaped more like the cervical vertebrae, being broader in the transverse dimension. The spinous process is similar to the seventh cervical process, being relatively longer and protruding more than the spinous processes of typical thoracic vertebrae. When the first thoracic spinous process is longer than that of the seventh cervical vertebra, it is known as the "vertebra prominens."

The ninth thoracic vertebra generally has one pair of demifacets, but often has two, in which case it is considered typical. The tenth thoracic vertebra generally has one complete pair of costal facets on the cephalic aspect of the body, but in those cases

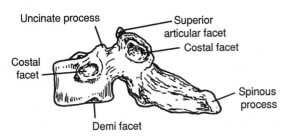

Figure 9.3. The first thoracic vertebra has *uncinate processes* on the cephalic surface, with one full *costal facet* on each side of the cephalic aspect of the body, for articulation with the first ribs, and one pair of *demifacets* in the caudal aspect, for articulation with the cephalic half of the second pair of ribs.

where the ninth has two pair of demifacets, the tenth may have one pair of demifacets. The eleventh thoracic vertebra typically has one complete pair of costal facets on the upper lateral part of the body and no facets on the ventrolateral aspect of the transverse processes.

The twelfth thoracic vertebra is considered a transitional segment, having characteristics of both the thoracic and lumbar regions. The body has one complete pair of costal facets for articulation with the twelfth pair of ribs, but no transverse facets, and protuberances on the distal aspect of the transverse process similar to the mamillary processes of the lumbar vertebrae (1). Acting as a bridge between the thoracic and lumbar regions, the last thoracic vertebra typically has superior articular facets like the other thoracic vertebrae, facing more in the coronal plane. The inferior facets correspond to those of the first lumbar vertebra and are oriented more in the sagittal plane (2). In the middle and upper portion of the thoracic spine, the more coronal facing facets provide stability against anterior translation. As they become more oriented in the sagittal plane, anywhere from the ninth to the twelfth thoracic segments, they provide stability against axial rotation (3).

The ribs of the typical thoracic vertebrae attach at two sites, one connecting the heads of the ribs with the bodies of the vertebrae and the other, the costotransverse joints, uniting the necks and tubercles of the ribs with the transverse processes. The joints at the heads of typical ribs are attached to adjacent vertebrae and to the intervertebral disc between them. The first, tenth, eleventh, and twelfth ribs typically each attach to a single vertebra.

The heads of the ribs are attached by the intraarticular, radiate, and capsular ligaments (Fig. 9.4). The intraarticular ligament separates the two articular facets on the head of the rib, attaching the rib head to the disc. This ligament divides the joint into two distinct parts. It is not found in the joints of the first, tenth, or twelfth costovertebral articulations, which are single synovial joints.

The radiate ligament connects the anterior part of the head of each rib with the sides of the bodies of adjacent vertebrae and the intervertebral disc between them. In the articulations of the first rib, the radiate ligament is attached to the body of the last cervical vertebra as well as the first thoracic. In the joints of the tenth, eleventh, and twelfth ribs, each of which attaches to a single vertebra, the radiate ligaments are connected to this vertebra and also the one above.

The fibrous capsules connect the heads of the ribs with the circumferences of the articular cavities. Some of the upper fibers pass through the intervertebral foramen to the back of the intervertebral disc, while the posterior fibers are continuous with the costotransverse ligament.

Figure 9.4. A, B, Ligaments of the thoracic spine.

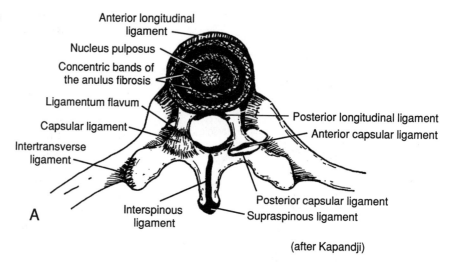

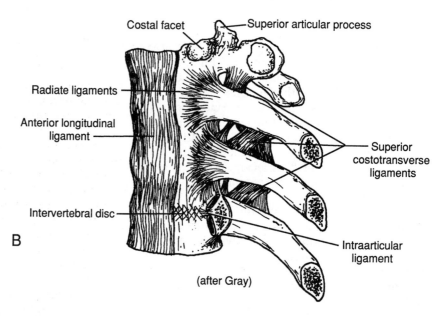

At the costotransverse joints, the tubercles of the ribs articulate with the reciprocal facets on the transverse processes of the corresponding vertebrae. Costotransverse articulations are not found in the eleventh and twelfth vertebrae. The costotransverse joints are united by the superior costotransverse and lateral costotransverse ligaments, as well as the fibrous capsule, which is attached to the circumference of the articular surfaces (4).

The sternocostal joints of the true ribs unite with the sternum (Fig. 9.5). These diarthrodial joints are reinforced by the radiate sternocostal ligaments and their fibrous capsules. The intraarticular ligaments are constant and found only between the second costal cartilages and the sternum. The first costocartilage is directly united to the sternum by a synchondrosis. The contiguous borders of the sixth, seventh, eighth, and sometimes the ninth and tenth articulate with each other by small, smooth, oblong-shaped facets. Each articulation is enclosed in a

thin, fibrous capsule, lined with synovial membrane and strengthened laterally and medially by interchondral ligaments.

The ligamentum flava and the anterior and posterior longitudinal ligaments are well developed in the thoracic region. Combined with the radiate and costotransverse ligaments, they provide considerable stability to the thoracic spine. The capsular ligaments in the thoracic region are thin and loose, providing little support against flexion. This capsular instability, in addition to the dorsal kyphosis produced by the wedge-shaped discs and vertebrae, cause the thoracic spine to be unstable in flexion (3). These characteristics may predispose to the flexion fixation commonly seen in the thoracic region.

Muscles of the Thorax

Muscles producing movement of the thorax include the respiratory muscles, the abdominal muscles, and the paraspinal muscles.

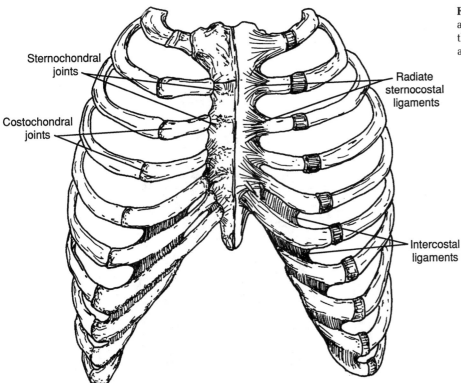

Respiratory Muscles

The respiratory muscles can be divided into the inspiratory muscles (which elevate the ribs) and the expiratory muscles (which depress the ribs and sternum). These categories may be further subdivided into primary and accessory muscles. The accessory muscles are active during deep respiration.

The diaphragm is considered the basic muscle of respiration, since it increases all three diameters of the thoracic cavity. When the diaphragm contracts, the central tendon, which is attached to the upper lumbar vertebra, increases the vertical diameter of the thorax. The transverse diameter is increased by the elevation of the lower ribs, and the anteroposterior diameter is increased by the elevation of the upper ribs, assisted by the sternum (2).

In addition to the diaphragm, the primary inspiratory muscles are the external intercostals, which arise from the lower border of each rib and are attached to the upper border of the rib below. Secondary muscles of inspiration include the sternocleidomastoideus; the scalenus anterior, medius, and posterior, which act as stabilizers of the cervical vertebral column; and the serratus anterior, latissimus dorsi, and pectoralis major and minor, when they act on the scapula and upper limb already in abduction. The serratus posterior superior and superior fibers of the iliocostalis also stabilize the upper thorax on deep inspiration.

The primary muscles of forced expiration are the internal intercostals, which depress the ribs. However, normal expiration is a passive process, due to recoil of the thorax assisted by gravity, air pressure, and the relaxation of the diaphragm, which reduces the size of the thoracic cavity.

Accessory expiratory muscles are extremely powerful and assist in forced respiration and clinically during the performance of Valsalva's maneuver. The additional expulsive force is aided by strong contraction of the muscles of the abdominal wall, particularly the oblique and transverse muscles and by the latissimus dorsi muscles, which contract suddenly and energetically with such efforts as coughing and sneezing. The muscles of the abdominal wall raise the intraabdominal pressure, which forces the relaxing diaphragm up and draws the lower ribs down and medial (4).

In the thoracolumbar region, the lowest fibers of the iliocostalis, longissimus, and serratus posterior inferior and the quadratus lumborum assist in forced expiration, which results in increased venous and cerebral spinal fluid pressure. Valsalva's maneuver utilizes forced expiration against a closed glottis and tight perianal sphincters to aid in diagnosing space-occupying lesions affecting the brain and spinal cord. Caution is advised in performing this maneuver, since the alteration in pulmonary and myocardial circulatory dynamics may cause myocardial ischemia. This test should not be employed on patients with heart disease (3).

Compression of the jugular veins may be used to enhance this procedure (Naffziger's test). The increased intrathecal pressure produced by this ma-

Figure 9.6. The *trapezius* and *rhomboid* muscles are powerful antigravity muscles that support the head and upper extremities during upright posture. Together with the *levator scapulae*, these muscles act as shoulder girdle stabilizers and are common sites of myofascial pain due to static loading, which occurs when the arms are extended for prolonged periods of time. These muscle syndromes are frequently mistaken for thoracic and radicular condition (see Chapter 12).

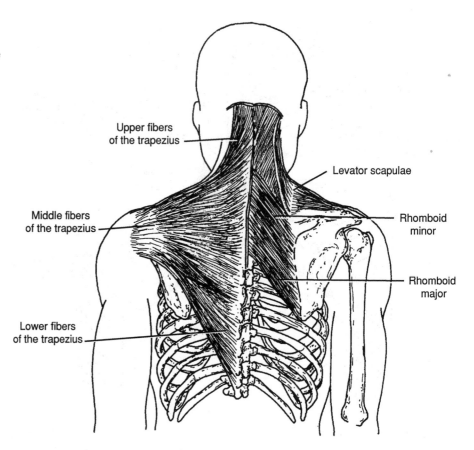

Upper fibers of the trapezius

Levator scapulae

Middle fibers of the trapezius

Rhomboid minor

Rhomboid major

Lower fibers of the trapezius

neuver greatly increases pain that has resulted from intervertebral disc prolapse with nerve impingement or pain due to intraspinal tumor. Coughing or sneezing produces a similar response because of the sharp rise in intrathoracic pressure during the pressure phase, which involves the closure of the glottis and the violent contraction of the intercostals and the accessory muscles of expiration, especially the abdominal muscles (2).

Muscles of the Abdomen

Muscles of the abdominal wall form a natural girdle that assists in forced expiration as well as offering support to the abdominal contents. Weak abdominal muscle tone leads to faulty body mechanics with sagging viscera and crowded organs. (Chapter 11). The most powerful expiratory muscles are those of the abdominal wall, the rectus abdominis, the internal and external obliquus, and the transversus abdominis. All of these muscles pull the lower ribs down and depress and narrow the costal arch (5). In forced expiration, when the muscles contract and the abdominal pressure is increased, the diaphragm is forced upward into the thoracic cavity, depressing and compressing the lower part of the thorax.

Paraspinal Muscles of the Thorax

The thoracic spinal musculature overlaps both the cervical and lumbar regions. The most prominent superficial muscle in this region is the trapezius, which extends into the cervical region. It is a powerful, antigravity muscle and, along with the rhomboid muscles, supports the head and upper extremities in upright posture (Fig. 9.6) (Chapter 11). These muscles are a common site of myofascial pain, frequently described as thoracic pain (Chapter 12).

The sacrospinalis (erector spinae) muscles lie in a groove on the side of the vertebral column and can easily be palpated as a fleshy mass flanked by a visible groove on the lateral border. This muscle inclines laterally, crossing the ribs at their angles. In the thoracic region, the erector spinae splits into three parts: the lateral iliocostalis, the intermediate longissimus, and the medial spinalis (Fig. 9.7).

The iliocostalis thoracis originates from the upper borders of the angles of the lower six ribs. It ascends to the upper borders of the angles of the upper six ribs and the posterior aspect of the transverse process of the seventh cervical vertebra.

The longissimus thoracis is the intermediate and largest of the sacrospinalis. In the thoracic region it is attached by rounded tendons to the tips of the transverse processes of all the thoracic vertebrae, and to the lower nine or ten ribs, between their tubercles and angles.

The most medial of the sacrospinalis, the spinalis thoracis, is barely a distinct muscle and is blended with the medial side of the longissimus thoracis. It

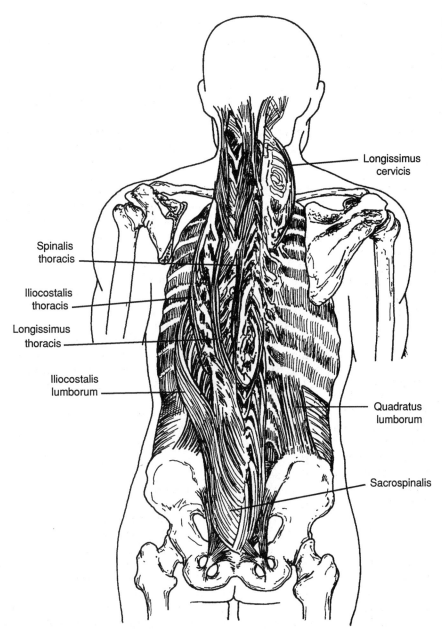

Longissimus
cervicis

Spinalis
thoracis

Iliocostalis
thoracis

Longissimus
thoracis

Iliocostalis
lumborum

Quadratus
lumborum

Sacrospinalis

is attached to the spine at the eleventh and twelfth thoracic and at the first and second lumbar vertebrae. These three muscle groups, as the name erector spinae implies, are extensors of the vertebral column, while the iliocostalis also laterally flex the spinal column.

The transverse spinalis muscles serve as stabilizers of the spinal column and function primarily as postural muscles (6) (Chapter 2). Their detailed patterns of activity and combinations are not fully understood at this time. In the thoracic region they consist of the semispinalis, thoracis multifidus, and rotatores thoracis.

The semispinalis thoracis arise by a series of tendons from the transverse processes of the sixth to the tenth thoracic vertebrae and insert onto the spines of the upper four thoracic and lower two cervical vertebrae. Their bilateral action extends the spine, while unilateral contraction rotates the vertebral bodies to the opposite side.

The multifidus attaches to all the transverse processes in the thoracic region and ascends obliquely and medially to attach to the entire length of the spinous process of one of the vertebrae above. The fasciculi vary in length. The most superficial extends from one vertebra to the third or fourth above. The next layer runs from one vertebra to the second or third above, while the deepest connects contiguous vertebrae. Their actions include lateral flexion and rotation.

The rotatores thoracis are located between the thoracic vertebra and are small and quadrilateral.

The rotatores are best developed in the thoracic spine and run deep to the multifidus. Each connects the upper and posterior part of the transverse process of one vertebra to the lower border and lateral surface of the lamina of the next vertebra above. As their name implies, they rotate the spine.

The interspinales are short, paired muscles between the spines of contiguous vertebrae on each side of the interspinous ligament. In the thoracic region, they are located between the first and second vertebrae and sometimes between the second and third, and the eleventh and twelfth vertebrae. The interspinales assist in extension of the spine.

The intertransversarii are small muscles spanning the transverse processes of the vertebrae. In the thoracic region they are present between the transverse processes of the last three thoracic vertebrae only and between the transverse processes of the last thoracic and the first lumbar vertebrae. The action of the intertranversarii is lateral flexion of the vertebrae.

Thoracic Innervation

The spinal muscles in the thoracic region are supplied by the dorsal rami of the spinal nerves. The other muscles of the thorax are supplied by the adjacent intercostal nerves. From the ventral rami, each nerve is connected with the adjoining ganglion of the sympathetic trunk by gray and white rami communicantes. The intercostal nerves are primarily distributed to the thoracic and abdominal walls. The first two nerves supply the upper limb as well as their thoracic branches. Two to six supply the thoracic wall only, while seven to twelve supply the thoracic and abdominal walls.

The first lumbar nerve is known as the subcostal because it lies inferior to the twelfth thoracic rib. It supplies the abdominal wall and the gluteal skin. The abdominal muscles are supplied by the ventral rami of the lower six thoracic and the first lumbar spinal nerves (7).

ANOMALIES OF THE THORACIC SPINE

Thoracic spinal anomalies include block vertebrae (congenital synostosis), sagittally cleft vertebrae (butterfly vertebrae), and hemivertebrae as found in other areas of the spine (Chapter 1). Thoracic spinous processes are frequently asymmetrical, and the tip of one or more may be congenitally deviated from the midline by as much as 0.5 cm (7).

Manipulative attempts at correction of these static "misalignments" can cause considerable discomfort to the patient and can be avoided by evaluating the motion of these vertebrae (7). Using motion palpation as the criterion for determining the site of application of manipulation avoids the pitfall of attempting to reposition an asymmetrical segment.

MOVEMENT OF THE THORACIC SPINE

The thoracic spine is the least mobile part of the spinal column. This is primarily due to the attachment of the rib cage, along with narrower discs and elongated spinous processes.

The thoracic spinous processes overlap much like shingles on a roof (7), with tips of the spinous processes lying nearly at the level of the subjacent vertebral lamina in the region of the middle seventh or eighth thoracic vertebral motion segments.

As with other areas of the spine, the amount and type of motion of the thoracic vertebral motion segments is determined by the angulation and spatial orientation of the facet joints. Orientation of the facet joints in the coronal plane decreases from approximately 20° in the upper thoracic region to 15° or less in the lower segments. The superior facets are oriented backward and slightly outward and upward with an angulation of approximately 60° to the medial sagittal plane.

This angulation facilitates rotation of the vertebral motion segments, which decreases from approximately 14° at the T1–2 vertebral motion segment to less than 5° at the T11–12 vertebral motion segment. The average rotation at T5–6 and T7–8 vertebral motion segments is 10° (8).

Coupled with rotation is lateral bending, which is greatest at the T11–12 motion segment, averaging between 13 and 14°, and least at T5–6, averaging 5°. It is generally 2–3° greater in the other vertebral motion segments.

Flexion and extension is the least from T1–2 through T5–6, averaging less than 5°. It approaches 8° at T7–8 through T9–10, reaching nearly 19° at the T11–12 (8) vertebral motion segment with the facets oriented more in the sagittal plane (Table 9.1). During extension, the articular facets limit motion, by bony impingement of the articular processes and by jamming of the spinous processes. The anterior longitudinal ligament becomes stretched, while the posterior longitudinal ligament, ligamenta flava, and interspinous ligaments relax.

During flexion, the spinous processes' interspace widens as the nucleus is displaced posteriorly and the articular surfaces of the inferior facets slide upward. Flexion is limited by tension on the interspinous ligament, ligamenta flava, the capsular ligaments, and the posterior longitudinal ligaments. The anterior longitudinal ligament then relaxes.

Anterior translation is limited by the coronal facets (2). The disc is compressed anteriorly and is expanded posteriorly.

Lateral flexion and rotation in the thoracic spine are coupled motions as in the other areas of the spine. On lateral flexion of the thoracic vertebrae, the facets on the side of flexion approximate with the superior facet sliding downward. On the contralateral side, the superior facets slide upward. Lateral flexion is limited by bony impingement of the ipsi-

Table 9.1 Differential Diagnosis

Condition	History & Symptoms	Diagnostic Indicators	Therapy
Pathological lesions			
Metabolic disorders			
Osteoporosis	Postmenopausal females & over 65 affected, back pain, increased dorsal kyphosis	Radiographs reveal thinning of the cortex & trabecular of vertebral body, concave endplates, "cod fish" vertebra	Nutritional supplements, activity, refer for hormone therapy if severe
Osteitis deformans (Paget's disease)	Back pain	Radiographs demonstrate exaggerated, bizzare bony trabeculae & bone expansion; heat-labile alkaline phosphatase high	Refer for medication
Diffuse ideopathic skeletal hyperostosis DISH, (Forestier's disease)	Over 50 affected, history of diabetes in 20% of cases, T7 through T12 most common sites, back pain, decreased ROM, stiffness	Radiographs demonstrate laminated new bone formation with ossification of the anterior longitudinal ligament	Gentle manipulation and mobilization where indicated.
Infectious disorders			
Costochondritis (Tietze's syndrome)	History of previous upper respiratory infection, chest pain increased by respiration, coughing, sneezing.	Tender nodular swelling of rib cartilage, especially the 2nd & 3rd ribs	Heat, vitamin supplementation; manipulation is contraindicated (see text)
Herpes zoster	Severe persistent pain following distribution of the intercostal nerve	Characteristic skin rash appears 2–14 days along course of at the intercostal nerve	Vitamin A & B supplementation
Pleurisy	Chest pain aggravated by breathing	Rales & friction rub on auscultation	Immobilization of respiratory movement with rib belt, refer for antibiotics
Ankylosing spondylitis (Marie Strumpell)	Late teens to 35 years affected, male more than female, back pain	Radiographic changes seen in sacroiliac joints, first vertebrae show square borders & marginal syndesmophytosis	Heat, mild exercise, manipulation when acute phase is past, refer for pain & antiinflammatory medication when severe
Tuberculosis	Young adults affected	Radiographic findings reveal disc and endplate destruction with resultant gibbus formation and ankylosis, loss of pedicle "eye" on AP projection	Refer for medication
Stress disorders			
Rib fracture	History of trauma or pathology, pain increased by respiration, ribs 4–7 most vulnerable	Radiographs reveal radiolucent bands	Immobilize & stabilize with a rib belt 6–8 weeks
Vertebral compression fractures	History of trauma or pathology, back pain, T12-L1 most vulnerable	Radiographs reveal vertebral wedging	Bed rest, body cast if pain is severe
Juvenile kyphosis (Scheuermann's disorder)	Onset at puberty, increased dorsal kyphosis, pain at the end of an active day, affects 3–4 adjacent vertebral bodies in mid & lower thoracic spine	Radiographs reveal irregularities along the vertebral borders (Schmorl's nodes), collapse of anterior vertebral body	Exercise, vitamin supplementation, cast or brace if severe, extreme case refer for surgery
Thoracic disc herniation	Males in 5th decade most affected, T11-12 most common site, back pain increased by neck flexion, coughing, straining; paresis & paresthesia of lower extremities, severe cases may show loss of sphincter control & paraplegia	Radiographs may reveal calcified disc, CT & MRI reveals disc herniation	Traction, refer for surgical decompression if pain is severe or patient exhibits advancing neurological deficits
Referred pain			
Coronary artery disease, myocardial infarction	Severe, prolonged crushing/ constricting pain, chest pain, ashen pallor, sweating, marked bradycardia, arrhythmia, drop in blood pressure, rapid weak pulse	Abnormal EKG, increased LDH, CPK	Refer to cardiologist

Table 9.1 *(Continued)*

Condition	History & Symptoms	Diagnostic Indicators	Therapy
Angina pectoris	Transient pain on exertion	Abnormal EKG, LDH, & CPK	Refer to cardiologist
Pericarditis	Substernal pain described as crushing heavy or squeezing	Tachycardia muffled heart sounds, low blood pressure, friction rub, EKG radiographs may show large, bottle-shaped heart shadow	Refer to cardiologist
Dissecting aneurysm	Severe excruciating chest pain of sudden onset, can begin in the back between shoulder blades	Shock, progressive obliteration of the pulses in the carotid then in arm & leg vessels, progressive increase in the width of aortic shadow on radiograph	Refer to cardiovascular consultant surgeon
Pulmonary embolus	Severe crushing substernal pain	Pallor & cyanosis, shock, rapid pulse, dyspnea	Refer to cardiologist or ER
Visceral conditions			
Diaphragmatic hernia	Substernal pain radiating to the substernal notch and throat, dysphagia, pain increased on recumbancy or on increased abdominal pressure	Radiographs reveal gastric or bowel gas above the level of the diaphragm	If severe, refer for surgery
Gall bladder disease	Pain referred to lower border of right scapula, attacks of nausea	Radiographs reveal gallstones; if radiopaque, cholecystography & diagnostic ultrasound necessary for radiolucent stones	If severe, refer for surgery
Biomechanical disorders Traumatic & movement syndromes			
Facet-joint fixation	History of unguarded movement, pain on respiration	Motion palpation reveals restricted facet joint motion	Manipulation (see text)
Costovertebral fixation	History of unguarded movement, pain on respiration	Motion palpation reveals restricted costovertebral joint motion	Manipulation (see text)
Facet-joint sprain	History of trauma, violent cough or sneeze, pain on respiration	Motion palpation reveals absence of fixation at site of pain	Immobilize with a rib belt
Costovertebral sprain	History of trauma, violent cough or sneeze, pain on respiration	Motion palpation reveals absence of fixation at site of pain	Immobilize with a rib belt
Muscle syndromes			
Shoulder strain	History of trauma, deep ache in shoulder & upper thoracic region, pain radiating into arm	Trigger points in shoulder-girdle muscles	Apply deep pressure to trigger points, physical therapy
Postural strain	History of static loading of apex extremity antigravity muscles, burning pain at the cervicodorsal junction radiates up and down spine	Trigger points in trapezius and rhomboid muscles	As above
Intercostal strain	History of trauma, pain on respiration	Trigger points in intercostal muscles	As above
Thoracic strain	History of trauma, posterior thoracic pain	Trigger points and spasm in paraspinal muscles	As above

lateral articular processes and by the contralateral ligamenta flava and intertransverse ligaments. Concomitant with lateral flexion of the vertebral motion segments, the widening of the intercostal spaces occurs on the contralateral side, with narrowing of the intercostal space on the side of flexion.

Rotation of each vertebral motion segment in the thoracic region is accompanied by a similar movement in the corresponding ribs. This rotation is limited by the attachment of the ribs to the sternum (2). Due to the orientation of the thoracic facets, minimal translation is coupled with rotation in this region. The axis of rotation is the point of intersection of perpendicular lines drawn from the facets (Fig. 9.8). This allows little rotation of the vertebral body and twisting of the intervertebral disc, instead of the shearing forces typically found in the lumbar region. This twisting allows for greater rotation in the re-

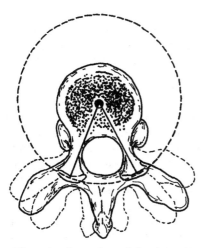

Figure 9.8. The axis of rotation of the thoracic vertebrae is the point of intersection from perpendicular lines drawn from the facets.

gion. The spinous processes move in a larger arc than the small ones in the lumbar spine.

The absence of shearing forces during rotation of the thoracic spine may contribute to the lower incidence of disc herniation in this region and produces relatively little change in the instantaneous axis of rotation in the thoracic vertebral motion segments.

The kinesiological characteristics of the upper thoracic spine are similar to those of the cervical region, while the kinesiological characteristics of the lower thoracic spine are similar to those in the lumbar region (9). This is most noticeable in the coupling patterns of each area. In the cervical and upper thoracic region, the spinous processes move toward the convexity of the curve with lateral bending, while in the lower thoracic region, the spinous processes move toward the concavity of the curve. The

transitional segment for this reversal is approximately T6 (9).

During lateral flexion of the thoracic column, the thoracic cage is lowered, the intercostal space narrowed, and the costochondral angle becomes smaller. On the contralateral side, the thorax is elevated, the intercostal space is widened, and the thoracic cage is enlarged. The thoracic cage greatly increases the length of the vertebral levers and movement of inertia, resulting in stability and resistance to motion in all planes (2).

Movement of the Thorax during Respiration

Respiratory excursion is a function of the combined movement of the ribs. Each rib possesses its own range and direction of movement, with the axis of movement lateral to the costotransverse articulation. When the shaft of the rib is elevated, the neck is relatively depressed. Due to the large difference in the length of the lever arms, small movements at the vertebral end are magnified at the anterior end.

The ribs not only slant downward and forward from their vertebral attachments, but are also oblique in relation to the transverse plane, so that the lateral aspect lies on a lower level than the vertebral or sternal attachments. The shafts of the ribs elevate and rise forward during expansion of the rib cage. Further expansion is provided by an elevation of the lateral portion of the rib, producing an increase in the transverse diameter of the chest. During inspiration, the upper ribs thrust upward like the movement of a bucket handle (10) (Fig. 9.9) increasing the anteroposterior diameter of the chest while the lower ribs open like calipers, which increases the lateral diameter of the chest (Fig. 9.10).

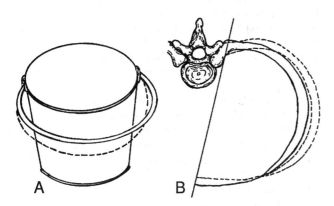

Figure 9.9. **A,** During inspiration the upper ribs are thrust upward, similar to movement of a bucket handle. **B,** This movement increases the anteroposterior diameter of the chest. (Adapted from Grice AS: A biomechanical approach to cervical and dorsal adjusting. In Haldeman S: *Modern Developments in the Principles and Practice of Chiropractic.* East Norwalk, CT, Appleton-Century-Crofts, 1979, p 352.)

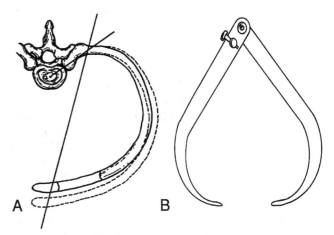

Figure 9.10. **A,** The lower ribs open the rib cage similar to **B,** the movement of calipers, increasing the lateral diameter of the chest during inspiration. (Adapted from Grice AS: A biomechanical approach to cervical and dorsal adjusting. In Haldeman S: *Modern Developments in the Principles and Practice of Chiropractic.* East Norwalk, CT, Appleton-Century-Crofts, 1979, p 352.)

The mobility of the ribs varies considerably. The first ribs are more fixed than the others, due to the weight of the upper extremities and the strain of the ribs beneath. Maximized on deep inspiration, movement of the first rib occurs about an oblique axis through the neck, while the shaft is displaced upward and laterally. The undersurface then faces more directly downward. Movement of the second rib is slight on quiet respiration. Mobility is increased successively down to the last two, which are freely moveable. Since these ribs have free anterior extremities and only costovertebral articulations with no intraarticular ligaments, they are capable of movement in all directions. When the other ribs are elevated, these are fixed by the quadratus lumborum muscle to form fixed points of action for the diaphragm.

THORACIC VERTEBRAL AND COSTOVERTEBRAL SYNDROMES

The ominous significance of thoracic pain can cause unnecessary worry when biomechanical joint dysfunction goes undiagnosed. The differential diagnosis of thoracic pain must of course consider coronary, pulmonary, and other origins of viscerosomatic pain. Referred pain from the viscera can mimic musculoskeletal disorders and should be ruled out before the chiropractor proceeds with manipulative therapy (Table 9.1).

Vertebral and costal joint dysfunction are often characterized by pain during respiration. As with all regions of the spine, areas of hypermobility must be avoided when applying a manipulative thrust. This is especially important in the thoracic region, since joints in this area are difficult to stabilize due to the constant respiratory excursion. While this can be a problem, the constant motion of the thorax is a beneficial factor in the prevention of degenerative joint disease, which is less severe in this area than in other areas of the spine.

Clinical Considerations

History and Etiology

The etiology of thoracic vertebral and costovertebral syndromes is generally a sudden, unguarded movement. The patient may have a history of explosive coughing or sneezing (11–13) or may report a sudden stabbing pain following lifting or reaching overhead (13). A crushing blow to the chest (such as occurs when a driver is thrown against the steering wheel during a motor vehicle accident) can also precipitate thoracic vertebral and costovertebral lesions. Patients with pronounced scoliosis are prone to articular fixation and compensatory hypermobility in this region. Fixation of the first and second ribs commonly accompanies whiplash injuries and traction injuries to the upper extremities (7). Work-related injuries resulting from carrying heavy weight on the shoulders or prolonged pulling (7) and hauling also produce joint dysfunction in this area. Lower rib lesions may also occur as a result of motor vehicle accidents involving a lap seat belt that restrains the pelvis while allowing the trunk to be thrown forward and rotated to one side (7).

Signs and Symptoms

Unilateral pain in the thoracic spine is the most common symptom of vertebral and costovertebral joint dysfunction (12). The pain is frequently described as sharp and stabbing, accentuated by deep inspiration, coughing, and sneezing (12). Lesions of the rib heads commonly accompany thoracic vertebral problems with characteristic intercostal muscle spasm. Common complaints are continuous soreness at the costovertebral angle, with pain radiating around to the lateral or anterior chest wall, resembling intercostal neuralgia (12). Absence of joint movement, determined by motion palpation, gives the most definitive diagnosis; however, prominence of the rib head and localized tenderness are also indicators of costovertebral fixation. Radiographic findings indicating retraction of the rib margin and asymmetry of the rib cage may also indicate rib fixation (13).

Thoracic Spine Examination

In addition to motion palpation of the thoracic vertebral and rib articulations, a limited number of orthopaedic tests are useful in diagnosing thoracic spine dysfunction.

Orthopaedic Tests of Thoracic Spine Dysfunction

Passive Neck Flexion

Soto Hall Test. With the patient placed in a supine position without a pillow, the doctor places one hand on the sternum and exerts light pressure to stabilize the thoracic and lumbar spine. The doctor then passively flexes the patient's neck with the other hand, which is placed under the occiput. Flexion of the head and neck produces a pull on the posterior spinous ligaments from the head caudally. A localized pain will be experienced at the level of a lesion such as a fracture of the spinous process or vertebral body (positive Soto Hall test). There will also be a localized pain at the level of a sprain or strain (14).

Lhermitte's Sign. A positive Lhermitte's sign (15) is elicited if the patient complains of a sudden, transient, shock-like sensation spreading down the spine and into one or several extremities. This sensation is an indication of spinal cord degeneration, cervical cord injuries, or multiple sclerosis. The patient that exhibits this sign should be referred for neurological evaluation.

Brudzinski's Sign. Meningeal irritation will cause the patient to flex the knees when the neck is flexed (Brudzinski's sign) (14).

Lindner's Sign. If neck flexion produces low back symptoms (Lindner's sign), there may be a localized vertebrogenic lesion of the low back (14).

Soft Tissue Palpation

Palpation of the thorax is important in ruling out muscle trigger points. Myofascial pain syndromes produce characteristic patterns of pain that are often mistaken for spinal lesions. Careful examination of the muscles of the thorax should be performed, especially in the trapezius, rhomboid, levator scapulae, serratus anterior, and intercostal muscles (Chapter 12).

Percussion

Percussion of the spinous processes is helpful in determining the level of the lesion (Chapter 5). When percussion produces an acute pain that rapidly subsides, it is indicative of traumatic joint pathology. A dull pain that disappears slowly suggests a fracture, neoplasm, or other bone disease (14). Radiologic evaluation is essential for a differential diagnosis.

Chest Expansion

Circumferential measurement of the chest should be included in examination of the thorax if ankylosing spondylitis is suspected. The circumference of the chest should expand, from expiration to inspiration, 1.5 to 2.5 inches for the male, and 1 to 1.5 inches in the female (14).

Indications for Thoracic Vertebral and Costovertebral Manipulation

Identification of vertebral and costovertebral fixation is most effectively determined by motion palpation. To palpate motion of the thoracic spine and ribs, the patient is seated in front of and facing away from the doctor. The patient's position is then controlled and stabilized by the doctor's nonpalpating hand, which is placed on the patient's contralateral shoulder, with the forearm lying across the upper thoracic area and the elbow contacting the patient's ipsilateral shoulder. The patient can then be flexed, extended, laterally flexed, and rotated by the stabilizing forearm and hand.

The level of vertebral motion segment fixation is determined by the full spine scan using the dorsum of the hand to palpate segmental motion, which is part of the routine spinal examination (Chapter 5). The restricted segment can then be further evaluated for movement restriction in flexion, extension, lateral flexion, and rotation, as well as for fixation of the ribs.

Manipulation of the Thoracic Spine and Ribs

Manipulation of the thoracic spine and ribs can be successfully performed with the patient prone, supine, or standing (16–25). The line of drive of the thrust for thoracic spine manipulation varies according to the angle of the facets and the motion that is being restored (Fig. 9.11).

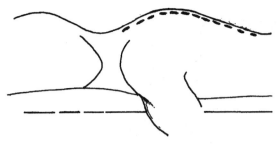

Figure 9.11. Orientation of the thoracic facets decreases from approximately 14° from the vertical at the T1-2 vertebral motion segment, to less than 5° at the T11–12 vertebral motion segment. The planes of the facets as well as the thoracic curve must be considered when determining the line of drive of the manipulative thrust, to avoid jamming the facets.

Contraindications for Manipulation of the Thoracic Spine and Ribs

There is a tendency by many doctors to be less specific in manipulation of the thoracic spine (9), but as with restoration of normal motion to any joint, the more specific the line of drive, the less force is required to release the fixation and the less trauma is imparted to the patient. The doctor should never employ more force than is necessary to restore motion, in order to avoid damage to the holding elements of the spine, including the discs, ligaments, and muscles. The most common conditions contraindicating manipulation of the thoracic region are rib fractures and sprains of the costochondral, costosternal, and interchondral joints.

Palpation of Thoracic Vertebrae Fixed in Extension

When a thoracic vertebra is fixed in extension, motion is restricted in the sagittal plane around the X-axis. With the patient seated in front of and facing away from the doctor, the palpating thumb is placed between the spinous processes. When the patient is passively flexed by the stabilizing hand, the spinous processes should separate. At the extreme of flexion, joint play is tested by pressing the spinous ventrally into forced flexion (Fig. 9.12). The normal articulation exhibits the springiness that is characteristic of joint play. When the vertebra is fixed in extension, the spinous processes do not open and the springiness of joint play is absent.

Manipulation of Thoracic Vertebrae Fixed in Extension (16, 18, 20–23)

With the patient prone, a knife-edge contact is taken between the spinous processes that do not open on flexion (Fig. 9.13). A thoracic roll or pillow may be used to create an apex at the involved segment. The doctor stands on either side of the patient in a low fencing stance, facing the patient's head.

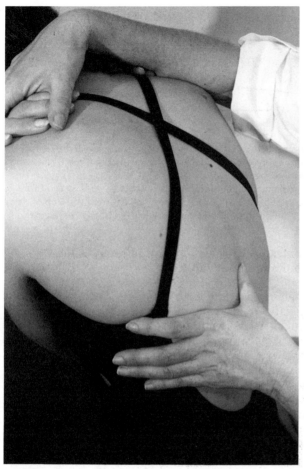

Figure 9.12. Joint play is tested at the extreme of flexion by pressing the spinous ventrally into forced flexion.

Skin traction is applied cephalad prior to contact, to take out tissue slack, and the stabilizing hand is placed on top of the contact hand, with the pisiform of the stabilizing hand placed in the anatomical snuffbox of the contact hand for reinforcement. The contact hand presses cephalad to the point of tension as the doctor's body weight is shifted cephalad.

The patient is then instructed to exhale, and at the point of maximum exhalation, the manipulative thrust is applied cephalad to release the fixation and allow the spinous processes to open. When the fixation occurs in the lower thoracic spine, the doctor is positioned more caudally. The thrust is then directed in an oblique ventral direction as well as cephalad.

When the fixation occurs in the upper thoracic region, the extra skin slack is tractioned cephalad, and the stabilizing hand exerts cephalic traction on the occiput instead of reinforcing the contact hand. The thrust with the knife-edge contact is then directed ventrally as well as cephalad. In all regions of the thoracic spine, a body drop is utilized to enhance the impulse of the manipulative thrust.

A bilateral knife-edge or hypothenar contact may also be taken on transverse processes, with a strongly cephalad thrusting vector. Manipulation of a thoracic vertebra fixed in extension can also be performed with the patient in the supine position (Fig. 9.14). The doctor assumes a low fencing stance facing the patient's head and reaches under the patient, on the same side or across and under the patient, to contact the level of fixation with fingers curled and the middle finger placed between the approximated spinous processes. The patient grasps the back of the neck with the hands, keeping the

Figure 9.13. Manipulation of a thoracic vertebra fixed in extension can be achieved with the patient prone and a knife-edge contact between the spinous processes.

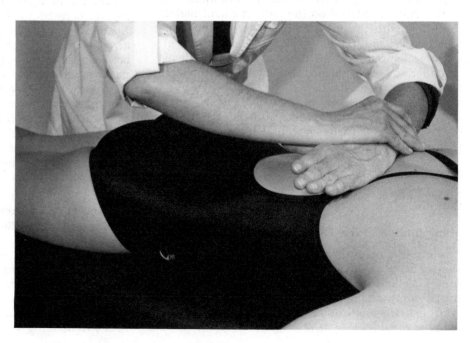

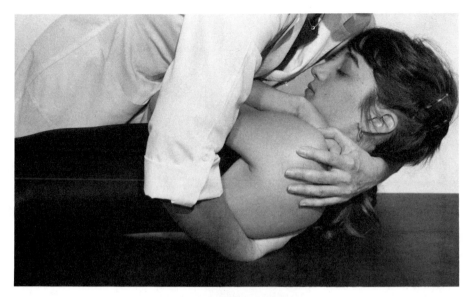

Figure 9.14. The doctor's hand acts as a fulcrum when manipulating a patient in the supine position. A thrust is directed through the patient's elbows, utilizing a chest contact and body drop.

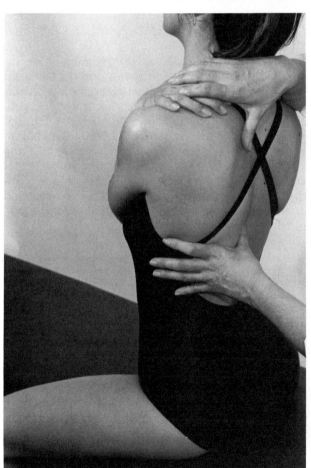

Figure 9.15. The spinous processes of a vertebra fixed in flexion will not close on extension.

sal direction on the patient's elbows, utilizing a chest contact and a body drop. The contact hand acts as a fulcrum, and by keeping the patient in flexion, the blocked spinous processes separate as the fixation is released.

This same principle can be applied with the patient standing against a padded wall and the doctor's hand acting as a fulcrum between the patient's spine and the wall. This method can be cumbersome if the patient is large, because the doctor loses the advantage of the body drop. When the doctor is larger than the patient, this can be an effective method to manipulate the thoracic spine. Repalpation of the manipulated vertebral motion segment should show the spinous processes separating as motion in the sagittal plane is restored.

Palpation of Thoracic Vertebrae Fixed in Flexion (18)

When a thoracic vertebra is fixed in flexion, motion is restricted in the sagittal plane around the X-axis. With the patient seated facing away from the doctor, the palpating thumb is placed between the spinous processes (Fig. 9.15). When the patient is passively extended by the stabilizing hand, the spinous processes should come together. If a vertebra is fixed in flexion, the spinous processes do not close on extension but remain fixed in flexion.

Manipulation of Thoracic Vertebrae Fixed in Flexion (16, 18, 20, 21, 23, 24)

With the patient prone and the doctor facing cephalad in a low fencing stance, a bilateral hypothenar contact is taken on the transverse processes of the fixed vertebra (Fig. 9.16). Skin slack is taken out prior to contact, by tractioning in a cephalad direction. Pressure is then applied in a ventral direction to the point of tension. Following maximum exhalation, a ventral thrust is made utilizing an impulse and a body drop.

elbows together and the forearms parallel. Alternatively, patients may cross their arms across the chest. The patient is then held in flexion with the stabilizing hand, while the doctor thrusts in the dor-

Figure 9.16. To manipulate a patient with a vertebra fixed in flexion in a prone position, a thrust is made with a bilateral hypothenar contact in a ventral direction.

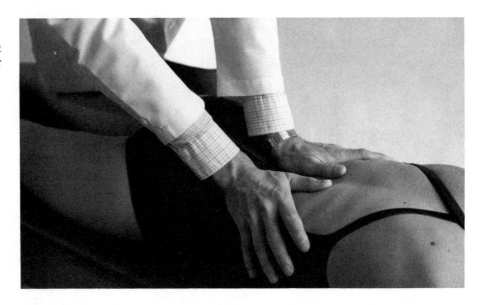

In the upper thoracic region the doctor may stand at the head of the patient facing caudally, and the thrust is made slightly ventral as well as in a caudad direction to accommodate the plane of the discs (i.e., perpendicular to the facet planes) (Fig. 9.11). In the lower thoracic region the thrust is slightly ventral as well as cephalad, according to the thoracic curve.

Manipulation of a thoracic vertebra fixed in flexion can also be accomplished with the patient supine (Fig. 9.17). The doctor assumes a low fencer stance, and the patient's arms are crossed or the hands are locked behind the neck, with the patient's arm on the side of the doctor's contact arm, inferior. The patient is then flexed, with the doctor's stabilizing hand behind the patient's head, and the other hand contacting the transverse processes of the inferior vertebra of the fixed motion segment. The fingers of the contact hand are curled and placed on the transverse process on one side, with a thenar and hypothenar contact on the other transverse process. The patient is then lowered with the stabilizing hand, and at the end point of patient exhalation, the thrust is made on the patient's elbows, utilizing a chest contact and a body drop, while the patient is extended over the contact hand, which acts as a fulcrum. The spinous processes of the manipulated vertebra should then close on repalpation of the previously fixed vertebral motion segment.

Figure 9.17. Manipulation of a thoracic vertebra fixed in flexion can be performed by extending the supine patient over the contact hand which acts as a fulcrum.

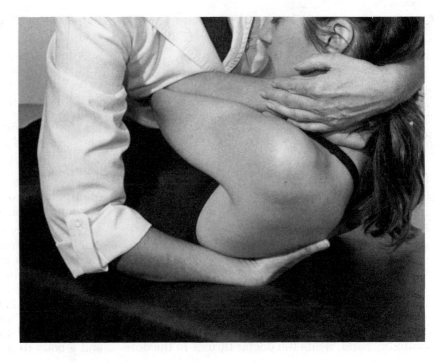

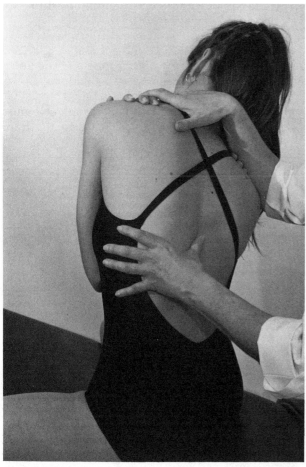

Figure 9.18. Loss of joint play, indicating lateral flexion fixation, can be palpated with the thumb placed against the side of the spinous process, while the patient is laterally flexed to the same side.

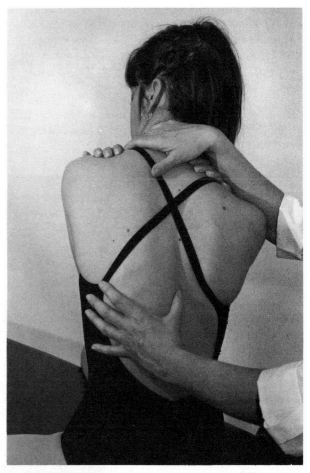

Figure 9.19. Palpation for a loss of rotation in a thoracic vertebra is determined with the palpating thumb pressed against the side of the spinous process, while the patient is rotated to the extreme range of motion on the contralateral side.

Palpation of Thoracic Vertebrae Fixed in Lateral Flexion and Rotation (18)

Because lateral flexion and rotation are coupled motions (Chapter 2), manipulation of the thoracic spine is generally designed to release movement restriction in both the coronal and horizontal planes around the Z and Y axes. Motion palpation will be described for each component of this coupled movement since one component may be more restricted than the others. By determining if one predominant component of this coupled movement is more restricted than the other, the line of drive of the thrust can be directed toward the predominant movement restriction more specifically, to release the fixation.

When a thoracic vertebra is fixed in lateral flexion, motion is restricted in the coronal plane around the Z-axis. With the patient seated and facing away from the doctor, the palpating thumb is placed against the side of the spinous process, and the patient is ipsilaterally flexed. In the lower thoracic spine the spinous processes move toward the thumb (Fig. 9.18).

As the contralateral facets separate, the normal articulation exhibits the springiness of joint play. When the vertebra is fixed in lateral flexion, the springiness of joint play is absent. In the upper thoracic spine the spinous processes move away from the thumb, and as the contralateral facets separate, joint play is also tested by springing the joint.

Lateral flexion to the opposite side is tested by placing the thumb on the other side of the spinous process, and the test for joint play is repeated by pressing on the spinous process and flexing the patient to the ipsilateral side. Absence of joint play indicates a fixation in lateral flexion. Since it is not possible by this method of motion palpation to determine the side of articular fixation, static palpation and x-rays are also useful in determining the side of the open wedge and cephalad transverse process which may become the contact point for the manipulation.

When a thoracic vertebra is fixed in rotation, motion is restricted in the horizontal plane around the Y-axis. With the patient seated and facing away from the doctor, the palpating thumb is placed against the side of the spinous process, and the patient is rotated to the extreme range of motion on the contralateral side (Fig. 9.19).

To determine whether the facet joints are fixed in rotation, joint play is tested by springing the spinous process further into rotation. Joint play on the opposite side is then tested by placing the thumb on the other side of the spinous process and rotating the patient to the extreme range of motion on the contralateral side.

Manipulation of Thoracic Vertebrae Fixed in Rotation and Lateral Flexion (16–23)

Rotational manipulation of the thoracic spine may be performed with the patient prone and the doctor standing on the side opposite the rotational restriction (Fig. 9.20). The doctor takes a broad stance facing the patient or faces slightly cephalad, and an inferior hand pisiform contact is made on the transverse process of the segment in question. The

Figure 9.20. Manipulation of a thoracic vertebra fixed in rotation can be performed with the patient prone. The pisiform of the stabilizing hand is placed in the anatomical snuff box of the contact hand for reinforcement.

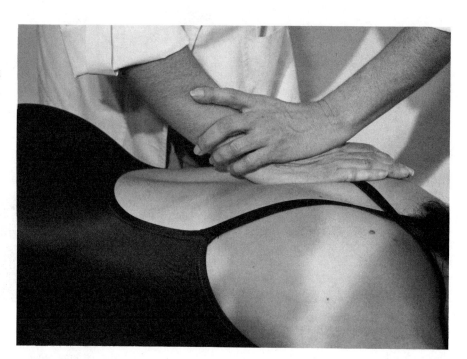

Figure 9.21. A crossed bilateral contact is commonly used to manipulate the supine patient with a rotational fixation in the thoracic spine.

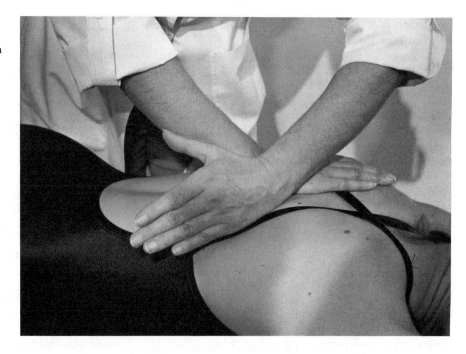

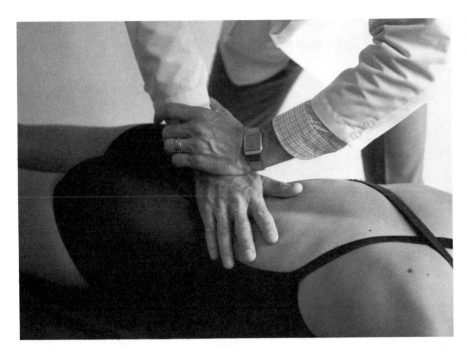

Figure 9.22. A spinous process contact can be used to restore rotation and lateral flexion in a fixed thoracic vertebra.

pisiform of the stabilizing hand is placed in the anatomical snuffbox of the contact hand for reinforcement, and a cephalad tissue pull is taken. At joint tension, a high-velocity thrust is given in a ventral and cephalad direction, paralleling the plane of the facet joints. Maximizing the cephalad component of the vector increases contralateral lateral bending.

This same manipulation may be done with a crossed bilateral contact, in which the stabilizing hand contacts the contralateral transverse process with a pisiform or thenar contact (Fig. 9.21). Lateral bending may thus be maximized by using a cephalad vector with the contact hand and a caudad vector with the stabilizing hand. This causes a torquing of the vertebra (i.e., lateral bending).

The spinous process may be used as a contact point, with the doctor facing the prone patient (Fig. 9.22). A pisiform contact is made on the side of the spinous process toward which rotation is to be restored. The fingers cross the spine, and a thrust is given medially after tissue slack is removed. Adding a cephalad or caudad component to the vector allows simultaneous restoration of lateral flexion.

An upper thoracic vertebra fixed in lateral flexion and/or rotation may be manipulated with the patient in a prone or sitting position, utilizing a thumb con-

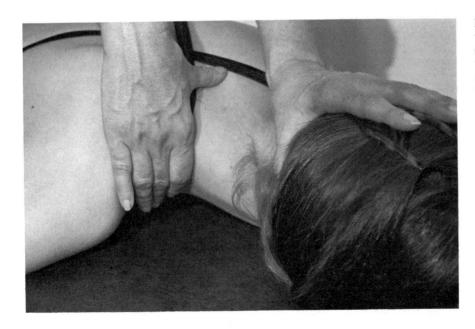

Figure 9.23. An upper thoracic vertebra fixed in lateral flexion and/or rotation may be manipulated with the patient prone (as above) or seated, by utilizing a thumb contact placed against the side of the spinous process.

Figure 9.24. A vertebra fixed in lateral flexion and/or rotation can be manipulated with the patient supine, by lowering the patient's body over the contact hand, which acts as a fulcrum. The patient is laterally flexed and rotated away from the side of thenar contact by the stabilizing hand.

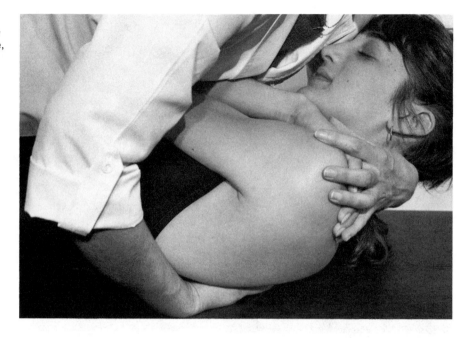

tact (Fig. 9.23). The thumb is placed against the side of the spinous process toward which lateral bending will occur. The stabilizing hand cups the contralateral side of the head and tractions cephalad as the head is laterally bent toward the contact hand. At proper joint tension, a high-velocity medial thrust is delivered with the thumb, as the stabilizing hand simultaneously tractions cephalad and laterally bends the head and cervicothoracic spine. Repalpation of the manipulated segment should reveal restoration of normal motion and end play.

Manipulation of a thoracic vertebra fixed in lateral flexion and rotation can also be performed with the patient in the supine position (Fig. 9.24). The doctor assumes a low fencer stance facing the patient's head and reaches under the patient on the same side or across and under the patient on the opposite side, contacting the more cephalad transverse process with the thenar eminence. The patient grasps the neck with the hands, keeping the elbows together and the forearms parallel. The patient is then flexed and laterally flexed away from the side of thenar contact, by the stabilizing hand. As the patient is lowered over the contact hand (which acts as a fulcrum) the doctor thrusts on the patient's elbows, utilizing a chest contact and body drop.

A vertebra fixed in lateral flexion and rotation can also be manipulated with the patient in side pos-

Figure 9.25. A vertebra fixed in lateral flexion and rotation can be manipulated with the patient in side posture facing the doctor, by using a double thumb contact.

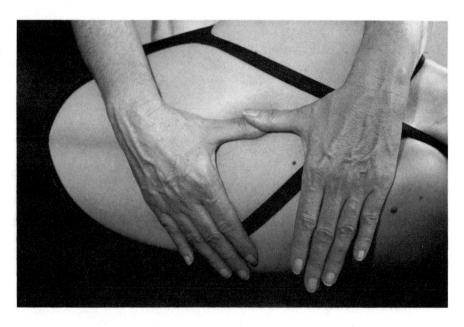

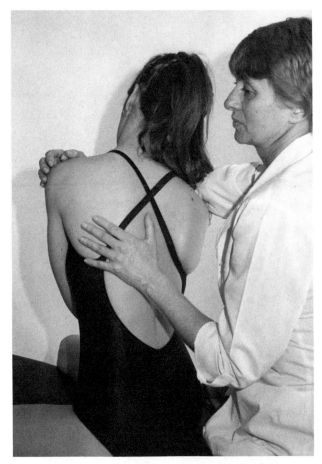

Figure 9.26. A vertebra fixed in rotation can be manipulated with the patient seated, by contacting the facet joint with a pisiform contact and further rotating the patient, giving a slight impulse to release the fixation.

ture, on the side contralateral to the fixation, facing the doctor (Fig. 9.25). The patient stabilizes himself by grasping the table. The doctor reaches over the patient and takes a double thumb contact on the spinous process of the fixed segment. The contact thumb is reinforced by the stabilizing thumb, and a thrust is made with a sharp impulse. The line of drive is medial with a slight cephalad torque, depending on which component of the coupled motion is more restricted. Repalpation of the manipulated segment should reveal normal joint play.

A vertebra fixed more in rotation than lateral flexion can be manipulated with the patient seated (Fig. 9.26). The patient is stabilized by the doctor's knee, which is placed against the patient's thigh, or by the patient straddling the table and gripping it with the knees. The patient's hands are then placed on the shoulders, and the patient is rotated to the extreme range of motion by the doctor's stabilizing arm, which reaches around the patient and contacts the patient's elbows. The doctor then contacts the facet joint with a pisiform contact and further rotates the

patient, giving a slight impulse to release the fixation. Lateral bending, flexion, or extension movements may be added as needed. Repalpation of the fixed vertebral motion segment should reveal normal joint play following manipulation.

Palpation of Costovertebral Fixation

There are two basic types of rib motion. The upper ribs move anteriorly and superiorly, much like the raising and lowering of a bucket handle (Fig. 9.9). This movement expands the thoracic cage in an anterior to posterior direction. The lower ribs move laterally, like opening calipers, and expand the rib cage from side to side (Fig. 9.10).

Motion Palpation for First Rib Fixation

First rib fixation can cause numbness of the upper extremities (Fig. 9.27A). Motion palpation of the first rib is performed with the patient seated and facing away from the doctor. The doctor's palpating fingers contact the first rib in the supraclavicular space. The patient's head is then extended and laterally flexed to the ipsilateral side (Fig. 9.27B). Normal movement of the first rib occurs around the X-axis in the sagittal plane, and the rib becomes more prominent as the neck is laterally flexed and extended to the ipsilateral side.

Manipulation of a First Rib Fixed in Flexion

The first rib is commonly fixed in flexion, with motion restricted in the sagittal plane around the X-axis. When the fixed rib is palpated for motion, it appears elevated and does not recede from the palpating finger as the neck is laterally flexed and extended. This restriction of movement is a common finding following hyperextension injuries of the cervical spine, because of the attachment of the scalene muscles.

To manipulate the first rib, the patient is placed prone, with the doctor standing on the side contralateral to the fixation in a low fencing stance. The contact hand reaches beyond the first rib and contact is made with the lateral aspect of the first metacarpal-phalangeal joint, moving back onto the first rib as the tissue slack is tractioned in a posterior, caudal, and medial direction (Fig. 9.28A). The stabilizing hand contacts the patient's occiput, and the head is rotated away and laterally flexed toward the side of fixation (Fig. 9.28B). As the contact hand tractions dorsally and the patient's head is rotated and laterally flexed further, the contact hand thrusts in a ventral and caudal direction, with a rolling action to the rib. A slight torque is introduced by pronation of both forearms, and both hands thrust simultaneously (25). Repalpation of the manipulated rib should reveal restored motion as the rib becomes less prominent on lateral flexion and rotation of the neck.

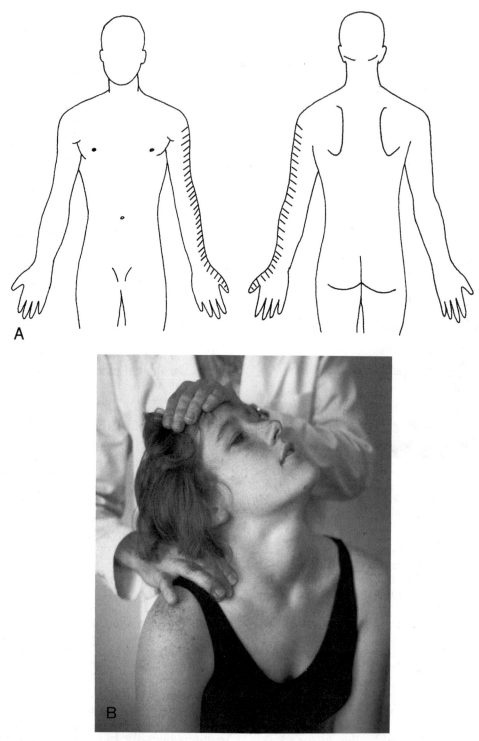

Figure 9.27. First rib fixation. **A,** Pain pattern of a patient with a first rib fixation. Major complaints were numbness (−) in the lateral aspect of the left upper extremities, including the thumb, and weakness of the left arm, forearm, and hand.

B, Palpation of first rib motion is monitored by contacting the first rib in the supraclavicular space and then extending and laterally flexing the patient's head.

Motion Palpation of Other Costovertebral Fixation

With the patient seated in front of and facing away from the doctor, the doctor's stabilizing arm reaches in front of the patient, grasping the back of the contralateral shoulder, with the biceps contacting the front of the shoulder. The patient's head is laterally flexed, and the patient maximally rotated

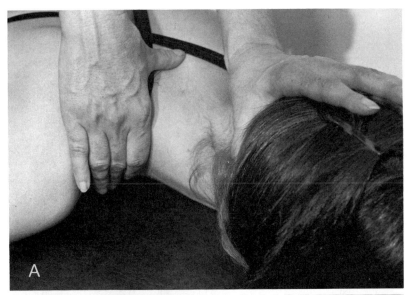

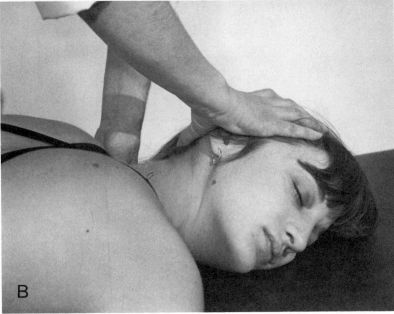

Figure 9.28. **A,** To manipulate the first rib, the doctor's first metacarpal-phalangeal joint contacts the rib. **B,** The stabilizing hand rotates the patient's head toward the contralateral side.

away from the side being palpated. The palpating thumb then slides out from the spinous process onto the angle of the rib. Motion of the costovertebral joint is then palpated, while the stabilizing hand flexes, extends, laterally flexes, and rotates the patient. Joint play can also be tested by springing the joint. The fixed rib will appear more prominent, and motion will be restricted.

Manipulation of Costovertebral Fixation

Costovertebral fixation causes complaints of stabbing pain accentuated by breathing (Fig. 9.29A). Palpation of a rib fixed in flexion reveals a narrow and deeper intercostal space above the rib and a wider but shallower intercostal space beneath. Movement of the rib is restricted in extension. To release a rib fixed in flexion, the patient is positioned supine with the arms crossed and the hands grasping the back of the neck. The arm on the side of fixation is placed underneath. The doctor stands on the contralateral side in a low fencing stance and reaches across the patient. The patient is flexed by the doctor's stabilizing hand, which is placed beneath the patient's neck. The fingers of the contact hand are flexed, and the thenar eminence is placed in the intercostal space above the fixed rib, contacting the posterior superior margin of the rib angle. The thrust is then made by the doctor's chest on the patient's arms. The contact hand acts as a fulcrum, with the thenar eminence exerting a rolling force directed caudad as the thrust is made (Fig. 9.29B). Repalpation should reveal restored motion to the manipulated rib.

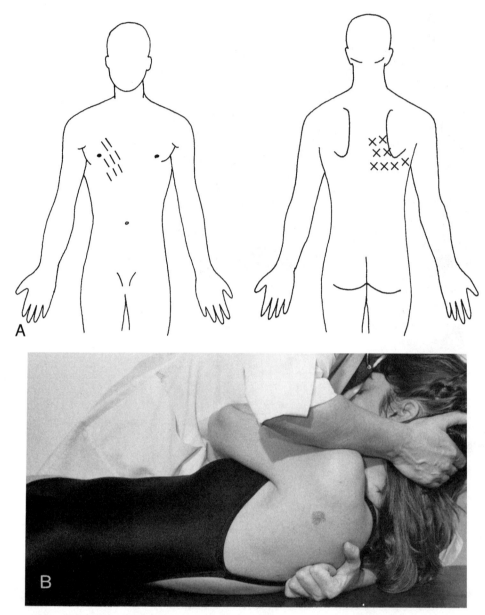

Figure 9.29. Costovertebral fixation. **A,** Pain chart of a patient with a midthoracic rib fixation, complaining of a stabbing pain in the anterior chest (\) and aching in the posterior thoracic region (×). **B,** To manipulate a costovertebral fixation with the patient supine, the thenar eminence of the doctor's contact hand is placed on the margin of the rib angle.

To manipulate a rib fixed in extension, the procedure is the same as that above, with the contact point on the posterior inferior margin of the rib angle. As the body drop is made, the contact hand rolls the fixed rib, lifting the rib into flexion. Repalpation should reveal restored motion. If motion is more restricted in lateral flexion and rotation, a slight torque can be introduced into the restriction, making the manipulation more specific.

To manipulate a costovertebral fixation with the patient prone, the doctor's low fencing stance is varied, depending on the direction of fixation. For a rib fixed in flexion the doctor faces caudally with a pisiform contact on the angle of the rib. Tissue slack is tractioned in a caudal direction and the stabilizing hand contacts the contralateral transverse process. The thrust is in a caudal direction with a torque directed into the resistance, to release any lateral flexion restriction.

When a rib is fixed in extension, the doctor faces cephalad in a low fencing stance. The tissue slack is tractioned cephalad to tension, and the line of drive of the thrust is cephalad, with a slight torque introduced to release any restriction in lateral flexion. A short body drop accompanies the thrust. Repalpation of the manipulated rib should reveal restored motion at the costovertebral articulation (Fig 9.30).

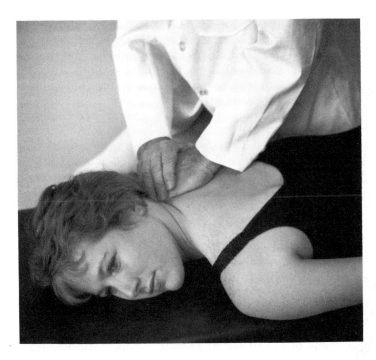

Figure 9.30. To manipulate a costovertebral fixation with the patient prone, the doctor's low fencing stance (above) is varied, depending on the direction of the fixation.

DIFFERENTIAL DIAGNOSIS OF THORACIC SPINE DISORDERS

In addition to vertebral and costovertebral joint dysfunction, a number of other conditions should be considered when diagnosing thoracic spine disorders.

Thoracic Disc Herniation

One of the most serious of these conditions is the herniated thoracic intervertebral disc. While the incidence of thoracic disc herniation is not as great as that of disc lesions in the cervical and especially in the lumbar spine, thoracic disc lesions do occur and can produce serious consequences, including paraplegia in the worst cases (26, 27). According to D'Ambrosia (15), thoracic disc herniation is "not a common disease by any estimation." He indicates that it occurs predominantly in males, with the highest incidence in the fifth decade. The T11-T12 vertebral motion segment is the site most frequently involved. Extrusion of a thoracic intervertebral disc compromises the function of the spinal cord, either by direct compression on the cord or indirectly by interruption of the vascular supply (28). Predisposing factors include previous injury, often of an insignificant degree (27), degeneration, and healed osteochondrosis (Scheuermann's disease) (21).

Clinical features may include vague back pain that is poorly localized. It may be referred unilaterally or bilaterally about the chest, abdomen, or lower extremities. Typically, the pain is intensified by neck flexion, coughing, or straining. It is usually relieved by recumbancy (27). Sensory deficits may include paresthesia and paresis of the lower extrem-

ities. Advanced cases exhibit paraplegia and loss of sphincter control.

The herniated thoracic disc frequently shows degenerative changes on radiographs, with calcification of the disc (19). Adjacent discs may also show calcification, and when the calcific shadow appears in the spinal canal, it is an indication of an extruded disc (27). Further diagnostic imaging is necessary to confirm suspected disc herniation, as at any level of the spine.

Stoddard (21) recommends intermittent manual traction of the spine, with the patient in the supine position. With the ankles strapped to one end of the table, he recommends six or seven pulls with the doctor's right hand tractioning the occiput, and the left hand gripping the chin. When the patient has relaxed, a stronger pull is applied, which he suggests may produce a painful click. This technique is not recommended where severe muscle guarding is palpable, where the symptoms are acute, or where hypermobility is present. Advancing neurological deficits are a contraindication to conservative chiropractic care, and these patients should be referred immediately for neurological evaluation (Chapter 4). Stoddard (21) observes that the acute phase of thoracic prolapse subsides more quickly than does disc herniation in the cervical and lumbar regions of the spine. The acute phase passes in approximately 10 days.

Juvenile Kyphosis (Scheuermann's Disease)

Juvenile kyphosis was first described by Scheuermann in 1920 as a fixed, arcuate deformity developing at puberty, caused by wedged-shaped changes in the vertebrae (20). This condi-

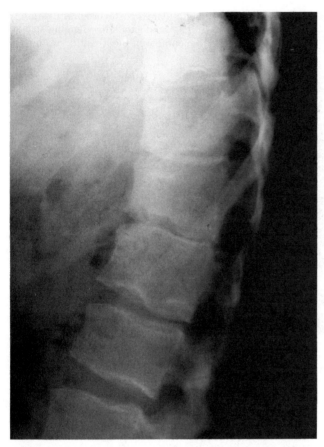

Figure 9.31. Early radiographic changes seen in cases of juvenile kyphosis (Scheuermann's disease) show irregularities of intervertebral disc material into the anterior vertebral bodies (Schmorl's nodes). Advanced changes are indicated by anterior body collapse with characteristic wedging of adjacent vertebrae.

tion has been variously described as vertebral epiphysitis, adolescent kyphosis, osteitis deformans juvenalis, and vertebral osteochondritis (7, 27, 29–32).

It is fairly common, affecting both males and females. The onset is usually at puberty, and the condition progresses during adolescence until vertebral growth has ceased in the later teens. It commonly involves the epiphyseal plates of three or four adjacent vertebral bodies of the mid and lower thoracic spine.

Despite the high incidence (up to 8.3%) (15), the etiology of this condition has not been established. Current theories on the pathogenesis of juvenile kyphosis include aseptic necrosis, low-grade infection, disc herniation (Schmorl's nodes), endocrine abnormalities, hereditary factors, vitamin deficiencies, fluoride toxicity, malnutrition, osteoporosis, mechanical factors, deficient calcification, and trabecular deficiencies of the spine (29).

Turek (27) outlines the sequence of pathology as follows:

1. Loss of disc substance through defects in the cartilaginous endplate into the body.
2. Excessive pressure on the cephalad and caudad surfaces of the body, mainly anteriorly.
3. Interference with ossification of the apophyseal ring by pressure.
4. Interference with endochondral ossification by pressure. Improper proliferation and maturation of the chondrocytes in the epiphyseal plate prevents normal bony replacement. This results in irregularity of the final bone endplates.
5. Wedge-shaped vertebra development because the maximum pressure and retardation of longitudinal growth is anterior.
6. Fixation of the involved portion of the spine due to loss of disc substance and replacement by fibrous tissue.

Clinical features include kyphotic deformity, with complaints of progressive back pain in 20 to 60% of patients (15). The pain is particularly common at the end of an active day. Previous attempts to encourage the patients to improve their posture have not been successful. Postural evaluation reveals an exaggerated kyphosis in the thoracic region, with a compensatory increase in the lumbar lordosis. Palpation and percussion of the spinous processes may produce local tenderness. Palpable paraspinal muscle spasm may also be present. The hamstring and pectoral muscles are tight (29, 31).

Radiographic examination (Fig. 9.31) in the early stages may show no abnormalities, but as the condition progresses, irregularities along the vertebral body and intervertebral disc border are seen, with protrusion of the disc material into the anterior vertebral bodies (Schmorl's nodes). As the anterior border of the vertebra is progressively weakened, the anterior body collapses, with characteristic wedging affecting several adjacent vertebrae. The intervertebral discs become narrowed and irregular. In advanced cases only a slit-like disc remains. Fusion of the apophyseal ring is delayed, uniting at 18 to 20 years of age or later. Ununited apophyses resemble limbic bones and should not be mistaken for fractures.

Mild cases of Scheuermann's disease may go unnoticed until identified in later radiographic examinations. Since the condition is self-limiting, treatment is aimed at the prevention of progressive thoracic kyphosis. In the early stages, exercises to strengthen the spinal extensors are beneficial (31). Reflex muscle spasm may be reduced by basic reflex technique (29), which applies a light contact to the sacrotuberous ligament (Chapter 7), or through deep-tissue massage (Chapter 12). Osseous manipulation should be limited to light thrusts to the area of involvement when concurrent fixations exist. Tight pectoral and hamstring muscles should be stretched (Chapter 22). Joint fixations due to the compensa-

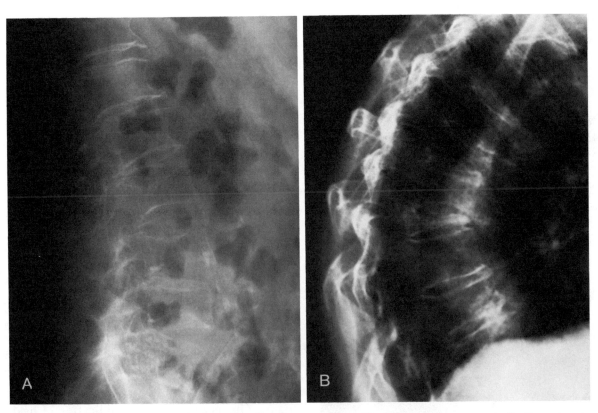

Figure 9.32. **A**, Typical "codfish" vertebrae are found in patients with vertebral collapse due to osteoporosis. **B**, Anterior compression fractures are common in the thoracic spine with advanced osteoporosis.

tory increase in the cervical and lumbar lordotic curves should be treated with manipulation. Jahn et al. (29) recommend tractional techniques and physical therapy as adjunctive therapies (Chapter 14), as well as nutritional supplementation including 40,000 IU of vitamin A daily for three months. Plaster body casts and modified Milwaukee braces are recommended during the painful phase in severe cases to help to prevent progressive deformity. Significant deformity and pain may require referral for surgical treatment.

Osteoporosis of the Spine

Osteoporosis of the spine involves a reduction in number and size of bony trabeculae, which weakens the vertebrae and results in deformity and pain (33). The spine, ribs, and pelvis exhibit the most prominent changes, and compression fractures of T-12 and L-1 are the most common complications involving the spine. There is a higher incidence in females, probably due to hormonal factors and inactivity. Schmorl and Junghanns (33) state that beyond age 65, over 65% of females and 20% of males show radiographic evidence of osteoporosis. Other etiological factors have been implicated including dietary deficiencies, malabsorption syndromes, iatrogenic steroid administration, and endocrine disorders.

Pathological changes include thinning of the cortex and trabeculae of the vertebral body. The supe-

rior and inferior body endplates may be concave from indentation by the intervertebral disc. In the thoracic spine, the bodies are compressed anteriorly, accentuating the dorsal kyphotic curve. Microscopically, the transverse trabeculae are absent, and the longitudinal trabeculae are depleted in number and size (27).

Clinically, the patient complains of ill-defined, aching back pain. A sudden sharp pain may occur with the slightest pressure, as the fragile bone succumbs and fractures. This may be provoked by minimal trauma such as bending, lifting, or raising a window. The affected portion of the spine is tender to palpation and percussion. If compression is extreme, a kyphotic point may be evident. Painful muscle spasm accompanies the acute phase, and the patient gradually becomes hunched. If the fracture occurs at multiple levels, the patient suffers a stepwise loss of height. Radiographs reveal the typical "codfish" vertebrae (15) (Fig. 9.32A). All patients who are susceptible to osteoporotic changes, due to age or history, must be evaluated radiographically before manipulation is attempted (Fig. 9.32B) (Chapter 4).

Conservative treatment includes bed rest for a short time while the patient is acute (27). Following this, activity is encouraged. Malabsorption deficits should be treated, and adequate protein, vitamin, and mineral requirements should be included in the diet. Severe cases may be referred for administration

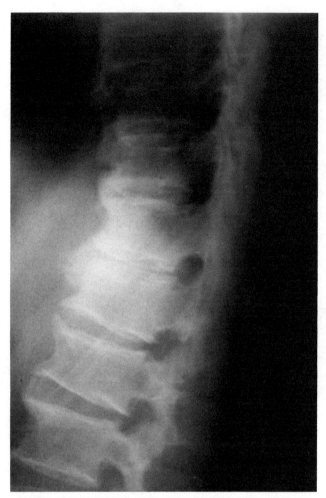

Figure 9.33. Characteristic radiographic findings seen in patients with diffuse idiopathic skeletal hyperostosis are laminated new bone formations along the anterior vertebral bodies.

of sex hormones, but this is not without side effects and should not be used as a substitute for more conservative therapies. Medical treatment may include intramuscular injection of liver extract, folic acid, vitamin B_{12}, and calcium lactate, in addition to dietary supplementation (27).

Diffuse Idiopathic Skeletal Hyperostosis (Forestier's Disease)

Diffuse idiopathic skeletal hyperostosis (DISH) is characterized by ankylosing vertebral hyperostosis. It occurs in patients over the age of 50 who develop ossification of the anterior and right lateral aspects of the vertebral column. It is generally not seen on the left due to the pulsating aorta. The most common sites of involvement are the middle and lower thoracic regions, usually T7–12. This ossification may take on a flowing appearance in the cervical region and produce osteophytes large enough to cause dysphagia.

The presenting symptoms are vertebral stiffness, back pain, and decreased range of motion. Peripheral musculoskeletal involvement with pain and stiffness of the extremity joints accompanies less than half of the cases. Radiographic findings include a distinct pattern of laminated new bone formation along the anterior and right lateral bodies (Fig. 9.33). Disc spaces are unaffected, distinguishing this condition from degenerative joint disease and ankylosing spondylitis (15). Patients should be tested for diabetes, which occurs concomitantly in over 20% of cases (34).

Costochondritis (Tietze Syndrome)

Costochondritis should not be confused with biomechanical joint dysfunction. This syndrome, characterized by a nodular swelling of the rib cartilage, is not amenable to manipulation, which can lead to further irritation of these joints if repeatedly applied. The patient commonly reports a history of an upper respiratory viral infection that becomes localized in the costochondral joints. The patient complains of pain in the chest accentuated by respiratory movement and coughing. Palpatory tenderness and swelling at the costochondral joints, especially of the 2nd and 3rd ribs, is seen clinically (30). Healing may be hastened by the application of heat and vitamin supplementation. A rib belt may be utilized to restrict respiratory movement.

Thoracic Myofascial Pain Syndromes

Most of the thoracic myofascial trigger points are found in the upper thoracic, paraspinal, accessory, and interscapular muscles. The antigravity muscles that support the pectoral girdle, including the trapezius, rhomboid, and levator scapulae, are among the most common harboring myofascial trigger points. This is primarily due to static loading of these muscles as the individual works for prolonged periods with the arms in elevated positions. The pain tends to be aggravated by fatigue, static load, and stress.

Shoulder girdle involvement must be differentiated from and is commonly mistaken for thoracic and cervical spine conditions. Trigger points must be differentiated from rib fixations since they produce similar symptoms, including pain on respiration (Chapter 12).

Ankylosing Spondylitis

Ankylosing spondylitis (Marie-Strumpell disease) is a form of polyarthritis characterized by progressive bony ankylosis of the sacroiliac and spinal joints. The disease is much more common in males than in females, with estimated ratios ranging from 9:1 to 15:1 (15, 31). The onset is usually between the late teens and 35 years of age. The etiology of ankylosing spondylitis is unknown, although hereditary factors are thought to be involved. It primarily affects the sacroiliac and apophyseal joints of the

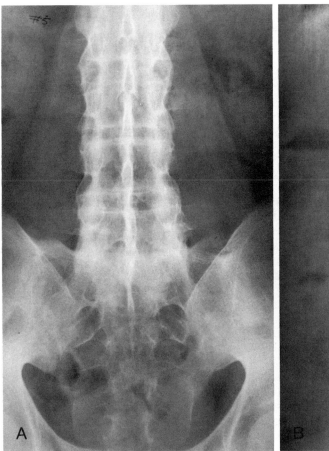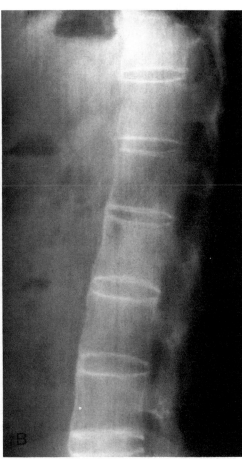

Figure 9.34. **A**, Early radiographic changes in patients with ankylosing spondylitis, as seen in the sacroiliac articulation irregularities and blurring of the subchondral body margins, with reactive sclerosis in both sides of the joint. **B**, Advanced changes seen in the thoracic spine include squared vertebral bodies and ossification of the anulus fibrosis, producing the characteristic "bamboo spine."

spine, but may involve the proximal joints of the extremities.

Ankylosing spondylitis is a systemic inflammatory disorder marked by synovial proliferation. The process also involves the surrounding fibers and ligaments, which may ultimately become ossified, leading to bony ankylosis. Beginning usually in the sacroiliac joints, the process spreads upward and may ultimately involve the intervertebral discs and the costovertebral and posterior facet joints.

Clinically, the patient presents with low back pain, often unrelieved by rest. There may be systemic complaints of fatigue, anemia, intermittent low-grade fever, anorexia, and weight loss. Marked loss of lateral flexion bilaterally is a consistent clinical finding (7, 34). Involvement of the costovertebral joints causes a significant decrease in chest expansion, with pain on deep breathing. As the spinal column becomes progressively stiffer, it also becomes more kyphotic. The disease process may arrest spontaneously at any stage, but with relentless progression the patients may become so ky-

photic that they cannot look straight ahead. The more severe cases may also involve the hip joints, and walking is extremely difficult.

Changes are first seen radiographically in the sacroiliac articulations, which show irregularities and blurring of the subchondral margins, with reactive sclerosis on both sides of the joint (Fig. 9.34A). Eventually these joints ossify. Vertebral erosions develop at the superior and inferior anterior aspect of the vertebral bodies, giving them a square appearance. Subsequent ossification of the anulus fibrosis of the intervertebral disc produces the characteristic radiographic appearance of the "bamboo spine" (Fig. 9.34B). Laboratory examination reveals mild anemia and an elevated ESR, with a positive HLA-B27 antigen in 80% of cases.

Manual treatment is aimed at relieving pain and preventing progressive flexion deformity. Maintenance of thoracic mobility is important (7), but forceful manipulation in the acute inflammatory phase is contraindicated (24, 34). Gentle manipulation and adjunctive soft-tissue therapy is not pre-cluded and may in some cases provide significant palliative effect (personal communication, P Solicito, 1989).

Referred pain from diseased viscera should always be considered with pain in the thoracic region. Viscerosomatic referred pathways are well recognized, with right subscapularis pain accompanying gallbladder disease, and left arm pain typical in cardiac patients. Thoracic joint problems commonly simulate visceral disease through autonomic nerve involvement as well. These somatovisceral reflexes can cause much confusion and needless anxiety when they are unidentified. Grieve (35) suggests that the incidence of counterfeit visceral symptoms is probably much higher than that of frank visceral disease. He recommends that vertebral segments be routinely examined whenever visceral pathology is under consideration, noting that the thoracic spine has a unique capacity for much mischief by way of referred pain.

Further discussion of visceral conditions related to the spine is found in Chapter 14. Undoubtedly the state of the spinal column affects the functional status of visceral organs. Because successful manual therapy can mask the pain of visceral pathology, which may remain uninfluenced by removal of muscle spasm caused by referred pain, true visceral pathology should be considered. Patients may have both visceral disease and a biomechanical disease of the spine in associated segments. In this situation the patient is best managed by cooperation between the medical specialist and the chiropractor (36).

References

1. Hildebrant RW: *Chiropractic Spinography: A Manual of Technology and Interpretation*, ed 2. Baltimore, Williams & Wilkins, 1985, p 101.
2. Kapandjii IA: *The Physiology of the Joints*, vol 3: *The Trunk and Vertebral Column*, ed 2. Translated by Honore. London, Churchill Livingstone, 1974, pp 130, 132, 134, 146, 164, 239.
3. White AA, Panjabii MM: *Clinical Biomechanics of the Spine*. Philadelphia, JB Lippincott, 1978, pp 236, 75.
4. Warwick R, Williams P: *Gray's Anatomy*, ed 35. Philadelphia, WB Saunders, 1973, pp 418–419, 510–513, 519.
5. Steindler A: *Kinesiology of the Human Body Under Normal and Pathological Conditions*. Springfield, IL, Charles C Thomas, 1973, p 215.
6. Donish EW, Basmajian JV: Electromyography of deep back muscles in men. *Am J Anat*, 133:25–36, 1972.
7. Grieve GP: *Common Vertebral Joint Problems*. New York, Churchill Livingstone, 1981, pp 14–16, 234–235, 242, 244–246.
8. White AA, Hirsch C: The significance of the posterior elements in the mechanics of the thoracic spine. *Clin Orthop* 81:2–14, 1971.
9. Grice AS: A biomechanical approach to cervical and dorsal adjusting. In Haldeman S: *Modern Developments in the Principles and Practice of Chiropractic*. East Norwalk, CT, Appleton-Century-Crofts, 1979, pp 352–353.
10. Fligg DB: Lateral recumbent rib adjustment. *JCCA* 28:277–278, 1984.
11. Vear HJ: *Notes for 263 Principles, Disorders and Syndromes of the Thoracic Spine*. Toronto, CMCC, Feb 1979, p 4.
12. Schoenholtz F: Conservative management of costovertebral subluxation. *ACA J Chiro* 17:S-76-S-79, p 14, 1980.
13. Maurer EL: The thoraco-costal facet syndrome with introduction of the marginal line and the rib sign. *ACA J Chiro* 13:S-151-S-164, 1976.
14. West HG: Physical and spinal examination procedures utilized in the practice of chiropractic. In Haldeman S: *Modern Developments in the Principles and Practices of Chiropractic*. East Norwalk, CT, Appleton-Century-Crofts, 1979, pp 280, 284, 286.
15. D'Ambrosia RD: *Musculoskeletal Disorders: Regional Examination and Differential Diagnosis*. Philadelphia, JB Lippincott, 1977, pp 217, 271, 273, 279, 287.
16. Peterson DH: *Western States Chiropractic College Adjustive Technique Manual*. Portland, OR, WSCC, 1988, pp 12–44.
17. Herbst RW: *Gonstead chiropractic science and art*. Sci-Chi Publications, 1971–1980, pp 81–92.
18. Schafer RC, Faye LJ: *Motion Palpation and Chiropractic Technique*. Huntington Beach, CA, Motion Palpation Institute, 1989, pp 159–164, 169–183.
19. Bovee MI, Burns JR, Carrigg PM, Harmon RO, Johnson MR, Kern DP, Swearingen TC, Willhite FS: *Adjusting Technique Manual*. Davenport, IA, Palmer College of Chiropractic, 1981, pp 143–159.
20. Bourdillon JF, Day EA: *Spinal Manipulation*. Los Altos, CA, Appleton and Lange, 1987, pp 156–162.
21. Stoddard A: *Manual of Osteopathic Practice*, ed 2. London, Hutchinson, 1983, pp 203–208, 210–211.
22. Maigne R: *Orthopedic Medicine, A New Approach to Vertebral Manipulations*. Springfield, IL, Charles C Thomas, 1972, pp 126–129, 358–360.
23. States AZ: *Spinal and Pelvic Techniques*. Lombard, IL, National College of Chiropractic, 1968, pp 47–56.
24. Maitland GD: *Vertebral Manipulation*, ed 4. London, Butterworth, 1977, p 210.
25. Stonebrink RD: Thoraco-costal adjustments and related supine techniques. *ACA J Chiro* 12:S-55-S-61, 1975.
26. Kumar R, Buckley TF: First thoracic disc protrusion. *Spine* 11:499–501, 1986.
27. Turek SL: *Orthopaedics: Principles and Their Application*, ed 3. Philadelphia, JB Lippincott, 1977, pp 1359, 1380, 1381, 1393, 1395.
28. Benson MKD, Byrnes DP: The clinical syndromes and surgical treatment of thoracic intervertebral disc prolapse. *J Bone Joint Surg (Br)* 57B:471–477, 1975.
29. Jahn WT, Griffiths JH, Hacker RA: Conservative management of Scheuermann's juvenile kyphosis. *J Manip Physiol Ther* 1:228–245, 1978.
30. Gartland JJ: *Fundamentals of Orthopaedics*, ed 2. Philadelphia, W B Saunders, 1974, pp 89, 217.
31. Salter RB: *Textbook of Disorders and Injuries of the Musculoskeletal System*. Baltimore, Williams & Wilkins, 1970, pp 183, 279.
32. Wiles P: *Essentials of Orthopaedics*, ed 3. Boston, Little Brown & Co, 1959, p 101.
33. Schmorl G, Junghanns H: *The Human Spine in Health and Disease*, ed 2. New York, Grune & Stratton, 1971, p 105.
34. Cyriax J: *Textbook of Orthopaedic Medicine*. vol 1: *Diagnosis of Soft Tissue Lesions*. Baltimore, Williams & Wilkins, 1975, pp 424, 430.
35. Grieve GP: Thoracic joint problems and simulated visceral disease. In Grieve GP (ed): *Modern Manual Therapy of the Vertebral Column*. New York, Churchill Livingstone, 1986, pp 377–395.
36. Inglis BD, Fraser B, Penfold BR: *Chiropractic in New Zealand: Report of the Commission of Inquiry*. Wellington, New Zealand, PD Hasselberg Government Printer, 1979, p 3.

CHAPTER 10

Disorders of the Cervical Spine

MERIDEL I. GATTERMAN, M.A., D.C.
DAVID M. PANZER, D.C.

Chiropractic treatment of the cervical spine has a relaxing effect on the spinal musculature and a loosening or antihypokinetic effect on spinal articulations, thereby affecting, in a curative manner, a number of ailments elicited by the cervical spine structures. (1)

The cervical spine is made up of two anatomically and functionally distinct regions. These two regions provide for a wide range of movement in all planes, allowing for almost pure rotation and lateral flexion in addition to flexion and extension of the neck (2). The cervical spine forms a long lever, with the head, weighing approximately 10% of the body weight, balanced at the top. This arrangement makes the cervical spine especially vulnerable to traumatic forces.

The primary structures protecting the spine are the muscles, ligaments, and joint capsules. These are the most common components damaged in neck injuries. Other soft-tissue injuries include disc rupture, direct trauma to the nerve roots, and compromise of the neurovascular bundle. Fracture and dislocations do occur, but by far the most common injury to the neck is joint sprain with articular locking and accompanying muscle strain. Joint sprain of the cervical spine is more complex and problematical than sprain of most other joints. The most common biomechanical pattern seen in the cervical spine is locking of the joints at either end of the lever arm, formed by the neck, with stretching of the ligaments in the middle of the cervical spine.

Although it has been suggested that the term "whiplash" be abandoned, it remains a thoroughly descriptive term (3) that applies to many cervical injuries. Because the head is situated at the end of an open chain, the forces generated in the upper cervical region are considerable when the head is unsupported. Any impact to the body when the head is not restrained will produce a whiplike action, jamming the upper and lower cervical joints while stretching the midcervical ligaments that protect the apex of the curve.

This stretching of the anterior and posterior longitudinal ligaments is thought to lead to premature degenerative changes seen in the midcervical spinal joints in posttraumatic (whiplash) victims (4). It is postulated that unreleased joint fixation in the vertebral motion segments of the upper and lower portions of the cervical spine perpetuates the elongation of the sprained ligaments in the midcervical region, making cervical manipulation of traumatic joint fixation the treatment of choice following whiplash injuries (5).

With joint fixation in one vertebral motion segment, compensatory hypermobility in adjacent segments is commonly seen (4, 6, 7). Untreated immobility of blocked motion after "whiplash" injuries tends to prolong symptoms (5) when the body strives to maintain its normal, overall range of cervical motion. Rapid improvement has been demonstrated 8 weeks after the accident with early mobilization of acute whiplash injuries (5).

ANATOMY OF THE CERVICAL SPINE

The seven cervical vertebrae are the smallest moveable vertebrae and are identifiable by their transverse processes, which are perforated by a foramen (foramen transversarii). The first, second, and seventh cervical vertebrae are atypical and will be considered separately.

Typical Cervical Vertebra

The typical cervical vertebra (Fig. 10.1) is wider than it is high, with a comparatively large vertebral foramina. Its superior surface (superior plateau) is

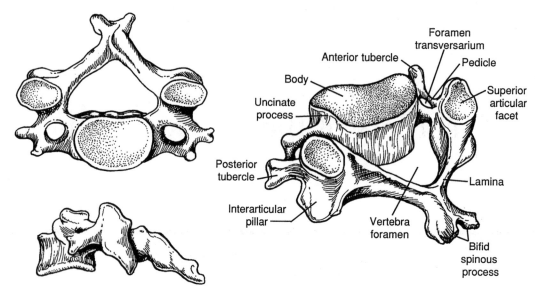

Figure 10.1. A typical cervical vertebra (C3-C6).

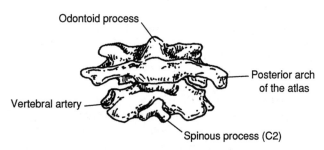

Figure 10.2. Atlas-axis complex (C1-C2 vertebral motion segment). The first and second cervical vetebrae account for 50% of cervical rotation. The *odontoid process* of the axis (C2) serves as a pivot for the ringlike atlas (C1).

raised laterally to form the uncinate processes. These projections harbor the corresponding articular facets in the lateral inferior plateau of the vertebra above, forming the uncovertebral joints (joints of Luschka) (8). Like other synovial joints they are of clinical significance because they are subject to degenerative changes. The anterior inferior surface of the body exhibits a lip that projects downward and fits together with the transversely concave superior surface of the vertebra below. This creates a saddle effect that limits lateral flexion and guides antero-posterior movement during flexion and extension.

The pedicles project somewhat laterally, as well as backward, and the lamina are angled from them in a medial direction. The spinous process is short and usually bifid. The articular pillars extend from the lamina-pedicle junction and support cartilage-lined facets above and below. The superior facets are oval and flat and are directed backward and upward, reciprocating with the similarly shaped inferior facets, which are turned forward and downward (9).

Atypical Cervical Vertebra

The atypical vertebrae of the cervical column are C1 (atlas), C2 (axis), and C7 (vertebra prominens). The first cervical vertebra has been named the atlas because it supports the "globe-like" head. It differs significantly from all other vertebrae in that it lacks a body. Its centrum fuses with the body of the axis to form a projecting pivot (the dens), around which the atlas rotates (Fig. 10.2).

It has no true spinous process, consisting of two large lateral masses connected anteriorly by a short anterior arch and posteriorly by a longer posterior arch. This ringlike structure is divided in two by the transverse ligament, which holds the dens of the axis in the smaller anterior compartment. The spinal cord and the meninges pass through the larger posterior compartment. The anterior arch is slightly curved with a small tubercle at the convexity of the external surface for the attachment of the anterior longitudinal ligament.

On the inner surface there is a small facet (fovea dentalis) that articulates with the odontoid process of the axis. The upper surface of each lateral mass bears a concave facet that faces upward and medially and articulates with the corresponding occipital condyle. The inferior surface of each lateral mass exhibits flat or slightly concave, almost circular facets, which articulate with the similar superior articular facets of the axis. The inferior facets face downward, medially and slightly backward. The medial aspect of each lateral mass has a small rough tubercle for the attachment of the transverse ligament.

The upper surfaces of the posterior arch show a wide groove posterior to each lateral mass, through which the vertebral artery winds. Occasionally, the groove is converted to a foramen (arcuate foramen) by a spicule of bone arching backward from the upper surface of the lateral mass (posterior ponticulum) (10, 11) (see Chapter 4). The first cervical nerve also lies in the groove between the artery and bone. The posterior atlantooccipital membrane attaches to the posterior arch behind the two grooves.

The highest pair of ligamenta flava attach to the lower margin of the posterior arch. The posterior tubercle represents the spinous process that provides for the attachment of the ligamentum nuchae. The two posterior recti capitus minor flank this. The wide transverse processes serve as long lever arms for the muscles that aid in rotation of the head. Attached superiorly are the rectus capitus lateralis in front of the superior oblique. At the tip, the inferior obliques attach, and laterally below, slips of the levator scapulae, splenius cervicis, and scalene medius are inserted (9).

The second cervical vertebra is named the axis, for it provides the pivot around which the atlas, and with it the head, rotates (Fig. 10.2). The dens (odontoid process) extends vertically upward like a tooth. A small oval facet on the front of the dens articulates with the fovea dentalis, the corresponding facet on the back of the anterior arch of the atlas. A groove on the posterior of the dens supports the transverse ligament of the atlas. The apex of the dens is pointed and joined to the apical ligament. Its sides are flattened where the alar ligaments attach.

Lateral to the dens are large oval facets that articulate with the inferior facets of the atlas. They lie considerably anterior to the inferior facets and do not form articular pillars like those found on other cervical vertebrae.

The vertical part of the longus colli muscles attach on each side of the midpoint of the anterior body, and the anterior longitudinal ligament connects to a downward projection on the lower border. The posterior longitudinal ligament and the membrane tectoria attach to the lower posterior border of the body. The pedicles are short, and the lamina thicker than in other cervical vertebrae, providing attachment for the ligamenta flava.

The large and powerful spinous process provides for the pull of muscles which extend, retract, and rotate the head. The inferior obliques arise on each side of the spine, with the rectus capitis posterior major attaching a little posterior to this. The ligamentum nuchae attaches to a gap at the apex of the spine, together with slips of the semispinalis, spinalis cervicis, interspinales, and multifidus. The transverse processes of the axis are small and the levator scapulae attach to the tip between the scalenus medius in front and splenius cervicus behind. The intertransverse muscles attach superiorly and inferiorly.

The transverse foramina are directed superolaterally to allow for lateral deviation of the vertebral arteries as they pass upward to the wider atlas. The inferior articular facets at the junction of the pedi-

cles and laminae face downward and forward, as do those of the typical cervical vertebra.

The seventh cervical vertebra is referred to as the "vertebra prominens" because the long spinous process protrudes at the lower end of the nuchal furrow. The first thoracic vertebra may be just as prominent or more so. The spinous process of C7, thick and almost horizontal, has the lower end of the ligamentum nuchae joined to it. The trapezius, rhomboideus major, serratus posterior superior, splenius capitis, spinalis cervicis, semispinalis thoracis, multifidus, and interspinales are all attached near the tip of the spine of C7. The transverse foramina are small, relative to the large transverse processes (and the vertebral arteries do not pass through the foramina normally).

Ligaments of the Cervical Spine

With the exception of the ligamentum nuchae, the ligaments stabilizing the lower cervical spine (C3-C7) are a continuation of those found in the thoracic and lumbar regions. The ligamentum nuchae (see Typical Vertebral Motion Segments, Chapter 1) is a fibroelastic membrane that forms an intermuscular septum in the neck and is homologous with the supraspinous and interspinous ligaments (Fig. 10.3A).

Superficially, it extends from the external occipital protuberance and external occipital crest to the spine of the seventh cervical vertebra, attaching to the posterior tubercle of the atlas and spines of the cervical vertebrae. This takes the form of a single rounded band, the funicular portion. Attached to the anterior surface of the funicular part is the lamellar portion, which also attaches to the spinous processes of all the cervical vertebrae, the posterior tubercle of the atlas, and intervening interspinous ligaments.

The ligamentum nuchae forms a septum for attachment of muscles of the two sides of the neck. It is less developed and contains fewer elastic fibers in bipedal man than in quadrupedal mammals. It is thought to contain proprioceptive receptors that participate in a connection between the nerves in the nuchal ligament and posterior cervical musculature by way of the spinal cord, assisting in head position and control (12).

The upper cervical complex composed of the occiput, atlas, and axis are anatomically and functionally unique, in comparison to the typical vertebral motion segments that make up the remainder of the spinal column. The supporting ligaments in this region are numerous and strong (Fig. 10.3B&C), and the articular structures are designed to provide a wide range of movement.

The paired atlantooccipital joints are symmetrical and mechanically linked, with reciprocally curved articular surfaces. The convex condyles of the occipital bone articulate with the concave superior articular facets of the atlas. Each atlantal facet is oval and

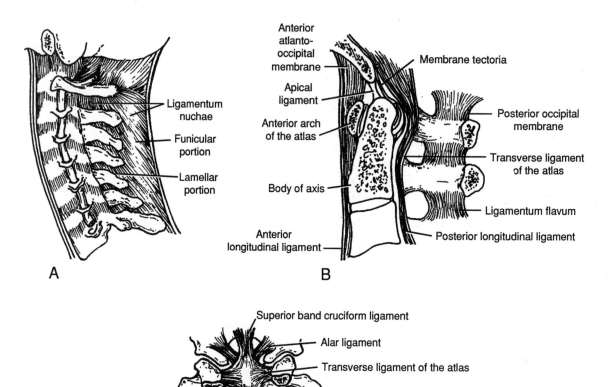

Figure 10.3. Ligaments of the cervical spine.

usually constricted about its middle, running obliquely, anteriorly, and medially.

The bones are united by the articular capsules and the anterior and posterior atlantooccipital membranes. The fibrous capsules are thickened posteriorly and laterally, but are thin and deficient medially.

The dense and broad anterior atlantooccipital membrane passes between the anterior margin of the foramen magnum above and the upper border of the anterior arch of the atlas below. It is continuous laterally with the capsular ligaments and is strengthened in front by the continuation of the anterior longitudinal ligament.

The broad but thin posterior atlantooccipital membrane is connected above to the posterior margin of the foramen magnum and below to the upper border of the posterior arch of the atlas. On each side it arches over the groove for the vertebral artery. The free border of the membrane, as it arches over the artery and first cervical spinal nerve, is sometimes ossified (see ''Posterior Ponticulus,'' Chapter 4).

Four joints comprise articulation of the atlas and axis. The paired, lateral atlantoaxial joints articulate

the inferior facets of the lateral masses of the atlas with the superior facets of the axis. Both articular surfaces are slightly convex in their long axes. The capsular ligaments are thin and loose and strengthened medially by an accessory ligament, which is attached to the body of the axis near the base of the dens and above to the lateral mass of the atlas near the transverse ligament. The two vertebrae are connected in front by a continuation of the anterior longitudinal ligament, which attaches to the anterior arch of the atlas and to the front of the body of the axis. A broad, thin membrane joins the lower border of the posterior arch of the atlas to the upper edges of the lamina of the axis, in series with the ligamenta flava. This membrane is pierced by the second cervical nerve.

The median atlantoaxial joints are formed by the pivot of the atlas around the dens of the axis. Anteriorly, the facet on the anterior surface of the dens articulates with the fovea dentalis on the posterior aspect of the anterior arch of the atlas. This articulation is surrounded by a weak, loose, synovial lined fibrous capsule.

Posteriorly, a second and larger synovial cavity (sometimes termed a bursa) lies between the carti-

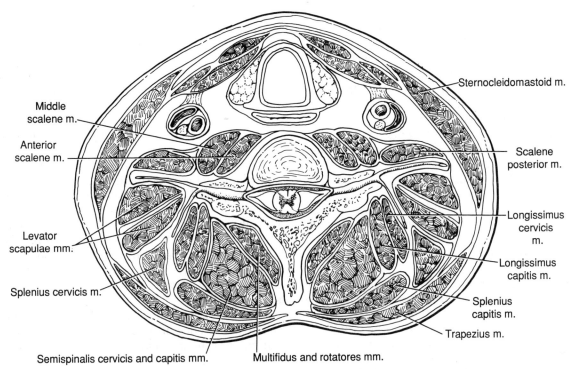

Figure 10.4. Cross-section of prevertebral and posterior muscles of the lower cervical spine. (Modified from Magee DJ: *Orthopedic Physical Assessment*, Philadelphia, WB Saunders, 1987.)

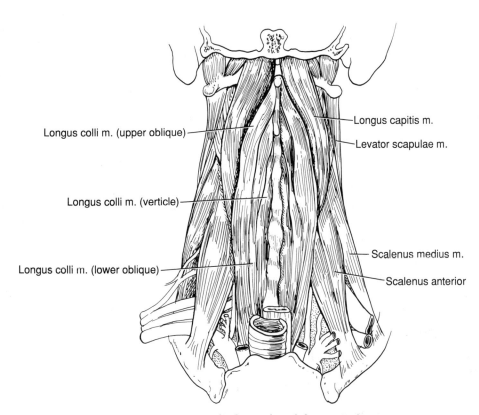

Figure 10.5. Prevertebral muscles of the cervical spine.

lage-covered inferior surface of the transverse ligament of the atlas, where it articulates with the posterior grooved surface of the dens.

The transverse ligament of the atlas is a thick, strong band that compartmentalizes the arch of the atlas and retains the dens in contact with the anterior arch. It is broader in the middle than at the ends and firmly attached on each side to a small tubercle on the medial surface of the lateral mass of the atlas. The anterior median surface is covered by a thin layer of articular cartilage.

It is reinforced by a small, longitudinal band attaching at the upper surface to the basilar portion of the occipital bone between the apical ligament on the membrana tectoria. The lower portion is attached to the posterior body of the axis. This crosslike arrangement gives rise to the name cruciform ligament of the atlas.

The apical ligament of the dens extends from the tip of the dens to the anterior margin of the foramen magnum, blending with the atlantooccipital membrane and upper longitudinal band of the cruciform ligament of the atlas (Fig. 10.3*B*). It retains traces of the notochord in its substance and is said to represent the core of the centrum of the proatlas vertebra.

The tectorial membrane is a broad, strong band situated within the spinal canal. It appears as a continuation of the posterior longitudinal ligament. It covers the posterior aspect of the dens and extends upward, attaching to the basilar part of the occipital bone.

The alar ligaments are two strong, rounded bands on each side of the upper part of the dens. They pass obliquely upward and laterally, attaching to the medial sides of the occipital condyles. The alar ligaments are relaxed on extension of the head but become taut on flexion, limiting this movement. Rotation is also checked by the alar ligament.

Muscles of the Cervical Spine (Tables 10.1, 10.2)

The efficiency of the neck muscles depends on the alignment of the cervical vertebral column. The head is held in equilibrium, balanced by the numerous prevertebral and posterior muscles of the neck (Fig. 10.4). The neck is flexed by bilateral contraction of the prevertebral muscles, which attach anterior to the cervical vertebrae (Fig. 10.5). Extension occurs with bilateral contraction of the posterior cervical muscles (Fig. 10.6 *A-D*). Rotation and lateral flexion are produced by combined unilateral contraction of the prevertebral posterior muscles.

ANOMALIES OF THE CERVICAL SPINE

Anomalies of the cervical spine range from minor to the much more serious malformations that are incompatible with life. Spinal dysraphism is a condition related to failure of formation of the dorsal elements during embryonic development. It ranges from spinal bifida occulta (absence of the posterior arch) to meningomyelocele, diastematomyelia, and dermal cysts.

The more severe anomalies are fatal in the cervical region, whereas the lesser ones may produce only a hairy nevus or radiologic bony anomalies. Isolated defects may appear at the base of the skull, but various combinations involving bone and nerves are more common. The frequent occurrence of these patterns and combinations suggests an interrelationship, if not a common cause.

Basilar impression is one of the most common congenital anomalies affecting the atlantooccipital region. It is an upward movement of the base of the skull in the region of the foramen magnum and is measured by the intracranial extension of the tip of the odontoid process (see Chapter 6). A line is drawn between the posterior edge of the hard palate to the posterocentral margin of the foramen magnum (Chamberlain's line). If the tip of the odontoid process is greater than 6 mm above this line, basilar impression is present. McGregor's line, which is drawn from the upper surface of the posterior edge of the hard palate to the most caudal point of the occipital curve, is another commonly used measurement (Chapter 6).

Clinical symptoms are due primarily to the involvement of neurologic structures. If long tract involvement is present, weakness and later spasticity may be present, depending on the duration of symptoms. Sensory defects are variable. Cerebellar ataxia and lower cranial nerve dysfunction can occur, causing dysphagia and dysarthria. Nystagmus and bizarre respiratory patterns may also occur, along with altered conciousness and periods of confusion. Treatment consists of surgical decompression (13).

Occipitalization of the atlas is a common anomaly of the upper cervical spine. Fusion usually occurs anteriorly, between the arch or rim of the foramen magnum. Though symptoms may not be present, the majority of these patients have some form of neurological abnormality due to the altered shape of the foramen magnum or an associated basilar impression. Neurological symptoms may include ataxia and numbness and pain in the limbs. Long-tract signs with hyperreflexia, Babinski response, spasticity, and weakness may occur. Neck pain may be present, along with abnormal head posture. Treatment is aimed at decompression of the affected structure (13).

The Arnold-Chiari malformation frequently occurs with other congenital malformations of the upper cervical spine. In this anomaly, the cerebellar tonsils and fourth ventricle project into the upper cervical canal. A syrinx, or dilatation of the central canal of the spinal cord, is commonly associated. In infants, hydrocephalus and frequently myelomeningocele are present along with the spinal cord compression. In adults, clinical signs and symptoms may develop slowly and tend to accentuate spinal cord dysfunction. Treatment for this condition is surgical (13).

Table 10.1 Muscles That Move the Head[a]

Muscle	Upper Attachment	Lower Attachment	Nerve Supply
Action: flexion of the head			
1. Rectus capitis anterior	Basilar part of occiput	Inferior lateral mass C1	C1, C2
2. Rectus capitis lateralis	Jugular process occiput	Transverse processes C1	C1, C2
3. Longus capitis	Basilar part of occiput	Transverse processes C3-C6, anterior bodies T1-T3	C1, C2, C3
4. Sternocleidomastoid (head in neutral or flexion)	Mastoid process, lateral 1/2 superior nuchal line	Manubrium of sternum, medial 1/2 superior clavicle	Accessory nerve & C2
Action: extension of the head			
1. Splenius capitis	Mastoid process & below lateral 1/3 superior nuchal line	Lower 1/2 ligamentum nuchae & spinous processes C7-T4	C4, C5, C6
2. Semispinalis capitis	Between superior & inferior nuchal line	Transverse processes C7, T1-T6 & articular processes C4-C6	C1-C8
3. Longissimus capitis	Posterior margin mastoid process	Transverse processes C3-T5	C6-C8
4. Spinalis capitis	Between superior & inferior nuchal line	Transverse processes C7,T1-T6	C6-C8
5. Trapezius	Medial 1/3 of nuchal line, ligamentum nuchae, lateral acromion & spine of scapulae	Spinous processes C1-T12	Accessory, C3-C4
6. Rectus capitis posterior minor	Medial 1/2 inferior nuchal line	Tubercle of posterior arch C1	C1
7. Rectus capitis posterior major	Lateral inferior nuchal line	Spinous process C2	C1
8. Obliquus capitis superior	Between superior & inferior nuchal line	Transverse process C1	C1
9. Obliquus capitis inferior	Transverse process C1	Spinous process C2	C1
10. Sternocleidomastoid (head in extension)	Mastoid process, lateral 1/2 superior nuchal line	Manubrium of sternum, medial 1/2 superior clavicle	Accessory nerve & C2
Action: rotation of the head (muscles contracting to one side)			
1. Trapezius (face moves to opposite side)	Medial 1/3 of nuchal line, ligamentum nuchae, lateral acromion & spine of scapulae	Spinous processes C1-T12	Accessory, C3, C4
2. Splenius capitis (face moves to same side)	Mastoid process & below lateral 1/3 superior nuchal line	Lower 1/2 ligamentum nuchae, spinous processes C7-T4	C4-C6
3. Longissimus capitis (face moves to same side)	Posterior margin mastoid process	Transverse processes C3-T5	C6-C8
4. Semispinalis capitis (face moves to same side)	Between superior & inferior nuchal line	Transverse processes C7, T1-T6 & articular processes C4-C6	C1-C8
5. Obliquus capitis inferior (face moves to same side)	Transverse process C1	Spinous process C2	C1
6. Sternocleidomastoid (face moves to same side)	Mastoid process, lateral 1/2 superior nuchal line	Manubrium of sternum, medial 1/2 superior clavicle	Accessory, C2
Action: lateral flexion of the head			
1. Trapezius	Medial 1/3 of nuchal line, ligamentum nuchae, lateral acromion & spine of scapulae	Spinous processes C1-T12	Accessory, C3, C4
2. Splenius capitis	Mastoid process & below lateral 1/3 superior nuchal line	Lower 1/2 ligamentum nuchae & spinous processes C7-T4	C4-C6
3. Longissimus capitis	Posterior margin mastoid process	Transverse processes C3-T5	C6-C8
4. Semispinalis capitis	Between superior & inferior nuchal line	Transverse processes C7, T1-T6 & articular processes C4-C6	C1-C8
5. Obliquus capitis inferior	Transverse process C1	Superior process C2	C1
6. Rectus capitis lateralis	Jugular process occiput	Transverse processes C1	C1, C2
7. Longus capitis	Basilar part occiput	Transverse processes C3-C6, anterior bodies T1-T3	C1-C3

[a]Modified from Magee DJ: *Orthopedic Physical Assessment*, Philadelphia, WB Saunders, 1987, pp 34–35.

Table 10.2 Muscles That Move the Neck[a]

Muscle	Upper Attachment	Lower Attachment	Nerve Supply
Action: flexion of neck			
1. Longus coli	Transverse processes C5-C6, anterior arch atlas, anterior bodies C2-C4	Bodies C5-C7, transverse processes C5-C6 & bodies T1-T3	C2-C6
2. Scalenus anterior	Transverse processes C3-C6	First rib	C4-C6
3. Scalenus medius	Transverse processes C2-C7	First rib	C3-C8
4. Scalenus posterior	Transverse processes C4-C6	Second and third ribs	C6-C8
Action: extension of the neck			
1. Splenius cervicis	Transverse processes C2-C3	Spinous processes T3-T6	C6-C8
2. Semispinalis cervicis	Spinous processes C2-C5 or C6	Transverse processes T1-T5	C1-C8
3. Longissimus cervicis	Transverse processes C2-C6	Transverse processes T1-T5	C6-C8
4. Levator scapulae	Transverse processes C1-C4	Superior angle scapula	C3-C4, C5 through dorsal scapular nerve
5. Iliocostalis cervicis	Transverse processes C4-C6	Angles third through sixth ribs	C6, C7, C8
6. Spinalis cervicis	Spinous processes C2-C5	Lower part of ligamentum nuchae & spinous processes C7 & T1-T2	C6-C8
7. Multifidus	Spinous processes C2-C5	Articular processes C4-C7	C1-C6, C7, C8
8. Interspinalis cervicis	Spinous processes C2-C7	Spinous processes C3-T1	C1-C8, accessory nerve
9. Trapezius	Medial 1/3 of nuchal line, ligamentum nuchae, lateral acromion & spine of scapulae	Spinous processes C1-T12	C3, C4, accessory nerve
10. Rectus capitus posterior major	Inferior nuchal line	Spinous process C2	C1
11. Rotatores brevis	Lamina C2-C5	Transverse processes C4-C7 & adjacent vertebrae	C1-C8
12. Rotatores longi	Lamina C2-C5	Transverse processes C4-C7 & one or two vertebrae below	C1-C8
Action: lateral flexion of the neck			
1. Levator scapulae	Transverse processes C1-C4	Superior angle scapula.	C3-C4, C5, through dorsal scapular nerve
2. Splenius cervicis	Transverse processes C2-C3	Spinous processes T3-T6	C6-C8
3. Iliocostalis cervicis	Transverse processes C4-C6	Angles third through sixth ribs	C6-C8
4. Longissimus cervicis	Transverse processes C2-C6	Transverse processes T1-T5	C6-C8
5. Semispinalis cervicis	Spinous processes C2-C5 or C6	Transverse processes T1-T5	C1-C8
6. Multifidus	Spinous processes C2-C5	Articular processes C4-C7	C1-C8
7. Intertransversarii	Lower transverse processes C1-C7	Upper transverse processes C2-T1	C1-C8
8. Scaleni	Transverse processes	Upper transverse processes C2-T1	C1-C8, accessory
9. Sternocleidomastoid	Mastoid process, lateral 1/2 superior nuchal line	Manubrium of sternum, medial 1/2 superior clavicle	C2
10. Obliquus capitis inferior	Transverse process C1	Spinous process C2	C1
11. Rotatores brevi	Lamina C2-C5	Transverse processes C4-C7 & adjacent vertebrae	C1-C8
12. Rotatores longi	Lamina C2-C5	Transverse processes C4-C7 & one or two vertebrae below	C1-C8
13. Longus coli	Transverse processes C5-C6, anterior arch atlas, anterior bodies C2-C4	Bodies C5-C7, transverse processes C5-C6 & bodies T1-T3	C2-C6
Action: rotation of the neck coupled with lateral flexion			
1. Levator scapulae (face moves to same side)	Transverse processes C1-C4	Superior angle scapula	C3-C4, C5, through dorsal scapular nerve
2. Splenius cervicis (face moves to same side)	Transverse processes C2-C3	Spinous processes T3-T6	C6-C8
3. Iliocostalis cervicis (face moves to same side)	Transverse processes C4-C6	Angles third through sixth ribs	C6-C8
4. Longissimus cervicis (face moves to same side)	Transverse processes C2-C6	Transverse processes T1-T5	C6-C8

Table 10.2 *(Continued)*

Muscle	Upper Attachment	Lower Attachment	Nerve Supply
5. Semispinalis cervicis (face moves to same side)	Spinous processes C2-C5 or C6	Transverse processes T1-T6	C-C8
6. Multifidus (face moves to opposite side)	Spinous processes C2-C5	Articular processes C4-C7	C1-C8
7. Intertransversarii (face moves to same side)	Lower transverse processes C1-C7	Upper transverse processes C2-T1	C1-C8
8. Scaleni (face moves to same side)	Transverse processes C2-C7	First and third ribs	C3-C8
9. Sternocleidomastoid (face moves to opposite side)	Mastoid process, lateral 1/2 superior nuchal line	Manubrium of sternum, medial 1/2 superior clavicle	Accessory, C2
10. Obliquus capitis inferior (face moves to same side)	Transverse process C1	Spinous process C2	C1
11. Rotatores brevis (face moves to same side)	Lamina C2-C5	Transverse processes C4-C7 & adjacent vertebrae	C1-C8
12. Rotatores longi (face moves to same side)	Lamina C2-C5	Transverse processes C4-C7 & one or two vertebrae below	C1-C8

*a*Modified from Magee DJ: *Orthopedic Physical Assessment*, Philadelphia, WB Saunders, 1987, pp 34–35.

Development of an anomalous ossification center in the atlantooccipital ligaments, which forms a bony arch called the posterior ponticulum (ponticulus posticus) (Figs. 1.10 & 4.4), originates from the embryonic dorsal arch of the proatlas (11). The resulting foramen is named the arcuate, or posterior atlantoid foramen, and contains the suboccipital nerves as well as the vertebral artery (10). Seen by some as an incidental finding of little clinical significance (14), it has been considered a factor in compromise of the vertebral arteries on rotation of the cervical spine and has been implicated in vertebrobasilar vascular accidents associated with cervical manipulation (15). In many cases, compromise is thought to result because of inequality in the size of the two vertebral arteries. A more detailed discussion of vertebral artery syndromes is included in Chapter 4. A few physical tests (15–17), combined with a careful review of the patient's history and radiographic screening, may be helpful in identifying patients at risk (18).

Congenital anomalies of the odontoid are uncommon and are usually discovered on radiographics following trauma. The trauma may initiate symptoms in the already compromised, but previously asymptomatic, segment. If they produce an abnormal atlantoaxial shift, they may produce serious neurological complication and even death from spinal cord pressure. Stability can be determined by lateral stress radiographs or by the use of tomography (14).

Odontoid anomalies include aplasia (complete absence), hypoplasia (partial absence), and the most common, os odontoideum (Fig. 1.11). Aplasia is extremly rare and the most serious of the three, with complete absence of the base of the odontoid. Hypoplasia most commonly takes the form of a short peg of odontoid projecting just above the C1-C2 facet articulations. Os odontoideum is seen as a round ossicle with a smooth, dense border of bone separate from the axis.

Clinically, the signs and symptoms of the three, aplasia, hypoplasia, and os odontoideum, are the same. When present, these include local neck symptoms, transitory episodes of paresis following trauma, and frank myelopathy secondary to cord pressure. Severity varies, and some patients remain asymptomatic. Neck pain, torticollis, and headache may be mechanical, due to local irritation of the atlantoaxial articulation. Neurological symptoms are due to displacement of the atlas, causing spinal cord compression. Surgical stabilization is indicated in the event of neurological involvement, instability greater than 5 mm anterior or posterior, progressive instability, or intractable neck complaints (19).

Klippel-Feil syndrome refers to persons with congenital fusion of several cervical vertebrae (Fig. 1.13). Clinically, the patient with Klippel-Feil syndrome may exhibit a short neck, a low posterior hairline, and limited range of motion in the neck. Occasionally these patients have associated facial asymmetry torticollis and webbing of the neck. Patients with single-level fusion or fusion of the lower cervical spine frequently have normal range of motion. With greater involvement, loss of lateral bending is seen. Sprengle's deformity, scoliosis, and an omovertebral bone often accompany Klippel-Feil syndrome (20). Surgical intervention may be necessary if marked compensatory hypermobility of adjacent segments leads to neurological involvement (21).

Cervical ribs and elongated transverse processes can both cause thoracic outlet syndrome, with compromise of the neurovascular bundle supplying the upper extremity. This occurs in about 10% of cases (21). A true cervical rib includes a head, neck, and body of the rib and most often an articulation to the transverse process of C7 like the thoracic ribs (21). Rarely are the symptoms serious enough to warrant

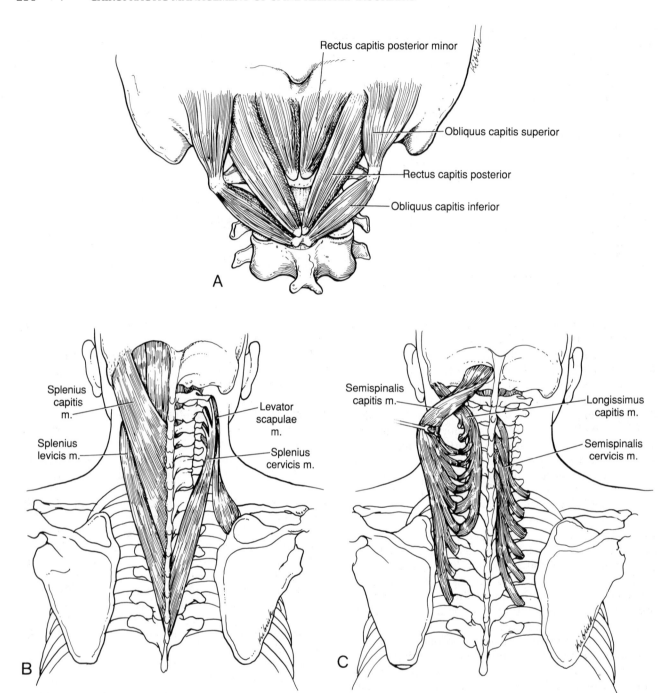

Figure 10.6. Posterior cervical muscles.

surgical excision of the cervical rib (see "Thoracic Outlet Syndromes").

MOVEMENT OF THE CERVICAL SPINE

The cervical spine is the most mobile area of the vertebral column, sacrificing stability for mobility. The individual geometry of the cervical vertebral motion segments allows for the wide range of movement, while the multiple layers of muscles provide motion in all orthogonal axes (22). The two anatomi-

cally and functionally distinct regions of the cervical spine are discussed separately.

Upper Cervical (Occipital-Atlanto-Axial) Complex

The upper cervical region, the occipital-atlanto-axial complex, is unique and contains the most intricate and highly specialized structures in the vertebral column (3). It is a transitional region between the globe-like skull and the typical segments of the remainder of the spinal column. The unique design

Figure 10.7. **A,** Cervical flexion starting with the chin tucked in (retraction) produces greater motion in the upper cervical spine than **B,** initiating flexion with the head erect. The overall range of motion remains the same. A patient x-rayed in flexion without first retracting the chin may be mistakenly reported to exhibit hypomobility of the upper cervical spine.

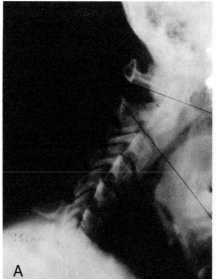 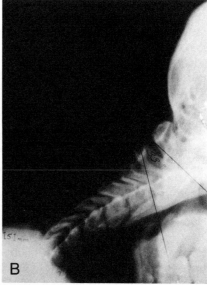

of the upper cervical vertebrae allows a wide range of motion, while offering protection for the spinal cord and vertebral arteries. The anatomical mechanism for axial rotation at C1-C2 places the instantaneous axis of rotation as close as possible to the spinal cord, permitting a wide range of movement without bony impingement on the spinal cord. The large vertebral canal of C2 (axis) also promotes freer movement in this region.

The safety zone of space between the anterior wall of the spinal canal of the atlas and axis, and the medulla is a constant that defines, according to Steele (23), the rule of thirds. This safety zone provides one-third cord, one-third odontoid, and one-third space (23). The unique design of the upper cervical segments also provides for protection of the vertebral arteries. This is achieved by the limited rotation at C0-C1, where the arteries enter the calvarium, in contrast to the large amount of axial rotation allowed at C1-C2.

Movement of the Occipital-Atlanto Joints

Movement at the occipital-atlanto joints (C0-C1) occurs primarily in the sagittal plane, producing flexion and extension. The two joints are mechanically linked by the convex occipital condyles that articulate with the cup-shaped atlanto facets. The condyles are ovoid and fit into the facets like eggs lying in spoons. The facets are tilted somewhat medially and are often constricted in the middle. During both flexion and extension of the occiput on the atlas, the condyles must slide on the lateral masses of the atlas. Steindler (24) reports 10 mm of forward and backward gliding during flexion and extension.

Fielding (25) found considerably more extension (about 25°) than flexion (about 10°). Earlier studies reported by Steindler (24) support this total range of motion with a combined flexion and extension of

approximately 35°. White and Panjabi (3) report significantly less (13°) average total flexion and extension at the occipital-atlanto joint, and Kapandji (2) estimates the total range of flexion and extension at this level to be 15°.

Jones (26) reports two patterns of total cervical flexion relative to chin position at the beginning of movement (Fig. 10.7A&B). Both patterns show paradoxical motion at C0-C1, with the occiput moving into extension on the atlas. Lane (27) considered this paradoxical motion to be a normal movement pattern. Cervical flexion starting with the chin tucked in (retracted) produces greater motion at the C0-C1 segment than flexion initiated with the head erect.

With the chin retracted, as flexion begins the lower cervical spine straightens, producing a straightening of the lordosis and a forward movement of the upper segment. With marked chin retraction, the midcervical segments angulate forward. As flexion continues in this pattern, the lordotic reversal progresses and the sharp angulation is lessened. The total flexion in the lower cervical spine is less with this particular motion than starting flexion without chin retraction.

Flexion of the cervical spine followed by chin retraction allows greater motion, in the lower cervical spine, with less angulation in the midcervical region and greater extension at C0-C1. Proper x-ray positioning is important, since failure to retract the chin first may be mistakenly reported as a lack of C0-C1 motion. The difference between these two patterns of movement may account for the variation in the reported range of movement of flexion at the C0-C1 level.

Extension at C0-C1 is limited by the tectorial membrane and by contact between the occiput and the posterior rim of the foramen magnum, the apex of the dens via an interposed bursa (28), and the occiput striking the posterior tubercle of the atlas.

Most authors agree that pure rotation cannot occur at the C0-C1 vertebral motion segment. A coupled movement combining rotation and lateral bending is possible when one condyle rides up anteriorly and laterally while the other slides and rocks posteriorly and medially. Bending to the left is thus associated with rotation to the right (25). The resultant position is described as an oblique tilt, which necessarily involves a lateral movement combined with rotation (29).

Jirout (30) refers to this as rotational synkinesis of the occiput and atlas on lateral inclination. He concluded that rotation of the head to the opposite side of lateral inclination can be taken for a dynamic stereotype that is more usual than rotation toward the side of inclination. This mechanism may be a source of joint fixaton when a camming effect is produced by asymmetrical or degenerated joint surfaces.

While Kapandji (2) describes the occipital-atlantal joint as an enarthrosis with 6 degrees of freedom and 3° each of lateral flexion and rotation, it appears that the osseous geometry permits only a coupled motion at these articulations.

Recent studies utilizing computerized tomography have clearly indicated rotation of the occiput on the atlas in normal subjects. Penning and Wilmink (31) reported a mean value of 1° rotation at this level. Dvorak, Panjabi, Gerber, and Wichmann (32) found 4.35° right and 5.9° left rotation at this joint. Dvorak, Hayek and Zehnder (33) stated that rotation at C0-C1 greater than 8° indicates hypermobility. They proposed that CT scans might be used not only for diagnosing hypermobility but also for diagnosing hypomobility of the upper cervical spine.

Rotation at the C0-C1 vertebral motion segment is checked by the alar ligaments. Panjabi and coworkers (34) found less motion on lateral bending (5.5°) at C0-C1 than on axial rotation (7.2°). Lateral bending at C0-C1 is primarily restricted by the structure of the articular surfaces. The muscles that move the head and neck are many and complex. Their attachments' nerve supply and action are outlined in Table 10.1.

Movement at the Atlantoaxial Joints

The pattern of motion between the atlas and the axis is primarily controlled by the geometry of the vertebral osseous structures. The mechanically linked four-joint complex lacks the disc of the typical vertebral motion segment. Instead, the odontoid process of the axis provides a pivot around which the ring of the atlas slides, supported by the transverse ligament.

The paired, lateral, atlantoaxial joints guide and restrict motion that is more complex than that of the typical vertebral motion segment. The shape and orientation of the fovea dentalis of the odontoid fur-

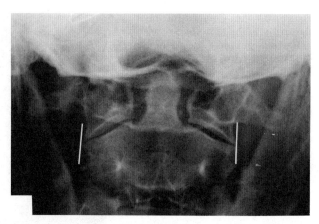

Figure 10.8. Atlantoaxial alignment. Normal alignment. (From Yochum TR, Rowe LJ: *Essentials of Skeletal Radiology.* Williams & Wilkins, Baltimore, 1986, p 256.)

ther guides the rocking motion as the atlantal ring rotates around the peg-like odontoid process. This forms the anterior median atlantoaxial articulation. The fourth atlantoaxial joint is formed medially, where the transverse ligament articulates with the posterior aspect of the odontoid process.

Rotation of the atlas around the Y-axis provided by the odontoid process is the major motion of the upper cervical region and constitutes 45–50% of the total range of rotation in the cervical spine (3, 25, 33).

The lateral atlantoaxial joints are classified as plane joints although they are not entirely flat. The superior facet of the axis is more convex than the inferior facet of the atlas, which has been described as both slightly convex and flat. The convexity is primarily due to the hyaline cartilage covering the articular facets (2, 3, 9, 22, 25, 27, 33).

The central atlantoodontoid joint is formed by the facet on the interior arch of the atlas, which articulates with the odontoid articular facet. The odontoid articular facet is convex anteroposteriorly and guides the ring of the atlas as it pivots around the odontoid process of the axis (2) (Fig. 10.8).

Rotational movement of the atlas on the axis is not that of a simple ring turning around a pivot, but rather a complex coupling of movement. This movement has been described as a screw-like action in which the atlas drops vertically by 2–3 mm. During right rotation, the left lateral mass moves forward while the right lateral mass moves backwards. Because of the convexity of the joint surfaces, a small spiral or helical action is described when the atlas translates vertically and the convex surfaces slide past one another. Coupled with rotation is a slight degree of ipsilateral lateral bending (35). The center of the odontoid process in the rotational position is found halfway between the lateral masses of the atlas (Fig. 10.8) and remains in contact with the anterior arch of the atlas, which is also the case in the neutral position of the normal cervical spine (31).

from above

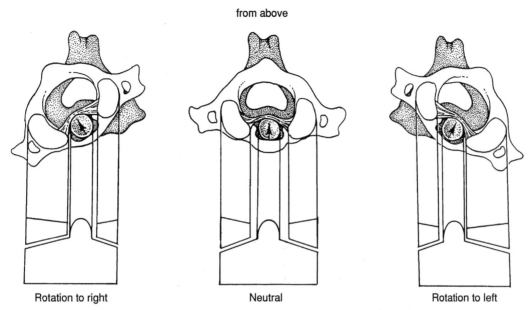

Rotation to right   Neutral   Rotation to left

Figure 10.9. Rotation of the atlas in relation to the axis. When C1 rotates to the left on C2, the right articular (lateral) mass of C2 moves forward. The concomitant posterior movement of the left lateral mass of C1 results in an apparent increase in the distance between the left lateral mass and the dens, as seen on anteroposterior radiograph. The oblique lateral mass appears to narrow as it is viewed on end. The right lateral mass appears wider because it is viewed broadside with an apparent narrowing of the distance between the atlas and the odontoid. The opposite is true for rotation to the left. (Modified from White AA, Panjabi MM: *Clinical Biomechanics of the Spine*. Philadelphia, JB Lippincott, 1978.)

The wall of the vertebral foramen of the atlas swings laterally to a considerable extent across the foramen of the axis, which decreases the opening of the spinal canal between these two segments and angulates the canal during rotation (6).

While the rule of thirds provides a wide margin of safety because of the larger vertebral foramen at this level, Grice (22) contends that additional rotation, ligamentous laxity, and/or pathomechanical motion may contribute to subtle trauma at this level, lending importance to rotational manipulation of the upper cervical spine. Radiological manifestation of atlantoaxial rotation, as seen through the open mouth (Fig. 10.9) with 15° of right rotation of the head, shows anteromedial rotation and upward shift of the left atlantoarticular mass, with an apparent medial approximation to the odontoid. The right atlantoarticular mass moves posteromedially and down, and its profile narrows with the concomitant widening of the profile of the left articular mass.

With the upward slide of the left atlantoarticular mass there is little or no apparent widening of the left atlantoaxial joint. The concomitant downward and posterior slide of the right atlantoarticular mass produces an apparent narrowing of the right atlantoaxial joint. Wortzman and Dewar (36) have reported the following radiographic changes with rotation to the right:

1. An approximation of the left atlantoarticular mass to the odontoid;

2. An apparent increase in width of the left atlantoarticular mass, with an apparent decrease in the width of the right atlantoarticular mass;

3. A slightly widened left atlantoaxial joint and a narrowed right atlantoaxial joint.

With a marked increase on rotation, an approximation of both atlantoarticular masses to the odontoid will be seen as they swing further around the pivot of the odontoid. Rotation of the lower cervical segments will also occur, as evidenced by the changed position of the spinous processes.

Anatomical asymmetry and patient positioning must be considered in evaluation of any spinal radiograph, since apparent positional changes are not pathognomonic of joint fixation. Of major importance is the position of the vertebral arteries as the atlas rotates (Fig. 4.1) (see Chapter 4). Selecki (37) noted that rotation of 30° caused kinking of the contralateral vertebral artery (i.e., right rotation narrows the left vertebral artery). As rotation progressed to 45°, kinking also occurred in the ipsilateral artery. Obstruction of the vertebral artery at the C1-C2 level on rotation of the head has been demonstrated by angiography.

This occlusion becomes clinically significant when it produces brain stem ischemia (38). Vertebrobasilar insufficiency is manifested clinically by a broad range of symptoms including ataxia, "drop attacks" vertigo, nausea, tinnitus, and visual disturbances. Stroke, secondary to brain stem ischemia, is the most serious consequence of this phenomena and is significant because of the implication that stroke can be produced by cervical manipulation (39) (Chapter 4). Grice (22) recommends that for C1-C2 rotation fixations the clinician should rotate the spine to 30° and then produce mild lateral flexion (3–5°) at the C1-C2 segment. He states, "This should produce optimal biomechanical rotational correction and should be less traumatic than full cervical rotation which has the possibility of stretching vital structures there."

Penning and Wilmink (31) found a mean value of 40.5° to either side on atlantoaxial rotation, with a range of 29–46°. This is consistent with Dvorak and coworkers, who found a mean value of 32.2° in 1985 (34) and 43.1° in 1987 (33). Panjabi reports a mean value of 38.9° in a 1988 study. Dvorak et al. (33) consider rotation at C1-C2 greater than 56° or a right-left difference greater than 8° to indicate hypermobility. They consider segmental rotation at C1-C2 of less than 28° to indicate hypomobility. Rotation to the right is checked by the tension of those fibers of the right alar ligament that are attached to the dens in front of the axis of movement and those of the left alar ligament that are attached to the process behind the axis of movement (29).

During flexion and extension at C1-C2, the anterior arch of the atlas moves up and down on the odontoid process, while the inferior facet of the lateral masses rolls and slides in the superior articular facet of the axis. The latter motion has been likened to the gliding of the femoral condyles on the tibial plateau (2). On flexion there is a separation between the posterior arch of the atlas and spinous process of the axis, and there is approximation on extension (25). Generally the width of the atlantoodontoid interspace diminishes during flexion (25). Panjabi et al. (34) reported a mean value of 11.5° flexion and 10.9° extension at the C1-C2 joint.

On lateral flexion, motion between the atlas and axis is also complex, with the atlas laterally displaced on the axis, producing a definite offset of the articular facets and an asymmetrical position of the atlas in relation to the odontoid process (40). Hohl (41) reported that with lateral tilting of the head there is 10 to 15° of atlantoaxial rotation combined with ipsilateral lateral gliding (translation) of the atlas. He noted that rotation is necessary to loosen the capsular ligaments so that lateral gliding can occur. He found 2–4 mm of articular offset. Penning (35) reported a mean value of lateral bending to one side of 10°, while Panjabi et al. (34) found it to be 6.7°.

Jirout (42) has reported that as the head tilts to one side there is a synkinetic rotation of the axis and inclination of the atlas to the opposite side. This results in projectional widening of the articular interspace on the side of inclination and narrowing on the opposite side, with frequent slight overlapping of the lateral parts of the respective articular processes. He concludes that this paradoxical move-

ment is the result of rotation of the axis beneath the atlas. On rotation of the head to the right the atlas moves on the axis (rotating to the right). On lateral flexion to the right the axis rotates to the right below the atlas. Therefore, during maximal lateral bending, the atlas is seen to rotate opposite to the other segments (35). This altered relationship between the atlas and axis occurs with lateral flexion because the axis rotates and laterally flexes following the coupled pattern of motion seen in the lower cervical spine (Fig. 10.10). The atlas, which is then caught in a pincer action between the occiput and axis, is forced laterally, translating toward the side of inclination.

Jones (26) has compared the atlas to a washer or bearing between the skull and spine, while Jirout (42) describes the atlas as a meniscus in the occipitoaxial dynamic system. Grice (22) concludes that the atlas has an intermediate linkage position and behaves largely in a passive manner. He states, "This intermediary role of C1 provides an ideal contact point for correcting many biomechanical aberrations and fixations and clearly is the reason why many techniques have developed around the C1 vertebral segment." Shapiro and coworkers (28) conclude that the atlantoaxial joint is a unique joint because the articular surfaces are convex with a horizontal orientation. This combination permits maximal motility (rotation) at the cost of stability.

Movement of the Lower Cervical Spine

Movement of the lower cervical spine is more typical of the remainder of the spine than is that of the specialized upper cervical segments. Flexion, extension, rotation, and lateral flexion all occur between the second and seventh cervical vertebra. In the lower cervical spine all five mobile sections, C2–C3 through C6–C7, show the same type of movement (35). Unlike motion at the interspace between the first and second cervical vertebrae (which can move independently), below the second cervical vertebra, motion at one interspace is generally accompanied by similar motion at other levels (43). This movement is governed by the zygopophyseal facet and uncovertebral joints (joints of Luschka).

Two strong coupling elements are seen in the lower cervical spine. Sagittal-plane motion (flexion-extension) combines translation and rotation (3), while lateral bending and rotation are coupled so that the spinous processes point in the opposite direction to that in which lateral bending takes place (toward the convexity) (3). This pattern is clearly present in the upper portion of the thoracic spine. It becomes weaker and changes in the middle and lower portion of the thoracic spine where the spinous processes rotate toward the concavity in the same direction in which lateral bending takes place (3). Movement in the lower cervical spine occurs chiefly in the sagittal plane (flexion, extension) (43). The joint surfaces of the articular processes lie in

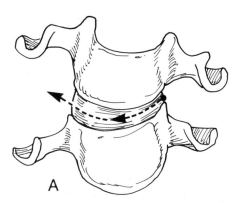

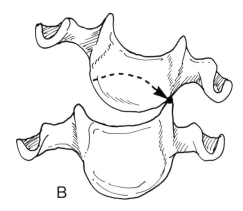

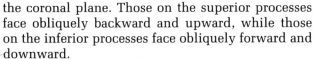

A   B

Figure 10.10. Lateral flexion of the cervical spine. **A,** Movement in the cervical spine during lateral flexion is guided by the uncinate processes. **B,** Without translation permitted by the disc, the upper cervical vertebra would jam on the uncinate process of the vertebra below. Translation is accompanied by lateral flexion and rotation, which produces a change in the instantaneous axis of rotation. Failure of this mechanism may lead to mechanical locking in the cervical spine. (Modified from Penning L, Wilmink JT: Rotation of the cervical spine. *Spine* 12:732–738, 1987.)

the coronal plane. Those on the superior processes face obliquely backward and upward, while those on the inferior processes face obliquely forward and downward.

Kapandji (2) reports that the obliquity is greatest between C2 and C3 (40–45°), progressively decreasing to 10° at C7–T1. During flexion, the upper vertebra glides forward on the articular processes of the vertebra below, and the vertebral body shifts foward. In extension, the opposite shift occurs. The inclination of the facets is responsible for the forward and backward shift of the vertebral body during flexion-extension (25). During flexion, the disc widens posteriorly, narrows anteriorly, and slides forward (43). The range of motion is dictated to some extent by the geometry and stiffness of the disc (3). As a consequence of the sliding motion, a step is formed along the ventral wall of the spinal canal in flexion, with dorsal bodies arranged like a flight of steps (44). In extension, the arrangement resembles a washboard pattern (45). In the neutral position, a line down the posterior bodies in normal spines forms a smooth arc (George's line) (see Chapter 6). At the extreme of flexion, the facets tend to be angled on each other, allowing the spinous processes to spread (26). Maximum extension produces a widening of the superior segment of the facet joints, with approximation of the spinous processes. Extension is limited by impingement of the spinous processes (26).

Range of segmental motion in the lower cervical spine is reportedly greatest at the C5–6 segment, approaching a mean value of 20°. The least segmental motion in the lower cervical spine is found at C7–T1, with a mean value of approximately 10° (44, 45). Values between 10 and 20° have been reported for the movement between the lower cervical motion segments (44, 45).

The interdependency, or coupling, of lateral flexion and rotation in the lower cervical spine can be explained by the oblique position of the intervertebral joints (2, 3, 35) and by the morphology of the vertebral body (uncinate processes) (8, 31). During lateral flexion, the inferior articular processes on the concave side glide downward and backward, while those on the convex side glide upward and forward (25). This movement causes the articular facets on the concave side to imbricate, while those on the concave side ride apart. White and Panjabi (3) conclude that "because these joints are oriented at about a 45° angle to the vertical in the sagittal plane, the lateral bending results in axial rotation." During lateral bending to the right, as the right facet of the superior vertebra moves down the 45° incline to the right, it is also displaced somewhat posteriorly. As the facet on the right moves up the 45° incline on the left, it is displaced somewhat anteriorly. This means that lateral bending to the right is coupled with rotation to the right (35).

Penning and Wilmink (31), utilizing computerized tomography to study rotation of the cervical spine, found that this coupling is not solely determined by the direction of the intervertebral joint spaces. Following the work of Hall (8), who theorized that the uncinate processes are essential for rotation, Penning and Wilmink (31) evaluated CT slices of the cervical spine, which they concluded support Hall's theory.

Hall (8) speculated that the cervical vertebrae are in a process of developing back into ball-and-socket diarthrodial joints. In a comparative anatomic study he noted that the uncinate processes are found on the cervical vertebrae of primates, marsupials, and rodents, who are obligatory or facultative bipeds. To look about, these animals require rotation of the neck, whereas quadrupeds use lateral flexion of the neck for the same purpose. He did not find uncinate processes in the dog (8). He noted that the cartilage-covered, ridge-like prominence on each side of the upper surface of the vertebra and the cartilaginous facet on the lateral edge of the immediately superior vertebra can easily move on each other, so that flexion and rotation to all sides is easily possible (8).

Penning and Wilmink confirmed this (31). They found that to avoid its lateral wall abutting the uncinate process of the vertebra below during lateral flexion, the superior vertebra performs a translation in a contralateral direction (31) (Fig. 10.10). Because the unciform process is located posteriorly on the edges of the vertebral bodies, this mechanism will only take place posteriorly. The axis of this motion must then be in the center of the upper vertebral body. Lateral flexion of the anterior bodies takes place with a center of motion in the neighborhood of the discs, with slight translation of the upper vertebrae into the direction of lateral flexion.

With anterior and posterior translational movements of the upper vertebra, with respect to the lower vertebra in opposite direction during lateral flexion, simultaneous rotation must occur. Rotation occurs in the direction of lateral flexion because, anteriorly, translation is toward the side of lateral flexion and posteriorly, from the side of lateral flexion.

Penning and Wilmink (31) report the following mean values for rotation in the lower cervical spine (C2–3 through C6–7): 3.0°, 6.5°, 6.8°, 5.4°, and 2.1°. This is consistent with other authors (3, 19) who reported the greatest lateral flexion and rotation at the C4–C5 and C5–C6 vertebral motion segments and the least at C6–C7. Jones (26) stated that "the increased function here has been considered the cause for early development of degenerative changes at this point."

BIOMECHANICAL DISORDERS OF THE CERVICAL SPINE

Biomechanical disorders of the cervical spine commonly result from trauma such as occurs with motor vehicle accidents, sports injuries, and falls (3). In addition to fracture and soft-tissue injury, segmental blockage can be precipitated by trauma to the cervical spine (46, 47). Compensatory segmental fixation from faulty postural habits (47) or from working in confined spaces frequently occurs. Even uncoordinated movements while stirring in sleep may lead to spontaneous blockage (47).

Especially common are fixations at the C1–2 vertebral motion segment. While the reaction of the atlantoaxial joints to minor injury that results in fixation of the joint is not understood (37), it is easily correctable with manipulation. It is a common clinical finding of practitioners of manipulation and accounts for a fair proportion of patients with symptoms about the neck and cranium and signs of limited rotation (47). Wortzman and Dewar (37) conclude that muscle spasm is not a factor, for the fixation persists in spite of cessation of signs and symptoms. This is supported clinically by the lack of response to muscle relaxants.

Injury is usually of a moderate nature, such as flexion-extension injury from rear-end collision or a relatively minor blow to the head. The high frequency, as seen in patients without trauma, also suggests a compensatory mechanism by which the head remains level in spite of unlevel segments below. Grieve (47) describes this as "a physiological necessity to normalize the head position and to adjust visual and equilibratory apparatus in correct orientation to the vertical and horizontals of the environment." This is in keeping with the body's constant attempt to maintain homeostasis.

Coutts (46) describes another mechanism whereby the rotation of the atlas is primary, with compensatory rotation in the lower part of the cervical spine. The dramatic response to manipulation of the atlas in patients with a variety of biomechanical distortions in other areas of the spine supports this mechanism and has led to a number of chiropractic techniques with theories based on it.

Coutts (46) describes the atlantoaxial articulations, when examined from the lateral aspect, as resembling the end view of the sterns of two boats placed keel to keel. In the neutral positon the convex surfaces oppose one another, with maximum separation of the joint provided by the convexity of the lateral masses. When the atlas is fully rotated, only the peripheral part of the articular cartilages are in contact, with a vertical drop of 2 to 3 mm. This drop may produce a camming mechanism whereby the atlas becomes fixed and is prevented from returning to its neutral position (Chapter 8).

ORTHOPAEDIC TESTS

Examination of the cervical spine must include the neck and upper extremity (48). Many of the symptoms that occur in the upper limb can originate from the neck and require differentiation. Referred pain from trigger points in the neck and upper back must not be mistaken for radicular pain and should not be dismissed as nonanatomical because they do not follow typical dermatome patterns (Chapter 12). Differentiation of nerve root, articular, and muscular syndromes requires careful testing to determine the site of origin of the patient's symptoms. Inappropriate care directed to the incorrect area often delays appropriate care and may aggravate the patient's condition and foster a chronic pain syndrome.

Distraction Test

The distraction test (Fig. 5.9) can be performed with the patient supine or seated, with one hand placed under the patient's chin and the other hand around the occiput. The examiner slowly tractions the patient's head. The result is considered positive if the pain is relieved or decreased when the head is lifted or distracted. It is indicative of joint fixation or pressure on nerve roots.

maintain maintenance

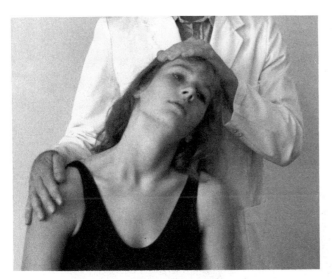

Figure 10.11. Shoulder depression test.

Foraminal Compression Test

The foraminal compression test (48) (Fig. 5.10) is performed with the patient seated. The patient is instructed to laterally bend and then extend the neck. The examiner carefully presses straight down on the head. A test result is positive if pain radiates into the arm on the side toward which the neck is laterally bent. The distribution of the pain and altered sensation can give some indication as to which nerve root is involved.

Shoulder Depression Test

The shoulder depression test (48) (Fig. 10.11) is performed with the examiner standing behind the seated patient. The patient's head is tilted to one side, and downward pressure is applied to the contralateral shoulder. If radicular pain is increased, it indicates irritation or compression of the nerve root, adhesions about the dural sleeves of the nerve roots and the adjacent capsules, or foraminal encroachments. This procedure places a tug on the nerve roots, and if there are adhesions or osteophytic changes, radicular pain is produced (49).

Shoulder Abduction (Fig. 10.12)

A decrease or relief of symptoms when the patient actively elevates the arm through abduction, so that the hand or forearm rests on top of the head, indicates a cervical extradural compression problem, usually at the C5–C6 area. Nerve root compression, epidural vein compression, or a herniated disc should be differentiated (48, 50).

Lhermitte's Sign

A sharp pain and "electric-shock" sensation into the upper or lower limbs on flexion of the neck is referred to as a positive Lhermitte's sign. It is indicative of dural irritation in the spine (48).

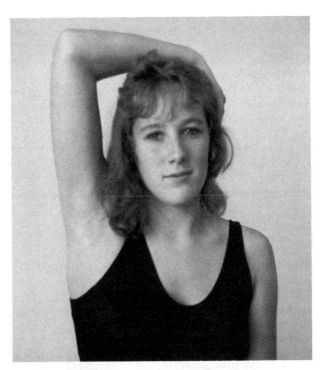

Figure 10.12. Shoulder abduction test.

Extension-Rotation Test

The extension-rotation test (Fig. 5.7) is performed with the patient supine, with the shoulders at the edge of the table and the neck extended over the end of the table. The patient is asked to actively extend the neck and rotate the head while keeping the eyes open. This position is held for a minimum of 15 seconds and repeated on the contralateral side. A positive test result includes nystagmus, blanching around the mouth, complaints of dizziness, nausea, or dyplopia. A positive test should be stopped immediately and is a contraindication for manipulation with the cervical spine in an extended and rotated position (see Chapter 4).

Sitting Extension–Rotation Test (Adson's Maneuver)

With the patient seated, the doctor palpates the radial pulse and directs the patient to extend the neck and turn the chin toward the side being tested (Fig. 10.13A). The patient is instructed to take a deep breath and hold it. A disappearance of the pulse with an increase in symptoms indicates neurovascular compression due to a decrease in the interscalene space, which can compress the subclavian artery and the lower components (C8 and T1) of the brachial plexus against the first rib (48, 51).

A modified Adson's maneuver (Halstead maneuver) (Fig. 10.13B) is performed as above, with the head rotated to the side opposite the one being tested while the tested extremity is tractioned downward (48).

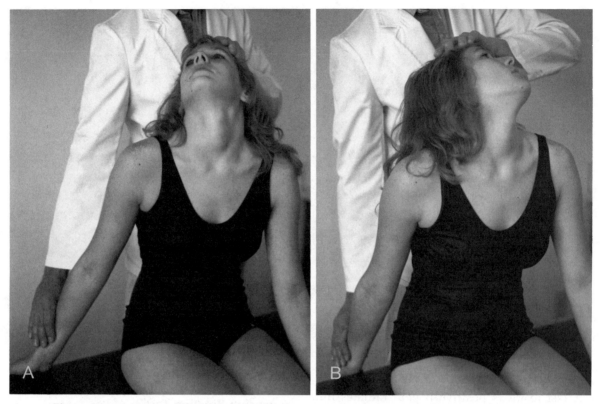

Figure 10.13. Sitting extension-and-rotation tests. **A,** Adson's maneuver. **B,** Halstead maneuver.

Military Posture Test (Eden's Test, Costoclavicular Syndrome Test) (Fig. 10.14)

The seated patient is instructed to draw the shoulders down and back and hold a deep inspiration while the doctor monitors the radial pulse. The test result is positive if weakening or loss of pulse occurs with an increase in symptoms, indicating pressure on the neurovascular bundle as it passes between the clavicle and first rib (costoclavicular syndrome) (51).

Hyperabduction Test (Wright's Test) (Fig. 10.15)

With the patient seated, the radial pulse is palpated from the posterior with the forearm extended. As the arm is hyperextended through a 180° arc, pressure on the brachial plexus and axillary vessels by the pectoralis minor tendon can diminish the pulse and increase neurological or vascular symptoms. A diminished or lost pulse without symptoms is considered a false positive and occurs in the majority of asymptomatic individuals (51).

MANIPULATION OF THE CERVICAL SPINE

Because of the relative ease with which an audible release can be achieved when manipulating the cervical spine, there is persistent temptation to assume a manipulation is a success because of the noise generated. Careful application of biomechanical principles often reveals this not to be the case, how-

ever, and a more specific criterion for success is required (52).

When motion is lost within a cervical joint in one or more axes, motion palpation will reveal the specific nature of the joint dysfunction, and an appropriate adjustment can be chosen to restore or improve the motion which is lost. Postmanipulative motion palpation serves as an indicator of the degree of success. The application of biomechanical principles to motion palpation and manipulation of the cervical spine is described by a number of authors (53–65).

Contraindications to Cervical Manipulation

Chief among the contraindications to cervical manipulation is a lesion or insufficiency in the vertebrobasilar system. Vascular integrity of the vertebrobasilar system should be evaluated using standard tests that combine rotation and extension of the upper cervical spine (see Chapters 4 and 5), as the most ominous complications of cervical manipulation arise from vertebrobasilar accidents. A careful history may be helpful in detecting abnormalities in this region, by indicating past incidents of transient ischemia or frank infarct. Family history and other vascular risk factors should be noted (15, 16, 18).

Other considerations that must be ruled out before undertaking cervical manipulation include: fracture, neoplasm, segmental instability, cervical disc herni-

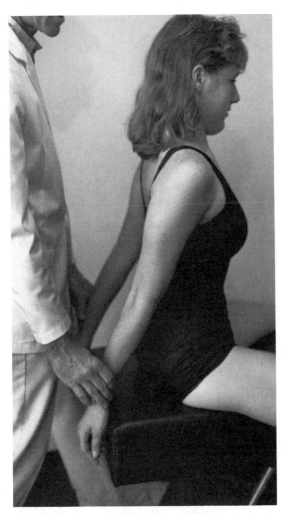

Figure 10.14. Military posture. (Eden's test for costoclavicular syndrome).

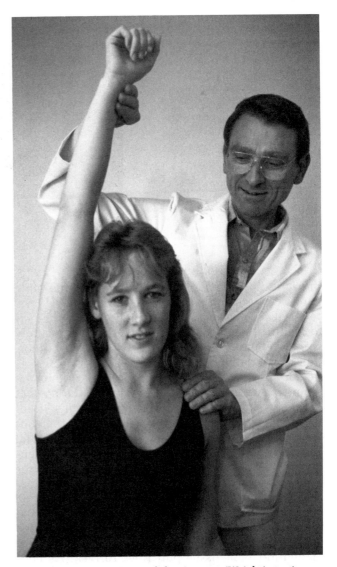

Figure 10.15. Hyperabduction test (Wright's test).

ation, parathyroid dysfunction, advanced osteoporosis, significant congenital anomaly, rheumatoid arthritis, and other upper cervical arthridites (15, 53). (see also Chapter 4).

Palpation of Cervical Vertebrae Fixed in Rotation (53, 55–57, 61, 65)

With the patient supine, the doctor stands or kneels at the head of the table with one hand cradled under the patient's head. The middle portion of the radial side of the index finger of the other hand is used to contact the ipsilateral articular pillar of the segment in question by taking a medial-to-lateral tissue pull (Fig. 10.16). As the segment is lifted in the direction of rotation and the head is guided to follow, the articular pillar should smoothly glide anteriorly in relation to the segment below in a stair-step fashion. A springy joint play should be noted at the conclusion of this movement.

Manipulation of Cervical Vertebrae Fixed in Rotation (53, 55, 58–61)

With the patient in the supine position and the doctor standing or kneeling at the head of the table, the cervical spine may be manipulated using the radial side of the index finger as a contact point (just as in the palpation). When rotational joint tension is perceived, a specific, rotational, high-velocity, low-amplitude thrust is delivered. It may be helpful to slightly laterally flex the cervical spine toward the side of contact to further isolate the segment in question and increase the specificity of the manipulation.

An alternative contact can be taken with the thumb on the ipsilateral articular pillar and the fingers resting lightly on the patient's jaw (Fig. 10.17A). After the joint is rotated into a position of tension, a specific rotational thrust is given to move

Figure 10.16. Palpation of cervical segmental rotation with the patient supine.

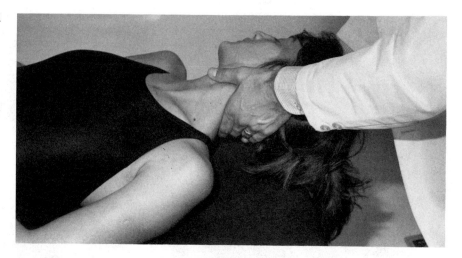

the joint in question while the nonmanipulating hand supports and guides the head.

Cervical rotational manipulation can also be performed with the doctor standing behind the securely seated patient. Contact is taken with the distal portion of the radial side of the index finger on the articular pillar, with the index finger reinforced by the other fingers as needed. The thumb of the contact hand rests against the side of the patient's head, while the other hand supports and guides the contralateral side of the head and cervical spine (Fig. 10.17B). As rotational tension is developed, a high-velocity thrust is delivered in a rotational vector away from the doctor, with a slight inferior-to-superior component to follow the facet planes.

With the doctor standing in front of the seated patient, a contact can be made with the palmar surface of the middle finger on the articular pillar, using a medial-to-lateral tissue pull (Fig. 10.17C). As both hands support the head and the contact hand pulls

the segment into rotation, the head is tilted toward the contact side to assist in isolating the specific segment in question. As specific joint tension is developed, a pulling, high-velocity, low-amplitude thrust is delivered in the direction of rotation (i.e., toward the doctor) with simultaneous upward distraction applied.

When restoring a loss of cervical rotation, the contact is generally taken on the posterior aspect of the articular pillar with the production of a posterior-to-anterior rotation as described in the previous examples. At times there may be loss of anterior-to-posterior rotation in the facet joints of the opposite side, which requires a specific contact. In this case, the doctor stands in front of the seated patient and cradles the side of the head and neck with one hand while the pisiform of the other carefully contacts the anterior portion of the transverse process of the segment to be rotated. As tension is generated in an anterior-to-posterior direction with the contact hand, a

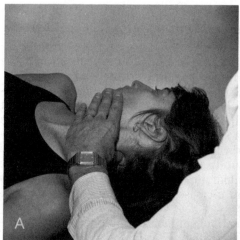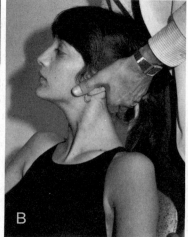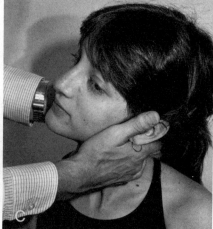

Figure 10.17. Manipulation of cervical vertebrae fixed in rotation may be done using the same contact as in the palpation (see Fig. 10.16). A thumb contact with the patient supine or

various contacts taken with the patient seated and doctor standing may also be utilized.

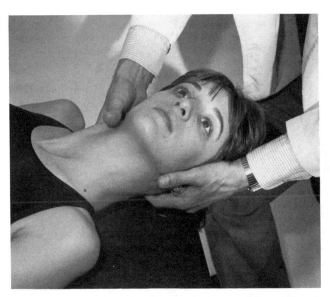

Figure 10.18. Palpation of cervical segmental lateral bending.

high-velocity thrust is delivered in the same direction to restore mobility to the restricted facet joint (3, 58).

Palpation of Cervical Vertebrae Fixed in Lateral Flexion (3, 56, 57, 61, 63, 65)

With the patient supine, the doctor stands or kneels at the head of the table, with one hand cradling the patient's head. The other hand contacts the lateral portion of the articular pillar of the segment in question with the middle portion of the radial aspect of the index finger (Fig. 10.18). As the head is translated toward the side of contact and the contact hand glides laterally to medially, specific lateral bending should be exerted around the contacting finger. The joints should be felt to curve around the palpating finger at each level, with a characteristic springiness felt at the end of the motion.

Manipulation of Cervical Vertebrae Fixed in Lateral Flexion (1, 54, 56–61, 65)

With the patient in a supine position, the radial side of the index finger may be used to contact the articular pillar of the segment in question, while the other hand supports and guides the head and cervical spine. As the contact hand generates specific joint tension in a lateral-to-medial direction, and the support hand counters that movement by bending the cervical spine around the contact, a high-velocity thrust is given with the contact hand in a lateral-to-medial and slightly superior-to-inferior vector.

Lateral flexion may also be restored with the doctor standing behind the securely seated patient (Fig. 10.19A). Contact is taken with the distal portion of the radial index finger on the lateral articular pillar, while the other hand supports and guides the head

and cervical spine. Specific joint tension is created by laterally bending the cervical spine around the contact finger, with a simultaneous lateral-to-medial push of the contact hand. When specific tension is developed at the fixated segment, a high-velocity thrust is applied in a lateral-to-medial and slightly superior-to-inferior direction.

The same manipulation can be performed with the doctor standing in front of the seated patient (Fig. 10.19B). Contact is taken with the palmar surface of the middle finger on the articular pillar, and both hands are used to cradle the neck and head. As the cervical spine is tipped toward the contact side, with the apex of the curve at the contact point, tension in a lateral-bending direction is created. A high-velocity thrust is delivered in a lateral-to-medial and slightly superior-to-inferior direction as the doctor pulls back.

With the patient prone and face down on a table with a cutaway nose piece, lateral flexion manipulation may be performed (Fig. 10.19C). Standing on the side opposite contact, the doctor reaches over the patient to contact the lateral articular pillar with the proximal portion of the radial aspect of the index finger, with the thumb draped over the posterior cervical spine. The other hand cradles the opposite side of the patient's head and rocks the head toward the side of contact, while the contact hand creates tension in a lateral-to-medial direction. A high-velocity impulse is given in a lateral-to-medial and slightly superior-to-inferior direction, with the support hand following through in the opposite direction.

Palpation of Cervical Vertebrae Fixed in Flexion (53, 57, 63, 65)

With the patient supine, the doctor stands or kneels at the head of the table and places the tips of the index fingers on the articular pillars of the segment in question (Fig. 10.20). A symmetrical vertical lifting is performed until the facet joints extend over the palpating finger and the characteristic springy end play is felt. This process may be facilitated by having the patient's head extend beyond the end of the examination table to allow greater extension.

While the previous technique allows for segmental extension and quick bilateral comparison, extension may also be checked one side at a time. The doctor contacts the supine patient's articular pillar with the radial portion of the index finger as the other hand cradles the patient's head and cervical spine. As the doctor lifts the segment in a straight posterior-to-anterior direction, the support hand allows the head to drop, thus allowing more extension. Having the patient's head off the table may be beneficial, and it is possible to combine a lateral flexion and/or rotational palpation with the unilateral extension palpation.

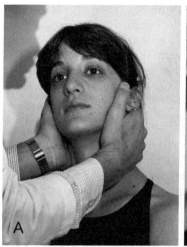 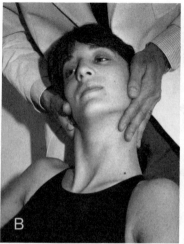 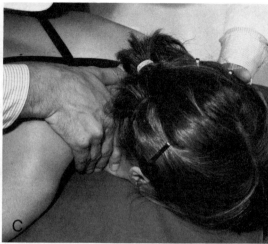

Figure 10.19. Manipulation of cervical vertebrae fixed in lateral bending may be done using the same contact as the palpation (see Fig. 10.18). **A,** A pull or **B,** push maneuver may be utilized with the patient seated and the doctor standing. **C,** The patient may be placed in a prone position.

Manipulation of the Cervical Vertebrae Fixed in Flexion (54, 56, 57, 59, 64)

With the patient supine and the doctor standing or kneeling at the head of the table, a contact is taken with the radial surface of the index finger on the articular pillar. Extension movement and tension are created by lifting the segment posterior to anterior as the support hand allows the patient's head to drop posteriorly. When appropriate tension is produced, a high-velocity, posterior-to-anterior thrust is administered.

Another method of restoring extension to a cervical motion segment involves the doctor standing behind the securely seated patient. Contact is made over the articular pillar with the distal radial surface of the index finger, as the other hand supports the head and cervical spine. As appropriate tension is generated by gliding anteriorly with the contact hand as the head and cervical spine glide posteriorly, a high-velocity, posterior-to-anterior thrust is delivered (Fig. 10.21).

Extension can also be restored with the patient prone and face down on a table with a cut-away nose piece. Contact is taken over the more fixated facet with the proximal portion of the index finger, and tension is generated by gliding the contact anteriorly as the support hand slightly rocks the head

Figure 10.20. Palpation of cervical vertebrae fixed in flexion.

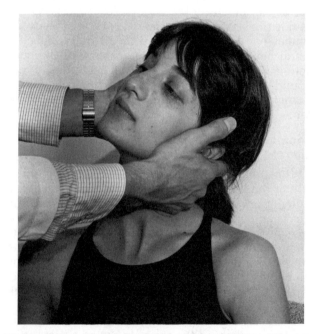

Figure 10.21. Manipulation of cervical vertebrae fixed in flexion may be done with the patient seated and the doctor standing, or utilizing the same contact as the palpation (see Fig. 10.20).

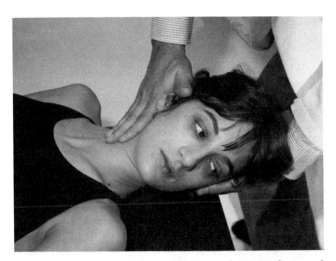

Figure 10.22. Position for palpation and manipulation of cervical vertebrae fixed in extension.

posteriorly. When appropriate joint tension is reached, a high-velocity, posterior-to-anterior thrust is delivered.

Palpation of Cervical Vertebrae Fixed in Extension (53, 63–65)

With the patient supine and the doctor standing or kneeling at the head of the table, the head is cradled by one hand and rotated to the ipsilateral side (Fig. 10.22). Since rotation will occur first in the upper cervical spine, with the atlas rotating on the axis approximately 25° before any other segment moves, modest rotation of the head will still leave the middle and lower cervical segments in a neutral position, facing anteriorly. Utilizing this fact, a broad contact is taken with the pads of the 2nd, 3rd, and 4th fingers over the anterior aspect of the transverse process of the cervical segment in question. The sternocleidomastoid muscle is either palpated through or pushed gently aside. Care is taken to avoid adjacent neurovascular structures as the contact hand pushes anterior to posterior, while the support hand lifts the head off the table. The procedure is repeated bilaterally. Spinous process separation may also be palpated as in the thoracic and lumbar spine, but this is often difficult in the midcervical spine.

Manipulation of Cervical Vertebrae Fixed in Extension (56, 58, 62, 64)

This manipulation can be done with the patient supine and the doctor standing or kneeling at the head of the table (Fig. 10.22). The head is cradled by one hand and rotated slightly ipsilaterally, while the other hand contacts over the anterior portion of the transverse process of the segment in question, utilizing a broad contact with the middle and distal palmar portions of the 2nd, 3rd, and 4th fingers. As appropriate tension is developed, with the fingers pressing posteriorly and the head being lifted off the

table, a high-velocity thrust is delivered in an anterior-to-posterior direction as the support hand lifts the head simultaneously. Variations of this technique are possible with the patient seated, combining flexion with rotation and/or lateral bending.

Palpation of the Occiput Fixed in Rotation (51, 53, 55, 63, 65)

With the patient seated or supine, the doctor places the tip of the index finger across the gap between the transverse process of the atlas and the ramus of the mandible. The doctor's other hand is placed on top of the patient's head to guide rotation. As rotation is passively induced, away from the side of contact, a distinct widening of the space between the mandible and atlas transverse process should be felt near the end of the range of motion. This movement of the mandible represents the movement of the occiput in relation to the atlas.

Manipulation of the Occiput Fixed in Rotation

Since rotation is a relatively minor component of atlantooccipital movement, it is usually not manipulated alone, but in conjunction with an accompanying fixation (see following descriptions). Recently, however, Szaraz (62) has described rotary manipulation of the atlantooccipital joint.

Palpation of the Occiput Fixed in Flexion (53–56, 63–65)

With the patient seated or supine, the doctor cradles the occiput and mastoids bilaterally with the palmar surface of the fingers, as the thumbs support the head laterally. A rolling movement is carefully produced to create extension at the atlantooccipital joint without involving adjacent cervical segments. This movement can be isolated more unilaterally by adding ipsilateral lateral flexion to the test (Fig. 10.23).

If desired, a fingertip may be placed between the atlas transverse process and mandibular ramus or mastoid to feel their interspace open or close respectively (Fig. 10.24). As the hands "roll" the occiput over the atlas, a distinct movement and springy endfeel should be perceived.

Manipulation of the Occiput Fixed in Flexion (54, 56, 57, 59, 61, 65)

With the patient seated or supine, the doctor contacts the mastoid on the most involved side using a pisiform, thenar, proximal index, or other contact (Fig. 10.23). The other hand supports the opposite side of the head, allowing the hands to gently but firmly squeeze the patient's head, to prevent slipping and allow good control. The occiput is then extended and laterally flexed toward the involved side until the point of fixation is reached. A high-velocity, low-amplitude thrust is then made, with a posterior-to-anterior, lateral-to-medial, and superior-to-

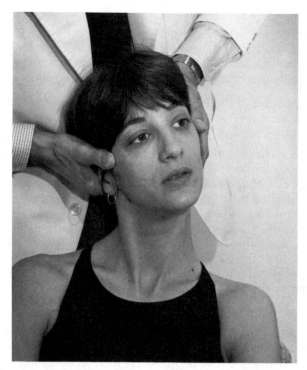

Figure 10.23. Palpation and/or manipulation of the occiput fixed in flexion, emphasizing unilateral movement by combining lateral flexion.

inferior vector. Care is taken to minimize rotation, to insure movement between the occiput and atlas.

An alternative technique employs the same vectors with the doctor facing the seated patient. The doctor contacts the inferior lateral surface of the occiput and the mastoid process with the palmar aspect of the middle finger, while the opposite hand stabilizes the contralateral occiput and temporal ar-

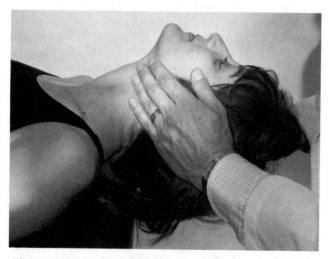

Figure 10.24. Palpation of the occiput fixed in flexion, with palpation of opening between atlas TP and mandibular ramus.

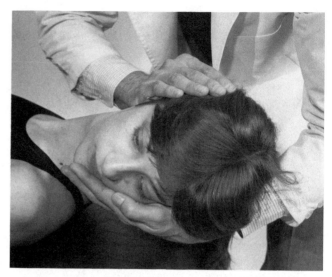

Figure 10.25. Unilateral palpation of the occiput fixed in extension.

eas. A high-velocity, low-amplitude "pulling" thrust is then delivered.

Palpation of the Occiput Fixed in Extension (52, 53, 56, 65)

With the doctor standing behind the seated patient, the palmar surface of the thumb may be used to contact the posterior inferior mastoid process on the side in question. The other hand stabilizes the vertex of the head and forehead, assisting in the production of flexion and slight lateral bending away from the contact hand. Simultaneously, the contact thumb lifts to cause flexion/distraction of the ipsilateral atlantooccipital joint.

This same movement can be reproduced with the doctor kneeling or squatting at the head of the supine patient. The occiput is cradled in both hands and is distracted and rolled into flexion, with isolation of one side by contralateral, simultaneous lateral bending (Fig. 10.25).

Both sides may be checked at once, if desired, by avoiding lateral bending, and a fingertip may be used to monitor changes in the interspaces between the atlas transverse process and the mastoid process or the mandibular ramus.

Another method involves the placement of the doctor's hands atop the patient's head, with fingers interlaced and the patient seated facing away from the standing doctor. The occiput is rolled into flexion, and its movement atop the cervical spine is noted (Fig. 10.26).

Manipulation of the Occiput Fixed in Extension (54, 56–58, 62)

Many manipulations exist to flex and/or distract the atlantooccipital joint, and a few examples will be given. With the patient supine and the head turned away from the side of fixation, the doctor

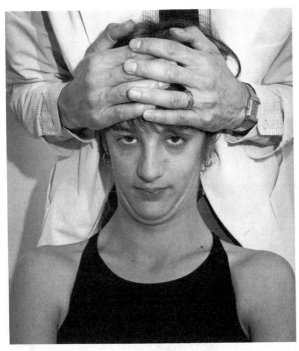

Figure 10.26. Position for sitting palpation and manipulation of the occiput fixed in extension.

stands at the head of the table on the side of restriction. The doctor's forearm supports the patient's head, with fingers cradling the patient's chin. The doctor's caudad hand then contacts the involved side, with a pisiform on the inferior lateral occiput near the mastoid. When proper joint tension is achieved, a high-velocity, low-amplitude thrust is delivered in a cephalic direction to distract the joint (Fig. 10.27A). This procedure may also be done with the involved joint down (i.e., contacting the uninvolved side). The occiput is then laterally flexed away from the involved side during the distractive thrust to maximize distraction. This will also produce lateral bending (Fig. 10.27B).

With the doctor standing behind the seated patient, the occiput may be flexed by placing overlapping fingers on the glabella, while the back of the patient's skull rests against the doctor's chest. As the doctor lifts the occiput superiorly using the chest contact, a scooping, caudad-and-posterior thrust is given after tension is achieved (Fig. 10.26).

Another flexion manipulation in which the doctor stands behind the seated patient is the occipital lift (Fig. 10.27C). The patient's head is rotated away from the more fixated side, and the doctor contacts the inferior border of the occiput near the mastoid with overlapping fingers. The side of the patient's head rests against the doctor's chest. Utilizing a lateral-to-medial scooping action, the doctor impulses upward, with arms lifting and knees extended to distract the occiput. This maneuver also improves lateral glide.

With the patient prone, the occiput can be flexed with the doctor utilizing a knife-edge (lateral hand) contact while facing cephalad. The noncontact hand reinforces the contact hand, and a cephalad vector is utilized with the doctor in a low fencer stance.

Palpation of the Occiput Fixed in Lateral Flexion (53, 56, 62, 65)

Lateral flexion is a component of most flexion and extension palpations and manipulations of the atlantooccipital joint, but it may also be considered independently. With the patient supine or sitting, the doctor's hands cup both sides of the occiput and roll the occiput into lateral flexion on the atlas (Fig. 10.28). Extreme care must be taken not to inadvertently move the cervical spine. Straight cephalad distraction during the procedure helps minimize cervical involvement.

Manipulation of the Occiput Fixed in Lateral Flexion (52–56, 58)

With the patient supine, the doctor stands at the head of the table. The patient's head is rotated so the side of restricted lateral bending is facing up. The doctor then uses the medial hand to cradle the underside of the head, while the pisiform of the other hand contacts the posterolateral occiput near the mastoid on the side that is turned up (Fig. 10.28). A high-velocity, low-amplitude, lateral-to-medial thrust is delivered when tissue tension is reached.

A flexion or extension manipulation may be chosen and applied with emphasis on lateral flexion (see Occiput, Flexion and Extension Manipulation).

Palpation of Atlas-Axis Movement (54, 55, 58)

Rotational movement of the atlas may be palpated in the manner as the other cervical segments (see Rotational Palpation) (Fig. 10.16), except that the posterior portion of the atlas transverse process is used as a contact point. Since rotation is the primary movement of the atlas-axis joint and the range of motion is so extensive, a large amount of anterior glide should be noted during palpation. Lateral glide is a much less dramatic motion, which can be palpated as the occiput is laterally flexed.

With bilateral index finger contacts, the atlas transverse process will be felt to glide toward the side of occipital lateral bending. A springy joint play should be noted, and the transverse process should glide back medially as pressure is applied on the side of lateral bending. Static positioning of the occiput-atlas-axis alignment should also be noted, as well as suboccipital muscle tone.

Manipulation of the Atlas Fixed in Rotation (54, 58, 59, 61, 62, 65)

With the patient supine and the doctor standing/ kneeling at the head of the table, the lateral portion of the index finger contacts the posterior portion of

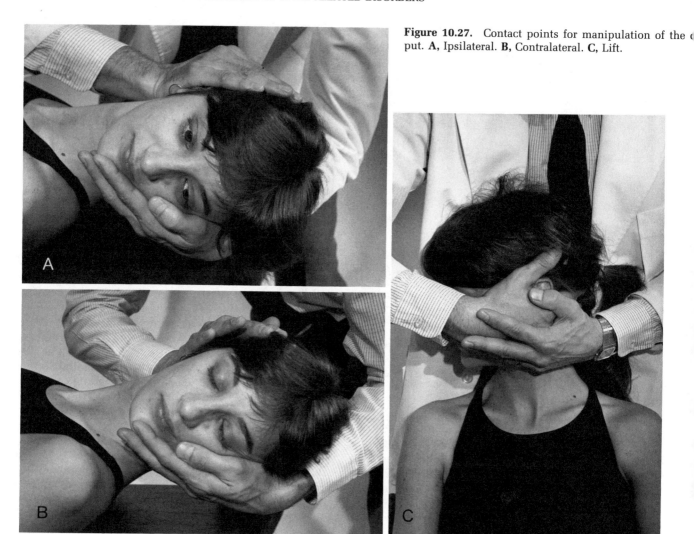

Figure 10.27. Contact points for manipulation of the o
put. **A,** Ipsilateral. **B,** Contralateral. **C,** Lift.

the atlas transverse process, after taking a medial-to-lateral tissue pull. When joint tension is achieved, a rotary anterior thrust is given.

This same adjustment could be made with the doctor standing in front of, or behind, the seated patient, as was true for rotational adjustments of the other cervical segments. Lateral bending may be combined to enhance preadjustive tension, thereby minimizing rotational stress to the vertebral artery.

Manipulation of the Atlas Fixed in Lateral Glide (54, 58, 59, 62)

With the patient supine, an index finger or pisiform contact is made over the lateral portion of the atlas transverse process, as the occiput is ipsilaterally laterally bent. While the other hand distracts the occiput, the contact hand thrusts medially to restore lateral glide. This could be done with the patient seated.

The patient may be placed on the side, with the head supported in a neutral position, allowing the atlas to "hang" freely underneath the supported oc-

ciput. A pisiform contact is made on the atlas transverse process, and a specific, high-velocity thrust is given in a medial vector with carefully measured depth and amplitude. A toggle recoil thrust may be delivered, which will mobilize the C0-C1 or C1-C2 joint.

DIFFERENTIAL DIAGNOSIS OF CERVICAL SPINE DISORDERS (Table 10.3)

"Whiplash" Injuries

"Whiplash" is not a diagnostic term, but rather a descriptive label that implies a mechanism of injury (3) whereby the body comes to a sudden stop followed by a sudden snap of the unsupported neck and head. The term "whiplash" has become controversial, and various authors have preferred to use hyperflexion, flexion, hyperextension, extension, acceleration and deceleration, as well as the commonly used cervical strain/sprain, when discussing this syndrome (6–73).

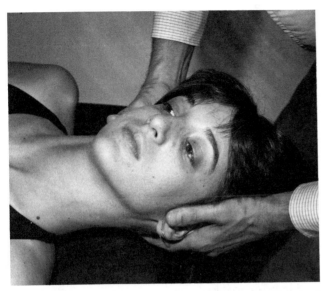

Figure 10.28. Position for palpation and manipulation of the occiput fixed in lateral flexion. The patient's head may also be rotated prior to lateral flexion.

Cailliet (66) suggests using hyperflexion or hyperextension to describe the reaction of the neck to the force, with deceleration or acceleration used to describe the mechanics of the force. He suggests that the extent of injury then be referred to as sprain or strain. Hohl (4, 71) discusses the injuries received in automobile accidents under the broad category of soft-tissue injuries. None of these terms give a specific diagnosis of the various structures involved.

The syndrome suffered as a result of the "whiplash" can include damage to cervical muscles, ligaments, discs, blood vessels, and nerves, as well as to osseous structures, which has been demonstrated experimentally (74). An accurate diagnosis of such injuries must be individualized and be based on the specific tissues that have been damaged. "Whiplash" in the following discussion is used to denote the mechanism of injury and is not suggested as a diagnostic term.

The syndrome produced by the whiplike action of the neck frequently consists of a complex array of symptoms from damaged structures that must be differentiated. Complicating the situation is the spectrum of psychosomatic illnesses and secondary gain that must be considered, since the vast majority of neck injuries result from motor vehicle accidents, which inherently have the potential for litigation. Fortunately there is now a body of scientific knowledge that helps the clinician understand the mechanism of injury, the anatomic basis for many of the resulting symptoms, and the prognosis for recovery (4, 67, 71–73).

The rotational and translational forces generated in the head and neck as a result of whiplash are much greater than that of the vehicle itself (70). In any motor vehicle collision, the unrestrained head first snaps in the direction of impact, then recoils in the opposite direction.

In rear-end collisions, even with a high seat back or head restraint, the neck is thrown into extension in proportion to the distance between the occupant's head and the supporting structure (70). As the victim's torso is forced backward into the seat back, the head and neck initially remain fixed, while the vehicle moves forward.

This initial inertia of the head is followed by extension of the cervical spine at the end of this rearward translation. After deflecting off the seat back or head restraint, the head rebounds forward, forcing the neck into flexion. In cars without head restraints, or with "head rests" in a low position, hyperextension occurs. If the head rest is not high enough, it may actually act as a fulcrum over which the cervical spine pivots (3). As the neck recoils forward, hyperflexion is stopped as the chin strikes the chest (67).

Head-on collisions cause a sudden, forceful flexion of the neck followed by recoil into extension. The unsupported body is thrown forward until it strikes something stationary such as the steering wheel, the dashboard, or the windshield (49).

A thorough history is necessary to evaluate the extent of sagittal plane forces, as well as forces in other planes. Asymmetric rotational forces may be introduced by the shoulder harness that restrains one shoulder, allowing the other to be forced forward during the hyperflexion phase of the "whiplash." The resultant shoulder girdle strain is a common clinical finding with motor vehicle accidents. Different structures will be injured if the victim is looking in the rearview mirror or stretching out the arm to protect others in the car at the time of impact. With the neck rotated 45°, the physiological range of extension is half of this range, and the posterior joints can be pushed beyond this physiologic range with resulting strain (67) and joint fixation.

The most serious injuries occur with the head forced into hyperextension (70) MacNab (67) states, "When the tone of the anterior cervical muscles is overcome, there is nothing to resist the extension movement of the neck, except the anterior longitudinal ligament and the anterior fibers of the annulus."

When the impact is from the side, a similar whiplash action occurs in the cervical spine, with the neck first snapped in the direction of the impact, followed by recoil in the opposite direction (49). Lateral flexion is limited, as the head strikes the shoulder (67) or side of the vehicle.

The biomechanical injuries seen clinically that result from the whiplash mechanism tend to follow a characteristic pattern. Cameron and Cree (75) report that torque and lofting of the head play an important role at the C1 and C7 vertebral segments during whiplash. It can be postulated that this torque and loft frequently produce fixation of the upper and lower cervical segments, while the middle segments

Table 10.3 Differential Diagnosis of Common Disorders of the Cervical Spine

Condition	History and Symptoms	Diagnosis Indicators	Therapy
Muscle syndromes			
Cervical strain	History of trauma (whiplash); neck pain radiating into the head, shoulders, and arms	Spasm and trigger points in neck muscles; pain on active ROM, no pain on passive ROM	Ischemic compression to trigger points, physical therapy & exercise (see Chapter 12)
Postural strain	History of forward head with static loading of neck extension muscles; pain radiating into neck, head, shoulders, & arms	Trigger points in extensor muscles of the neck	Ischemic compression to trigger points, physical therapy, exercise & postural retraining (see Chapter 12)
Biomechanical disorders			
Facet joint fixation	History of unguarded movement or trauma, pain in neck	Motion palpation reveals restricted vertebral motion segment fixation	Manipulation (see text)
Cervical joint facet sprain	History of trauma, pain, and stiffness of neck, protective muscle spasm; pain may radiate to occiput & into shoulders	Motion palpation reveals absence of joint fixation; stress radiographs reveal hypermobile vertebral motion segments once muscle spasms reduced	Immobilize with cervical collar when acute; exercise
Cervical disc herniation	Pain in neck & shoulder radiating down the arm in the distribution of involved nerve root; paresthesia, numbness, tingling & sensory and reflex deficits	Loss of reflex and sensation and muscle weakness; enhanced imagery necessary for diagnosis (MRI, CT scan)	Refer severe cases for surgical evaluation; moderate cases may respond to specific, gentle manipulation, immobilization, physical therapy, and exercise
Inflammatory disease			
Rheumatoid arthritis	Neck pain, progressive pain of myelopathy, neurologic manifestation that may be subtle (i.e., easy fatigability or difficulty in walking with sensory loss or gross paralysis)	Radiographs reveal osteoporosis, hypermobility, dislocations, and subluxations of the cervical spine; atlantoaxial dislocation may occur with lysis of transverse ligaments; flexion-extension views necessary for accurate evaluation; 3 mm gap between anterior atlas & odontoid; forward subluxation is 4–5 mm significant; Positive rheumatoid factor	Manipulation contraindicated in cases of vertebral segmental instability; immobilization & referral for surgical stabilization
Ankylosing spondylitis	Predominantly seen in males; stiffness, spinal pain, muscle pain, & loss of chest expansion	High ESR and HLA-B27 during active phase; radiographs demonstrate a progressive loss of segmental motion with ossification of the ligaments & disc spaces; disc spaces are not narrowed as in DJD; ligamentous laxity above rigid segments may be seen with atlantoaxial occipital dislocation	Gentle mobilization, heat, mild exercise, manipulation when acute phase is past; refer for pain & antiinflammation medication when severe
Spondylosis & spondyloarthrosis	Neck pain & stiffness; decrease in range of motion; pain may refer to interscapular, shoulders, & occipital regions	Radiographs reveal decreased disc height, osteophytes, sclerosis of vertebral body endplates, decreased facet/uncovertebral joint spaces with osteophytes and sclerosis	Manipulation, traction, exercise; cervical collar may benefit when acute

become hypermobile due to ligamentous sprain that occurs at the apex of the cervical curve (Fig. 10.29). Rib fixation is commonly seen in the upper dorsal segments. Jackson (49) reports that the greatest amount of injury occurs at the C4–5 to C5–6 segments; Cameron and Cree (75) relate this to the torque occurring at C1 and C7 which, they note, explains the frequent midcervical distraction injuries.

Dislocation of the posterior facets with or without cord injury may occur, and in severe cases, fracture of the posterior elements of the vertebrae as they are forced apart have been noted (69). Compression fracture of the vertebral bodies (Chapter 2) can occur and may not be visualized in early radiographs, becoming evident when more compression and healing have occurred (49).

Whiplash injuries to neurological structures include contusion of the brain and spinal cord. Damage to the cortex and cerebellum may occur from a contrecoup as the brain hits the inner table of the skull, as well as from a direct blow to the skull (3). Gay and Abbott (72) report the mechanics of the concussion in hyperflexion injuries as a sudden mechanical deformity and pressure on the frontal and temporal lobes of the brain when forward movement of the brain is arrested against the anterior walls of the skull, as the head and neck are whipped backward.

Damage to the spinal cord is produced by a combination of hyperextension and backward shearing forces (72). Marar (76) found that the cord is damaged in an anteroposterior direction by the squeezing effect produced between a backward-subluxating vertebral body at the disc space level or through a complete fracture of the vertebral body just below the pedicle anteriorly and an infolded ligamentum flava posteriorly. Trauma to the cord may also occur as the result of edema as well as transection.

Electroencephalographic abnormalities have been demonstrated in patients following whiplash injuries (77). Jackson (49) suggests that injury to the brain and to the brain stem may be the result of a pressure gradient created by pressure build-up or by shearing forces and mass movements of the intracranial contents. Vascular insufficiency may also be produced by constriction or occlusion of one or both vertebral arteries within the transverse foramina.

If the head is rotated at the time of impact, the shearing force may fracture a vertebral arch or posterior facet. The lateral masses of the atlas and axis may suffer compression fractures, and a transverse process fracture may occur on the side of rotation. Ligaments on the contralateral side from rotation may be torn, causing dislocation of the atlas or axis (49). More commonly seen are rotational fixations of the atlas or the axis (Fig. 10.8). Described by Jacobson and Adler (78) in 1956 as a pathologic fixation in a position within the normal range of motion, this condition was described in detail by Coutts (46) in 1934. Wortzman and Dewar (37) report that rotational fixation is usually of a moderate nature, such as occurs in a flexion-extension injury in a rear-end collision.

Injuries caused by side collision may produce strain of the lateral neck muscles and tearing of the alar and atlantoaxial ligaments and upper joint capsules (Fig. 10.3). If severe, a wedging of the lateral

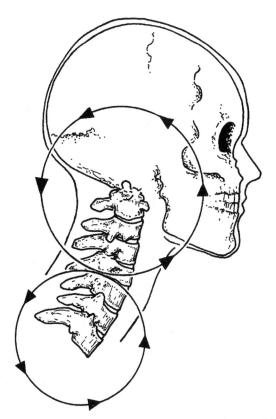

Figure 10.29. The elements of torque at C1 and C7 and lofting of the head may produce fixation of the upper and lower cervical segments. The middle segments become hypermobile due to the ligamentous sprain that occurs at the apex of the cervical curve. (Modified from Cameron BM, Cree CMN: A critique of the compression theory of whiplash. *Orthopedics* 2:127–129, 1960.)

Hyperextension injuries caused by rear-end collisions frequently strain the "anterior strap" muscles (scalene and sternocleidomastoideus). If the head is rotated and tilted to one side, the torsional effect causes greater damage on one side than on the other (49). Forceful hyperextension injuries may produce traction on the anterior longitudinal ligament, which sprains the fibers attached to the intervertebral disc. An avulsion fracture may occur as a piece of bone is torn from the inferior margin of the vertebral body (71). Rupture of the underlying annulus may occur, with displacement of nuclear material (74). Compressive forces on the posterior structures may produce avulsions of the capsular ligaments, as in folding or creasing of the interlaminar ligaments and damage to the articular cartilage as the posterior joints are jammed together (69). Extension with compression can produce a crushing of the posterior elements of the vertebra (69).

Hyperflexion injuries caused by head-on collisions may tear or stretch the nuchal ligaments, the capsular ligaments of the Luschka and posterior facet joints, the interspinous ligaments, and the other posterior ligaments of the neck (Fig. 10.3).

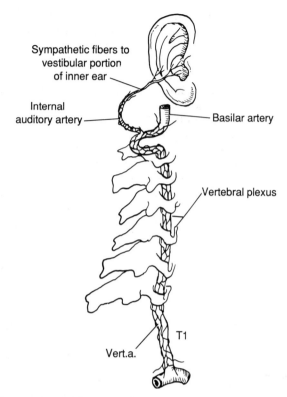

Sympathetic fibers to
vestibular portion
of inner ear

Internal
auditory artery

Basilar artery

Vertebral plexus

T1

Vert.a.

Figure 10.30. The cervical sympathetics accompanying the vertebral arteries are vulnerable to injury as they are pulled backward against the posterior wall of the bony rings formed by the transverse foramen. (Modified from Jackson R: *The Cervical Syndrome*, ed 4. Springfield, IL, Charles C Thomas, 1977, p 179.)

aspect of a vertebral body and its associated lateral mass can occur (69).

Direct traumatic insult to the nerve roots produces inflammation in the dural sleeves and perineural tissues, which may result in fibrosis. Adhesions between the dural sleeves and the adjacent capsular structure may prevent normal motion of nerve roots (49). Irritation of the cervical sympathetics gives rise to a variety of symptoms. Sympathetic ganglion damage (71) as well as damage to sympathetic fibers in the spinal cord is thought to be responsible for these symptoms. Cervical sympathetic nerve irritation may occur by reflex stimulation as well as by direct trauma. Because of their close proximity to the vertebral arteries, the cervical sympathetics are particularly vulnerable to injury (Fig. 10.30). The vertebral arteries and the encircling sympathetic nerves within the transverse foramen may be subjected to trauma as they are pulled backward against the posterior wall of their bony rings, or by subluxation or fracture of the adjacent bony structure, or injury to adjacent soft tissues (49).

Grieve (47) compares the mechanism of "whiplash" injury to multiple "sprained ankles" in the neck, with the added complications of nerve root and plexus traction injury, meningeal irritation, tearing of ligaments and muscle fibers, and trauma to blood vessels and lymphatics. He notes that the overall effect is an upset of sensitive structure and delicately balanced function.

History

The patient with "whiplash" most commonly gives a history of minor to moderately severe rear-end collisions (3) or other types of vehicular crashes, such as a head-on or side collision. Occasionally the patient suffering from "whiplash" presents with a history of a fall. A sideways fall on the outstretched arm can produce a lateral "whiplash" effect on the cervical spine. A blow such as from a swinging object (49) may also produce "whiplash."

It is important to obtain as much information as possible about the injury. The direction of force, position and relationship of the head and spine, and state of tension of the neck muscles all help to determine the location of stress. The position of the patient at the time of impact should be noted. Was the patient looking straight ahead or positioned with the head or body turned? Was the patient driving? Was the arm outstretched? Did the head or another body part strike something? Did something loose in the vehicle strike the patient? Was the patient wearing a seat restraint (lap type or combined lap-shoulder harness), and what was the nature of the head support? Was there loss of consciousness or mental confusion? Was the patient thrown from the car? What were the relative sizes of the involved vehicles, make of the vehicles, and type of suspension in the injured party's vehicle? What was the approximate speed involved? Was the patient's foot down hard on the brake pedal or floor board? Was the seat torn loose? Did the backrest break away? Had there been a previous or old neck injury? The answers to these questions all aid in the assessment of the severity of injury in addition to indicating which structures are involved.

Symptoms of "Whiplash" Injury

Patients suffering from whiplash injuries complain of a large variety of symptoms, typically much broader than other neck injuries. Frequently they are not aware of significant injury immediately following the accident, but after a few minutes develop a feeling of discomfort in the neck, associated with some degree of nausea (69). A feeling of tightness and stiffness gradually ensues, and after several days a broad symptom complex may develop (3). Patients treated immediately following whiplash should be informed that they may gradually feel worse for several days, to prevent them from thinking the treatment has made them worse. After 72 hours, a gradual decrease in symptoms can be expected. The most common complaints are neck pain with limited motion (Fig. 10.31).

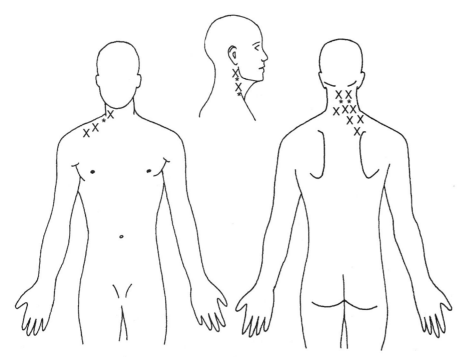

Figure 10.31. Typical pain chart of a patient following whiplash injury. Trigger points (*) in the scalene and posterior cervical muscles refer pain (×) in this pattern.

Neck pain may occur at the back, front, and sides of the neck (49). The pain may radiate into the shoulders and arms to the fingers. The radiation may be unilateral or bilateral. Chest and back pain may also be present. The character of pain may be described as burning, sharp, throbbing, or stabbing, or as a dull ache. A deep, aching or dull pain is common with joint lesions. Nerve irritation produces a stabbing or lightning-like pain that radiates in specific patterns. A sharp, localized pain may indicate a fracture. Throbbing pain is indicative of vascular involvement (70).

Headaches are a frequent complaint with cervical spine disorders (49). The pain may be at the back of the head, the top of the head, or in the temple area (49). It may be unilateral or bilateral, intermittent or constant, localized or generalized. Muscle contraction headaches are generally associated with occipital pain, or pain radiating to the frontal area (Fig. 10.32). These so-called tension headaches may be caused by spasm, injury, or inflammation to the muscles or myofascial connection to the cranial periosteum. The greater and lesser occipital nerves may be irritated by the clinically contracted muscle or by irritating substances (bradykinins, proteolytic enzymes, etc.) that accompany inflammation. Ischemia may accompany chronic muscle spasm, activating a reflex whereby the pain-spasm-pain cycle becomes chronic. Vascular headaches may occur in patients with head injuries, but they represent a small fraction of those patients suffering from headaches as a result of "whiplash."

Stiffness following injury usually limits motion in the direction opposite to that of the muscle spasm. Weakness of the muscles of the neck, arms, and

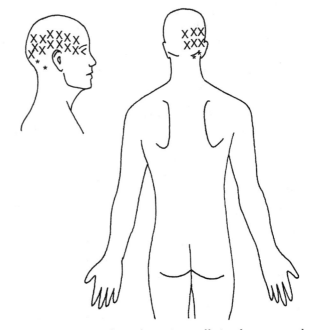

Figure 10.32. Pain chart of a patient suffering from a muscle contraction headache. Trigger points (*) in the cervical muscles refer pain (×) cephalad.

hands may be noted by the patient, and the patient often complains of difficulty balancing the head or the neck because of weakness of the neck muscles (49). Complaints of loss of grip strength and things slipping from the hands are common.

Sensory complaints include numbness and tingling, frequently without actual demonstrable hypesthesia or sensory changes. Numbness of the neck, shoulders, arm, forearm, and fingers may be the result of nerve root irritation or compression, circulatory embarrassment, or referral from trigger points in the strained muscles (49, 79).

Visual disturbances are frequent following trauma to the neck. Blurred vision is a common complaint, and usually of short duration. It may be due to damage to the vertebral arteries or may reflect damage to the cervical sympathetic chain (67). Other complaints can include "eye strain," fatigue, diplopia, and photophobia (47).

Occasionally symptoms of irritation of the sympathetic nerve supply in the neck occur. This can produce dilation of one pupil with irritation of the sympathetic fibers surrounding the internal carotid arteries and their branches to the eye. Horner's syndrome is occasionally seen due to sympathetic ganglion damage around the sixth cervical level (67, 69).

Feelings of instability or dysequilibrium with a tendency to list to one side have been reported (47). Disruption of the proprioceptive system from injury to muscles and joints of the cervical spine or vasospasm or vasodilation with edema affecting labyrinth function may result in dizziness, unsteadiness, or lightheadedness (67). Dysphagia (complaints of difficulty in swallowing) and other laryngeal disturbances, with compulsive clearing of the throat (47), may be the result of swelling of the anterior neck structures or to retropharyngeal hematoma. The latter can be seen on routine lateral radiographs as forward displacement of the air shadow of the pharynx. Dysphagia, occurring after the passage of several weeks, is usually emotional in origin (67).

Complaints of dyspnea or shortness of breath may be the result of pain in respiratory muscles. Heart palpitations (tachycardia) from irritation of the fourth nerve root or irritation of the cardiac sympathetic supply should be investigated thoroughly. Vertebrobasilar arterial insufficiency can precipitate drop attacks or black out sensations. Nausea and vomiting and complaints of irritability, insomnia, and lightheadedness may also be noted.

Low back pain is frequently reported in cases of moderate to severe injury resulting from rear-end collisions, and occasionally a patient complains of leg symptoms. Sprains of the lumbar region may occur from acute flexion of the low back at the time of the accident (72) (see Chapter 8) and are frequently overlooked initially because of the more severe cervical complaints at the onset.

Grieve (47) stresses the vulnerability of the "whiplash" victim to rough handling. He describes this as a highly reactive "brittleness" during the early stages. He notes that this is quite different from the irritability of a single peripheral joint. He states, "If the badly injured whiplash patient is handled vigorously with careless movement, the exacerbation can be very severe with headaches of hideous intensity, bizarre visual upset, psychic distress amounting to abject misery and cervical pain of frightening viciousness." He notes further that the "brittle" stage may last for a week or up to 3 months and may return for a few days in the following months if the patient is badly jolted or given unnecessary vigorous treatment. This fragility, along with the wide variety of presenting symptoms, should not label the patient as psychoneurotic and should be thoroughly investigated.

What appears to be a minor vehicular collision may produce a varied pattern of symptoms that can be understood by careful evaluation of the structures that can be damaged. It is not possible to determine the type or extent of soft-tissue damage by estimating the cost of auto damage (70). Fortunately, with appropriate management, the prognosis for the vast majority of these patients is favorable.

Objectively, the acute signs of whiplash injury include muscle tenderness, spasm, and restricted motion (67, 77). A few hours to a few days after the injury, when most patients are usually seen, there is tenderness and swelling in the anterior neck region (anterior strap muscles) and often palpable spasm in the trapezius muscle, accompanied by variable restriction of neck motion (4, 71). The splenius capitis muscles are frequently strained, especially if the head and neck are somewhat rotated at the time of impact (79). The sternocleidomastoid muscle resists forceful backward movement and, along with the scalene muscles, is commonly injured by hyperextension and lateral flexion injuries (79).

Frequently overlooked are trigger points in the posterior scalene muscle at the attachment to the second rib. These trigger points are difficult to locate because they pass beneath the levator scapulae, which must be pushed aside at the point where the levator scapulae emerges from the anterior, free border of the upper trapezius (79). Superior fixations of the first rib are commonly found in patients suffering from "whiplash" injuries and are frequently associated with trigger points in the anterior scalene muscles. If the thoracic lumbar paraspinal muscles are stiffened at the time of impact, the sudden acceleration or deceleration may rapidly stretch these muscles, activating trigger points. The trapezius muscle and the levator scapulae check rein flexion and are frequently strained in accidents involving forceful hyperflexion (79).

A careful evaluation of the many muscles (Tables 10.1 and 10.2) supporting the neck and head should be performed. This is the most complex area of the spine, and strain of various combinations of muscles should not be overlooked. As with any acute muscle strain following injury due to whiplash, trigger points are not too readily palpable. The generalized muscle spasm and swelling may mask the trigger points, which become much more apparent as the spasm and swelling subside (Chapter 12).

In the presence of cervical nerve root irritation, the upper extremity reflexes may be hyperactive im-

Table 10.4 Radiographs Recommended for Whiplash Injuries

View	Differentiation
AP open-mouth	Alignment and integrity occiput, atlas, dens
Lower cervical antero-posterior	Fracture, dislocation, alignment
Lateral (neutral)	Straightening of curve, fracture, dislocation, baseline for templating motion
Lateral flexion and extension	Segmental motion
Right and left oblique	Narrowing of foramen or fractured lamina
Pillar views	Fracture of lateral masses

mediately following an injury. After a few days they become hypoactive, provided there is no spinal cord involvement. Sensory changes may be found anywhere along the cervical nerve-root distribution. Soon after an injury, hyperesthesia may be present, which changes to hypoesthesia after a short time (49). Pupillary dilation may be present which indicates irritation of the sympathetic nerve supply (49).

Irritation of the sympathetic nerve supply gives rise to vasoconstriction of the arteries that are supplied by sympathetic fibers, and is indicated by a wide blood-pressure variation between arms. A 10- to 20-point difference can be produced by cervical spine disorders (49). Spasm in the scalene muscles may cause diminution or obliteration of the radial pulse when the head is tilted and rotated to the opposite sides (see Thoracic Outlet Syndromes).

Vertebral motion segments may be blocked anywhere in the spine with "whiplash" injuries, but most common are upper cervical fixations (22, 37, 46, 47, 78), followed by fixation at the C7-T1 vertebral motion segment, and first costovertebral articulation.

Radiological Findings of "Whiplash"

The clinician must be prepared to evaluate the clinical and radiographic pictures as a whole, and clinical findings must be correlated with the radiographs. Gross derangements sometimes give rise to minimal symptoms and clinical findings, whereas minimal derangements may cause severe symptoms and marked clinical findings. Radiologic examination is essential following trauma to the cervical spine to determine appropriate therapy. It is necessary to rule out fractures, dislocations, pathologic conditions, and anomalies where manipulative therapy is contraindicated (15) (Chapter 4). Gore et al. (80) note that "it is important to realize that although roentgenographic abnormalities represent structural changes in the spine, they do not necessarily cause symptoms."

Routine radiographs following cervical trauma (Table 10.4) should include the neutral lateral, AP open mouth, and AP lower cervical initially. Flexion and extension laterals and right and left obliques should be added after thorough scrutiny of the initial views to rule out fracture or severe ligament damage. These seven views comprise the Davis series. Right and left AP lower cervical pillar views should be added if compressive fractures of the articular pillars are suspected.

Radiographs of patients following "whiplash" accidents are frequently read as normal except for loss of physiological cervical lordosis. A considerable number of rear-end collision victims have a cervical curve flattening or reversal. While loss of lordosis can be caused by muscle spasm, Hohl (71) suggests that a flattened cervical spine is probably a normal variation in most cases. He notes that "dynamic studies, including flexion-extension views are likely to persuade the careful observer, in cases of flattening or curve reversal, that no serious condition exists if the expected movement is demonstrated at each level."

Rechtman and coworkers (81) found that the sharply reversed cervical curve appears to indicate a degree of structural damage. Hohl (71) notes that when there is an existing sharp reversal of the cervical curve, the flexion-extension films usually fail to indicate normal mobility at the involved level. If the reversal occurs over more than one segment, he concludes that there is a lesser degree of injury and the flexion-extension views show relatively normal motion. Alterations of the cervical curve without injury have been noted frequently in association with degenerative disc narrowing and spur formation, and the straightening or reversal is not particularly significant after soft-tissue injury if segmental fixation is not seen (71). Congenitally tall articular pillars also produce an apparent straight cervical spine, which cannot be considered clinically significant (82).

Occult fractures after neck injury should be suspected in patients with persistent severe restriction of neck movement that may have not been apparent on initial films. Repeat films and views of the articular pillars may be necessary to see the lateral masses. Cervical fractures can be categorized according to the mechanism of injury, flexion-extension, lateral flexion, rotation, or compression (28) (see Chapter 2). Classification according to stability is the foremost consideration since unstable fractures require prompt referral for neurological and surgical evaluation. Unstable fractures pose a serious threat in the cervical region because of the possibility of spinal cord defects that can result in quadraplegia and even death.

While fracture of the occipital condyle is considered rare (70), it can have serious consequences. Anderson and Montesano (83) reported six cases in the four years prior to 1988, in addition to 20 other cases reviewed in the literature. They noted that four of the six cases treated had presented with avulsion fractures of the occipital condyle, which

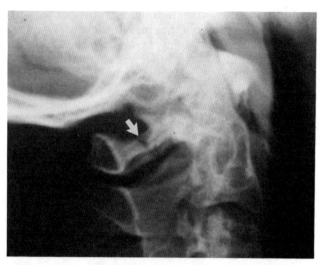

Figure 10.33. Fracture of the posterior arch of the atlas. (From Yochum TR, Rowe LJ: *Essentials of Skeletal Radiology.* Baltimore, Williams & Wilkins, 1987, p 431.)

are potentially unstable since loss of integrity of the alar ligaments may coexist (80).

The most common fracture of the atlas occurs in the posterior arch during marked hyperextension (Fig. 10.33). The posterior arch of the atlas is compressed between the occiput and the larger, sturdier, posterior arch of the axis, causing the atlas to fracture at the weakest point in the ring, where it is grooved by the vertebral arteries. Stability can be assessed by flexion-extension radiographs (Chapter 6), provided there is no neurological deficit.

Bursting of the ring of the atlas can occur with a direct blow to the vertex of the head. The downward vector of force on the skull has a bilateral chisel effect. The occipital condyles are forced downward, causing a bursting fracture with bilateral lateral displacement of the lateral masses of the atlas (28) (Fig. 2.24).

Described by Jefferson in 1920 (84), this classic compression fracture is characterized by disruption of the atlas ring in four places, two anteriorly and two posteriorly. Lateral displacement of both lateral masses with respect to the dens may be seen on a true anteroposterior radiograph, with the spinous process of the axis in the midline. Posterior displacement of the fragments may be seen on lateral flexion, but a CT scan allows a more accurate diagnosis.

Fracture of the dens may occur with or without dislocation of the atlas. In hyperflexion injuries, the dens is displaced anteriorly with the atlas; in hyperextension injuries the dens is displaced posteriorly with the atlas. In adults, fracture of the dens without dislocation of the atlas occurs more or less transversely through the base of the dens at or above the level of the superior articular facets. In young children, the fracture is an epiphyseal separation within the body of the axis below the level of the facets.

Differentiation from os odontoideum may occasionally present a problem, particularly if the fracture was overlooked initially. The presence of a normal-shaped dens helps to differentiate pseudoarthrosis from an os odontoideum.

Fracture of the arch of C2, classically referred to as the hangman's fracture (Fig. 10.34), occurs with hyperextension and distraction (85). A similar fracture can be produced by vertical compression and extension in motor vehicular accidents where the driver's chin strikes the rim of the steering wheel, due to the sudden oblique force delivered to the hyperextended head from above and behind while the cervical spine is in forward flexion. The fracture line at the pars interarticularis is vertical, horizontal, or oblique and is best visualized on lateral radiographs. When both pedicles are fractured, the body of C2 slides anteriorly, while the posterior arch is fixed by the inferior articular process, producing a traumatic spondylolisthesis of the axis. This fracture may or may not produce neurological symptoms (3).

Fractures of the body of C2 at the anterior-inferior margin are commonly due to an hyperextension injury. With forced hyperextension, the spinous and articular processes are squeezed together and act as a fulcrum, which results in the rupture of the anterior longitudinal ligament. This can result in a small bone chip separating from the anterior rim of the axis at the point of rupture of the anterior longitudinal ligament.

Compression fractures of the cervical vertebrae are thought to be due to flexion injuries (69) (Fig. 2.25). A simple compression fracture with minimal deformation suggests a lower force than a vertical compression fracture with a central depression (3). These fractures may or may not produce neurological deficit. More severe is the "tear-drop" fracture (Fig. 10.35), in which one vertebral body is crushed by the vertebral body above in such a manner that the anterior part of the involved centrum is not only compressed, but completely broken away. The triangular fragment seen at the anteroinferior border of the involved vertebra has been compared to a "tear drop," hence the name tear-drop fracture. This fracture can produce severe neurological deficit, as it is commonly associated with posterior ligamentous disruption, and should be referred for neurological evaluation.

Lateral flexion injuries can produce unilateral wedging or fracture of the vertebra, with or without neurological deficit. In addition to wedging of the vertebral body, unilateral facet dislocation or fracture of the lateral masses on one side with ligamentous sprain and rupture may occur on the contralateral side. These injuries may be complicated by brachial plexus lesions as well as lesions of the spinal cord (86). Neurological deficits may range in severity from rapidly resolving (15 seconds to several minutes or hours) including pain, paresthesia, and paralysis, to complete unresolving tetraplegia (3).

Figure 10.34. Fracture of the arch of C2 (hangman's fracture). (From Yochum TR, Rowe LJ: *Essentials of Skeletal Radiology.* Baltimore, Williams & Wilkins, 1987, p 433.)

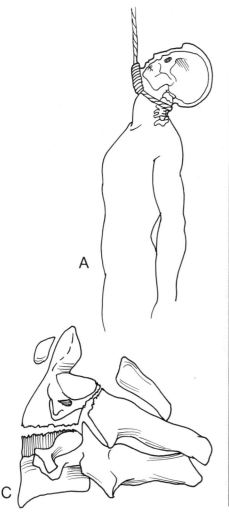

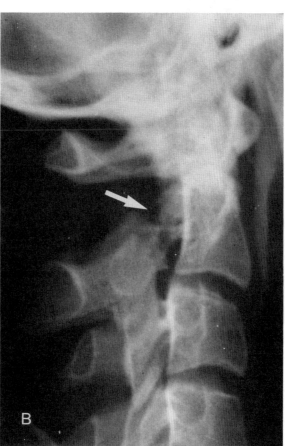

Fractures of the posterior elements of a cervical vertebra without compression can occur, but extension without compression usually produces minimal bony injury (69). Extension with compression will produce a crushing of the posterior elements of the vertebra. The inferior facets above the point where the forces are resolved are impacted. Fractures of the pedicles may result in dorsal displacement of the lateral masses and spinous processes. With extreme extension, fractures of the spinous processes and lamina of the vertebra are common, due to the direct contact of one spinous process upon another (69).

Dislocations of the cervical spine can be more serious than fractures, because they almost always result in cord compression as well as nerve root compression with loss of motor and sensory function. Forceful flexion of the neck may cause complete disruption of the transverse ligament of the atlas, with complete forward dislocation of the head and atlas on the axis. This results in marked compression of

the spinal cord and is usually incompatible with life. Dislocation of the posterior facets can also occur with sudden forceful flexion. Displacement of the inferior facets forward over the superior facets of the adjacent vertebra may cause compression of the spinal cord, which results from narrowing of the intervertebral and vertebral foramen. Forceful hyperextension can produce posterior dislocation, however, these dislocations often reduce themselves without radiographic evidence that they have occurred.

Management of "Whiplash" Injuries

Treatment of patients suffering from "whiplash" injuries must be individualized, based on the mechanism of injury, symptomatology, examination, and radiographic findings (49). A thorough history, along with a careful physical and appropriate radiographic examination, gives the patient confidence in the physician in the face of a variety of puzzling and disturbing symptoms (71).

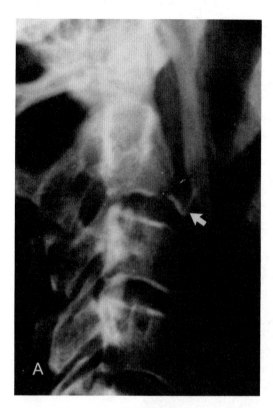

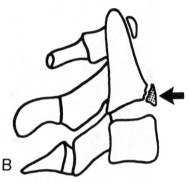

Figure 10.35. Tear-drop fracture. (From Yochum TR, Rowe LJ: *Essentials of Skeletal Radiology*. Baltimore, Williams & Wilkins, 1987, p 434.)

Treatment should be based on the severity of the injury. The basic treatment for mild to moderately severe injuries in the acute phase is protection of overstretched muscles and ligaments. Patients with fractures and/or dislocations should be referred for determination of stability and neurological evaluation.

Restricting movement of the neck with a cervical collar limits the motions that cause pain (68). Pain produced by muscle spasm, which is a protective mechanism following an acute injury, can be reduced by restricting motion of the injured part. In most cases, soft collars that offer head support increase comfort and allow for some motion, which is necessary for adequate circulation to the injured structure. It should be remembered that immobilization is the enemy of joints, which are designed for motion and require movement to be healthy (Chapter 3).

Gay and Abbott (72) recommend that patients wear a comfortable cervical collar support for about 2 weeks. They consider it important for the patient to wear the collar intermittently. Following this, the collar is worn when the patient is likely to jar the neck, or at the end of the day, when fatigue of the neck muscles is most pronounced. It should be worn when traveling in motor vehicles during the first 6 to 8 weeks, to prevent serious reinjury to vulnerable tissues that may be further traumatized by sudden stops. A second whiplash injury during the healing stage often does much more damage than the first, even when minor, because the protective structures of the neck have not yet healed.

Use of the collar should never be prolonged without appropriate exercise. Prolonged immobilization leads to contracture of soft tissues and limited range of motion, muscular atrophy, and psychologic dependence (64, 83). Cailliet (66) warns that excessive or complete immobilization allows organization of extravasated blood and edema fluid, shortening of contracted muscle, thickening of periarticular tissue, muscle atrophy, and equally important, psychological and physiological fixation.

The cervical collar should be designed to hold the neck in an optimal position for healing of injured skeletal, ligamentous, and capsular structures (49), and the neck should be held straight with the chin tucked in. Immobilization in hyperextension causes further stretching of the anterior longitudinal ligament and allows the posterior ligaments to heal in a shortened position with narrowing of the intervertebral foramen (49).

Bed rest may be necessary for 24–72 hours in moderately severe cases but should not be prolonged (72). Macnab (74) points out that to avoid iatrogenic neurosis, the patient should be taught to live with minor discomfort. Treatment should not be perfunctory, yet at the same time the doctor must never overtreat the patient. Treatment should not interfere with the patient's daily routine. Patients should be told that if they restrict activities because of fear of harm, they are mistaken. In the majority of instances, the patient can return to work within 3 to 7 days. Patients should be given instructions on how to avoid extension strain to the neck during activities of daily living (49) and, most importantly, must be told the difference between hurting themselves and harming themselves (67).

Analgesics may be necessary for pain relief, but muscle relaxants have not proven advantageous (3). Ice applied to the paracervical structures for 20 minutes each hour or two, for the first 36–48 hours, provides an anesthetic effect. Hot, moist heat applied for 10 minutes at intervals after 48 hours reduces muscle spasm (68). Gentle massage, manual traction, and a rolled towel placed under the occiput may also be used to reduce muscle spasm. Ultrasound is also useful in reducing the discomfort produced by muscle spasm and swelling found in acute patients (Chapter 12).

Gentle mobilization and manipulation of joint fixation should be implemented as soon as possible, once contraindications have been ruled out (Chapter 4) (5, 87). Patients who have not had a course of manipulation prior to the injury may be apprehensive, and it is better to wait several days in these cases, until swelling and spasm have been reduced. Patients who have received the benefit of previous manipulation may expect manipulation on the first visit. In these cases, gentle manipulation can be advantageous. When the acute phase (characterized by spasm, swelling, and inflammation) has passed, the patient will begin to complain more of weakness. This usually occurs after several weeks.

An exercise program should be instituted early in the management of patients suffering from whiplash injuries. Stretching exercises should be graduated and not performed beyond the subpain level, to prevent reflex muscle spasm. The object of exercise is to elongate the soft tissues to their normal range, minimize the periarticular fibrosis contracture of the zygapophyseal joint, regain the normal length of the muscle, and by muscular action, increase circulation to the deep neck tissues (87).

By improving flexibility and muscle tone, posture and neck function can be improved. The patient should be instructed in full usage of motion exercises. Isometric exercises, which require no joint motion, are advantageous and can be performed with varying degrees of rotation to the left and right, lateral flexion to the left and right, as well as flexion and extension with the head resisting pressure exerted by the hands (73).

Activities should be modified to prevent undue stress of injured tissue, which delays healing. Proper total body posture should be stressed including avoidance of any prolonged position, maintenance of mobility, and avoidance of acute or prolonged extension of the neck with minimal prolonged hyperflexion. The patient should be encouraged to hold the head up and back, with the chin in and the neck flat (66).

Patients should be instructed to avoid sleeping prone, which places constant strain on the neck because of the sustained rotation of the neck and hyperextension of the lumbar spine. Sleeping with one or both arms above the head may compromise the circulation to the upper extremities and produce sleep dysesthesia. A cervical (contour) or soft down pillow insures proper positioning of the neck, avoiding strain on the back or side of the neck. Prolonged sitting in a slumped position with the head "poked" forward should also be avoided. Using headphones is preferable to cradling the telephone on one shoulder for prolonged telephone conversations.

A gradual return to recreational activities should be encouraged, and patients reassured that they are not disabled by their injuries. Once the acute condition has abated, usually 4 to 6 weeks, as evidenced by a decrease of symptoms, negative physical findings, and a fuller range of motion, the physician can consider the condition chronic (68). Lasting symptoms are most often intermittent neck ache, stiffness, and headaches, as well as interscapular pain and upper extremity pain and numbness (71).

Often there is little to be found on physical examination, however, careful palpation of these patients in many instances reveals unresolved trigger points in muscles that have been strained. Trigger points are frequently difficult to find initially, because of overlying swelling and muscle spasm. Much pain and disability can be prevented by appropriate treatment of these muscle syndromes (Chapter 12).

Routine manipulation long into the chronic phase can prolong muscle syndromes, by initiating reflex muscle spasm that returns to protect injured joints. A long course of repeated manipulation that brings only one to two hours of relief following treatment is contraindicated and fosters a dependency on passive treatment that offers no lasting benefit to the patient. Rather, treatment directed at reduction of muscle syndrome symptoms, including ischemic compression and active stretching, resolves many of the chronic symptoms.

A period of control for a minimum of 3 to 4 months should be established whereby periodic checkups, treatment when necessary, and reevaluation will provide active follow-up. After this, the patient is advised to receive treatments on an "as needed" basis (PRN). Emotional reactions, which sometimes occur following injury due to "whiplash," should not be discounted on the basis of psychoneurosis or secondary gain. Brain damage and frustration over unrecognized organic injuries can lead to considerable psychic distress. White and Panjabi (3) state, "there is no doubt that some of the intracranial lesions may account for, or at least contribute to, some of the bizarre local symptoms, as well as some of the psychoneurotic problems that are often associated with this disease complex."

Acknowledgment that the mental distress is real, and in most cases will disappear with time, is often all that is necessary to allow the involved structures to heal. Reassurance is often necessary to restore the emotional equilibrium of these patients and to reduce the further somatization of complaints, which can result from pain and impaired function. Anxiety is a powerful psychic force that may be as disabling as a severe physical handicap. Prolonged psychic distress may be due to other organic dysfunctions, substance abuse, concurrent domestic problems, or personality disorder. Referral for neurological evaluation or psychometric testing is recommended for an appropriate diagnosis if any of these conditions is suspected.

Multiple prognostic factors play a role in the successful recovery of victims of "whiplash" injuries (4, 73). Clinical, psychosocial, and medicolegal factors must all be considered. Clinical findings that influence patient recovery, in addition to severity of injury, include congenital anomalies and prior injury. Hohl (4) notes significant positive correlation between poor results and findings of numbness or pain in one or both upper extremities, sharp reversal of the cervical lordosis visible on radiographs, and restricted motion at one interspace, as shown by flexion-extension radiographs.

Both congenital block vertebrae and reduced spinal canal size have been identified as poor prognostic indicators by Foreman and Croft (70). Norris and Watt (88) found that preexisting degenerative changes, no matter how slight, appear to alter the prognosis adversely.

This was not supported by Gore and coworkers (89), who found no statistically significant relationship between the presence of degenerative changes on the initial and final films and the levels of pain reported by the patient, nor between changes in roentgenographic abnormalities and changes in pain. They also noted that the sagittal diameter or change in sagittal diameter did not relate to the severity of pain reported and that reversal of cervical lordosis was not related to the presence or absence of degenerative change. They further reported that anterior osteophyte formation was the only roentgenographic finding that was more common in those with neck pain. According to their study, two-thirds of the 205 patients evaluated had a favorable long-term result, while one-third had unfavorable results, with pain that interfered to some extent with their life-style.

This is consistent with other studies of patients with neck pain (4, 73, 74), including Hohl (71), who found that 39% of patients with preexisting degenerative changes of the neck had residual symptoms after an average of 7 years. Greenfield and Ilfeld (73) reported that interscapular or upper back pain prognosticated a less favorable result.

Patients suffering from "whiplash" injuries have been characterized as hysterical, neurotic, or dishonest. Others have been accused of developing symptoms following "coaching" to build a case for litigation. While secondary gain is no doubt a factor in a few cases, not all patients with ongoing complaints are simply seeking large settlements. Gotten (90) reported a dramatic difference in the time lost from work before and after settlement. In many cases, this may mean that the settlement occured near the end point of medical care, when the patient had become medically stationary. His hypothesis that illness was used as a means of implementing psychological adjustments that had been postponed or unfulfilled because of financial difficulties may have basis in some, but is not universal to all, "whiplash" victims.

The adversarial system including patients, attorneys, and insurance carriers is subject to abuse by all parties. Patients are seen to feign illness or magnify symptoms for secondary gain (Chapter 4). Equally damaging to the system as well as to the patient, is the attorney who encourages the doctor to falsify records and prolong time loss and treatment in an attempt to magnify the severity of injury in order to gain a larger settlement.

Not without culpability are doctors who render unnecessary treatment and foster disability by magnifying the patient's impairment. MacNab (74) states that "above all (the physician) must take care not to fan the flames of hostility that these patients so commonly exhibit and thereby initiate, aggravate, or perpetuate a financially motivated exaggeration of symptoms."

Equally damaging to patients are representatives of insurance carriers who prematurely close claims or badger patients to settle before maximum medical improvement has been reached. Fortunately, the majorty of patients suffering "whiplash" injuries recover in a timely manner with little or no impairment when appropriate chiropractic management has been implemented.

Cervical Strain

The most common form of neck injury is cervical strain. Muscle strain occurs with overstretching or overuse. Traumatic cervical strain can be caused by a fall, a direct blow to the head, or as a part of "whiplash" injury. Traumatic cervical strain occurs when a sudden, unguarded movement stretches and tears muscle fibers (91). The resulting inflammation is the muscular component observed in "whiplash" injuries.

A mild cervical strain produces pain and spasm that lasts only a few days. Moderately severe strains exhibit trigger points characteristic of myofascial pain syndromes and chronic muscle strain. Treatment is directed to interruption of the pain-spasm cycle by ischemic compression, massage, and stretching exercises (Chapter 12).

Chronic muscle spasm also occurs with faulty posture that requires sustained eccentric contraction of the posterior neck muscles when the neck is flexed for prolonged periods of time. This sustained contraction produces traction at the site of muscle insertion, leading to pain and tenderness. The attachment of the neck extensor muscles is a common site of chronic muscle strain that causes the common "tension" headache (66). The muscles that attach to the occiput at the site of emergence and passage of the superior occipital nerve, produce irritation that refers pain across the top and side of the head to the frontal area (66). Sustained muscle contraction creates intramuscular pressure, which paradoxically shuts off the blood flow required for oxygenation and elimination of catabolites. The resulting pain-spasm-pain cycle is self-sustaining. Alternating contraction and relaxation is necessary for painless, nonfatiguing muscular activity. Sustained muscle contraction interferes with this normal cycle.

Some persons react to stress by hypertonicity of voluntary muscles (72). Triggering factors include anxiety, depression, and repressed hostility (92). Longer-lasting relief is achieved when treatment is directed at both the "muscle" tension and the underlying psychological trigger mechanism.

Sustained muscle contraction can be the result of muscle splinting of hypermobile joints, secondary to adjacent articular fixation. These cases respond readily to manipulation of the fixed joint determined by motion palpation. Routine, repeated, nonspecific manipulation, which often affects hypermobile joints rather than adjacent fixed joints, should be avoided since it brings no lasting benefit. In cases without joint fixation, therapy directed to the muscle spasm (rather than manipulation of the hypermobile joint) is more lasting (Chapter 12).

Torticollis

Torticollis is a rotational deformity of the cervical spine. The most commonly seen form of torticollis (wryneck) is produced by spasm in the sternocleidomastoid following an upper respiratory infection or exposure to a cold draft (91). The patient holds the head to one side in an attempt to relax the muscle. Bilateral involvement is seen occasionally, with almost total restriction of neck motion. Treatment consists of moist heat, ultrasound, massage, and ischemic compression. The condition typically resolves in 2 to 3 days. It should be differentiated from a rotary subluxation fixation (46, 47, 66, 78) by motion palpation (55). Rotary subluxation fixation is readily amenable to manipulation.

Congenital torticollis is observed at birth, with unilateral tightness of the sternocleidomastoid muscle. Frequently a fibrous tumor is found within the muscle. Spasmodic torticollis is characterized by spontaneous intermittent or persistent muscle contractions producing the typical wryneck deformity (91). The condition is resistant to conservative therapy, requiring surgical nerve section (91).

Cervical Sprain

Sprain, by definition, is injury of ligamentous structures. A severe injury with ligamentous tears may produce partial or complete loss of stability. These cases should be referred for surgical evaluation. Ligamentous soft-tissue injuries may encompass discs and articular capsules as well as the supporting ligaments of the articulations. By far the most common cause of cervical sprain is "whiplash" injury. Severe blows to the head with the head in flexion, extension, or lateral flexion may cause tearing of the cervical ligamentous and capsular structures.

The extent of the cervical injuries produced by falls depends upon the direction and amount of force applied to the neck. Forward falls usually produce hyperextension of the neck, causing tearing of the anterior longitudinal ligament. If the head is forced to one side, tears and traction injuries may occur on the side that makes contact with the ground. If the head is forced forward, traction injuries of the posterior ligaments can occur. Forceful pulls or thrusts on the arms may cause a snapping of the neck, with resulting sprain of the cervical ligamentous structures. Sports injuries, such as occur in football and diving, are common causes of cervical sprain (49).

Ligamentous sprain produces an inflammatory reaction that can heal with scar tissue that is less elastic and less functional if inflammation persists. Immobilization of joints or functional inactivity results in stasis of circulation and is a common cause of posttraumatic joint stiffness (49). Because of the meager blood supply to ligamentous and capsular structures, it is important to avoid complete immobilization of sprained joints. A small amount of movement in injured joints (rather than complete immobilization) reduces the inflammation by dispersing the products of tissue breakdown from the site of injury, reducing the risk of fibrous arthrosis (93). The patient should be encouraged to move the joints within the normal range of movement while avoiding excess movement.

It is essential that joint fixation in articulations adjacent to sprained joints be manipulated or mobilized. This allows the sprained joints to heal in an optimal length of time, avoiding a compensatory mechanism that results from an attempt by the sprained joints to take over the function of the fixed areas of the neck (49). Radiographic evidence of ligamentous sprain as well as joint fixation can be determined by flexion-extension studies (Chapter 6).

Isometric neck exercises can be introduced within 2 weeks of injury, and patients encouraged to return to their normal work and recreational activities as soon as possible. Repair of injured capsular and ligamentous tissue is slow, taking up to 6 to 8 weeks (49). During this period, the patient must be careful to avoid overstretching the damaged ligaments, without restricting the joints from normal range of motion.

Degenerative Joint Disease in the Cervical Spine

Degenerative changes occur in the cervical spine in the intervertebral discs (spondylosis) and the posterior zygapophyseal joints (cervical arthrosis). In addition, the paired joints of Luschka more commonly exhibit marked degeneration (8, 21, 47).

The stages of degeneration in the lower cervical spine follow a similar pattern to that of the lumbar re-

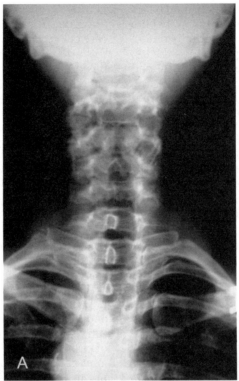

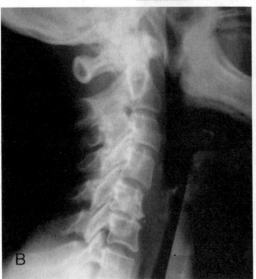

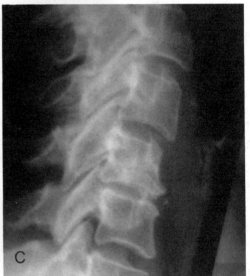

Figure 10.36. Degenerative changes of the cervical spine. **A,** AP Cervical. Note the spurs projecting from the apophyseal joints and C6 uncinate process. **B,** Neutral lateral. Disc space narrowing associated with endplate spondylophytes and an intercalary bone. **C,** Close-up of **B**. The lucency through C5 is due to unicinate arthrosis.

gion (94) (Chapter 8). Disc degeneration between C2 and C7 with loss of disc thickness progresses from a stage of dysfunction to one of instability. In the early stages, the contact between uncinate processes of the vertebral body below and the beveled lower edge of the vertebra above increases. As this process proceeds, instability increases, with horizontal fissures extending transversely inward, ultimately breaking through to meet, often dividing the cervical disc in two.

Stability returns as the degeneration reaches a further stage. With further degeneration and destruction of the intervertebral disc, there is a much closer approximation of the vertebrae. The uncinate processes are no longer vertically directed with a sharp upper margin. Instead, the uncus is flared out laterally in opposition, with similarly horizontally oriented changes in shape and extent of the corresponding lower edge of the vertebra above. The articular cartilage degenerates and becomes narrower (8). These changes are

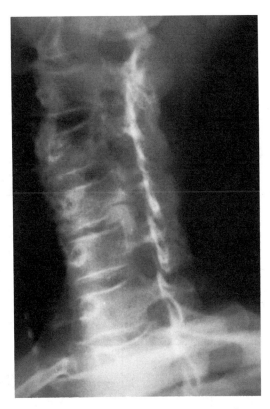

Figure 10.37. Foraminal osteophyte encroachment.

clearly recognizable in the AP radiographs as pointed and frequently spur-like or hump-like bony protuberances (Fig. 10.36).

Because the uncinate processes approximate the transverse processes of the superior vertebrae with progressive disc thinning, the lateral radiograph often reveals a horizontal lucency superimposed over the vertebral body. This lucency is called a "mock" effect because it simulates a fracture. It is imperative to recognize this lucency as the result of severe uncovertebral arthrosis and not to erroneously call it a fracture.

During these stages of degeneration, the uncinate process changes from a vertical ridge with a clearly defined superior margin to an oblique shelf with a flattened superior surface. At the same time, a fissure extends transversely from one side of the intervertebral region to the other (8). Hall (8) states that "during these changes of the disc and the Luschka joint, the joint between the bodies of the vertebrae is altered from a fibrocartilaginous amphiarthrosis, to a ball and socket shaped diarthrosis." This is seen as early as the third decade (47).

The most common segments to be affected by degenerative changes are the C5–6 and C6–7, which, like the lower lumbar segments, are particularly mobile and in the area of maximal lordosis. Salter (94) states that "in the cervical spine there is little room in the intervertebral foramen for exit of the nerve roots; consequently subluxation and osteophytic formation in

the posterior facet joints readily compress these roots, particularly after any injury with its soft tissue swelling." Foraminal osteophytic encroachment from the anterior is due to uncinate process hypertrophy, while encroachment from the posterior is due to zygapophyseal arthrosis (Fig. 10.37).

Cervical Disc Herniation

Disc herniation is much less common in the cervical spine than in the lumbar spine; however, it may occur as a dramatic event in the degenerative process for the same reasons and in the same manner as in the lumbar region (Chapter 8). The more common type of herniation is posterolateral, and frequently it compresses a nerve root. Relatively uncommon and more serious is central herniation that compresses the spinal cord (94).

Cervical Radiculopathy

Cervical radiculopathy is defined as pain in the distribution of a specific cervical nerve root as a result of compressive pathology, whether from disc herniation, spur formation, or hypermobility states (95). Kelsey et al. (96) found a strong predilection for disc herniation among individuals who lift heavy objects, in cigarette smokers, and in divers, with a borderline propensity among those who operate vibrating equipment or ride in cars for prolonged periods. Cervical disc herniation is most common at C5–6, followed by C6–7, C4–5, C3–4, and C7–T1 (50, 97, 98).

Most persons over the age of 60 exhibit evidence of degenerative disc disease and degenerative joint disease in the cervical spine visualized on radiographs (94). Dillin (95) reports that 82% of patients over 55 show evidence of disc degeneration, with little correlation between symptomatic and asymptomatic groups and structural change on radiographic examination. Many of these patients remain asymptomatic, while others exhibit only mild stiffness of the neck. With cervical nerve-root encroachment, however, a variety of symptoms can appear, including pain in the neck and shoulders as well as pain down the arm in the distribution of the involved nerve root (brachialgia). The radicular pain may be accompanied by pain into the upper anterior and posterior chest and paresthesia in the form of numbness or tingling.

The onset of symptoms is often gradual, but can be acute, particularly when an injury is added to the preexisting degenerative changes (94). The pain is accentuated by movement of the neck and by coughing, sneezing, and straining. The discomfort is severe at night and interferes with sleep, with the patient seeking relief by sleeping in the upright position. Movement of the head, especially toward the side of pain, increases the discomfort.

Clinically, the findings include marked muscle spasm and limitation of active and passive movement, particularly toward the side of the lesion. Cervical lordosis is reduced, and localized tenderness is felt over the involved disc space slightly to one side of the mid-

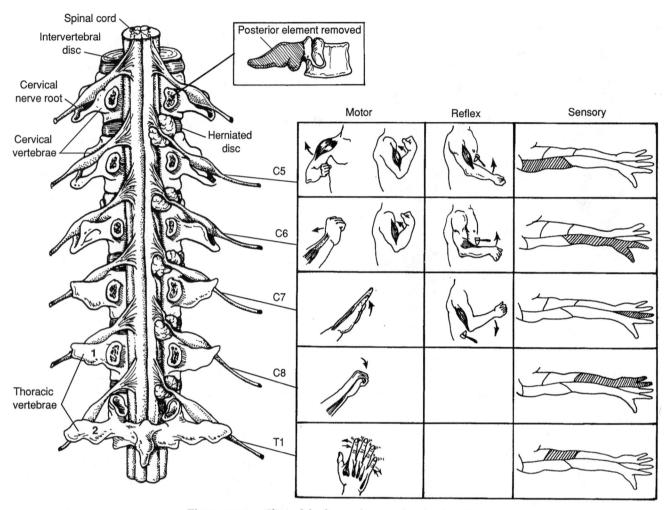

Figure 10.38. Clinical findings of cervical radiculopathy.

line (91). Often, marked relief of radicular pain is obtained by abduction of the affected shoulder (shoulder abduction test) (50). Distraction of the head or neck brings a decrease or relief of pain when pressure on the nerve root is reduced (48). Foraminal compression can increase nerve-root pressure, and the test result is positive when pain radiates into the arm or the side to which the head is laterally flexed and compressed (50).

Identification of the symptomatic level is based on correlation of clinical findings (Fig. 10.38) with MRI or CT scans. Diminished biceps reflex and diminished skin sensation in the thumb and index finger with weakness of the deltoid and biceps muscles is indicative of compression of the sixth cervical nerve root from either osteophyte or disc herniation at the C5–6 level.

Compression of the seventh cervical nerve root from either osteophytes or disc herniation at the C6-C7 level produces a diminished triceps reflex, diminished skin sensation in the index and middle finger, and weakness of the triceps muscle.

Sensory and motor deficits with asymmetric reflexes should be referred for a neurological evaluation.

Compression of the spinal cord from a central disc herniation with lower extremity symptoms requires immediate referral for surgical evaluation. It is important to differentiate compression neuropathies of the upper extremity from other conditions that can produce shoulder and arm pain. More commonly seen are myofascial pain syndromes with persistent trigger points that refer pain into the upper extremity (Chapter 12). The nebulous thoracic outlet syndrome is often implicated with a variety of presentations. EMG and nerve conduction velocity tests are necessary to identify entrapment syndromes such as carpal tunnel syndrome. Tumors, inflammatory conditions, toxic and allergic conditions, in addition to visceral and vascular lesions must be differentiated.

Conservative management of cervical radiculopathy is effective for the majority of patients in the absence of advancing neurological and motor deficits. Pain relief is afforded by local rest provided by a cervical collar (94). Gentle manipulation may prove beneficial (60, 64) as does intermittent cervical traction (94). Prompt referral for decompression is necessary in cases with severe pain, advancing sensory or motor deficits, and lower extremity symptoms (94).

Thoracic Outlet Syndrome

Thoracic outlet syndrome is a term coined by Rob and Standeven (99) in 1958 to describe problems of the shoulder girdle, caused by compression of the neurovascular bundle. It is just as nebulous a term as the popular "whiplash" syndrome and refers to a symptom complex caused by a variety of etiological factors. Liebenson (100) states that the symptoms are largely caused by the brachial plexus being compressed or irritated and that the vascular component has been largely overrated. Grieve notes that, in the biomechanical sense, the cervicodorsal region of the spine is an area where the most mobile region of the vertebral column is physically interdependent with a region of major vascular and neurological "traffic" and a transitional area that is developmentally restless, with anomalies of skeletal and soft tissue common (47).

Thoracic outlet syndrome should not be considered a diagnosis of exclusion. The key to diagnosing thoracic outlet syndrome is recreation of the patient's symptoms by careful testing and positioning of the involved arm (100). Turek (91) warns that multiple factors may be operative, with compression within the costoclavicular space generally common to all. He further warns that all inciting and contributing factors must be clearly defined before a definite diagnosis can be established.

A greater incidence of thoracic outlet syndrome has been noted in middle-aged women, particularly those with esthenic builds and poorly developed axial and shoulder girdle muscles (101). Other predisposing factors include vigorous occupations and weight lifting that result in increased muscle build (101). Undue tightness of the scalene muscles and tight pectoral muscles that become chronically contracted due to the weight of heavy breasts in some women have been suggested as an etiological factor by Phillips and Grieve (102). A higher incidence has also been found in cash register operators, typists, packers, and assembly line workers (103), due to the awkward work posture and repetitive motion that produces continuous muscle tension.

Congenital factors including cervical ribs, bifid clavicles, elongated transverse processes at C7, bony protuberances of the first rib, and abnormal insertion of the scalenus medius on the first rib have also been implicated (104). Traumatic causes of thoracic outlet syndromes include clavicular fracture and subacromial dislocation of the humeral head. Occasionally trauma to the upper thorax may unduly stretch a portion of the brachial plexus and/or thrombose the artery or vein. Arteriosclerosis in older individuals (fifth to sixth decades) may produce ischemic symptoms with minimal compression (104).

Commonly seen in chiropractic practice are patients with a history of trauma leading to hypertonicity and trigger points in the scalene muscles, cervical motion segment fixation, and fixation of the first ribs, all of which produces symptoms associated with thoracic outlet syndrome. Lewit (105) noted that manual functional diagnosis frequently reveals movement restriction of the cervicothoracic spine and first ribs with concomitant muscle spasm in patients without any structural abnormalities who exhibit symptoms associated with thoracic outlet syndrome.

The most common symptoms of thoracic outlet syndrome are numbness and tingling of the fingers and, less frequently, the forearms and hands. Aching pain with weakness and fatigue of the arm is also common. The symptoms are often bilateral. The pain radiates from the neck and shoulder down the arm, forearm, hand, and fingers. Paresthesia is most often perceived in the C8 and T1 distribution, distally to the fourth and fifth fingers. Numbness, most frequently involving the fingers and less frequently the hands and forearm, may be noted (104). Ischemic symptoms include numbness, coldness, weakness, and discoloration (104). Patients may also report dropping objects from the hand (79). Headaches have been reported as presenting symptoms of thoracic outlet syndrome (105, 106). Edema of the hand occurs occasionally, over the dorsum of the hand and base of the four fingers (79), especially on awakening in the morning.

A thorough clinical examination is necessary to identify the site of neurovascular compression. Motion palpation reveals fixations of the cervical and thoracic spine and ribs, which readily respond to manipulation (100, 102). The autonomic nerve supply to the upper limb is derived from segments as far caudally as T8 (102), making fixation of the thoracic vertebral motion segments responsible for some shoulder, arm, and hand symptoms (Chapter 9). Rarely are more than one or two treatments necessary when the offending segment is mobilized, relieving the compressive segments and the concomitant edema in cases where joint fixation is the perpetuating factor.

Radiographs of the cervical spine and upper thoracic region will readily identify anomalous cervical ribs and elongated transverse processes, as well as malalignment of clavicular fractures, or bony exostoses. It is important to rule out apical lung tumors as well as inflammatory or other neoplastic disease. Phillips and Grieve (102) note that arthritis of the synovial joints of the cervical spine and radiological evidence of disc degeneration are age-related findings and need not diminish the credibility of a diagnosis of thoracic outlet compression.

The cervical rib is a supernumerary rib that arises from the seventh and rarely the sixth or fifth cervical vertebrae (Fig. 10.39). It is frequently bilateral (91), and may be palpable as a bony prominence at the base of the neck. Failure to palpate the rib does not rule out cervical rib involvement, since a fibrous band may be the offender (91). A cervical rib is not necessarily implicated as the cause of thoracic outlet syndrome, since only 5–10% of patients with a cervical rib are symptomatic (100).

Symptoms caused by a cervical rib are accentuated by downward displacement of the shoulder girdle

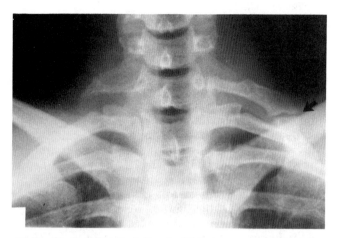

Figure 10.39. Cervical ribs. **A,** AP lower cervical. There is a complete cervical rib present at C7 on the right side. An attenuated cervical rib is present at C7 on the left side. **B,** Lower cervical. There is a cervical rib with an accessory articulation (*arrow*). A small cervical rib is also noted on the opposite side. (From Yochum TR, Rowe LJ: *Essentials of Skeletal Radiology.* Baltimore, Williams & Wilkins, 1987, p 111.)

when fatigued or when carrying a heavy object (91). A cervical rib narrows the thoracic outlet and can compress both the brachial plexus and the subclavian artery between the clavicle and the rib during elevation and retraction (94) of the arm (hyperabduction syndrome). A positive Wright's test result (100), indicated by a loss of radial pulse and development of neurological symptoms on hyperabduction of the arm to 180°, can be produced by neurovascular compression between the clavicle and cervical, or first rib, or by pressure on the axillary artery and veins under the pectoralis minor tendon and coracoid process (100).

Mild to moderate cases of cervical rib syndrome can be treated conservatively. According to Turek (91), elevation of the shoulder girdle releases tension on the brachial plexus and the axillary artery. He recommends exercises designed to increase the tone of the trapezius and levator scapulae muscles, while avoiding activities requiring lifting. An armrest to support the shoulder girdle in an elevated position can also prove helpful. If symptoms are incapacitating and fail to respond to conservative therapy, then surgical removal of the rib is recommended (91).

The scalene muscles without a cervical rib can be responsible for pressure on the neurovascular bundle, with consequent clinical symptoms (104). The interscalene triangle, a normally occurring space between the anterior scalene anteriorly and the scalenus medius posteriorly, with the first rib forming the inferior border of the triangle, permits passage of the brachial plexus and the subclavian artery. A cervical rib or structural variation with a more posterior attachment of the scalenus anterior to the first rib demands greater angulation from the subclavian artery so that it can clear the rib (104). A conjoined insertion of the scalenus medius and scalenus anterior can further compromise the subclavian artery and lower trunk of the plexus. The scalene muscles vary considerably in both their insertion into the first rib and the arrangement of their fibers (104).

Travell and Simons (79) note that when trigger point activity in the scalenus anterior or medius elevates the first rib, fibers of the lower trunk must angulate more sharply over the rib. This angulation also wedges the subclavian artery more tightly against the lower trunk. While the modified Adson maneuver tests the susceptibility of the neurovascular bundle to compression, by tensing the anterior scalene and elevating the first rib when the neck is extended and the face rotated to the unaffected side, identification of the muscles involved is achieved by palpating for trigger points. Specific trigger-point compression, stretching exercises, and improved posture and body mechanics provides lasting relief (79) (Chapter 12). Thoracic outlet syndrome produced by scalene muscle involvement is a common sequelae of "whiplash injuries."

Entrapment of the axillary arteries and brachial plexus can occur where they pass beneath the coracoid process, posterior to the pectoralis minor and between the clavicle and the first rib. When the arm is abducted and externally rotated at the shoulder (79), the artery, vein, and nerves are bent and stretched around the pectoralis minor muscle close to its attachment and are likely to be compressed if the muscle is firm and tautened by trigger points. Rather than relying on the hyperabduction test (Wright's maneuver), which produces a diminished radial pulse in 83% of normal individuals (91, 102), palpation for trigger points gives a more accurate indication of involvement of this muscle.

Simons and Travell (79) note that one rarely finds active trigger points in the pectoralis minor without active trigger points in the pectoralis major. The anterior deltoid, sternocleidomastoid, and sternalis muscle are also commonly involved (79). In addition to ischemic compression of the trigger points, stretching of the involved muscles prevents recurrence of the syndrome (79).

Pressure between the clavicle and first rib (costoclavicular syndrome (91)) can be produced by holding the shoulders downward and backward. This exaggerated military posture can produce obliteration of the radial pulse when the position is held with deep inspiration (Eden's test (51)), as does longitudinal traction on the arms (102). Like other neurovascular compression tests, an exaggerated military position causes a dampening of the pulse in many normal people, and in the absence of reproducible symptoms is meaningless.

Costoclavicular syndrome can be produced by carrying heavy backpacks and by trigger points in the subclavicular muscle. These trigger points refer pain into the upper extremity on the same side. The pain travels down the front of the arm and along the radial side of the forearm. It frequently skips the elbow and wrist but affects the radial half of the hand, the dorsal and volar aspects of the thumb, index, and middle fingers. Inactivation of the trigger points brings prompt relief. Susceptible individuals can gain relief when carrying backpacks by insuring that the weight is carried on the pelvic girdle rather than the shoulders.

Phillips and Grieve (102) suggest that thoracic outlet "syndrome" might well be chased out of the literature because it initiates a wild goose chase for a simple site of impingement. It is not a definitive diagnosis with a precise diagnosis dependent on a comprehensive examination and identification of those structures from which symptoms can arise.

Complicating the differentiation is the possibility that the patient's symptoms are caused by lesions other than those of the shoulder or upper spine. Complex postural distortion may ultimately lead to clavicular displacement, narrowing the thoracic outlet (100). Phillips and Grieve (102) implicate faulty posture with increased upper dorsal lordosis, rounded shoulders, and the head pushed forward lifting the upper ribs forward and moving the clavicle caudally to impinge the neurovascular centers. They conclude that the relief afforded patients with upper limb symptoms by scalene muscle release, mobilization of spinal segments, pectoral stretching, and shoulder mobilization lays to rest the idea that trespass or impingement is the essential lesion in thoracic outlet syndrome.

Conservative chiropractic management of thoracic outlet syndrome must be as comprehensive and complete as this complex syndrome warrants. Liebenson (100) concludes that "with the knowledge we have today, its management by conservative procedure is universally accepted."

Double Crush Syndrome

While chiropractors traditionally place emphasis on the "special lesion" at the site of nerve entrapment, it must be remembered that nerve fibers compressed at one level become especially susceptible to damage further distally (107). The coexistence of nerve entrapment can be any combination of: the cervical nerve root, the peripheral nerve in the thoracic outlet, the elbow tunnel, or the carpal tunnel (108). Physiologically, damage to the nerve proximally can reduce the "metabolic safety margins" of the nerve axon to compressive insult distally (109).

Upton and McComas (109) found a high incidence (70%) of concurrent cervical/thoracic nerve root entrapment with electrodiagnostically proven neuropathy (either carpal tunnel syndrome or ulnar neuropathy). They considered the following condition as evidence of cervical/thoracic root lesions: (a) radiological demonstration of cervical spondylosis or other vertebral abnormalities; (b) complaints of pain and stiffness of the neck; (c) previous history of neck injury commonly of the hyperextension "whiplash" type as a result of rear-end motor vehicle accidents; (d) clinical evidence of sensory abnormalities corresponding to dermatomes, rather than peripheral nerve distribution; or (e) EMG evidence of denervation of peripheral nerves supplied by the related nerve roots (i.e., median, ulnar, etc.).

While a double crush syndrome need not be due to a singular traumatic incident (110), a whiplash injury to the neck when the victim firmly grasps the steering wheel to "brace for the impact" can produce a "crush-crush" mechanism (108).

A proximal axonal lesion may render the distal aspect of the neuron more susceptible or vulnerable to subsequent pressure injury from frank or microtraumatic incidents. The high incidence of carpal tunnel syndrome produced by industrial situations with concurrent nerve root compromise is significant (108).

The pathophysiology of the double crush syndrome is thought to be due to interruption of axoplasmic flow from sufficient collector damage producing neuronal impairment. Interruption of trophic substances secreted within the neuron perikaryon, which are transported along the axon, produces a loss of functional integrity of the axon, rendering it susceptible to distal focal insults that then cause denervation.

Patients more commonly present to chiropractors with cervical complaints, with secondary complaints of numbness or pain in the median or ulnar distribution of the hand. The extremity symptoms are frequently more prominent at night. The onset of neck pain may be insidious or related to a specific traumatic event. Questioning will often reveal repetitive insult to the upper extremity or pectoral girdle from occupational or recreational activity (108).

Examination of the cervical spine (Chapter 5), including neurovascular compression tests and radiographic evaluation of the cervical spine, helps to determine the location of neurological insult, but differential diagnosis frequently depends on EMG studies, which are always indicated when significant neurological deficit is found.

Surgical intervention can be prevented in those cases when the proximal neurological involvement is due to a manipulable lesion in the cervical, upper thoracic, or costovertebral articulation. A two-week trial of chiropractic manipulation is recommended for patients with suspected double crush syndrome, since significant reduction of the central spinal lesion has been demonstrated to reduce the necessity for surgical intervention in those patients whose proximal neuropathy is caused by restricted joint motion (108).

Cervicogenic Headache

It is widely recognized by practitioners of spinal manipulative therapy that headaches arising from functionally blocked cervical articulations respond favorably to manipulation (111–123). Cervicogenic headaches can also occur from muscle hypertonicity when there is normal mobility or hypermobility, in which case massage and ischemic compression are appropriate therapies.

As with other biomechanical lesions of the spine, it is essential to assess the movement patterns of the cervical spine as well as the soft-tissue pathology when

Table 10.5 Differential Diagnosis of Headaches

	Migraine, Classic	Migraine, Common	Migraine Variants	Cluster Headache	Vasculitis	Muscle Contraction (Tension)	Posttraumatic	Fibromyalgia
Location	Unilateral, preceded by focal aura	Unilateral, may switch sides	Variable	Orbital/retroorbital	Focal or unilateral	Occipitofrontal, frontotemporal, or holocranial, neck	Dull or throbbing	Occipital or occipito-temporal, neck and shoulder region
Pain character	Throbbing, stabbing, vise-like	Throbbing, stabbing, vise-like	Throbbing or none	Excruciating, may be stabbing	Throbbing	Dull, nonthrobbing, stiff muscles	Dull or throbbing	Superficial tenderness
Frequency	Random or periodic	Random or periodic	Random or periodic	Daily for weeks or months, often same time of day			Daily or nearly daily	
Duration	Hours to 1–2 days	Hours to days	Hours to days	Minutes to hours		Few to several hours	Often constant dull pain with episodic superimposed throbbing	Days to weeks
Temporal factors	May see increased tendency at ovulation or menses, rarely awakens			Often awakens from sleep		May be relieved with rest/sleep		
Precipitating factors	Change in attitude, weather change, fatigue, bright light, missed meals, possible food triggers, estrogens			Alcohol, smoking	Cocaine, systematic vasculitis such as lupus, et al. amphetamines	Stress, emotional conflict, depression	Head trauma or cervical strain	Stress
Associated symptoms	Aura of odor, numbness, clumsiness of extremity, aphasia or visceral disturbances lasting usually 20–30 minutes, followed by severe pain, nausea, vomiting	Nausea, vomiting, photophobia, sonophobia, dizziness, autonomic instability	Neurologic deficits lasting longer than aura would, may or may not be permanent, may be confused		Photophobia, focal neurologic deficits—transient or permanent	Neck or scalp tightness	Reduced attention/concentration, mood swings, memory difficulties, dizziness, tinnitus, irritability	Normal ESR, fatigue, muscle aching, stiffness
Treatment	Vasoconstrictors, analgesics, antinauseants, prophylaxis with tricyclic antidepressants, β-blockers, calcium, ice			Ergots, oxygen; prevention with methyseride, lithium, Tegretol, steroids		Manipulation, trigger point therapy, physical therapy, massage, ice, biofeedback, minor analgesics, nonsteroidal antiinflammatory agents, muscle relaxants, antidepressants	Manipulation, trigger point therapy, physical therapy, nonsteroidal antiinflammatory agents, tricyclic antidepressants	Manipulation, trigger point therapy, heat, massage, nonsteroidal anti-inflammatory agents, tricyclic antidepressants
Other	Calcium channel blockers or tricyclic antidepressants, may be hereditary, female predominance, often prone to motion sickness, hysterectomy does not cure			90% affected are male		May have features of vascular h/a—throbbing pain, may be designated tension-vascular (see text)	See text	See Chapter 11

*Courtesy of Christina Peterson, M.D. 1989.

Rheumatic	Psychogenic	Giant Cell Arteritis	Sinus	Temporomandibular Joint (TMJ)	Structural Tumor	Structural Aneurysm	Hypertension	Pseudotumor Cerebri	Miscellaneous 1) Allergy 2) Hangover 3) Eyestrain
Occipital, neck shoulder girdle	"All over"	Temporal or other cranial	Nasal region		Diffuse or local		Occipital, frontal, or vertex		1) Vertex or hatband 2) Migraine-like 3) Frontal
Superficial tenderness	Constant, "just an ache," or may be described in vivid terms	Boring, burning, or jabbing pain, superficial tenderness Intermittent over several months	Gnawing or pressure pain	Nonthrobbing	Gradual, progressive worsening Daily	Throbbing or sudden, severe, excruciating pain	Generalized, holocranial, or "hatband" distribution		
	"All the time"								1) 2–3 hours
Prevents sleep			Increases as day goes on		Worse in morning or upon reclining, may awaken at night		May Awaken 4–6 am, improves as day goes on, worse reclining	Worse in AM, improves as day goes on, worse reclining	
Cold, damp weather			Infection, nasal polyps, deviated septum				BP >200 systolic >110 diastolic	Tetracycline, steroids, vitamin A deficiency or excess, obesity	1) Seasonal allergies 2) Alcohol 3) Use of eyes
Low-grade fever, rheumatoid arthritis features, raised ESR	Lack of response to medication, lack of insight into feelings	May see stroke symptoms, jaw claudication, fever, weight loss, night sweats, transient visual loss, tender at temples	Fever, pain when chewing	TMJ crepitus or "click" dental malocclusion, stress, jaw clenching, bruxism	Vomiting, focal neurologic deficits, personality change, dysequilibrium	May have double vision, rigid neck, declining level of consciousness		Visual disturbance	1) Nasal congestion, watery eyes
Heat, massage, nonsteroidal antiinflammatory agents	Psychotherapy, avoid narcotic	Steroids	Antibiotics, surgical draining	Manipulation, trigger point therapy, minor analgesics, nonsteroidal antiinflammatory agents, relaxation training, biofeedback, dental or oral surgery	Surgery or radiation	Intensive care, support, cerebroselective channel blockers, surgery, analgesics	Antihypertensive agents, upright position	Acetazolamide, steroids, serial lumbar punctures	1) Antihistamine, desensitization 2) Fluids, fructose, minor analgesics 3) Correct vision
	History of abuse is often present, personal or family history of alcoholism or depression	Age >60, elevated ESR, anemia	Rare, often overdiagnosed	Infrequent cause of headaches					1) Food allergies very rarely cause headaches 2) Rare cause of headaches

treating cervicogenic headaches. The biomechanical diagnosis is based on movement evaluation determined by motion palpation, as well as flexion-extension and lateral bending radiographs.

An accurate history and clinical examination are necessary to obtain a pathological classification and differential diagnosis (Table 10.5). Vernon (111) classifies vertebrogenic headaches as muscle contraction, migraines, and mixed. Barbuto (121) stresses the multifaceted etiologies of head pain and the interaction involving somatic, neurogenic, vascular, and autonomic components.

While vertebrogenic headaches often disappear dramatically after manipulation of the upper cervical spine, it must be realized that this may be palliative therapy only and no more than a mechanical aspirin. To prevent recurrences, evaluation of the factors causing overstressing of these joints is necessary (122). They may include occupational factors such as prolonged, forward bending (dentists), static loading of the neck and upper back (typists, CRT operators, and assembly-line workers), and working with the arms outstretched or raised overhead (hairdressers and carpenters).

Triggering factors may include anxiety, depression, hostility, poor posture, occlusal problems, and ocular disorders (123). Functional disturbance can arise from chronic occupational overuse syndromes from static muscle loading, degenerative and traumatic joint instability, myofascial hypertonicity from chronic postural faults, congenital anomalies, and rheumatoid arthritis (121). Posttraumatic headache is a common finding with "whiplash" syndrome and other neck injuries and must be thoroughly evaluated.

The differential diagnosis of benign headaches should only begin after ruling out more threatening conditions including intracranial disorders, neoplasm, infections, and ocular disorders (Table 10.5). Barbuto (121) lists the following red-light warnings of organic disease:

1. Episodic fainting in relation to headache;
2. Abrupt onset of a severe headache for the first time;
3. Neurological abnormalities associated with headache;
4. Elevation in body temperature associated with headache;
5. Onset of headache after age 50;
6. Headaches associated with an increase in pressure (coughing, bending, valsalva, coitus);
7. History of recent blood pressure elevation;
8. Personality change;
9. Headache following history of head trauma;
10. Disturbance of pulse rate and respiration;
11. Constant sensory disturbances;
12. Onset of visual field defects.

Prompt referral for neurological evaluation is paramount in cases where red-light warnings suggest organic disease or an intracranial etiology. Cailliet (87)

warns that headaches that persist and do not respond to conservative measures or that elicit unusual symptoms and/or findings should be referred for thorough neurologic consultation. The majority of chronic headaches encountered in chiropractic practice are resolved using clinical methods rather than laboratory procedures. While there is substantial support in the clinical literature that chiropractic management of cervicogenic headaches is the treatment of choice, the role of manipulation is largely undervalued and frequently sought as a last resort, the patient having been unresponsive to all previous forms of treatment.

Muscle Tension Headaches

To successfully treat muscle tension headaches, it is necessary to determine if the muscle hypertonicity is primary or secondary to joint hypermobility or joint fixation (115). Primary muscle hypertonicity is frequently caused by acute, traumatic muscle strain or microtraumatic or chronic postural strain. The most common cause of headaches resulting from acute muscle strain is described under "whiplash" injuries.

Traumatic injuries to the cervical spine cause spasm, with inflammation of the paraspinal muscles as well as irritation of the myofascial connections to the cranial periosteum. The nerve roots can be entrapped with these irritated tissues (87). Chronic postural strain aggravated by occupational stress frequently occurs when individuals assume slumped posture with "poked" head and cervical hypolordosis. Frequently the postural muscles are statically loaded and under continuous eccentric contraction while the arms are used in a repetitive manner. These postures are assumed daily by office and assembly-line workers.

The chronic irritation of the tendinous periosteal junctions produces low-level chronic foci of tenderness and local occipital or nuchal and suboccipital pain (111). The chronically stretched muscles also respond with low-level hypertonicity and trigger points in the region of the muscle spindles (myofascial pain syndromes) (Chapter 12). These trigger points in cervical muscles can refer pain in a cephalad direction following constant, muscle-specific patterns. The resulting headache may be due to the pain referred from the trigger points or from secondary entrapment of accompanying neurovascular structures. Appropriate trigger-point release by ischemic compression and specific muscle stretching is described in Chapter 12. Postural retraining and modification of the workplace are often necessary to prevent reccurrence.

Muscle spasm and splinting secondary to joint hypermobility occur with the arthrokinetic reflex (124). The intraarticular nociceptors, when irritated by mechanical or chemical stimuli produced by local joint pain, initiate arthrogenic muscle spasm with referred pain, as a consequence of activation of convergent neurons (125). This same athrokinetic reflex can also be triggered by joint fixation or hypomobility.

The role played by joint dysfunction in the production of headaches is widely underestimated, and the role of manipulation greatly undervalued in the relief of these headaches. Motion palpation is used to determine movement restriction of fixed vertebrae (Chapter 6). Lewit (115) notes that the majority of cases of movement restriction (blockage) occur between the occiput and atlas. Jirout (126) found headaches in 90% of individuals with C2-C3 dysfunction, and Bogduk (127) reported upper cervical hypomobility as the major cause of headache previously termed "muscle contraction type."

Jull (128) concludes that the incidence of cervical involvement in benign headaches is underestimated. He found joint hypomobility in 96 headache patients, with the incidence at C0-C1 and C1-C3 slightly higher than that at C1-C2. He notes a rapid decrease in the incidence of comparable joint signs below C3-4.

Edeling (129) found unrecognized cervical headaches that were only diagnosed in retrospect when they responded to mobilization, having been unresponsive to all previous treatments, which were appropriate to other diagnoses. Jull (128) reported that in 55% of the population studied, those who suffered from headaches exhibited a greater incidence of upper cervical joint stiffness than the asymptomatic group.

Vascular headaches (migraine) of vertebrogenic origin can occur through several mechanisms. Osteophytes on the facet joints and uncovertebral joints can encroach upon the vertebral artery, vertebral nerve, and sympathetic plexus. Joint fixation or hypermobility in posttraumatic states can lead to irritation of both the sympathetic plexus and superior cervical ganglion (49). Vernon (111) postulates that disturbed somatoautonomic reflexes can be responsible for disordered cerebrovascular tone. Studies supporting manipulative therapy for the treatment of migraines have not been exhaustive, but Parker, Topling, and Pryor (130) noted a success rate for manual therapy in migraines to be 47% after 20 months.

Vernon (111) proposes a headache model based on severity, which interfaces with the vertebrogenic model (Table 10.5). He notes that a lower order of this mechanism is expressed by muscle contraction headache with a higher order of activation of the same mechanism producing an increase in severity expressed as the migraine phenomenon (111). He concludes the following three categories of headache sufferers:

1. Those in whom the vertebrogenic component is etiological. This group ideally will derive primary benefit from spinal manipulative therapy.
2. Those in whom the vertebrogenic component is secondary but synergistic. This group ideally could benefit from spinal manipulative therapy in conjunction with other therapeutic measures.
3. Those in whom there was a negligible vertebrogenic component and for whom manipulation would provide no benefit.

Vernon (111) reports a success rate of 75-90% in a typical treatment regime of spinal manipulation averaging 9 to 10 treatments for relief of benign headaches.

CONCLUSION

Mechanical lesions of the cervical spine have a profound effect because of the diversity and richness of cervical spine innervation. The arthrokinetic reflexes that underlie static and dynamic posture, when disturbed, may have an extensive reflex effect upon muscle tone in the neck, trunk, and limbs. The enormous variability of the vertebrobasilar vascular system makes it particularly vulnerable to mechanical aberrations, which can produce bizarre and widespread clinical features involving cranial and facial areas in addition to the trunk and all four limbs (47). Manipulation of cervical spine fixations normalizes disturbed function and may bring relief from a wide spectrum of pain syndromes and symptom complexes.

References

1. Hiviid H: Functional radiography of the cervical spine. *Ann Swiss Chiro Assoc* 3:36–65, 88–96, 1965.
2. Kapandji IA: *The Physiology of the Joints*, vol 3: *The Trunk and Vertebral Column*, ed 2. London, Churchill Livingstone, 1974, pp 174–176, 180–181, 184, 200.
3. White AA, Panjabi MM: *Clinical Biomechanics of the Spine.* Philadelphia, JB Lippincott, 1978, pp 65–66, 71–75, 82–85, 113–114, 123–166, 199.
4. Hohl M: Soft tissue injuries of the neck in automobile accidents: factors influencing prognosis. *J Bone Joint Surg* 56A:1675–1681, 1974.
5. Mealy K, Brennen H, Fenelon GCC: Early mobilization of acute whiplash injuries. *Br Med J* 8:656–657, 1986.
6. Fielding JW: Normal and selected abnormal motion of the cervical spine from the second cervical vertebra to the seventh cervical vertebra base on cineradiography. *J Bone Joint Surg* 46A(8): 1779–1782, 1964.
7. Sandoz R: A classification of locations subluxations and fixation of the cervical spine. *Ann Swiss Chiro Assoc* 6:217–276, 1976.
8. Hall MC: *Luschka's Joint.* Springfield, IL, Charles C Thomas, 1965, pp 5, 10, 43–46, 127.
9. Warwick W: *Gray's Anatomy*, ed 35. Philadelphia, WB Saunders, 1973, pp 234–236.
10. Berlin L: Unusual foramina, pseudoforamina and developmental defects of bone. *Am J Roentgentol Radiol Ther Nucl Med* 91:1089–1103, 1964.
11. Epstein BS: *The Spine: A Radiological Text and Atlas*, ed 4. Philadelphia, Lea & Febiger, 1976, pp 65–66, 157.
12. Fielding JW, Burstein AH, Frankel VH: The nuchal ligament. *Spine* 1:3–14, 1976.
13. Raynor RB: Congenital malformation of the base of the skull. In Baily RW: *The Cervical Spine.* Philadelphia, JB Lippincott, 1983, pp 147–155.
14. Henderson DJ: Radiographic Evaluation of the Upper Cervical Spine. In Vernon H: *Upper Cervical Syndrome Chiropractic Diagnosis and Treatment.* Baltimore, Wiliams & Wilkins, 1958, p 29.
15. Gatterman MI: Contraindications and complications of spinal manipulative therapy. *AJA J Chiro* 15:75–86, 1981.
16. George PE, Silverstein HT, Wallace H, Marshal M: Identification of the high risk pre-stroke patient. *ACA J* 15:26–28, 1981.
17. Steven AJ, Doppler JE: Sonography and neck rotation. *Manual Med* 1:49–53, 1984.
18. Henderson DJ, Cassidy JD: Vertebral artery syndrome. In Vernon H: *Upper Cervical Syndrome Chiropractic Diagnosis and Treatment.* Baltimore, Wiliams & Wilkins, 1988, p 204.

19. Hensinger RN: Congenital anomalies of the odontoid. In Baily RW: *The Cervical Spine.* Philadelphia, JB Lippincott, 1983, pp 164–173.

20. Pizzutillo PD: Klippel-Feil Syndrome. In Baily RW: *The Cervical Spine.* Philadelphia, JB Lippincott, 1983, pp 174–187.

21. Schmorl G, Junghanns H: *The Human Spine in Health and Disease,* ed 2. New York, Grune & Stratton, 1971, pp 58, 97, 200–203, 414.

22. Grice AS: Normal mechanics of the upper cervical spine. In Vernon H: *Upper Cervical Syndromes.* Baltimore, Williams & Wilkins, 1988, pp 86–87, 97.

23. Steele HH: Anatomical and mechanical consideration of the atlanto-axial articulations. *JBJ Surg* 50:1481, 1968.

24. Steindler A: *Kinesiology of the Human Body,* ed 4. Springfield, IL, Charles C Thomas, 1973, p 147.

25. Fielding JW: Cineroentgenography of the normal cervical spine. *JBJ Surg* 39A:1280–1288, 1957.

26. Jones MD: Cineradiographic studies of the normal cervical spine. *Calif Med* 93:293–296, 1960.

27. Lane G: Cervical spine: its movement and symptomatology. *J Clin Chiro Arch Ed* 1:128–145, 1971.

28. Shapiro R, Youngberg AS, Rathmor SLG: The differential diagnosis of traumatic lesions of the occipito-atlanto segment. *Radiol Clin North Am* II:505–526, 1973.

29. Worth DR, Selvick G: Movements of the craniovertebral joints. In Grieve GP: *Modern Manual Therapy of the Vertebral Column.* New York, Churchill Livingstone, 1986, p 54.

30. Jirout J: Rotational synkinesis of occiput and atlas on lateral inclination. *Neuroradiology* 21:1–4, 1981.

31. Penning L, Wilmink JT: Rotation of the cervical spine. *Spine* 12:732–738, 1987.

32. Dvorak J, Panjabi M, Gerber M, Wichmann W: CT-functional diagnostic of the rotatory instability of upper cervical spine, part 1: an experimental study on cadavers. *Spine* 12:197–205, 1987.

33. Dvorak J, Hayek J, Zehnder R: CT-functional diagnosis of the rotatory instability of the upper cervical spine, part 2: an evaluation on healthy adults and patients with suspected instability. *Spine* 12:726–731, 1987.

34. Panjabi M, Dvorak J, Duranceau J, Yomamoto I, Gerber M, Rauschning W, Bueff HV: Three-dimensional movements of the upper cervical spine. *Spine* 13:726–730, 1988.

35. Penning L: Normal movements of the cervical spine. *Am J Roentgenol* 130:317–325, 1978.

36. Wortzman G, Dewar FP: Rotary fixation of the atlantoaxial subluxation. *Radiology* 90:479–487, 1968.

37. Selecki BR: The effect of rotation of the atlas on the axis: experimental work. *Med J Aust* 56:1012–1015, 1969.

38. Barton JW, Margolis MT: Vertebral artery occlusion. *Neuroradiology* 9:117–120, 1975.

39. Miller RG, Burton R: Stroke following chiropractic manipulation of the spine. *JAMA* 229:189–190, 1974.

40. Hohl M, Baker HR: The atlanto-axial joints roentgenographic and anatomial study of normal and abnormal motion. *J Bone Joint Surg.* 46:1739–1752, 1964.

41. Hohl M: Normal motion in the upper portion of the cervical spine. *J Bone Joint Surg* 46-A(8):1777–1779, 1964.

42. Jirout J: Synkinetic contralateral tilting of atlas and head on lateral inclination, part II. *Manual Med* 1:121–125, 1985.

43. Fielding JW: Normal and selected abnormal motion of the cervical vertebra to the seventh cervical vertebra based on cineradiography. *J Bone Joint Surg* 46A(8):1280–1287, 1964.

44. Penning L: Nonpathological and pathologic relationships between the lower cervical vertebrae. *Am J Roentgenol Radiol Ther Nucl Med* 91(5):1036–1050, 1964.

45. White AA, Panjabi MM: The basic kinematics of the human spine: a review of past and current knowledge. *Spine* 3:12, 1978.

46. Coutts MB: Atlanto-epistropheal subluxations. *Arch Surg* 29:297–311, 1934.

47. Grieve G: *Common Vertebral Joint Problems.* New York, Churchill Livingstone, 1981, pp 88, 129–130, 206–208, 213, 222–223, 880.

48. Magee DJ: *Orthopedic Physical Assessment,* Philadelphia, WB Saunders, 1987, pp 25, 34–35.

49. Jackson R: *The Cervical Syndrome,* ed 4. Springfield, IL, Charles C Thomas, 1977, pp 46, 64, 75, 89, 95–97, 100, 105–109, 145, 150, 160–163, 181–182, 188–189, 269, 294, 297, 309–331.

50. Davidson RI, Dunn EJ, Metzmahn JN: The shoulder abduction test in the diagnosis of radicular pain in cervical extradural compressive monoradiculopathies. *Spine* 6:441–446, 1981.

51. Schafer RC: *Chiropractic Physical and Spinal Diagnosis.* Oklahoma City, Associated Chiropractic Academic Press, 1980, VIII-24.

52. Gatterman MI: Indications for spinal manipulation in the treatment of back pain. *ACA J Chiro* 16:51–65, 75–80, 116–119, 1982.

53. Peterson DH, Panzer DM, Muhlemann D: Biomechanics Palpation Manual. Portland, OR, Western States Chiropractic College, 1987, pp 56–67, 71–72, 76–77, 88–94, 250–260, 359–384.

54. Peterson DH: *Adjustive Technique Manual.* Portland, OR, Western States Chiropractic College, 1987, pp 12–13, 23–24, 63–68, 82–94, 103–112, 121–122, 127–130, 133–134, 137–139.

55. Fligg B: Motion palpation of the upper cervical spine. In Vernon H: *Upper Cervical Syndrome.* Baltimore, Williams & Wilkins, 1988, pp 113–123, 199–203, 242–247, 342–344.

56. Herbst RW: Gonstead Chiropractic Science & Art. (Seminar notes) Sci-Chi Publications, 1981, pp 17, 177–180, 242–247, 256–260.

57. Bovee ML, Burns JR, Carrigg PM, Harmon RO, Johnson MR, Kern DP, Swearingen TL, Willhite FS: Adjusting Technique Manual. Davenport, IA, Palmer College of Chiropractic, 1981. pp 10–12, 69–80, 82–121, 201.

58. Grice A: A biomechanical approach to cervical and dorsal adjusting. In Haldeman S: *Modern Developments in the Principles and Practice of Chiropractic.* East Norwalk, CT, Appleton-Century-Crofts, 1980, pp 110–111, 331–358.

59. States AZ: *Spinal and Pelvic Techniques.* National College of Chiropractic, 1968, pp 21–28, 33–38.

60. Maigne R: *Orthopedic Medicine: A New Approach to Vertebral Manipulation.* Springfield, IL, Charles C Thomas, 1972, pp 215, 328–338.

61. Stoddard A: *Manual of Osteopathic Technique.* London, Hutchinson, 1980, pp 46–47, 51, 106–107, 112–118.

62. Szaraz ZT: Adjustive and manipulative techniques. In Vernon H: *Upper Cervical Syndrome.* Baltimore, Williams & Wilkins, 1988, pp 120, 122, 124–138, 177–180.

63. Schafer RC: *Clinical Biomechanics: Musculoskeletal Actions and Reactions.* Baltimore, Williams & Wilkins, 1987, pp 354–356.

64. Bourdillon JF, Day EA: *Spinal Manipulation.* Los Altos, Appleton and Lange, 1987, pp 83–84, 90–91, 168–175.

65. Maitland, GD: *Vertebral Manipulation.* Boston, Butterworth, 1977, pp 44–47, 49–54, 192–196, 198–200.

66. Cailliet R: *Neck and Arm Pain.* Philadelphia, FA Davis, 1964, pp 40, 44, 61, 78, 84.

67. MacNab I: The "whiplash syndrome". *Orthop Clin North Am* 2(2), 1971.

68. Jahn W: Acceleration and deceleration injury. *JMPT* 1:95–102, 1978.

69. Whitly JE, Forsyth HF: The classification of cervical spine injuries. *Am J Roentgenol* 83:633–644, 1960.

70. Foreman SM, Croft AC: *Whiplash Injuries: The Cervical Acceleration Deceleration Syndrome.* Baltimore, Williams & Wilkins, 1988, pp 35, 58, 62, 65, 76.

71. Hohl M: Soft tissue neck injuries. In Baily RW: *The Cervical Spine.* Philadelphia, JB Lippincott, 1983, pp 282–287.

72. Gay JR, Abbott KH: Common whiplash injuries of the neck. *JAMA* 152:1698–1704, 1953.

73. Greenfield J, Ilfeld FW: Acute cervical strain: evaluation and short term prognostic factors. *Clin Orthop* 122:196–200, 1977.

74. MacNab I: Acceleration injuries of the cervical spine. *J Bone Joint Surg* 46-A:1797–1799, 1964.

75. Cameron BM, Cree CMN: A critique of the compression theory of whiplash. *Orthopedics* 2:127–129, 1960.

76. Marar C: The pathogenesis of damage to the spinal cord. *J Bone Joint Surg* 56A:1655–1662, 1974.
77. Torres F, Shapiro SK: Electroencephalograms in whiplash injury: a comparison of electroencephalographs. *Arch Neurol* 5:40, 1961.
78. Jacobson G, Adler DC: Examination of the atlanto-axial joint following injuries with particular emphasis on rotational subluxation. *Am J Roentgenol* 76:1081–1094, 1956.
79. Travell JG, Simons DA: *Myofascial Pain and Dysfunction: The Trigger Point Manual.* Baltimore, Williams & Wilkins, 1983, pp 189, 205, 299, 335, 350, 353, 357, 361, 594, 603, 605.
80. Gore DR, Sepic SB, Gardner GM: Roentgenographic findings of the cervical spine in asymptomatic people. *Spine* 11:521–524, 1986.
81. Rechtman AM, Borden AGB, Gershon-Cohen J: The lordotic curve of the cervical spine. *Clin Orthop* 20:208, 1961.
82. Peterson C, Wei T: Vertical hyperplasia of the cervical pillars: another look at the straight cervical spine. *ACA J Chiro* 21:78–79, 1987.
83. Anderson PA, Montesano PX: Morphology and treatment of occipital condyle fractures. *Spine* 13:731–736, 1988.
84. Jefferson G: Fracture of the atlas vertebra: report of four cases and a review of those previously recorded. *Br J Surg* 7:407, 1920.
85. Elliott JM, Rodgers LF, Wisinger JP: The hangman's fracture. *Radiology* 104:303, 1972.
86. Roaf R: Lateral flexion injuries of the cervical spine. *J Bone Joint Surg* 45B:36–38, 1963.
87. Cailliet R: *Soft Tissue Pain and Disability.* Philadelphia, FA Davis, 1984, pp 83, 130, 136.
88. Norris SH, Watt T: The prognosis of neck injuries resulting from rear-end vehicle collision. *J Bone Joint Surg* 65B:608–611, 1983.
89. Gore DR, Sepic SB, Gardner GM, Muriaz MP: Neck pain: A long-term follow-up of 205 patients. *Spine* 12:1–11, 1987.
90. Gotten N: Survey of one hundred cases of whiplash injury after settlement of litigation. *JAMA* 162:865–866, 1956.
91. Turek SL: *Orthopedics: Principles and Their Application,* ed 3. Philadelphia, JB Lippincott, 1977, pp 78, 740, 744, 780, 791, 799–804.
92. Trott RH: Tension headache. In Grieve GP: *Modern Manual Therapy of the Vertebral Column.* New York, Churchill Livingstone, 1986, pp 336–341.
93. Salter RB, Hamilton HW, Wedge JH, Tile M, Torode IP, O'Driscoll SW, Murnaghas JJ, Saringer JH: Clinical application of basic research on continuous passive motion for disorders and injuries of synovial joints: a preliminary report of a feasibility study. *J Orthop Res* 1:325–342, 1984.
94. Salter RB: *Textbook of Disorders and Injuries of the Musculoskeletal System: An Introduction to Orthopedics, Rheumatology, Metabolic Bone Disease, Rehabilition and Fractures.* Baltimore, Williams & Wilkins, 1970, pp 22, 216, 218–219, 603.
95. Dillin W, Booth R, Cuckler J, Balderston R, Simeone F, Rothman R: Cervical radiculopathy: a review. *Spine* 11:988–991, 1986.
96. Kelsey J, Githens, Walter SD: An epidemiological study of acute prolonged cervical intervertebral disc. *J Bone Joint Surg* 66A:907, 1984.
97. Lunsford LO, Biosorette DJ: Anterior surgery for cervical disc disease. *J Neurosurg* 53:12, 1980.
98. Henderson C, Hennessay R: Posterolateral foraminatomy as an exclusive operation technique for cervical radiculopathy a review of 846 conservatively operated cases. *Neurosurgery* 12:504, 1983.
99. Rob CG, Standeven A: Arterial occlusion complicating outlet compression syndrome. *Br Med J* 2:709, 1958.
100. Liebenson CS: Thoracic outlet syndrome: diagnosis and conservation management. *JMPT* 11:493–499, 1988.
101. Young HA, Hardy DG: Thoracic outlet syndrome. *Br J Hosp Med* 29:457–459, 1983.
102. Phillips H, Grieve GP: The thoracic outlet syndrome. In Grieve GP: *Modern Manual Therapy of the Vertebral Column.* New York, Churchill Livingstone, 1986, pp 359–364, 368.
103. Sallston J, Schmidt H: Cervicobrachial disorders in certain occupations with special reference to compression in the thoracic spine. *AM J Ind Med* 6:45–52, 1984.
104. Lord JW, Rosotti L: *Thoracic Outlet Syndromes, Clinical Symposia.* Summit, NJ, CIBA, 1971, pp 3–32, 306.
105. Lewit K: Impaired joint motion, function and entrapment syndrome. *Manual Med* 16:45–48, 1978.
106. Raskin NH, Howard MW, Ehrenfeld WK: Headaches as the leading symptoms of the thoracic outlet syndrome. *Headache* 25:208–226, 1985.
107. Sunderland, S: *Nerves and Nerve Injuries,* ed 2. Edinburgh, Churchill Livingstone, 1978.
108. Hansen DT: Double crush syndrome. *Pac NW J Clin Chiro* 3:11–13, 1983.
109. Upton AKM, McComas AJ: The double crush in nerve entrapment syndromes. *Lancet* 2:359–360, 1973.
110. Massey EW, Riley TH, Pleet AB: Co-existent carpal tunnel syndrome and cervical radiculopathy (double crush syndrome). *South Med J* 74:957–959, 1981.
111. Vernon H: Vertebrogenic headache. In Vernon H: *Upper Cervical Syndrome.* Baltimore, Williams & Wilkins, 1988, pp 164, 170–174, 178, 182–184.
112. Palmer DD: *The Chiropractic Adjuster: The Science, Art and Philosphy of Chiropractic.* Portland, Portland Printing House, 1910, pp 34, 526, 914.
113. Guillo F: The differential diagnosis and therapy of headaches. *Ann Swiss Chiro Assoc* 12:121–166, 1961.
114. Valenti E: The occiput-cervical region. *Ann Swiss Chiro Assoc* 4:225–232, 1969.
115. Lewit K: Pain arising from the posterior area of the atlas. *Eur Neurol* 16:263–269, 1977.
116. Shoenholtz F: Conservative management of cervical tension cephalgia. *ACA J of Chiro* 13:549–552, 1979.
117. Henderson DJ: Significance of vertebral dyskinesia in relation to the cervical syndrome. *JMPT* 2:3–15, 1979.
118. Droz JM, Crot F: Occipital headaches: statistical results in the treatment of vertebrogenous headaches. *Ann Swiss Chiro Assoc* 8:127–136, 1985.
119. Rig SY: Upper cervical vertebrae and occipital headache. *JMPT* 3:137–141, 1980.
120. Vernon H, Thamic MSI: Vertebrogenic migraine. *J Can Chiro Assoc* 29:20–24, 1983.
121. Barbuto LB: Differential diagnosis of headaches. In Vernon H: *Upper Cervical Syndrome: Chiropractic Diagnosis and Treatment.* Baltimore, Williams & Wilkins, 1988, pp 141–151.
122. Fisk JW: *The Painful Neck and Back.* Springfield, IL, Charles C Thomas, 1977, p 48.
123. Trott: Tension headache. In Grieve GP: *Modern Manual Therapy of the Spinal Column.* New York, Churchill Livingstone, 1986, pp 336–341.
124. Wyke SD: Articular neurology: a review. *Physiotherapy* 58:94–99, 1972.
125. Kellgren JH: On the distribution of pain arising from deep somatic structures with charts on segmental pain areas. *Clin Sci* 4:35–46, 1939.
126. Jirout J: Comments regarding the diagnosis and treatment of dysfunction in the C2-C3 segment. *Manual Med* 2:16–17, 1985.
127. Bogduk N: Headaches and cervical manipulation. *Med J Aust* 66:65–66, 1979.
128. Jull GA: Headaches associated with the cervical spine: a clinical review. In Grieve: *Modern Manual Therapy of the Spinal Column.* New York, Churchill Livingstone, 1986, pp 315–329.
129. Edeling J: The abandoned headache syndrome. In Grieve GP: *Modern Manual Therapy of the Spinal Column.* New York, Churchill Livingstone, 1986, pp 330–335.
130. Parker GB, Topling H, Pryor DS: A controlled trial of cervical manipulation for migraine. *Aust NZ J Med* 3:589–593, 1978.

CHAPTER 11

Postural Complex

DAVID M. PANZER, D.C.
SCOT G. FECHTEL, B.S., D.C.
MERIDEL I. GATTERMAN, M.A., D.C.

Posture is the biomechanical interaction between organism and gravity (1).

Human posture is based on an erect column of functional segments, better designed for movement than for standing still. Standing is in reality movement upon a stationary base, with postural sway being an integral component of the upright stance. Optimal posture allows for pain-free movement with a minimum of energy expenditure and is a sign of vigor and harmonious control of the body (2). Goldthwait (3) has described good posture as one in which the head is held erect, the chest is forward, the shoulders drawn back, and the abdomen retracted. This definition encompasses more than just the aesthetic aspect of posture, because it implies a relationship of the parts of the body to each other, which is the most favorable one for optimal functioning of the respiratory, circulatory, and digestive systems (4).

Good posture is not a simple static alignment of body parts like so many inert blocks; rather it is a dynamic and complex biomechanical interaction between organism and gravity (1). The counterforces to the pervasive pull of gravity are made more efficient by good body alignment, but because the living body is in constant motion, the biomechanical forces of muscles, ligaments, and bones must be considered. Even with the recumbency of sleep, the body frequently changes position, with good postural support being essential for good spinal hygiene. An unphysiologic mattress hampers breathing and impedes visceral functioning.

In addition to the emphasis on the spine as a dynamic organ of posture, the chain-link concept of spinal biomechanics is vital to the understanding of spinal biomechanics (Chapter 2). Conventional medical opinion, according to Jones (5), largely considers that each symptom arises from a defect of local origin. Chiropractors instead emphasize that postural distortion regularly gives rise to a generalized pattern of symptoms, with localized foci producing diffuse effects.

Knee pain, for example, can be the result of pelvic distortion when the ipsilateral sacroiliac joint is locked in flexion. This distortion produces a posterior rotation of the iliac crest (flexion), which causes a pull at the insertion of the sartorius muscle at the knee. The resulting knee pain disappears with manipulation of the sacroiliac joint.

Leg length discrepancies inherently affect spinal biomechanics, which often can be improved with shoe lifts or foot orthotics. The effects of functional scoliosis can frequently be minimized by careful postural evaluation and correction through exercise, braces, and lifts. The importance of pelvic tilt must be emphasized in relation to spinal curves and an increase in lumbar lordosis. Often back pain can be relieved by exercises that affect the offending link in the chain, not always at the site of the most severe discomfort.

POSTURAL DEVELOPMENT

The most significant difference between biped posture and quadruped posture is the specialization of the limbs, one pair for progression and one pair for prehension. This specialization plays an important part in the human postural complex, and as the infant matures there is a progression through the quadrupedal phase to the bipedal stance.

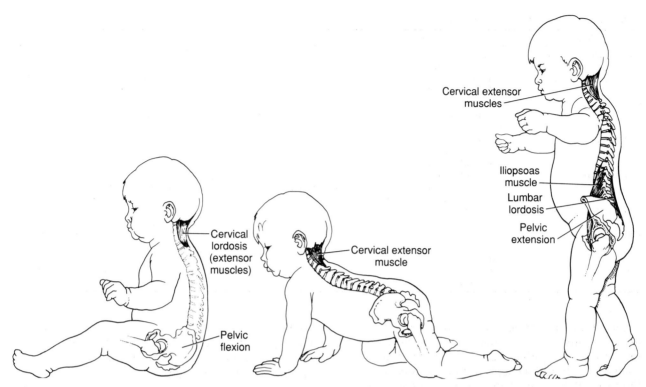

Figure 11.1. Cervical curve development. **A,** *Cervical lordosis* appears as the *extensor muscles* become stronger as the infant begins to sit. **B,** It is further accentuated when the child begins to creep. **C,** The lumbar curve develops around the end of the first year as the child begins to stand and attempts to walk. The *iliopsoas* by its attachment to the lumbar spine and the femur pulls the lumbar spine into lordosis. The pelvis is then held in extension as opposed to flexion (fetal position).

Spinal Curves

The newborn has a single "C"-shaped curve throughout the entire spine, with the convexity to the posterior. The first lordotic curve with the convexity to the anterior begins to form during the first 6 to 8 weeks, from the action of the cervical muscles. These posterior erector muscles gradually increase the cervical lordosis as the child raises the head in the early confrontations with gravity. This ongoing battle with the force of gravity continues throughout life as the primary source of stress on the body. As the infant begins to sit and hold the head erect, these cervical extensor muscles become stronger, increasing the cervical lordosis (Fig. 11.1A). This is accentuated even more as the child raises the head while creeping (Fig. 11.1B).

The second lordotic curve develops in the lumbar spine around the end of the first year, as the child begins to stand and attempts to walk. As the child stands, the iliofemoral band is stretched, tilting the pelvis forward. The lumbar lordosis is thus produced largely by the failure of the hip flexors to stretch and elongate (Fig. 11.1C). As the hips extend to assume the erect posture, the iliopsoas, by its attachment to the lumbar spine and the femur, causes a forward traction in the lumbar spine, producing the anterior convexity or lordosis.

The upright adult exhibits a balanced posture based on the physiological curves, with the convexity to the anterior in the cervical and lumbar regions and the convexity to the posterior in the thoracic and sacral regions. Maintenance of this elongated "S" depends on the continuous and harmonious synchronization of the numerous postural muscles (Table 11.1). The posterior paraspinal muscles tend to increase the lumbar lordosis, while the anteriorly placed abdominal muslces tend to augment the thoracic kyphosis. Loss of the spinal curves is found with muscle spasm and is a frequent finding with acute injury to the spine.

The shape and extent of the spinal curves also depends upon the configuration of the vertebrae and discs, which in turn have been shaped by the stress of muscle pull. The lumbar curve reaches from the last thoracic vertebra to the lumbosacral angle, with the convexity of the lower three segments greater than that of the upper two. It is caused mainly by the greater depth of the anterior parts of the intervertebral discs and is enhanced by the shape of the vertebral bodies (6).

The thoracic curve reaches from the second to the twelfth thoracic vertebra and is caused by the greater depth of the posterior part of the vertebral bodies (3).

The cervical curve is the least marked and may be absent in some normal individuals. It begins at the

Table 11.1 Primary Postural Muscles

Region	Muscle	Action
Posterior lower extremity	Soleus	Plantar flexion
	Gastrocnemius	Knee extension
Anterior lower extremity	Quadriceps	Knee extension
	Tibialis anterior	Dorsiflexion
Pelvis	Iliopsoas	Pelvic extension
	Gluteus maximus	Pelvic flexion
	Hamstrings	Pelvic flexion
Anterior trunk	Rectus abdominus	Trunk flexion
	External oblique	Together trunk flexion
	Internal oblique	Together trunk flexion
Posterior trunk	Sacrospinalis	Trunk extension
	Short postural muscles, multifidus, rotatores, interspinales & intertransversaries	Stabilize vertebral motion segments
Upper extremities	Trapezius	Stabilize scapulae
	Rhomboids	Stabilize scapulae
Anterior neck	Longus colli	Flexion of the head and neck
	Longus capitis	
	Recti capitis	
Posterior neck	Splenius capitis	Extension of the head and neck
	Splenius cervicis	

second thoracic vertebra and ends at the atlas. It is less pronounced, with relatively shorter pedicles, longer articular pillars, and less angulation of the facets. This should be kept in mind when evaluating the cervical curve in trauma victims, since a shallow or straight cervical spine may be normal for that individual (Chapter 10).

Spinal Curves and Pelvic Tilt

The human spinal curves in the upright position depend upon the angle of the sacral base, which in turn depends upon pelvic tilt. In the neutral position of the pelvis, the anterior superior iliac spines (ASIS) are in the same vertical plane as the symphysis pubis (7) (Fig. 11.2A). With anterior pelvic tilt, the ASIS move anterior to the symphysis pubis in

the vertical plane and increase the sacral base angle. The ASIS move posterior to the symphysis pubis in the vertical plane with posterior pelvic tilt, decreasing the sacral-base angle.

Because the spine is balanced on the sacrum like a flexible rod, movement of the sacral base affects the spinal curves. Anterior pelvic tilt (Fig. 11.2B) increases the lumbar lordosis, thoracic kyphosis, and cervical lordosis, while posterior pelvic tilt decreases the spinal curves (Fig. 11.2C). Anterior pelvic tilt puts increased weight on the posterior facet joints, which may produce back pain (Chapter 8).

Posterior pelvic tilt exercises reduce excessive lumbar lordosis. These exercises are a fundamental part of patient education utilized to alter poor pos-

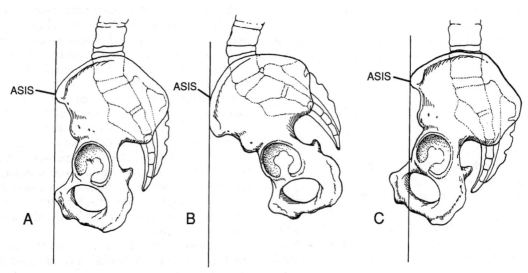

Figure 11.2. A, The *ASIS* are in the same vertical plane as the symphysis pubis when the pelvis is in the neutral position. **B,** With anterior pelvic tilt, the *ASIS* move anterior to the symphysis pubis in the vertical plane, increasing the lumbar lordosis. **C,** The *ASIS* move posterior to the symphysis pubis in the vertical plane when the pelvis is tilted posteriorly, decreasing the lumbar lordosis.

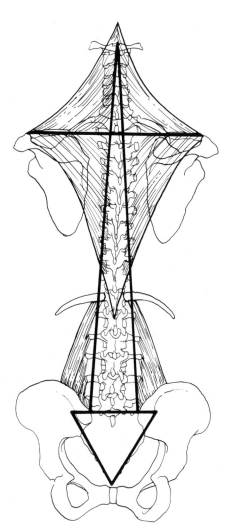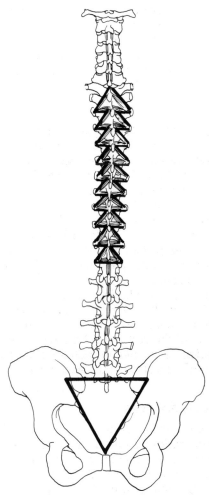

Figure 11.3. **A,** The general form of the spinal column is two isosceles triangles supported by the paraspinal muscles, which serve as guy wires. **B,** The short intersegmental (trans- versospinalis) muscles provide postural stabilizers between segments.

tural habits. Patients can be taught to decrease lumbar lordosis by flattening the back against the floor and tightening the gluteus muscles. Adding partial curl-ups with the knees bent (crunches) will then strengthen the abdominal muscles. A decreased lumbar lordosis will be benefited by extension exercises (Chapter 8). A loss of cervical lordosis can be restored through use of a cervical pillow or rolled towel placed under the supine cervical spine in addition to cervical extension exercises. Normalization of spinal curves depends on optimal movement of all vertebral motion segments, which is enhanced by manipulation, and exercise alone may not restore postural integrity until joint fixations are released through manipulation.

The curvature of the vertebral column increases its resistance to axial compression forces. Biomechanically, the resistance of a curved column is directly proportional to the square of the number of curvatures plus one. Applying this formula to the

vertebral column with the lumbar, thoracic, and cervical curves yields a spinal resistance to axial compression ten times greater than that of a straight column (8),

$$(3^2 + 1 \text{ or } 9 + 1 = 10).$$

Spinal Morphology

The spinal column viewed from the posterior (coronal plane) is relatively straight. A very slight right thoracic (physiological) curve is considered normal and is thought to be due to the position of the aorta (4). The vertebral segments are progressively wider toward the caudal end, with bodies consistently increasing in mass to sustain the weight of the trunk and upper extremities. From the first sacral segment to the last coccygeal segment their mass gradually decreases (9). This gives the spinal column the general form of two isosceles triangles (Fig. 11.3).

The elongated triangle formed by the spine balances the inverted-triangle-shaped sacrum that functions as a keystone wedge between the ilia (Chapter 7). These two triangles are stabilized by the paraspinal muscles that form guy wires providing an efficient support system in both static and dynamic posture (Fig. 11.3).

Spinal Length

The average spine is 25 inches (63.5 cm) long in the female and 28 inches (71.1 cm) long in the male. Approximately one-fourth of the length is formed by the intervertebral discs. The spine normally shows a variation in length from morning to evening due to postural compression. This shortening may be as much as three-fourths inch (2 cm). This decrease in length ordinarily corrects itself with normal sleep, but there is a gradual loss that is not regained. The average person loses approximately 1 inch (2.54 cm) in a normal life span.

This shortening is due to dehydration of the discs, which lose their hydrophilic property (see Chapter 8). An additional decrease in height may occur due to compression of the vertebrae. This actual shortening of the spine is further accentuated by the increase in spinal curvatures that accompanies aging (9).

PHYSIOLOGY OF POSTURE

Upright posture is an active process and is the result of the cooperation of a number of reflexes, many of which have a tonic character. Many parts of the central nervous system contribute to the function of posture (10). Human posture is the result of moment-by-moment modification of neuronal circuits that are responsible for response patterns. Some of these patterns are present at birth, and others appear as the nervous system develops. These stereotypical responses in the form of human reflexes include the stretch reflex, flexion reflex (withdrawal reflex), extension reflex, extensor thrust, and the positive supporting reflexes, crossed extensor reflex, righting reflex, etc.

The postural reflex patterns result in a coordination of many joint movements and combinations of muscle actions including contraction of prime movers, relaxation of antagonists, and supportive contraction of synergists and stabilizers. These muscles must be regulated with regard to their contraction intensity, speed, duration, and sequential changes in activity.

The integrative function is predominantly automatic and unconscious and results from the incessant shifting of the center of weight, known as postural sway. This postural shift is controlled by the asynchronous rotation of motor units, which is characteristic of postural contraction (11). Postural corrections are continuously mediated by the myotatic stretch reflex. Posture is further mediated by the vis-

ual, labyrinthine, and neck-righting reflexes and by the interplay of joint reflexes.

Postural Receptors

Postural receptors include the sensory nerve endings that respond to various stimuli relating to the body's position in space. These receptors may be classified as exteroceptors and interoceptors. Exteroceptors receive and transmit stimuli that come from outside of the body and include those monitoring touch and sight. Postural interoceptors are known as proprioceptors and receive impulses from the tissue directly concerned with musculoskeletal movements (12).

Postural Exteroceptors

Cutaneous Receptors

Cutaneous receptors initiate many of the fundamental inborn reflexes. The most significant cutaneous reflex involved in upright posture is that initiating the supporting reaction. A very slight touch to the pads of the foot is sufficient to evoke a strong tonic extension of the lower limb. Known as the extensor thrust reflex, this response is a spinal reflex and can be elicited in the hind limb of a dog with a completely transected spinal cord.

This reflex is also known as the "magnet reaction," since a very slight touch to the pads of the foot is sufficient to evoke a strong tonic extension of the whole hind limb. Even if dorsiflexion of the foot or toes is carefully avoided by keeping the fingers only just in contact with the foot, the slowly extended foot appears to be drawn after the receding fingers by some magnetic force. Touching the sole of an infant's foot elicits this response, and when placed with the soles on the floor, the infant extends the legs, simulating upright posture.

Visual Righting Reflexes

Visual feedback is used to orient the head and body correctly with the environment and is especially important when other sensory input is deficient (11). To accommodate this optical reflex, the head must balance squarely on the neck. The high incidence of upper cervical fixation may be in part due to the body's attempt to maintain the eyes level with the horizon in response to an unleveling farther down the spine. Individuals whose eyes are not level in their skull, due to congenital defects or birth trauma, adopt a voluntary postural misalignment in order to bring their eyes into a level relation.

This compensatory mechanism has been duly noted by a number of chiropractors (Chapter 10). Prolonged upper cervical joint fixation is a common cause of tension headaches, and whether compensatory to unleveling below or primary (commonly the result of flexion/extension injuries), this condition responds readily to manipulation (Chapter 10).

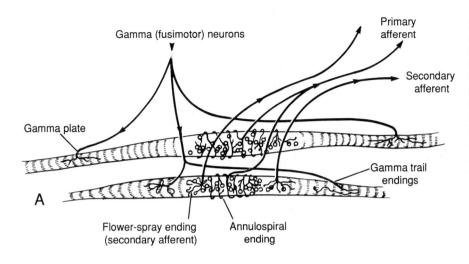

Gamma (fusimotor) neurons

Primary afferent

Secondary afferent

Gamma plate

Gamma trail endings

A

Flower-spray ending (secondary afferent)

Annulospiral ending

Figure 11.4. **A,** Neuromuscular spindles are highly specialized sense organs lying parallel to **B,** the extrafusal (contractile muscle) fibers. A muscle spindle is comprised of a fluid-filled capsule containing small intrafusal muscle fibers. (Modified from Gowitzke BA, Milner M: *Understanding the Scientific Bases of Human Movement,* ed 2. Baltimore, Williams & Wilkins, 1980.)

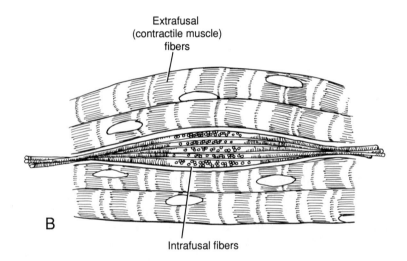

Extrafusal (contractile muscle) fibers

B

Intrafusal fibers

Postural Interoceptors (Proprioceptors)

Proprioceptors receive impulses from muscles, tendons, and joints as well as from capsules, ligaments, and other fibrous membranes. The proprioceptors are responsible for transmitting a constant flow of information from these structures to the spinal cord and brain, especially the cerebellum. They provide information regarding the degree, direction, and rate of change of muscle tension. The proprioceptors include the muscle spindle, Golgi tendon organs, pacinian corpuscles, Ruffini end-organs, labyrinthine receptors, and tonic neck receptors (12).

Muscle Spindles

Neuromuscular spindles (Fig. 11.4*A*) are highly specialized sense organs found interspersed among the bundles of contractile muscle fibers (Fig. 11.4*B*). They may be found throughout the mass of the muscle but tend to be more concentrated in the central portion. Muscle spindles are sensitive to change in muscle length and respond to both constant length

(as in maintained posture) and changing length (as during movement). The spindle activity reflects both the rate of change in length (phasic response) and the ultimate length achieved and maintained (tonic response).

The muscle spindles lie parallel to the contractile muscle fibers (extrafusal fibers). Each spindle is a tiny fusiform capsule (about 1 mm long) that contains two kinds of specialized muscle fibers, known as intrafusal fibers. The outer, multinucleate, intrafusal fibers are known as nuclear-bag fibers and are pericapsular and larger than the inner nuclear-chain fibers. Their nuclei are centrally located in a baglike area, which gives the bag fiber its name. The smaller nuclear-chain fibers are named for the single-file, chain-like arrangement of the nuclei in the slender, noncontractile central portion.

The sensory innervations of the intrafusal fibers of the spindle that respond to changes in muscle length are of two kinds. Primary endings, also called annulospiral endings because they are wrapped around both nuclear-bag and nuclear-chain fibers,

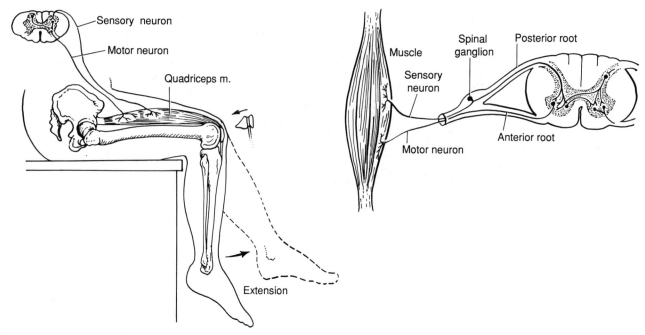

Figure 11.5. The stretch reflex. **A,** The most commonly cited example of the stretch reflex occurs with momentary shortening of the *quadriceps muscle* following stretch of the patellar tendon by tapping it with a reflex hammer. **B,** The central terminal branch of the *sensory neuron* synapses directly with the dendrites of the *motor neuron* which innervate the same muscle fibers that were stretched, creating a two-neuron reflex arc.

are tonically responsive to muscle length and phasically responsive to rate of change of length (velocity). They are classed as Ia fibers in size and are among the fastest conducting of all nerve fibers. Secondary endings are also known as flower-spray endings because of their shape and are associated almost exclusively with nuclear-chain fibers. Secondary endings are responsive only to tonic muscle length. They are classed as type II fibers and are slower conducting than Ia primary afferents (Chapter 12).

Stretch Reflex

The knee jerk is most typically cited as an example of the stretch reflex (Fig. 11.5). Tapping the patellar tendon momentarily stretches the quadriceps muscles and their spindles. This results in activation of the primary Ia afferents that monosynaptically facilitate the homonymous α-motoneurons, causing the quadriceps to shorten and the leg to extend. The shortening of the quadriceps shuts off the primary afferents, causing excitation of the α-motoneurons to cease and the leg to drop.

A description of the "simple stretch reflex" is not complete without mention of reciprocal innervation. For the quadriceps to be able to shorten, the antagonist hamstrings must at the same time (reciprocally) relax. This is accomplished via the primary afferents from the stretched spindles, which excite the homonymous (agonist) motoneurons in addition to stimulating inhibitory interneurons that in turn inhibit the motoneurons of the antagonist muscle (hamstrings).

Motor innervation of the spindles' intrafusal fibers is provided by small, primarily γ-sized motoneurons. They are more accurately referred to as fusimotor neurons because they are not all γ-sized. Their cell bodies are found in the ventral gray horns of the spinal cord along with the α-motoneurons supplying the homologous extrafusal muscle fibers. Two types of fusimotor neurons have been identified. They are different in structure, function, and pharmacological response. It has been suggested that the fusimotor neurons supplying nuclear-bag fibers are faster-conducting, have a dynamic (facilitating) action on the stretch reflex, and terminate in endings known as γ-plates, while fusimotor neurons supplying nuclear-chain fibers terminate as γ-trailendings, are slow-conducting, have a static or tonic response, and tend to inhibit the stretch reflex.

The practical function of fusimotor action on intrafusal fibers and in turn on spindle function is to take up the slack produced by the shortening of extrafusal fibers. Thus, rather than having a proprioceptive "silent" period during a muscle contraction that "unleads" the primary (annulospiral) afferents, fusimotor contraction of the polar ends of intrafusal fibers restretches the central regions and reactivates the primary afferents. This provides continuous, uninterrupted information to the central nervous system about the length of the muscle. Activation of the fusimotor system comes from supraspinal motor control centers and is not part of the stretch reflex circuitry.

The neuromuscular circuitry that provides continuous information to the central nervous system about muscle length and which maintains appropriate tension on opposite sides of a joint is referred to in engineering terms as a servo- or feedback mechanism. The most commonly cited servomechanism is the thermostat that maintains room temperature within certain predetermined limits.

Maintenance of erect (standing) posture is accomplished by a neuromuscular servomechanism. For example, an anterior displacement (sway) of the body's center of gravity stretches the spindles in the calf muscles (particularly the soleus) and initiates a myotatic (stretch) reflex contraction in the stretched muscles, which brings the body back over the ankle joint. Shortening of the muscle simultaneously removes the stretch on the spindles and reduces facilitation of the homonymous motor neurons. In calm standing, respiratory movements are the chief perturbations to vertical posture. As mentioned above, most of the slack in the postural servomechanism is taken up by the fusimotor system, so that small deviations require only small corrections, and balance is imperceptibly maintained, primarily by the soleus muscle.

The integration of the various neuromuscular signals that maintain vertical posture in the presence of anterior-posterior oscillations has been mathematically described in terms of the body as an "inverted pyramid" (4). Although an obvious oversimplification, this model permits analysis of the various components of upright posture.

Golgi Tendon Organs

The Golgi tendon organ is another specialized receptor incorporated into the gross muscle structures. Unlike the neuromuscular spindle, the Golgi tendon organ has an inhibitory effect on its own muscle by way of the homonymous α-motoneuron. It consists of nerve endings enclosed in a connective-tissue capsule embedded in the musculotendinous junction.

These organs are stimulated by stretch, primarily produced by contraction of the muscle in whose tendon they are situated. They may be excited by strong, passive stretch, but they are much more sensitive to the tension of the muscle contraction. Generally, Golgi tendon organs facilitate flexors and inhibit extensors (i.e., antigravity muscles). They have a protective inhibitory effect on their own muscle when its tension is excessive to the point of danger.

Afferent sensory impulses from the tendon organs are transmitted by large, rapidly conducting, type Ib nerve fibers. These fibers transmit signals both into local areas of the cord and by way of the spinocerebellar tracts into the cerebellum. The local signal is believed to excite a single inhibiting interneuron

that in turn inhibits the anterior motor neuron supplying the active or stretched muscle.

Joint Receptors

Pacinian corpuscles, Ruffini endings, and other joint proprioceptors are found in the ligaments and capsules surrounding the joints. Pacinian corpuscles are found also in muscle fascia and adjacent connective tissue. These receptors are activated by pressure and by changes in joint position. Their sensitivity is such that a change of 2° in joint angle is sufficient to alter their rate of discharge (11).

Joint receptors, especially those of the interphalangeal joints of the feet, contribute to the positive supporting reflexes along with the spindles of the interosseous muscles (11). A complex combination of stimuli processed by the cord facilitates the appropriate stretch reflexes of extensor muscles.

This process converts the limb into a firm, yet compliant, pillar. If the phalanges are squeezed together or flexed instead of being abducted, all the joints of the limb flex, thus reducing support. When any one of the three joints of a limb is flexed, the other two joints also flex. Conversely, when one of the joints is extended, the other two also extend. Compression of the limb as in weightbearing through reflex activity evokes extensor muscle contraction. Traction, as in hand suspension, produces flexion (11).

Postural sway to one side decreases the angle on the side of sway, while increasing the angle on the contralateral side. These actions evoke corrective responses in the abductor and adductor muscles of the hips and inverters or everters of the feet, which counteract the sway (11). In the spine, receptors in the joints of the vertebral motion segments, pelvis, and shoulders are coordinated to produce synchronous muscle action to support the body. Kinesthetic sensation from impulses arising in the joint receptors are projected by multisynaptic pathways to the sensorimotor cortex, which coordinates the appropriate motor response.

GRAVITY LINE

To maintain equilibrium in the standing position with the least expenditure of energy, the articulated parts of the spine and lower extremities must be aligned, with the center of gravity of each segment balanced above the joint upon which its weight impinges. To determine postural alignment, a plumb line representing the gravity line is used to analyze deviations from the midline. The only fixed point in upright posture is the base, where the feet are in contact with the floor.

The plumb line is then dropped to coincide with the fixed base. In a lateral view of an ideally aligned posture (Fig. 11.6A), starting at the base, the plumb line should coincide with the following points:

1. Slightly anterior to the lateral malleolus;

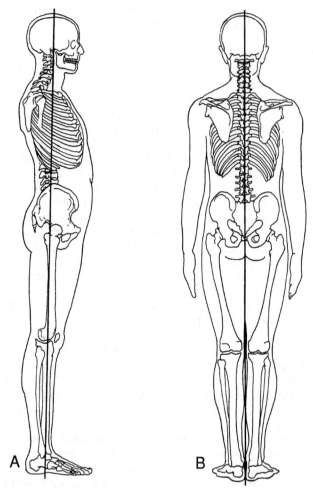

Figure 11.6. Ideally aligned erect posture. **A,** Lateral view. **B,** Posterior view.

2. Slightly anterior to the axis of the knee joint;
3. Bodies of the lumbar vertebrae;
4. Shoulder joint;
5. Bodies of most of the cervical vertebrae;
6. External auditory meatus;
7. Slightly posterior to the apex of the cervial curvature (7).

Viewed from the posterior, starting with the fixed point midway between the heels, the plumb line will be equidistant from the following parts:

1. Medial aspects of the heels;
2. Medial aspects of the legs;
3. Medial aspects of the thighs;
4. Scapulae.

It will coincide with the midline of the trunk and head (Fig. 11.6B). The head should not be tilted or slanted, the shoulders' level not elevated or depressed. The scapulae should be in the neutral position, with the medial borders essentially parallel and about 3 to 4 inches apart. The pelvis should be level with the posterior superior iliac spines in the

same transverse plane. The hips should be in the neutral position, not abducted or adducted, with the lower extremities in good alignment, not bowed or knock-kneed. The feet should be parallel or slightly turned out. The outer malleolus and outer margin of the sole of the foot should be in the same vertical plane, so that the foot is not pronated or supinated (7).

To maintain equilibrium in a standing position with the least expenditure of energy, optimal body alignment is desirable. Optimal alignment is rarely achieved, rather it is only closely approached, momentarily, as the body sways on its stationary base.

There is no single best posture for all individuals. For each person the best posture is one in which the body segments are balanced in the position of least strain and maximum support. To the chiropractor, the kinetic posture should be of greater clinical significance than the static alignment of body parts that, after all, are designed for movement.

POSTURAL MUSCLES

To prevent excessive postural sway or actual falling, muscular contractions of the sacrospinalis are necessary to provide dynamic guy wires that prevent overbalancing of the trunk. Strong plantar flexion, particularly due to increased tension in the soleus, is essential to counteract forward sway. Any considerable backward swaying of the trunk above the pelvis induces contraction of the psoas major muscle. The major postural muscles are outlined in Table 11.1. Stabilization of the upper extremities depends on the action of the middle trapezius and rhomboid muscles on the scapulae (Fig. 9.6).

Phasic and Tonic Muscles

Muscles are broadly classified as tonic or phasic on the basis of function. The tonic antigravity or postural muscles exhibit the continuous low level of contractile activity required to maintain a given posture. They contain proportionately more red, slow-contracting muscle fibers with a richer supply of hemoglobin (myoglobin), giving them a darker appearance and providing for long-continued contraction. The more rapidly contracting phasic muscles used in motor skills contract more rapidly and contain a larger proportion of white fibers.

Neck Reflexes

The neck reflexes arise from stimulation of the joint proprioceptors in the cervical spine, especially in the atlantooccipital articulations. They respond to cervical movement when the head is bent forward, backward, sideward, and rotated. The neck reflexes are present at birth and persist postnatally in a sterotypical manner referred to as tonic neck reflexes (13). These compulsive responses become less apparent as motor development proceeds. Between the sixth and eighth week, they begin to assume their more mature form of neck-righting reflexes.

The tonic neck reflexes, however, do not completely disappear in the adult. Their circuits remain intact, with their pattern of synaptic facilitation and inhibition altered by responses modified through motor developments into more useful patterns.

Typical tonic neck reflexes include responses to flexion, extension, and rotation of the neck. Flexion of the neck evokes flexor facilitation of the upper limbs, with extension of the lower limbs. Extension of the neck produces extension of the upper limbs and flexion of the lower limbs. Rotation of the head facilitates extension and abduction of the limbs on the same side, and flexion and abduction of the contralateral limbs. This posture is similar to the fencer's en garde position and that assumed when swimming the side stroke.

The afferents for these reflexes take their course through the upper three cervical posterior roots. An additional tonic neck reflex is produced with ventral pressure on the C7 vertebral prominence. Known as the vertebral prominens reflex, relaxation of the four limbs is produced with such pressure (10).

The head-righting movements play an important part in maintaining and regaining balance. These movements occur in combination with the equilibrium movements to bring about proper alignment of the head, center of gravity, and base of support.

It seems reasonable that injuries of the neck, such as those following the "whiplash phenomenon," interfere with the integration of limb movements into the total body patterns, since simple labyrinth and neck reflexes are concerned at all times with such movements. Upper cervical joint fixation has been known to cause a variety of seemingly bizarre symptoms, which are relieved by manipulation in patients suffering from upper cervical joint fixation (Chapter 10).

INDIVIDUAL POSTURAL VARIATIONS

Individual postural variations are related to age and somatotype as well as to psychogenic factors, primarily the individual's self-esteem. Postural changes occur as a natural progression of the life cycle. From the quadruped position of the creeping infant (Fig. 11.1), the young child assumes the upright posture. This phase is characterized by the protruding abdomen and relatively straight spine. This later develops into the adult spine with the lordotic cervical and lumbar regions and the kyphotic thoracic area. With aging, comes a noticeable increase in the thoracic kyphosis, which is primarily due to the generalized osteoporosis that occurs with aging (Chapter 9). This is more pronounced in the postmenopausal female and can be minimized through good preventive nutrition and regular exercise.

SOMATOTYPES

While considered insignificant by some, a person's somatotype has a noticeable bearing on posture and hence on bodily processes. These constitutional differences were discussed by Hippocrates, who related a tendency toward different diseases to the predominance of one or another type of body fluids. Later thinkers held that there is a relationship between the body type and the temperament (Table 11.2).

Kretchmer, a German psychiatrist, and later Sheldon, an American psychologist, classified body builds into three main body types (14) (Fig. 11.7). Goldthwait, (15) an American orthopaedic surgeon, also described three main body types, stating that "individuals of different body types show different susceptibility to various disease." While Kretchmer classified the body into three main types, he also discussed a fourth category or mixed type. The pyknic type he characterized as short and plump with rounded chest and shoulders. These individuals were described as social, friendly, and lively. The asthenic individual was described as tall, slender, narrow, and elongated with a serious, quiet, solitary personality. The athletic type is well-developed with a body mass proportionate to body height. His fourth category, the dysplastic group, is a contradictory or incompatible mixture of different body types.

Sheldon (14) postulated a constancy of somatotype for any individual over time. He also stated that there are not discrete, "either/or" body types, but rather continuous dimensions of variations. Following this thinking, he suggested that physique can be rated on a number of dimensions, rather than just categorized. His third principle asserts a relationship between morphogenotype (biological structures) as measured in the individual's somatotype (the rating of the physique) and personality dynamics as expressed in temperament. Sheldon based his classification on photographs of 4000 nude college men seen from the front, back, and side. He developed a system of measuring and classifying the structural aspects of individuals and distinguished three main components of physique, which he called endomorphy, mesomorphy, and ectomorphy.

Endomorphs exhibit a roundness of figure and softness of muscle, mesomorphs a predominance of bone and muscle, and ectomorphs a linearity and delicacy in the structures of the body. Sheldon decided that there are no clearly separate and distinct body types with no transition or intermediate forms, but rather continuous distributions of components.

If the extremes of each body type are placed at the angles of an isosceles triangle, the contribution of each component to an individual's physique can be measured in a systematic and objective way (14) (Fig. 11.8). The contribution of each component is rated on a seven-point scale, and the contribution of the three components is defined as the person's somatotype. Sheldon (14) expressed a person's somatotype as a series of three numerals, each expressing

Table 11.2 Comparison of Somatotype Characteristics

	Type I	Type II	Type III
Author			
Kretchmer	Asthenic	Athletic	Pyknic
Sheldon	Ectomorph	Mesomorph	Endomorph
Goldthwait	Slender	Intermediate	Stocky
Characteristic			
Appearance	Tall, slender	Well-developed	Short, plump
Personality	Introverted	Competitive	Extroverted
Socialization	Solitary	Physically active	Sociable
Subcostal angle	<70°	70–90°	>90°
Recreational activities	Running, swimming, cross-country skiing	Football, downhill skiing, contact sports	Volleyball

the approximate strength of one of the primary components in a physique. The first numeral he referred to endomorphy, the second to mesomorphy, and the third to ectomorthy. On his 7-point scale a 7–1–1 is the most extreme endomorph, a 1–7–1 is the most extreme mesomorph, and a 1–1–7 is the most extreme ectomorph. The 4–4–4 falls at the midpoint of the scale with respect to all three components.

A close relationship was found by Sheldon between the somatotype and temperament (16). Endomorphs, he found, tend to be jovial and pleasure loving, mesomorphs to be vigorous and aggressive, and ectomorphs to be introverted and inhibited. The three body types described by Kretchmer and Sheldon are similar to those described by Goldthwait, although not totally equivalent.

Figure 11.7. Female and male somatotypes.

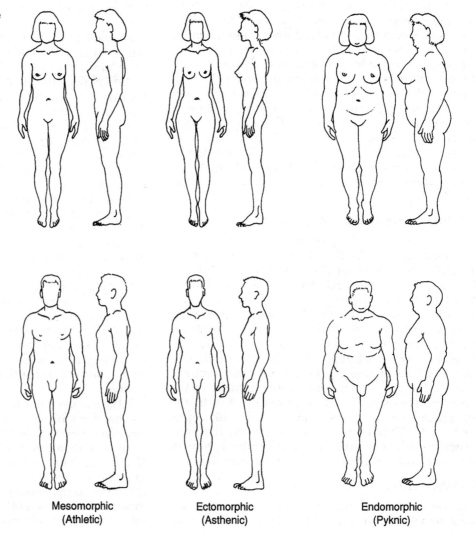

Mesomorphic
(Athletic)

Ectomorphic
(Asthenic)

Endomorphic
(Pyknic)

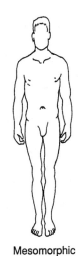

Mesomorphic

Figure 11.8. A person's physique can be measured systematically and objectively by placing the extremes of each body type at the angles of an isosceles triangle and then rating the components on a seven point scale. The contribution of the three components is defined as the person's somatotype.

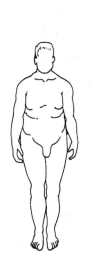

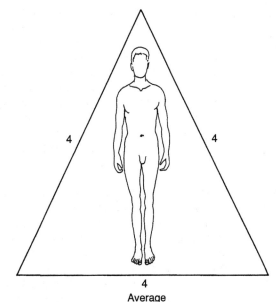

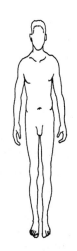

Endomorphic

4

4

4

Average

Ectomorphic

Based on varying anatomic features, Goldthwait's classification emphasizes body mechanics and the position of the organs in the body relative to their function.

Goldthwait's intermediate type corresponds somewhat with Kretchmer's athletic type and Sheldon's mesomorph. According to Goldthwait, this body type is characterized by a torso of moderate length and breadth with a subcostal border forming an angle between 70 and 90°. The thorax is full and moderately rounded, with the diaphragm high and a generous space for the viscera below. The postural habits differ in the three classes, with a proper adjustment and relationship of the various body parts most easily maintained in the intermediate type. This type exhibits normal spinal curves with visceral placement such that optimal function is promoted. Well-defined masses of fat provide protection and support around the viscera. Like

Kretchmer's athletic type, these individuals exhibit a well-developed body mass, proportionate to body height.

The slender type, with a subcostal angle less than 70°, is characterized as tall, slender, and sparsely built. These individuals have loose ligamentous attachments, with a range of motion from 15 to 30° more than the average. The torso is longer and narrower, and the rib articulations with the spine commonly show a greater range of motion than usual. The entire spine is lighter and more slender and has been described as the "industrial back," being more susceptible to strain and sprain injuries.

The stocky type is a heavily built individual, with the joints deeply set and the articular ligaments short. The total range of motion is often from 10 to 20° less than in the intermediate type. The subcostal angle is frequently greater than 90°, with the neck short and thick in proportion to the body length.

The vertebrae are large and heavy, with a relatively short lumbar spine and very little lumbar lordosis.

Posturally, the slender type exhibits an increased lumbar lordosis and anterior pelvic tilt. There is generally an exaggerated thoracic kyphosis, with the head poked forward. The ribs and clavicles tend to droop and there is inadequate support of the shoulders, so that they appear rounded. There is also more extensive downward displacement of viscera, with these individuals being more prone to visceroptosis. The stocky type tends to withstand postural strain more readily, due to heavier bones, thicker muscles, shorter ligamentous attachments, and decreased joint motion (15).

An understanding of somatotypes is useful for counseling patients in both their occupational and recreational activities. Individuals with ligamentous laxity are prone to joint injuries and are a poor risk for jobs requiring repetitive bending and lifting. Recommendation of exercises should take into consideration the suitability of the activity for the patient's somatotype. Ectomorphs tend to enjoy and excel at solitary sports such as distance running, swimming, and cross-country skiing. Mesomorphs have a high need for activity and enjoy contact sports such as football and downhill skiing. The endomorph may enjoy social activities more. While each of us has some characteristics of each somatotype, we generally have more characteristics of one of them.

PSYCHOLOGICAL FACTORS AFFECTING POSTURE

Posture and self-esteem are so interwoven that it is often difficult to determine which is the cause and which is the effect. Posture is "organ language," and emotions are reflected in one's posture (17). The healthy, self-assured individual exhibits an evenly balanced, free-wheeling posture, while emotionally disturbed persons appear to carry the "weight of the world" on their shoulders. Much can be discerned about emotions by careful observation of a person's carriage. Consider the number of expressions that represent somatization of the individual's feelings. For example, we refer to an unpleasant emotional situation as a "headache," a "pain in the neck," or "a backbreaker."

Patients suffering from shyness or abuse often exhibit poor posture, with the shoulders rounded as if reverting to the fetal position. This posture is readily observed in the young female who attempts to hide her developing breasts by rounding the shoulders and slouching forward (17). It becomes even more apparent in the heavy-breasted female who must fight the additional anterior weight to maintain her upright posture. These women frequently exhibit the "V" sign or "V"-shaped indentations in the shoulders from the constant pressure of bra straps. Such women frequently suffer from chronic thoracic spine and rib fixation, most commonly in the area of the bra line.

POSTURE MODIFICATION

Postural modification depends on accurate diagnosis (7, 18) and patient cooperation. Many postural faults can be modified through exercise (17, 19) while others may be corrected by simple changes in workplace and activities of daily living. Postural evaluation requires astute observation of patients as they walk, sit, and move about, in addition to the traditional standing analysis. Deviation from ideally aligned erect posture can be assessed by a variety of devices including plumb lines, posture guides, and inclinometers. Three-dimensional analysis has been developed by Johnston (20). Segmental alignment, flexibility, and muscle length and strength can be efficiently recorded on a body mechanics examination chart (Fig. 11.9).

Shortened agonists must be stretched before resistive exercise can be optimally effective (19). Postural kyphosis of the thoracic spine is often secondary to tightness in the anterior structures. Strengthening of the postural stabilizers (rhomboids and middle trapezius) is futile without adequate stretching of the agonistic pectoralis muscles. These exercises correct not only an excessive kyphotic curve, but help to align "poked head" and "rounded shoulders," which are the most commonly seen postural aberrations. These changes may only be possible with manipulation to release accompanying thoracic fixation.

Modification of the workplace so that the eyes are looking forward rather than downward is also necessary for lasting relief from postural strain. Psoas stretching is necessary when increased anterior pelvic tilt is creating excessive lumbar lordosis, another common postural fault (17). Strengthening the abdominal muscles and pelvic extension without adequate psoas stretches will have little lasting effect when the psoas muscle continues to pull the lumbar spine forward.

The happy backpacker knows the importance of carrying the weight low on the pelvis, thereby preventing increased lumbar lordosis and strain on the upper back and shoulders. The modern mother who transports her child in a carrier on her back prevents much backache. Slinging a child on the hip is a common cause of sacroiliac dysfunction as the hip is "hiked" to balance the weight. Carrying a child in front accentuates thoracic kyphosis.

Optimal balance of the physiologic curves creates effortless, nonfatiguing posture that is painless to the individual who can remain erect for reasonable periods of time (17). Frequent change of position prevents painful states and increases efficiency, and should be encouraged in the workplace. The effects of structural abnormalities can be minimized by emphasis on good body mechanics, which is important for an aesthetically pleasing appearance and essential for good health.

BODY MECHANICS EXAMINATION CHART

Name...Cl. no. ....Doctor ....

Diagnosis...Date of 1st Ex.......................

Onset ....Date of 2nd Ex.....................

Occupation...Height ....Weight.........................

Handedness.....................Age ....Sex ....Leg length: Left ....Right ....

PLUMB ALIGNMENT

Side view: Lt...Rt..

Back view: Deviated lt...Deviated rt..

SEGMENTAL ALIGNMENT

	Feet	Hammer toes		Hallux valgus		Low ant. arch		Ant. foot varus
		Pronated >		Supinated		Flat long. arch		Pigeon toes
	Knees	Med. rotat. >		Lat. rotat.		Knock-knees		Tibial torsion
		Hyperext. >		Flexed		Bow-legs		
	Pelvis	Leg in postural add.		Rotation		Tilt		Deviation
	Low back	Lordosis		Flat		Kyphosis		Operation
	Up. back	Kyphosis		Flat		Scap. abducted		Scap. elevated
	Thorax	Depressed chest		Elevated chest		Rotation		Deviation
	Spine	Total curve		Lumbar		Dorsal		Cervical
	Abdomen	Protruding		Scars		....		....
	Shoulder	Low		High		Forward		Med. rotated
	Head	Forward		Torticollis				

TESTS FOR FLEXIBILITY AND MUSCLE LENGTH

Forward bending......................Bk...........H.S........G.S.........

Arm overhead elevation: Lt. ....Rt. ....

Hip flexors: Lt. ....Rt. ....

Tensor fas. lata.: Lt. ....Rt. ....

Trunk extension:..

Trunk lat. flex.: To lt...........................To rt. ....

TREATMENT

Infra-red: ....

Massage: ....

Moist Heat:......................................

Paraffin Bath: ....

Diathermy: ....

Exercises:

F. L. Pelvic tilt ....

B. L.: Pel. tilt and breath. ....

Pel. tilt and leg sl. ....

Head and sh. raising ....

Pectoral stretch ....

Straight leg-raise ....

Hip flex. stretch ....

Sd. L.: Stretch ....tensor ....

Sit.: Forward bending

To stretch low bk. ....

To stretch h. s. ....

Wall-sitting

Middle trapezius ....

Lower trapezius ....

St.: Foot and knee ex. ....

Wall-standing

Other exercises:..

L	MUSCLE STRENGTH TESTS	R	R Date L
	Mid. trapezius		
	Low. trapezius		
	Back extensors		
	Glut. medius		
	Glut. maximus		
	Hamstrings		
	Hip flexors		
	Tib. posterior		
	Toe flexors		

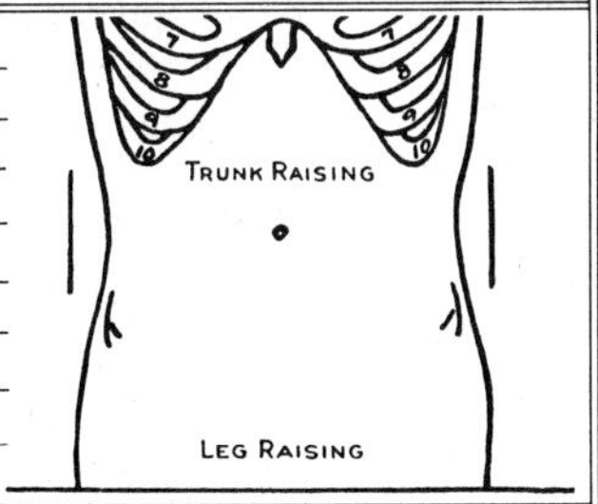

TRUNK RAISING

LEG RAISING

Left	SHOE CORRECTION	Right
	(Wide Heel) Inner wedge (Narrow heel)	
	Level heel raise	
	Metatarsal support	
	Longitudinal support	

NOTES:...

....

....

....

Support: ....

Figure 11.9. Body mechanics examination chart. (From Kendall HO, Kendall FP, Wadsworth GE: *Muscle Testing and Function*, ed 2. Baltimore, Williams & Wilkins, 1971, p 29.)

Table 11.3 Prevalence of Scoliosis by Degree[a]

Author(s)	No. of Patients	Patients with Curvatures (%)			
		>5°	>10°	>20°	>30°
Bruszewski & Kamza	15,000	3.8	3.0	0.46	0.15
Rogala et al.	14,999	4.3	—	0.3	0.3
Kane	75,290	—	—	—	0.13
Patynski et al.	5000	—	2.6	—	0.12
Shands & Eisberg	50,000	1.9	1.4	0.3	0.29
Strayer	928[b]	—	5.0	2.0	0.75

[a]From Bunnell WP: The natural history of idiopathic scoliosis. *Clin Orthop* 229:20–25, 1988.
[b]All female.

SCOLIOSIS

With the traditional emphasis placed on the spine in chiropractic, anomalies of spinal structure assume great importance. Scoliosis is the major alteration of both structure and function that occurs in the spine. While most spinal curves only affect the patient's appearance, a progressive scoliosis will affect the function of all organs within the rib cage and will impact the patient's ability to sit, stand, and walk.

Scoliosis was defined by Lovett (21) as a lateral curvature in the normally straight vertical line of the spine. Lovett indicated that any series of vertebral spinous processes that showed a constant deviation from the midline and were accompanied by twisting was a scoliosis, when viewed from the anterior to the posterior. Such a curve can be transient, when due to muscle spasm (see following discussion of functional scoliosis), or may be permanent and due to structural or pathological conditions. By far the greatest number of severe spinal curvatures are labeled idiopathic, since no identifiable cause can be located with the level of our current knowledge (Table 11.3).

Cailliet (22) pointed out that any scoliosis in a spine with the potential for continued growth must be considered to have the possibility for curve progression. Although current evidence suggests that it is possible to predict which curves have the highest probability of progression, there remains a need for diagnosis and appropriate follow-up.

The training and tools of the chiropractic physician warrant a role in the conservative management of static or slowly progressive scoliosis. Traditional modes of physical treatment of spine curves are within the scope of chiropractic practice. However, the role of spine manipulation in the treatment of idiopathic scoliosis is not yet defined and remains controversial.

Perhaps the most exciting development in scoliosis treatment is lateral electrical surface stimulation (23). This device stimulates the patient's muscles during sleep to pull the spine into a more appropriate alignment. Early results in curve reduction are encouraging (24). This method has been combined with spine manipulation with promising results in one patient (25).

Idiopathic scoliosis is commonly seen in chiropractic practices. Therefore, the practicing chiropractor must be familiar with the syndrome and be able to evaluate patients to determine which can be treated conservatively and which will require surgical stabilization.

Etiology of Scoliosis

In one sense, the etiology of scoliosis is very complex. This is because many diseases, injuries, and traumas can promote spine curvature development. However, scoliosis that can be treated conservatively is of the idiopathic type. This simplifies matters for the chiropractic physician. If examination discloses severe congenital anomalies, tumors, bony disease, or instability from trauma, the patient should be referred for definitive treatment.

If the patient has idiopathic scoliosis, the progression of the curve should be determined. With curves that progress more than 1° per month or are greater than 50° (Cobb measurement), surgical correction is in order (26). Slowly progressive curves offer a reasonable probability for successful treatment with conservative measures. In addition, those stable curves with painful sequelae respond to physical measures.

Classification of Scoliosis

The etiological classification of scoliosis has been established by the Scoliosis Research Society (Table 11.4). Chiropractic physicians should be able to identify which general category the patient fits into. Specific diagnosis of genetic, neurologic, or oncogenic factors that may be producing a structural scoliosis can be made by an appropriate specialist. Structural scoliosis due to osseous anomalies will be observed by the chiropractor through radiographic examination, and when appropriate, these patients can be referred to an orthopaedic surgeon specializing in scoliosis treatment. The nonstructural scolioses will be seen in the chiropractic office also. Other than for those curves caused by tumors or inflammatory conditions, conservative chiropractic treatment is appropriate (see the following section).

The group of curves most reasonably treated by outpatient, conservative means are the juvenile and adolescent idiopathic types. This group of patients

Table 11.4 Etiological Classification of Scoliosis[a]

Structural Scoliosis
I. Idiopathic
  A. Infantile
    1. Resolving
    2. Progressive
  B. Juvenile (3–10 years)
  C. Adolescent (>10 years)
II. Neuromuscular
  A. Neuropathic
    1. Upper motor neuron
      a) Cerebral palsy
      b) Spinocerebellar degeneration
        1) Friedreich's disease
        2) Charcot-Marie-Tooth disease
      c) Syringomyelia
      d) Spinal cord tumor
      e) Spinal cord trauma
      f) Other
    2. Lower motor neuron
      a) Poliomyelitis
      b) Other viral myelitides
      c) Traumatic
      d) Spinal muscular atrophy
        1) Werdnig-Hoffmann
        2) Kugelberg-Welander
    3. Dysautonomia (Riley-Day)
    4. Other
  B. Myopathic
    1. Arthrogryposis
    2. Muscular dystrophy
      a) Duchenne (pseudohypertrophic)
      b) Limb-girdle
      c) Facioscapulohumeral
    3. Fiber type disproportion
    4. Congenital hypotonia
    5. Myotonia dystrophica
    6. Other
III. Congenital
  A. Failure of information
    1. Wedged vertebra
    2. Hemivertebra
  B. Failure of segmentation
    1. Unilateral (unsegmented bar)
    2. Bilateral
  C. Mixed
IV. Neurofibromatosis
V. Mesenchymal disorders
  A. Marfan's
  B. Ehlers-Danlos
  C. Others
VI. Trauma
  A. Fracture
  B. Surgical
    1. Postlaminectomy
    2. Postthoracoplasty
  C. Irradiation
VII. Extraspinal contractures
  A. Post empyema
  B. Post burns
IX. Osteochondrodystrophies
  A. Diastrophic dwarfism
  B. Mucopolysaccharidoses (e.g., Morquio's syndrome)
  C. Spondyloepiphyseal dysplasia
  D. Multiple epiphyseal dysplasia
  E. Other
X. Infection of bone
  A. Acute
  B. Chronic
XI. Metabolic disorders
  A. Rickets
  B. Osteogenesis imperfecta
  C. Homocystinuria
  D. Others
XII. Related to lumbosacral joint
  A. Spondylolysis and spondylolisthesis
  B. Congenital anomalies of lumbosacral region
XIII. Tumors
  A. Vertebral column
    1. Osteoid osteoma
    2. Histiocytosis X
    3. Other
  B. Spinal cord (See Neuromuscular)

Nonstructural Scoliosis
I. Postural scoliosis
II. Hysterical scoliosis
III. Nerve root irritation
  A. Herniation of nucleus pulposus
  B. Tumors
IV. Inflammatory (e.g., appendicitis)
V. Related to leg length discrepancy
VI. Related to contractures about the hip

[a]Modified from Yochum TR, Rowe LJ: *Essentials of Skeletal Radiology.* Baltimore, Williams & Wilkins, 1986, p 226.

includes those with continued bone growth, slowly progressive curves, and minimal cosmetic and functional deformity. They have the highest likelihood of cessation of curve progression, improvement in the biomechanical properties of the spine, and minimal permanent symptoms.

All other types of curves (and patients) should be rigorously evaluated to assess the probability that conservative treatment will be beneficial, prior to referral for surgical care. It is not in the patient's best interest to pursue a course of conservative therapy when the outcome can be expected to be poor. Further, delaying definitive treatment for these patients will only result in increased curves, worse biomechanical faults, and greater cosmetic deformity—clear transgression of Hippocrates' admonishment to "do no harm"!

A common lexicon simplifies, reduces errors in, and increases communication. For this reason the Scoliosis Research Society has published a glossary of terms related to scoliosis (Table 11.5) (27).

Clinical Considerations

Once physical examination has suggested a spinal curve (e.g., unlevel pelvis, unlevel shoulders, axial rotation of body, unlevel scapulae, rib hump (Fig. 11.10), radiographic examination is undertaken. The definitive radiograph is the 14 × 36 or "full-spine" size obtained in the posteroanterior direction while the patient is weightbearing (Fig. 11.11).

The posterior-to-anterior direction is chosen to reduce the exposure of growing organs to ionizing radiation. It should be particularly noted that the most radiosensitive organ is the maturing breast. It is, therefore, wise to add appropriate shielding in this area for adolescent females.

The full-spine size gives a complete picture of all portions of the patient's spine. Weightbearing allows an understanding of the impact of gravity on the curve.

Table 11.5 Glossary of Scoliosis Terms[a]

Adolescent scoliosis—Spinal curvature presenting at or about the onset of puberty and before maturity.

Adult scoliosis—Spinal curvature existing after skeletal maturity.

Angle of thoracic inclination—With the trunk flexed 90° at the hips, the angle between the horizontal and a plane across the posterior rib cage at the greatest prominence of a rib hump.

Apical vertebra—The most rotated vertebra in a curve; the most deviated vertebra from the vertical axis of the patient.

Body alignment, balance, compensation—1) The alignment of the midpoint of the occiput over the sacrum in the same vertical plane as the shoulders over the hips. 2) In roentgenology, when the sum of the angular deviations of the spine in one direction is equal to that in the opposite direction.

Cafe au lait spots—Light brown, irregular areas of skin pigmentation. If sufficient in number and with smooth margins, they suggest neurofibromatosis.

Cervical curve—Spinal curvature that has its apex from C1 to C6.

Cervicothoracic curve—Spinal curvature that has its apex at C7 or T1.

Compensatory curve—A curve, which can be structural, above or below a major curve that tends to maintain normal body alignment.

Congenital scoliosis—Scoliosis due to congenitally anomalous vertebral development.

Curve measurement—1) Cobb method: Select the upper and lower end vertebrae. Erect perpendiculars to their transverse axes. They intersect to form the angle of the curve. If the vertebral endplates are poorly visualized, a line through the bottom or top of the pedicles may be used. 2) Ferguson method: The angle of a curve is formed by the intersection of two lines drawn from the center of the superior and inferior end vertebral bodies to the center of the apical vertebral body.

Double major scoliosis—A scoliosis with two structural curves.

Double thoracic curve (scoliosis)—A scoliosis with a structural upper thoracic curve, a larger, more deforming, lower thoracic curve, and a relatively nonstructural lumbar curve.

End vertebra—The most cephalad vertebra of a curve whose superior surface, or the most caudad one whose inferior surface tilts maximally toward the concavity of the curve.

Fractional curve—A compensatory curve that is incomplete because it returns to the erect. Its only horizontal vertebra is its caudad or cephalad one.

Full curve—A curve in which the only horizontal vertebra is at the apex.

Functional curve (nonstructural curve)—A curve that has no structural component and that corrects or overcorrects on recumbent side-bending roentgenograms.

Genetic scoliosis—A structural spinal curvature inherited according to a genetic pattern.

Gibbus—A sharply angular kyphos.

Hysterical scoliosis—A nonstructural deformity of the spine that develops as a manifestation of a conversion reaction.

Idiopathic scoliosis—A structural spinal curvature for which no cause is established.

Iliac epiphysis, iliac apophysis—The epiphysis along the wing of an ilium.

Iliac epiphysis sign, iliac apophysis sign—In the anteroposterior roentgenogram of the spine, when the excursion of ossification in the iliac epiphysis (apophysis) reaches its ultimate medial migration, vertebral growth may be complete.

Inclinometer—An instrument used to measure the angle of thoracic inclination or rib hump.

Infantile scoliosis—Spinal curvature developing during the first 3 years of life.

Juvenile scoliosis—Spinal curvature developing between the skeletal age of 3 years and the onset of puberty.

Kyphos—A change in the alignment of a segment of the spine in the sagittal plane, which increases the posterior convex angulation.

Kyphoscoliosis—Lateral curvature of the spine associated with either increased posterior or decreased anterior angulation in the sagittal plane in excess of the accepted norm for that region. In the thoracic region 20–40° of kyphosis is considered normal.

LESS—Lateral electrical surface stimulation.

Lordoscoliosis—Lateral curvature of the spine associated with an increase in anterior curvature or a decrease in posterior angulation in the sagittal plane in excess of normal for that region. In a thoracic spine, where posterior angulation is normally present, less than 20° would constitute lordoscoliosis.

Lumbar curve—Spinal curvature that has its apex from L1 to L4.

Lumbosacral curve—Spinal curvature that has its apex at L5 or below.

Major curve—Term used to designate the larger(est) curve(s), usually structural.

Minor curve—Term used to refer to the smaller(est) curve(s).

Myogenic scoliosis—Spinal curvature due to disease or anomalies of the musculature.

Neurogenic scoliosis—Spinal curvature due to disease or anomalies of nerve tissue.

Osteogenic scoliosis—Spinal curvature due to abnormality of the vertebral elements and/or adjacent ribs, acquired or congenital.

Pelvic obliquity—Deviation of the pelvis from the horizontal in the frontal plane. Fixed pelvic obliquities can be attributable to contractures either above or below the pelvis.

Primary curve—The first or earliest of several curves to appear, if identifiable.

Rib hump—The prominence of the ribs on the convexity of a spinal curvature, usually due to vertebral rotation, best exhibited on forward bending.

Skeletal age, bone age—The age obtained by comparing an anteroposterior roentgenogram of the left hand and wrist with the standards of the Gruellich and Pyle Atlas.

Structural curve—A segment of the spine with a fixed lateral curvature. Radiographically, it is identified in supine, lateral, side-bending films by the failure to correct. They may be multiple.

Thoracic curve—Scoliosis in which the apex of the curvature is between T2 and T11.

Thoracogenic scoliosis—Spinal curvature attributable to disease or operative trauma in or on the thoracic cage.

Vertebral endplates—The superior and inferior plates of cortical bone adjacent to the intervertebral disc.

Vertebral growth plate—The cartilaginous surface covering the top and bottom of a vertebral body which is responsible for the linear growth of the vertebra.

Vertebral ring apophyses—The most reliable index of vertebral immaturity, seen best in the lateral roentgenograms or in the lumbar region in side-bending anteroposterior views.

[a]Modified from the Terminology Committee of the Scoliosis Research Society: A glossary of scoliosis terms. Spine 1(1):57–58, 1976.

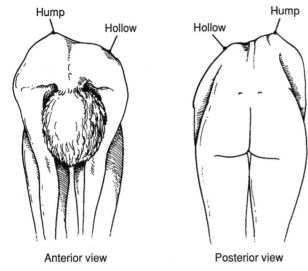

Figure 11.10. The Adams forward-bending test shows a rib rotational prominence (rib hump) when viewed from **A,** the front and **B,** the back.

This film can be supplemented with lateral-bending films to determine the flexibility of the curve (Chapter 6). Flexibility of the curve has been implicated as one measure of the risk of progression (28).

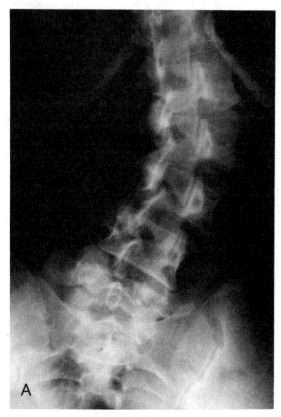

Figure 11.11. Radiograph of a 25-year-old female with idiopathic scoliosis. (From Yochum TR, Rowe LJ: *Essentials of Skeletal Radiology.* Baltimore, Williams & Wilkins, 1986, p 229.)

Additionally, coned-down or local views can improve the clarity of individual vertebrae and thus improve pathological diagnosis.

Characterization of the curve comes from the PA full-spine radiograph. The curve is named by the area(s) of the spine involved (Fig. 11.12). The apex vertebra is defined as that which is most rotated, or the most deviated vertebra from the vertical axis of the patient.

To evaluate the curve over time, a common method of analysis is needed. The Cobb method appears most reliable (29) (Fig 6.23) between observers, is simple to learn and apply, and does not detract from the spine image on the radiographs (Chapter 6). The topmost vertebra involved in the curve is identified by either assessing the angle into the concavity of the curve or by identifying the segment that has begun to return to the normal direction. The vertebra most inclined to the concavity of the curve is the topmost segment. The most inferior segment is then identified by the same method. A horizontal line is drawn along the superior endplate of the superior vertebra. Similarly, the inferior endplate of the bottommost vertebra is determined. Then perpendicular lines are drawn from the horizontal lines. The angle of intersection of the perpendicular lines describes the scoliosis. For future assessment, the top- and bottommost vertebrae should be identified and recorded. When later films are obtained, the same vertebral levels must be used to measure the curvature so that reliable comparisons can be made.

Rotation of the vertebral segments involved in the curvature is associated with cosmetic and functional deformity. The greater the rotation, the greater the rib deformity, the consequent rib hump, and the functional limitation in spine movement and cardiovascular compliance. A simple method of assessing the relative movement of the vertebra was published by Nash and Moe (29). This method uses the same 14 × 36 PA radiograph as that obtained for the Cobb measurement. Identification of the pedicle shadows of the spinal segments involved in the curve yields rotational information. As the segment rotates in the horizontal plane, the pedicle shift toward the convex side. Noting the degree of rotation at each evaluation of the curvature will allow accurate assessment of progression in both the sagittal and the horizontal planes. Since the progression of the curvature is the index to treatment, this is a critical evaluation.

Prediction of Curve Progression

Will a given curve progress? This question has been given rigorous evaluation. Retrospective studies of pre–skeletally mature scoliosis patients have been reported by Mannherz et al. (30), Suh and MacEwen (31), Bunnell (32), Picault et al. (33), and Weinstein (34), and in the post–skeletally mature by Ascani et al. (35). Bunnell (36) evaluated the clinical

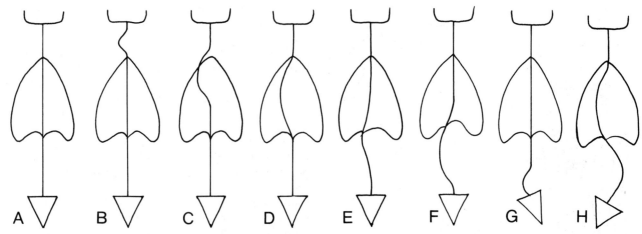

Figure 11.12. Classification of scoliosis according to location. **A,** Normal spine. **B,** Cervical (C1-C6). **C,** Cervicothoracic (C7-T1). **D,** Midthoracic (T2-T11). **E,** Thoracolumbar (T12-L1). **F,** Lumbar (L2-L4). **G,** Lumbosacral (L5-S1). **H,** Double lumbar and thoracic. (From Yochum TR, Rowe LJ: *Essentials of Skeletal Radiology.* Baltimore, Williams & Wilkins, 1986, pp 227.)

factors used as indicators of curve progression (Table 11.6).

For ease of assessment, three factors have been identified as most consistent indicators of the risk of curve progression. They are curve angle (Cobb measure), Risser sign, and chronological age. These represent essentially the magnitude and maturity of the curve. For curves between 20 and 30°, Lonstein and Carlson (37) constructed a nomogram using these three measures and a risk of progression curve. Using the nomogram, a percentage of incidence of progression can be determined. The risk of progression curve was calculated from a simple formula:

$$\text{Progression factor} = \frac{\text{Cobb angle} - 3 \times \text{Risser sign}}{\text{Chronological age}}.$$

The nomogram suggests that a value for this equation greater than 1.4 is associated with a percentage incidence of progression greater than 30. Another equation designed to predict the magnitude of curve progression was presented by Yamauchi and co-workers (27). Their formula was designed to predict, within 10°, the progression of the given curve

$$Y = 7.7 + 0.132X_1 + 0.258X_2 - 0.258X_3 - 0.295x_4 - 1.620X_5$$

where
Y = expected progression (in degrees);
X_1 = standing Cobb angle (in degrees);
X_2 = percentage rotation of the apical vertebra
X_3 = deviation of the apical vertebra (in millimeters);
X_4 = Risser's expected correction: (standing Cobb − supine Cobb) × 3 (in degrees);
X_5 = maturation of the iliac apophysis: Risser sign + 1.

A prediction of 0° can be interpreted to mean that a given curve will advance no more than 10° degrees, while a prediction of 10° will lead to an expectation of progression of 20° or more.

Subjecting an asymptomatic patient with a low likelihood of progression to treatment is a disservice, while not treating a patient with a high expectation of progression is similarly inappropriate. Since the progression of the curve in a given patient cannot be determined with high accuracy, these factors give the clinician a yardstick with which to measure the aggressiveness of follow-up. A curve with a low prediction of progression may be evaluated again in a year, while a patient with a high expectation of progression should be evaluated in 3 months. Bunnell (36) has calculated the risk curve of progression (Table 11.7).

Treatment of Scoliosis (Fig. 11.13)

With the advent of large-scale school screening programs for scoliosis, statistics concerning the frequency of this problem have accumulated. Ohtsuka

Table 11.6 Scoliosis Progression[a]

Parameter	Risk of Progression
Rapid growth phase	Prior to menarche about 50%, in postmenarche girls about 20%
Risser stage less than II	Risk is 3:1
Sex	Female to male ratio is 8:1 for curves over 30%
Curve magnitude	20° curves have a risk of 20%
	30° curves have a risk of 60%
	50° curves have a risk of 90%
Curve pattern	Thoracic curves at highest risk
	Lumbar curves at lowest risk
	Thoracolumbar curves have intermediate risk
	Double major curves the same as thoracic

[a]Modified from Bunnell WP: The natural history of idiopathic scoliosis. *Clin Orthop* 229:20–25, 1988.

Table 11.7 Risk of Curve Progression[a]

Curvature	Age (years)		
	10–12	13–15	>16
<20°	25%	10%	0%
20–30°	60%	40%	10%
30–60°	90%	70%	30%
>60°	100%	90%	70%

[a]From Weinstein SL: In Bunnell WP: The natural history of idiopathic scoliosis. *Clin Orthop* 229:20–25, 1988.

and coworkers (38) reported results of screening 1.24 million Japanese school children over an 8-year period. The incidence of curves in excess of 15° ranged from 0.07% of 5th grade boys and 0.44% of girls in the same year of school to 0.25% of boys and 1.77% of girls in the second year of junior high school.

The Chiba University Medical School's supervised program began with visual screening of students in the standing, forward-flexed posture, looking at rib-hump asymmetry, then had formal Moire topography screening during the 5th-grade year. Positive Moire students were evaluated by low-dose spinal radiography. Positive low-dose radiography patients were evaluated with normal spine-imaging studies, and the appropriate treatment recommended.

These findings are consistent with other reports (36) and indicate that a large group of school children can be expected to be forwarded from school screening programs for evaluation of spinal curvature. The chiropractor interested in this problem is well-equipped to complete the evaluation and prescribe appropriate treatment (39).

The clinical examination consists of the standard screening tests with radiographic confirmation. Clinical examination includes physical parameters, Moire topography, and integrated shape and imaging system (ISIS) (40) screening (for those physicians in centers so equipped). Since ionizing radiation exposure must be minimized, especially in adolescents, the nonradiographic examinations are advised for screening and clinical follow-up in the low-risk patient. In addition, new methods of radiographic examination reduce exposure by one-half and reduce cost significantly (41).

In the adult with 45° or more of curvature and cardiopulmonary complications, surgical referral is mandatory. For adults with less than 45° and mechanical pain, the usual conservative treatment is appropriate (42). This would include spine manipulation for identified fixation of joint motion, physical therapeutic modalities such as heat, ultrasound, and electrical stimulation, as well as bracing. In the context of late-adult-onset back pain, particularly with stenotic symptoms, the clinician should be aware of the onset of scoliotic curves due to severe degenerative joint disease (43). These patients appear to have rapid progression of their curves and may require surgery to stabilize them.

Patients with idiopathic scoliosis who have not reached skeletal maturity must be evaluated for the risk of curve progression using the methods described above. Children with curves of less than 20° can be followed at 3- to 6-month intervals, nonradiographically (44). If progression of deformity is observed, radiographic confirmation should be obtained, and treatment instituted. It should be noted that the variation in measurement in Cobb-method analysis of spinal radiographs is 2.5°, therefore, given the additional errors in spinal radiography, only changes of 5° between successive films should be considered significant (45).

Curves of between 20 and 39° should be assessed with radiographs at 3- to 6-month intervals. It is noted that roughly 80% of these curves will progress. Curves in the 25 to 35° range with 50% side-bending flexibility are appropriate candidates for lateral electrical surface stimulation (46) (Table 11.8). Late results from a multicenter trial of LESS suggest that compliance remains a significant concern. Progression of the curve more than 5° warrants discontinuing LESS and instituting brace treatment.

Lateral electrical surface stimulation is an easy-to-use, nighttime therapy. The ScoliTron instrument has been developed and marketed for this purpose. The instrument stimulates muscles with a low-amperage current and cycles on and off during the treatment time. The treatment is designed to be utilized while the patient sleeps. It appears to be well tolerated. Pad placement is determined by the apex of the scoliotic curve. A line is drawn from the apex to the midaxial line, and pads are placed equidistant from the line, in the midaxial line. The pads should be separated by 4 to 6 inches. They are taped in place before each treatment and removed posttreatment, on a daily schedule. The effectiveness of the placement can be assessed radiographically if necessary. Treatment time is 8 hours, the normal adolescent sleep requirement. Excess treatment time is not harmful. Patient compliance with the treatment regimen can be evaluated through the use of an accessory instrument, the Interrogator. Normal consideration of the skin response to the adhesive should be employed. Multicenter evaluation of this treatment regime has documented its effectiveness (47).

It should be noted that orthotic treatment for pain differs from that directed to stabilizing or correcting spinal curvature. Bracing is used in pain treatment to reduce pain by limiting the motion of the injured part and allowing the reparative process of inflammation to continue unhampered. Orthotic treatment for spinal curvature is a dynamic process. The full scope of the kinematics of brace treatment is beyond this chapter, and the interested reader is referred to other texts, such as that by White and Panjabi (48).

Spinal mobility is an area of continuing biomechanical research, particularly the variation between scoliotic and normal spines (49). A well-con-

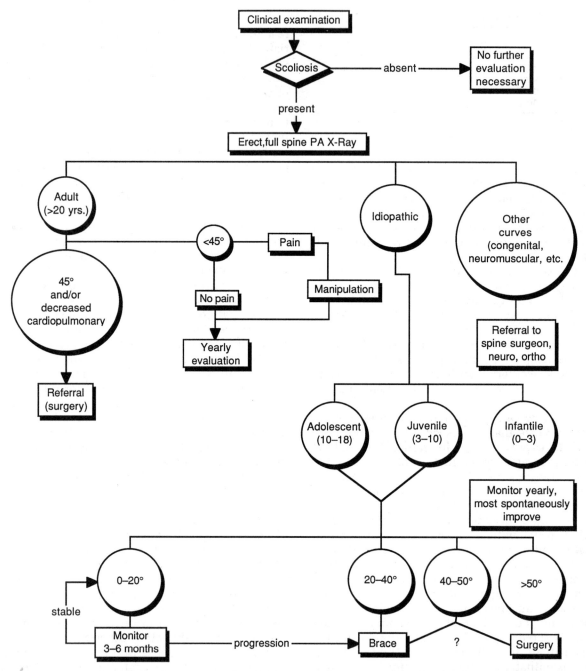

Figure 11.13. A general guide for the treatment of scoliosis. (Modified from Nykoliation JW, Cassidy JD, Arthur BE, Wedge JH: An algorithm for the management of scoliosis. *J Manip Physiol Ther* 9:1–14, 1986.)

structed spinal orthotic fixes the top and bottom of the curve and applies force to the apex of the curve in an attempt to derotate and straighten the spine. A properly designed and fitted brace must reduce the Cobb measurement of the curvature in the weightbearing radiograph from 30 to 50% to be considered adequate to halt curve progression (50). If this level of correction is not obtained, the brace must be rebuilt. Chiropractic practitioners interested in scoliosis treatment should become acquainted with the orthotists in their area, and with the reputation of each orthotist for production of adequate braces.

Initial brace correction of 75% of the curve measurement can be obtained. Although a variety of types of braces exist, the primary two are the Milwaukee and Boston appliances. These are active braces, providing pressure areas and relief areas. A passive, total-contact brace is available, known as the Wilmington plastic jacket. Active brace treatment is preferred for curve correction in nonsurgical treatment.

Table 11.8 Response of Curves to Electrical Stimulation[a]

Curve Pattern and Size	Number of Curves	Average Pretreatment Curve (degrees)	Initial Response Curve (degrees)	Average Post-treatment Curve (degrees)	Average Follow-up Curve (degrees)
Single thoracic					
20–29°	12	24 (20–29)	25 (18–36)	32 (20–44)	32 (20–44)
30–39°	6	34 (31–39)	32 (24–38)	45 (39–52)	45 (39–52)
Single thoraco-lumbar-lumbar					
20–29°	7	24 (20–28)	23 (20–28)	27 (18–34)	28 (18–34)
30–39°	1	30	30	34	34
Double major thoracic					
20–29°	21	25 (20–29)	26 (14–40)	36 (20–58)	37 (18–58)
30–39°	14	33 (30–36)	34 (25–42)	42 (30–52)	42 (31–52)
Double major thoracolumbar-lumbar					
20–29°	25	24 (20–29)	24 (17–33)	32 (16–50)	33 (16–50)
30–39°	8	32 (30–35)	27 (19–32)	35 (27–43)	34 (25–43)

[a]From *Clin Orthop* 229:109, 1988.)

The effectiveness of brace treatment remains under scrutiny (51–53). If progression of the curve continues while the patient undergoes brace treatment, consideration of surgical treatment must be undertaken.

There is little probability that curves in the 40 to 50° group will be benefited by brace treatment. Occasionally, brace treatment will halt progression of the curve or may be useful to maintain a curve until skeletal maturity and subsequent surgical management can be accomplished. Curves greater than 50° should have immediate surgical assessment. The likelihood that these curves will progress to cardiopulmonary complications is extremely high. In addition, the cosmetic deformity is great, except in compensated double curves.

Evaluation of brace treatment shows improvement in the cosmetic appearance of patients (54). Curve progression is halted but not improved in the majority of patients. Thus, the correction of scoliotic spinal deformity has not yet been attained. Aspegren and Cox (25) have reported a case utilizing spinal manipulation and electrical stimulation combined with LESS to maintain spine flexibility. The patient demonstrated curve cessation at 9-month follow-up, but not significant reduction. Physical therapy intervention was begun at 3 times per week for 3 weeks, then was reduced to a treatment of every 2 weeks. Both long-term follow-up and large-scale patient trials are required before this additional treatment regimen can be reliably recommended.

Until then, the role of the chiropractor in the conservative management of scoliosis should include (a) accurate diagnosis; (b) appropriate and timely nonradiographic clinical follow-up; (c) radiographic confirmation of curvature status when indicated; (d) advice about improvement in general health measures (e.g., manipulation, diet to provide high-level nutrient support for growth, and exercise to maintain flexible spines and strong paraspinal and support musculature); (e) institution of treatment including LESS or brace; (f) appropriate treatment monitoring and follow-up until spine maturity; and (g) referral to specialist consultation for confirmation of treatment appropriateness or surgical assessment, when indicated.

The clinician must remember that no matter what course of treatment is undertaken, the psychologic impact upon the patient is great (55). Therefore, the diagnosis and prognosis should not be presented in an exaggerated fashion. The clinician should approach the patient in a truthful and helpful fashion and be aware of all aspects of the patient's physical and psychologic health during evaluation and treatment.

FUNCTIONAL SCOLIOSIS

While the distortion associated with idiopathic or structural scoliosis can be quite obvious, nonstructural or functional scoliosis is a less dramatic but common clinical entity that is easily overlooked. Functional scoliosis is usually defined as an abnormal lateral curvature of the spine, which is flexible and disappears during flexion or side-bending movements (56–58). Functional scoliosis is generally much less progressive than idiopathic scoliosis and may be correctable by treating the underlying cause (58–64).

The classification of functional scoliosis is summarized below:

Table 11.9 Low Back Pain Associated with Leg Length Inequality[a]

Investigators	LBP Patients (N)	Controls (N)	LLI (mm)	LLI Incidence (%) LBP	Control
Giles & Taylor	1186	50	≥10	18.3	8
Stoddard	100	50	≥12.5	17	8
Rush & Steiner	1000	100	≥11	15	4
Henrard et al.	—	50	≥10	—	8
			≥5	75.4	43.5
Friberg	653	359	≥10	30.1	15.6
			≥15	11.7	2.2
Giles	300	—	≥10	13	—
Fisk & Baigent	206	—	≥12.5	6	—
Nichols	108	1007	≥10	22	7

[a]Compiled from Giles LGF, Taylor JR: Low back pain associated with leg length inequality, *Spine* 6:510–512, 1981; Stoddard A: *A Manual of Osteopathic Technique*, London, Hutchinson Medical Publications, 1959; Rush WA, Steiner HA: A study of lower extremity length inequality, *Am J Roent* 56:616–623, 1946; Henrad J-C1, Bismuth V, DeMolmont C, Gaux J-C: Unequal length of the lower limbs: measurement by a simple radiological method: application to epidemiological studies, *Rev Rhum Mal Osteoartic* 41:775–779, 1974; Friberg O: Clinical symptoms and biomechanics of lumbar spine and hip joint in leg length inequality, *Spine* 8:643–650, 1983; Giles LGF: Leg length inequalities associated with low back pain, *JCCA* 20:25–32, 1976; Fisk JW, Baigent ML: Clinical and radiological assessment of leg length, *NZ Med J* 81:477–480, 1975; Nichols PJR: Short leg syndrome, *Br Med J* 18:1863–1865, 1960.

I. Compensatory
   A. Leg length inequality (LLI)
   B. Pelvic unleveling secondary to pelvic subluxation/fixation
   C. Anatomical asymmetry
II. Postural
   A. Muscular imbalance
   B. Handedness
   C. Habitual
III. Transient
   A. Antalgic
   B. Inflammatory
   C. Traumatic

Anatomic Leg Length Inequality

Anatomical leg length inequality (LLI) is an important cause of functional scoliosis, but its overall clinical significance has been debated. Some authors have found little or no relationship between LLI and low back pain. Hult (65) concluded that an LLI of up to 3.72 cm was not associated with low back pain. Papaioannau and Kenwright (66) found that even though 6 of 23 subjects with LLI had structural scoliosis, none had degenerative disease or low back pain. More recently, Gross (67) studied runners and found that an LLI of less than 2.5 cm "did not appear to have a deleterious effect on function in marathon runners." It should be noted that these studies relied on measurements obtained with the patient in a supine static position.

Contrary to the above, many authors have found a significant correlation between LLI and low back pain. Giles and Taylor (68) found an 8% incidence of LLI of 10 mm or more in a control, compared to an 18.3% incidence in a low back pain group. These figures are in general agreement with those of other investigators (69–74) (Table 11.9). All of these studies used radiographic methods to determine LLI, with the exception of Nichols (75) who used clinical findings. Aside from back pain, Giles and Taylor (76) found that an LLI of 10 mm or more was associated with a higher incidence of structural asymmetry in the vertebral bodies of the lumbar vertebrae. Early appearance of traction spurs were also noted, suggesting asymmetric degeneration of the intervertebral discs. Degenerative joint disease of the hip has been noted to occur more frequently on the side of the long leg (72, 77, 78).

Causes of Leg Length Inequality Resulting in Compensatory Scoliosis

   A. Lower Extremity
     1. Asymmetrical growth of tibia or femur
     2. Previous fracture
     3. Immobilization, especially during growth years
     4. Foot pronation or supination
     5. Femoral neck deformity of hip rotation
     6. Knee meniscectomy
     7. Radiation therapy
   B. Pelvis
     1. Sacroiliac subluxation/fixation
     2. Lumbosacral subluxation/fixation
     3. Asymmetrical pelvic size (small hemipelvis)
   C. Spine
     1. Quadratus lumborum, psoas, or sacrospinalis imbalance
     2. Upper cervical subluxation/fixation

Given the significance of anatomical LLI, questions arise about the significance of functional LLI and its association with altered biomechanics and potential pain production. Functional LLI occurs when the apparent length of anatomically equal legs is made unequal due to a functional problem or a change in the alignment of an adjacent anatomical structure. For example, if the left ilium is fixed in a flexed position and/or the right ilium is fixed in relative extension, the relative position of the acetabulae changes, causing the left leg to appear short and the right leg to appear long (57, 58, 79–85).

The ilium fixed in a flexed position has been termed a "PI" (posterior inferior) ilium, using the

Table 11.10 Clinical Findings with Sacroiliac Subluxation

	Iliac Crest (standing)	Trochanter (standing)	Iliac Crest (prone)	Leg Length (supine/prone)	Leg Length (sitting)	PSIS (prone)	ASIS (supine)	Lumbar Scoliosis
Flexed ilium (PI)	Low	Level	High	Short	Long	Posterior inferior	Posterior superior	Ipsilateral
Extended ilium (AS)	High	Level	Low	Long	Short	Anterior superior	Anterior inferior	Contralateral
Anatomical leg length deficiency	Low	Low	Level	Short	Short	Level	Level	Ipsilateral
Unilateral quadratus lumborum or paraspinal spasm	High	Level	High	Possibly short	Even	Superior	Superior	Contralateral

posterior superior iliac spine (PSIS) as a reference point. The "AS" ilium is an ilium fixed in extension. The degree of functional leg length inequality that results from these malpositions depends on the degree of malposition and the range of motion of the patient's sacroiliac joints. As the ilium flexes, the following occurs:

1. PSIS moves posteriorly and inferiorly;
2. ASIS and ipsilateral pubis move superiorly;
3. Acetabulum moves anteriorly, laterally and slightly superiorly, causing functional shortening of the leg;
4. Iliac crest rotates slightly superiorly;
5. Sacrum moves relatively anteriorly and inferiorly on the ipsilateral side.

When the patient is standing, the pelvis is low on the PI side because of weightbearing on the short leg (58). An ipsilateral lumbar scoliosis generally results (57, 84, 86). Since most of the acetabular movement is in an anterolateral direction, there is minimal change in the palpable relative height of the greater trochanters. In contrast, with a simple anatomical LLI, there is a one-to-one relationship between drop in pelvic height and drop in trochanteric height. These and related findings are summarized in Table 11.10.

The anterior position of the acetabulum, which contributes to the functional leg shortening of a PI ilium, causes a change in leg length as the patient goes from a supine to a sitting position (58, 81, 87). As the patient sits, the relatively short leg becomes the long leg, because the anterior acetabular position adds leg length when the femur is flexed perpendicular to the trunk (i.e., 90° hip flexion) (Fig. 11.14, Table 11.10). This test is thus a valuable quick-screening test for pelvic obliquity. If simple anatomical LLI is present, no change in relative leg length will occur during the change from the supine to the sitting position.

Use of the above clinical criteria is extremely valuable to the diagnosis of pelvic subluxation and the differentiation of anatomical and functional LLI (Table 11.10). If an anatomical discrepancy is diagnosed, it can be quantified by a standing radiograph. Error and distortion can be minimized by directing the central ray through the level of the femur heads

(89), but many mathematical formulas have been developed to compensate for projectional distortion (83, 89–91).

Since it is possible for the pelvis to cause functional leg length change, the capacity exists for the pelvis to compensate for anatomical LLI (58, 92, 93). When this occurs, the standing iliac crest height will be more level than the trochanter height (Fig. 11.15), and the scoliosis is reduced. In this situation it may be inadvisable to correct the pelvic subluxation, unless shoe-lift therapy is being contemplated, since removal of the compensation would increase the scoliosis.

More frequent than compensation, however, is some variation of the basic distortion pattern first described by Lovett and Logan and expanded by Carver, Illi, Janse and others (94, 95). In the standing posture, this basic pattern includes the following:

1. Low trochanter and ilium on the side of the shorter leg;
2. Inferior and anterior tipping of the sacral base on the side of the shorter leg;
3. Lumbar scoliosis with convexity to the side of shorter leg;
4. Lumbar vertebral rotation toward the longer leg side (i.e., spinous process rotation into the concavity of the curve) if segments are freely moveable.

The frequency of this pattern was evaluated in 53 functional scoliosis patients by Vernon and Bureau (94). They observed that all of these parameters occurred with significant frequency except for the lumbar vertebral rotation, which was variable. Cyriax (63) and Barge (64) have reported that rotation of L5 can cause lateral pelvic tilt that is correctable by lumbar manipulation.

Having observed the relationship of anatomical and functional LLI to low back pain, the question is how small a difference in leg length inequality is significant. Travell and Simons (96) state that "a discrepancy of 0.5 cm (³/₁₆ in), if uncorrected, can perpetuate myofascial trigger points, e.g., in the quadratus lumborum after trigger points have been activated by gross or obscure trauma." They also state (96) that any discrepancy of 5 mm or more should be corrected (by shoe lift) if low back symp-

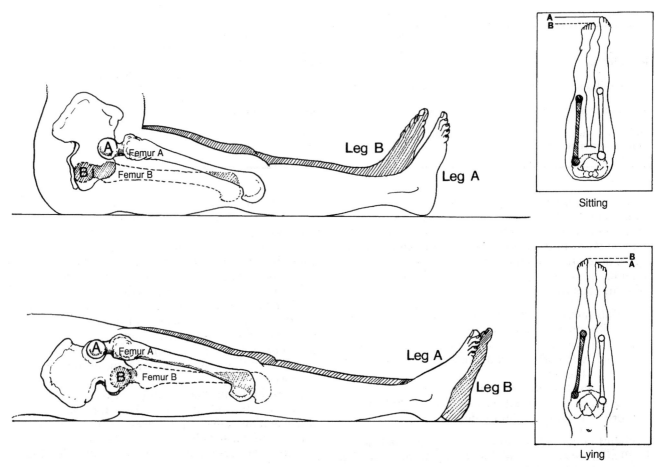

Figure 11.14. Relative changes observed in functional leg length during change from supine to sitting when a simple sacroiliac subluxation/fixation is present. *Leg A* represents the side of the PI ilium (flexion malposition) and *leg B* the AS ilium (extension malposition). Because of the relative anterior displacement of the actetabulum resulting from the flexed ilium (and opposite for the extended ilium), the leg that is functionally short reverses as the patient sits and the hip joint is flexed to 90°.

toms coexist and that a discrepancy of 1.3 cm (½ inch) or more should be corrected, even in the absence of symptoms.

Travell and Simons (96, 97) emphasize the quadratus lumborum as "by far the most commonly overlooked source of low back pain" and speak of trigger points in this muscle as being an effect of an unlevel pelvis and a potential cause of functional LLI. They (96) and others (98, 99) have also observed myofascial pain syndrome occurring in the scalenes, levator scapulae, upper trapezius, sternocleidomastoideus, and the muscles of mastication as a result of pelvic unleveling. Headaches are also mentioned as a potential result of this sequence.

Giles (73) agreed that a 5-mm LLI is clinically significant. Greenman (59) stated that any sacral base unleveling of greater than 4 mm was clinically significant, and Sharpe (77) found an LLI of over ½ inch to be clinically significant. Subotnick (84) considers correction necessary when leg length discrepancy is ⅛ inch or greater, when associated imbal-

ance symptoms exist. Schafer (58) observes that, if prolonged walking or standing does not aggravate a low back pain syndrome, it is unlikely that a small LLI is a significant factor in the syndrome. Clinical assessment of relatively small differences in leg length has been shown to be reliable (100, 101).

Cervical Causes of Functional Scoliosis

In addition to the more obvious causes of functional scoliosis already mentioned, the cervical spine may serve as a primary cause of a functionally short leg and/or scoliosis. As early as 1934, Coutts (102) noted that upper cervical subluxation can result in spinal distortion. Vernon (103) observes that postural imbalances can occur as a result of alteration of the proprioceptive input the cervical spine supplies to the cerebellum, vestibular nuclei, cuneatus, etc. Sandoz (104) observed the relationship that the mechanoreceptors responsible for the tonic neck reflexes have with the rest of the spine. These receptors are located between occiput, atlas, and axis. Sandoz states that in the presence of

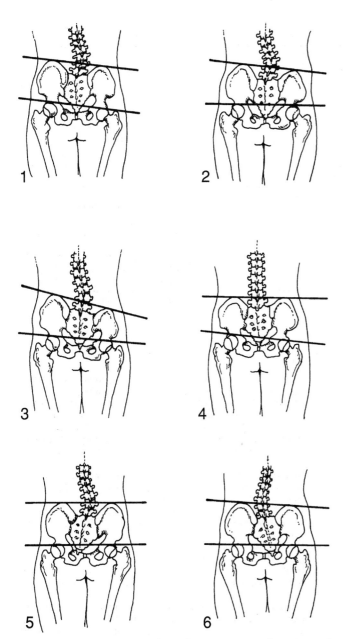

Figure 11.15. Common clinical presentation of anatomical leg length inequality (LLI) and/or pelvic subluxation/fixation observed with the patient standing. **1,** Uncomplicated LLI. Note that intercrestal and intertrochanteric lines are parallel. **2,** Uncomplicated sacroiliac subluxation/fixation, i.e., left AS ilium (extension malposition) and/or right PI ilium (flexion malposition). Functional shortening of the right leg results in lowering of the ipsilateral iliac crest. **3,** LLI (right short leg) with right PI and/or left AS ilium. **4,** LLI (right short leg) with left PI and/or right AS ilium, i.e., compensation. **5,** Sacral fixation. Note pelvis and trochanters are level. **6,** Sacral fixation with opposing pelvic tilt.

mechanical dysfunction, these mechanoreceptors are capable of producing secondary derangement in the rest of the spine, the pelvis, and even the lower extremities by creating imbalance in muscle tone between the left and right sides (103). Cervical joint

receptors have also been described by Wyke (105) and Vernon (103).

Lewit (86) has observed correction of pelvis distortion and associated scoliosis by manipulation of the upper cervical spine. It is observed in chiropractic practice that an LLI is associated with primary upper cervical dysfunction (101, 106–108), and a test has been described by Thompson (109), Shambaugh et al. (101) and O'Keefe (110) which can help to determine cervical involvement. Relative leg length is monitored as the patient rotates the head to each side. Change of relative leg length during this maneuver suggests possible primary cervical involvement (111, 101).

Treatment of Leg Length Inequality

Treatment of leg length inequality (LLI) depends on careful clinical and radiographic evaluation of the patient to determine the degree of anatomical versus functional discrepancy. If anatomical difference predominates, then shoe-lift therapy is appropriate. Generally, this is done with a heel lift that adds length to the short leg, although shoes may also be altered by adding to the sole of the short leg and/or subtracting height from the longer side (58, 59). The amount of correction is determined by the difference in femur head heights on the radiograph or by the amount of correction needed to bring the sacrum or L5 level. This will usually correlate clinically with palpable and observable leveling of the iliac crests.

Amount of Lift

Logan (95) and Steinbach (112) have shown that a 1:2:4 ratio exists between the lumbar spine, the sacrum, and the plantar heel. According to this ratio, raising the heel 8 mm will raise the ipsilateral sacral base 4 mm and the ipsilateral lumbar spine 2 mm. This formula is helpful in determining the amount of correction needed to achieve a desired amount of elevation of the sacrum or L5. Since a one-to-one relationship exists between the heel and femoral head height, lift size should be chosen accordingly when simple femur head leveling is desired.

Most authors agree that this should be done in increments rather than all at once (58), and it is generally considered safer to lift slightly less than the measured discrepancy to avoid overcorrection (58, 113, 114). Gonstead (83), however, advocates using a lift matching the full discrepancy. For a discrepancy greater than approximately 10 mm, it is advisable to add half of the correction to the sole of the shoe or also subtract height from the opposite heel (58, 59, 114) (see Table 11.11).

As previously mentioned, opinions differ about exactly how much anatomical discrepancy requires application of a lift. This is summarized in Table 11.12 (58, 59, 68, 72, 83, 84, 96, 115, 117).

Table 11.11 Treatment of Leg Length Inequality: Common Distortions and Related Shoe Lift Applications[a]

Type	Lateral Distortions Ipsilateral Application	Contralateral Application
Lumbar scoliosis (convexity)	Heel lift	Sole lift or heel drop
Sacral anteroinferiority	Heel lift	Sole lift or heel drop
Sacral posterosuperiority	Sole lift or heel drop	Heel lift
Iliac anterosuperiority	Sole lift or heel drop	Heel lift
Iliac posteroinferiority	Heel lift	Sole lift or heel drop
Unilateral pelvic anteriority	Sole lift or heel drop	Heel lift
Unilateral pelvic posteriority	Heel lift	Sole lift or heel drop
Unilateral low femur head	Plantar lift	
Unilateral short ischium	Ischial lift	

Type	Anteroposterior Distortions Application
Sprung back (lumbar)	Bilateral heel lifts
Kissing spines (lumbar)	Bilateral sole lifts or heel drops
Lumbar hyperlordosis	Bilateral sole lifts or heel drops
Lumbar flattening	Bilateral heel lifts
Fixed pelvic anterior tilt	Bilateral sole lifts or heel drops
Fixed pelvic posterior tilt	Bilateral heel lifts

[a]Modified from Schafer RC: *Clinical Biomechanics Musculoskeletal Actions and Reactions*, ed 2. Baltimore, Williams & Wilkins, 1987, p 618.

Table 11.12 Leg Length Inequality Requiring Lift Therapy[a]

Author	Leg Length Inequality
Subotnick	≥3 mm (⅛ inch)
Greenman	>4 mm sacral base unleveling
Giles & Taylor	>5 mm
Friberg	>5 mm
Travell & Simons	≥5 mm—(back pain)
	≥13 mm (½ inch)—(no back pain)
Gonstead	>6 mm (¼ inch)
Schafer	>6 mm
Cailliet	≥19 mm (¾ inch)
Anderson	>19 mm

[a]Compiled from Subotnick SI: Limb discrepancies of the lower extremity (the short leg syndrome), *JOSPT* 3:11–16, 1981; Greenman PE: Lift therapy, use and abuse, *JAOA* 79:238–250, 1979; Giles LGF, Taylor JR: Low back pain associated with leg length inequality, *Spine* 6:510–512, 1981; Friberg O: Clinical symptoms and biomechanics of lumbar spine and hip joint in leg length inequality, *Spine* 8:643–650, 1983; Travell JG, Simons DG: *Myofascial Pain and Dysfunction: The Trigger Point Manual*, Baltimore, Williams & Wilkins, 1983; Herbst RW: *Gonstead Chiropractic Science and Art*, Sci-Chi Publications, 1981; Shafer RC: *Clinical Biomechanics Musculoskeletal Actions and Reactions*, ed 2, Baltimore, Williams & Wilkins, 1987; Cailliet R: *Scoliosis Diagnosis and Management*, Philadelphia, FA Davis, 1975; Anderson VW: *Modern Trends in Orthopedics*, East Norwalk, CT, Appleton-Century-Crofts, 1972.

POSTURE AND MECHANICAL STRESS OF THE SPINE

Faulty posture creates mechanical stress and weakness of the human spine. It has an insidious effect upon the articulations of the vertebral column (117). Mechanical stress upon an area of the spine is likely to produce distortion at the vertebral segment that is an apex or a transition within the compensatory rotatory scolioses (117). Uncompensated distortions are often accompanied by upper cervical fixations that result from maintenance of the head in proper relation to the environment. Descending compensatory effects of the spine in response to upper cervical fixations also recur. In either case, manipulation of the offending primary site is essential if postural retraining is to be effective (117).

References

1. Michele AA: *Iliopsoas Development of Anomalies in Man.* Springfield IL, Charles C Thomas, 1962, p 384.
2. Metheny E: In Rasch PJ, Burke RK: *Kinesiology and Applied Anatomy: The Science of Human Movement*, ed 5. Philadelphia, Lea & Febiger, 1974, p 451.
3. Goldthwait JE: The opportunity for the orthopedist in preventive medicine through education work on posture. *J Orthop Surg* 14:443, 1916.
4. Steindler A: *Kinesiology of the Human Body Under Normal and Pathological Conditions.* Springfield, IL, Charles C Thomas, 1955, pp 126, 227, 364.
5. Jones L: *The Postural Complex Observations as to Cause, Diagnosis and Treatment.* Springfield, IL, Charles C Thomas, 1955, p 5.
6. Warwick R, Williams PL: *Gray's Anatomy*, ed 35, Philadelphia, WB Saunders, p 248.
7. Kendall HO, Kendall FP, Wadsworth GE: *Muscle Testing and Function*, ed 2. Baltimore, Williams & Wilkins, 1971, pp 18–19, 22, 201–239.
8. Kapandji IA: *The Physiology of the Joints*, ed 2. London, Churchill Livingstone, 1974, vol 3, p 20.
9. Winterstein RW: *Chiropractic Spinography: A Manual of Technology and Interpretation*, ed 2. Baltimore, Williams & Wilkins, 1985, p 91.
10. Magnus R: Physiology of posture. *Lancet*, 2:531–536, 1926.
11. Gowitzke BA, Milner M: *Understanding the Scientific Bases of Human Movement*, ed 2. Baltimore, Williams & Wilkins, 1980, pp 277–278, 305–306, 311.
12. Wells KF, Luttgens K: *Kinesiology: Scientific Basis of Human Motion*, ed 6. Philadelphia, WB Saunders, 1926, p 58.
13. McCouch GP, Deering ID, Ling TH: Location of receptors for tonic neck reflexes. *J Neurophysiol* 14:191–195, 1951.
14. Pervin LA: *Personality: Theory, Assessment & Research.* New York, John Wiley & Sons, 1970, pp 10–13.
15. Goldthwait JE, Brown LT, Swain LT, Kuhns JG: Essentials of body mechanics. In *Health and Disease*, ed 5. Philadelphia, JB Lippincott, 1952, pp 8–29.
16. Sheldon WH: Constitutional factors in personality. In Hunt JV (ed): *Personality and Behavior Disorders.* New York, Ronald, 1944, pp 526–549.
17. Cailliet R: *Low Back Pain*, ed 2. Philadelphia, FA Davis, 1968, pp 14, 16, 58–71.
18. Brunnstrom S: *Clinical Kinesiology.* Philadelphia, FA Davis, 1979, pp 235–281.

19. Buswell J: Exercises in the treatment of vertebral dysfunction. In Grieve GP: *Modern Manual Therapy of the Vertebral Column*. Edinburgh, Churchill Livingstone, 1986, pp 834–838.

20. Johnston CM: A report of findings and observations regarding the use of the posturometer and posturizer. *JCCA*, 1964, pp 10–13.

21. Lovett RW: *Lateral Curvature of the Spine and Round Shoulders*, ed 2. Philadelphia, P Blakiston's Son, 1913, p 44.

22. Cailliet R: *Scoliosis Diagnosis and Management*. Philadelphia, FA Davis, 1975, p 2.

23. Axelgaard J, Brown JC: Lateral electrical surface stimulation for the treatment of progressive idiopathic scoliosis. *Spine* 8:242–260, 1983.

24. Brown JC, Axelgaard J, Howson DC: Multicenter trial of a noninvasive stimulation method for idiopathic scoliosis: a summary of early treatment results. *Spine* 9:382–387, 1984.

25. Aspegren DD, Cox JM: Correction of progressive idiopathic scoliosis utilizing neuromuscular stimulation and manipulation: A case report. *J Manip Physiol Ther* 10:147–156, 1987.

26. Rinsky LA, Gamble JG: Adolescent idiopathic scoliosis. *West J Med* 148:182–191, 1988.

27. The Terminology Committee of the Scoliosis Research Society: A glossary of scoliosis terms. *Spine* 1(1):57–58, 1976.

28. Yamauchi Y, Yamaguchi T, Asaka Y: Prediction of curve progression in idiopathic scoliosis based on initial roentgenograms: a proposal of an equation. *Spine* 13:1258–1261, 1988.

29. Nash CL, Moe JG: A study of vertebral rotation. *J Bone Joint Surg (Am)* 5(2):223, 1969.

30. Mannherz RE, Betz RR, Clancy M, Steel HH: Juvenile idiopathic scoliosis followed to skeletal maturity. *Spine* 13:1087–1090, 1988.

31. Suh PB, MacEwen GD: Idiopathic scoliosis in males: a natural history study. *Spine* 13:1091–1095, 1988.

32. Bunnell WP: The natural history of idiopathic scoliosis before skeletal maturity. *Spine* 11:780–783, 1986.

33. Picault D, DeMauroy JC, Mouilleseaux B, Kiana G: Natural history of idiopathic scoliosis in girls and boys. *Spine* 1:777–778, 1986.

34. Weinstein SL: Idiopathic scoliosis natural history. *Spine* 11:780–783, 1986.

35. Ascani E, Bartolozzi P, Logroscina CA, Marchetti PG, Ponte A, Savini R, Travaglini F, Binazzi R, Di Silvestre M: Natural history of untreated idiopathic scoliosis after skeletal maturity. *Spine* 11:784–789, 1986.

36. Bunnell WP: The natural history of idiopathic scoliosis. *Clin Orthop* 229:20–25, 1988.

37. Lonstein JE, Carlson JM: The prediction of curve progression in untreated idiopathic scoliosis during growth. *J Bone Joint Surg* 66:1061–1071, 1974.

38. Ohtsuka Y, Yamagata M, Arai S, Kitahara H, Minami S: School screening for scoliosis by the Chiba University Medical School screening program: results of 1.24 million students over an 8-year period. *Spine* 13:1251–1257, 1988.

39. Nykoliation JW, Cassidy JD, Arthur BE, Wedge JH: An algorithm for the management of scoliosis. *J Manip Physiol Ther* 9:1–14, 1986.

40. Weisz I, Jefferson RJ, Turner-Smith AR, Houghton GR, Garris JD: ISIS scanning: a useful assessment technique in the management of scoliosis. *Spine* 13:405–408, 1988.

41. Manninen H, Kiekara O, Soimakallio S, Vainio J: Reduction of radiation dose and imaging costs in scoliosis radiography: application of large-screen image intensifer photofluorography. *Spine* 13:409–412, 1988.

42. Bradford DS: Adult scoliosis current concepts of treatment. *Clin Orthop* 229:70–87, 1988.

43. Grubb SA, Lipscomb HJ, Coonrad RW: Degenerative adult onset scoliosis. *Spine* 13:241–245, 1988.

44. Keller RB: Nonoperative treatment of adolescent idiopathic scoliosis. In *American Academy of Orthopaedic Surgeons Instructional Course Lectures* 38:129–135, 1989.

45. Goldberg MS, Poitras B, Mayo NE, Labelle H, Bourassa R, Cloutier R: Observer variation in assessing spinal curvature and skeletal development in adolescent idiopathic scoliosis. *Spine* 13:1371–1377, 1988.

46. Sullivan JA, Davidson R, Renshaw TS, Emans JB, Johnston C, Sussman M: Further evaluation of the Scolitron treatment of idiopathic adolescent scoliosis. *Spine* 11:903–906, 1986.

47. McCollough NC: Nonoperative treatment of idiopathic scoliosis using surface electrical stimulation. *Spine* 11:802–804, 1986.

48. White AA, Panjabi MM: *Clinical Biomechanics of the Spine*. Philadelphia, JB Lippincott, 1978.

49. Poussa M, Harkonen H, Mellin G: Spinal mobility in adolescent girls with idiopathic scoliosis and in structurally normal controls. *Spine* 14:217–219, 1989.

50. Kehl DK, Morrissy RT: Brace treatment in adolescent idiopathic scoliosis and update on concepts and techniques. *Clin Orthop* 229:34–43, 1988.

51. Chase AP, Bader DL, Houghton GR: The biomechanical effectiveness of the Boston brace in the management of adolescent idiopathic scoliosis. *Spine* 14:636–642, 1989.

52. Winter RB, Lonstein JE, Drogt J, Noren CA: The effectiveness of bracing in the nonoperative treatment of idiopathic scoliosis. *Spine* 11:790–791, 1986.

53. Emans JB, Kaelin A, Bancel P, Hall HE, Miller ME: The Boston bracing system for idiopathic scoliosis follow-up results in 295 patients. *Spine* 11:792–801, 1986.

54. Weisz I, Jefferson RJ, Carr AJ, Turner-Smith AR, McInerney A, Houghton GR: Back shape in brace treatment of idiopathic scoliosis. *Clin Orthop* 240:157–163, 1989.

55. Kahanovitz N, Weiser S: The psychological impact of idiopathic scoliosis on the adolescent female: A preliminary multi-center study. *Spine* 14:483–485, 1989.

56. Grimes HA: Scoliosis. *J Arkansas Med Soc* 71(11):375–379, 1975.

57. Magee DJ: *Orthopedic Physical Assessment*. Philadelphia, WB Saunders, 1987, pp 221, 383.

58. Schafer RC: *Clinical Biomechanics Musculoskeletal Actions and Reactions*, ed 2. Baltimore, Williams & Wilkins, 1987, pp 578, 607–610, 614, 617–619.

59. Greenman PE: Lift therapy, use and abuse. *JAOA* 79:238–250, 1979.

60. Cyriax E: Some common postural deformities and their treatment by exercise and manipulation. *Br J Phys Med* 2(6):202–207, 1938.

61. Darr A: Should I prescribe a heel lift? *ACA J Chiro* 5(2):511–512, 1968.

62. Carver W: *Carver's Chiropractic Analysis*. Oklahoma City, Semco Color Press, 1921, p 582.

63. Cyriax E: On lateral tilts of the pelvis in children. *Br J Child Dis* 30:274–281, 1933.

64. Barge FN: *Scoliosis*. Davenport, Bawden Printing, 1981, pp 17–49.

65. Hult L: Cervical, dorsal, lumbar spine syndromes. *Acta Orthop Scand Suppl* 17:35, 1954.

66. Papaioannau M, Kenwright J: Scoliosis associated with limb length inequality. *J Bone Joint Surg* 64A:69–53, 1982.

67. Gross RH: Leg length discrepancy in marathon runners. *Am J Sports Med* 11:121–124, 1983.

68. Giles LGF, Taylor JR: Low back pain associated with leg length inequality. *Spine* 6(5):510–512, 1981.

69. Stoddard A: *A Manual of Osteopathic Technique*. London, Hutchinson Medical Publications, 1959, p 212.

70. Rush WA, Steiner HA: A study of lower extremity length inequality. *Am J Roent* 56:616–623, 1946.

71. Henrard J-Cl, Bismuth V, DeMolmont C, Gaux J-C: Unequal length of the lower limbs: measurement by a simple radiological method: application to epidemiological studies. *Rev Rhum Mal Osteoartic* 41:775–779, 1974.

72. Friberg O: Clinical symptoms and biomechanics of lumbar spine and hip joint in leg length inequality. *Spine* 8(6)643–650, 1983.

73. Giles LGF: Leg length inequalities associated with low back pain. *JCCA* 20:25–32, 1976.
74. Fisk JW, Baigent ML: Clinical and radiological assessment of leg length. *NZ Med J* 81:477–480, 1975.
75. Nichols PJR: Short leg syndrome. *Br Med J* 18:1863–1865, 1960.
76. Giles LGF, Taylor JR: Lumbar spine structural changes associated with leg length inequality. *Spine* 7(2):159–162, 1982.
77. Sharpe CR: Leg length inequality. *Can Fam Physician* 29:333–336, 1983.
78. Gofton JP, Trueman GE. Studies in osteoarthritis of the hip (part II): osteoarthritis of the hip and leg length disparity. *Can Med Assoc* 104:791–799, 1971.
79. Fowler C: In Grieve GP (ed): *Modern Manual Therapy of the Vertebral Column.* New York, Churchill Livingstone, 1986, pp 805–814.
80. Grieve GP (ed): *Modern Manual Therapy of the Vertebral Column.* Churchill Livingstone, 1986, p 467.
81. DonTigny RL: Function and pathomechanics of the sacroiliac joint. *Phys Ther* 65:35–44, 1985.
82. Gitelman R: In Haldeman S: *Modern Developments in the Principles and Practice of Chiropractic.* East Norwalk, CT, Appleton-Century-Crofts, 1980, pp 286, 307.
83. Herbst RW: *Gonstead Chiropractic Science and Art.* Sci-Chi Publications, pp 25–38, 1981.
84. Subotnick SI: Limb discrepancies of the lower extremity (the short leg syndrome). *JOSPT* 3(1):11–16, 1981.
85. Bourdillon JF: *Spinal Manipulation,* ed 3. East Norwalk, CT, Appleton-Century-Crofts, pp 21–23, 62, 1982.
86. Lewit K: *Manipulative Therapy in the Rehabilitation of the Locomotor System.* Boston, Butterworth, 1985, pp 49–54, 62.
87. Saunders HD: *Evaluation, Treatment and Prevention of Musculoskeletal Disorders.* Minneapolis, Viking, 1985, p 24.
88. Giles LGF, Taylor JR: *Spine* 8(6):643, 1988.
89. Winterstein JF: *Chiropractic Spinography.* Wheaton, IL, Kjellberg, 1970.
90. Hildebrandt RW: *Chiropractic Spinography.* Des Plaines, IL, Hillmark, 1977, pp 214–226.
91. Phillips RB: The use of x-rays in spinal manipulative therapy. In Haldeman S: *Modern Developments in the Principles and Practice of Chiropractic.* East Norwalk, CT, Appleton-Century-Crofts, 1980, p 194.
92. Gillet H, Liekens M: Belgian Chiropractic Research Notes. Huntington Beach, Motion Palpation Institute, 1981.
93. Bourdillon JF: *Spinal Manipulation,* ed 4. East Norwalk, CT, Appleton-Century-Crofts, 1987.
94. Vernon H, Bureau J: A radiographic study of the incidence of low sacral base and lumbar lateral curvature related to the presence of an apparent short leg. *JCCA* 27(1):11–15, 1983.
95. Logan VF, Murray FM (eds): *Textbook of Logan Basic Methods* (from the original manuscript by HB Logan). St Louis, Logan Chiropractic College, 1950.
96. Travell JG, Simons DG: *Myofascial Pain and Dysfunction: The Trigger Point Manual.* Baltimore, Williams & Wilkins, 1983, pp 104–107.
97. Travell JG: The quadratus lumborum muscle: an overlooked cause of low back pain. *Arch Phys Med Rehabil* 57:566, 1976.
98. Liebenson CS: Thoracic outlet syndrome: diagnosis and conservative management. *JMPT* 11(6):493–499, 1988.
99. Sallstrom J, Celegin Z: Physiotherapy in patients with thoracic outlet syndrome. *Vasa* 12:257–261, 1983.
100. DeBoer KF, Harmon RG, Savoie S, Tuttle CD. Inter- and intra-examiner reliability of leg length differential measurement: a preliminary study. *JMPT* 6(2):61–66.
101. Shambaugh P, Sclafani L, Fanselow D: Reliability of the Derefield-Thompson test for leg length inequality and use of the test to demonstrate cervical adjusting efficacy. *JMPT* 11(5):396–399, 1988.
102. Coutts MB: Atlanto-epistropheal subluxations. *Arch Surg* 29:297–311, 1934.
103. Vernon H: *Upper Cervical Syndrome: Chiropractic Diagnosis and Treatment.* Baltimore, Williams & Wilkins, 1988, pp 79–80.
104. Sandoz R: Some reflex phenomena associated with spinal derangements and adjustments. *Am Swiss Chiro Assoc* 7:45–65, 1981.
105. Wyke B: Neurology of the cervical spinal joints. *Physiotherapy* 65(3):72–76, 1974.
106. Seeman DC: CI subluxations, short leg and pelvic distortions. *J Aust Chiro Assoc* 2:1–5, 1979.
107. Seeman DC: CI problems, short leg and pelvic distortions. *Upper Cerv Monogr* 2(5):1–5, 1978.
108. Gregory RR: A model for the supine leg check. *Upper Cerv Monogr* 2(6):1–5, 1979.
109. Thompson JC: *Derefield-Thompson Leg Check.* Davenport, Palmer College of Chiropractic, 1973.
110. O'Keefe JJ: *Thompson Technique Reference Manual.* Elgin, Williams Manufacturing, 1984.
111. West HG: Physical and spinal examination procedures utilized in the practice of chiropractic. In Haldeman S: *Modern Developments in the Principles and Practice of Chiropractic.* East Norwalk, CT, Appleton-Century-Crofts, 1980, pp 286–287.
112. Steinbach LL: *Spinal Balance and Spinal Hygiene.* Pittsburgh, LL Steinbach, 1957.
113. Cox JM: *Low Back Pain Mechanism, Diagnosis and Treatment,* ed 4. Baltimore, Williams & Wilkins, 1985, p 124.
114. Danbert RJ: Clinical assessment and treatment of leg length inequalities. *JMPT* 11(4):290–295.
115. Anderson WV: *Modern Trends in Orthopedics.* East Norwalk, CT, Appleton-Century-Crofts, 1972, pp 1–22.
116. Cailliet R: *Scoliosis Diagnosis and Management.* Philadelphia, FA Davis, 1975, p 40.
117. Homewood EA: *The Neurodynamics of the Vertebral Subluxation,* ed 3. St. Petersburg, FL, Valkyrie, 1977, pp 52, 195.
118. Yochum TR, Rowe LJ: *Essentials of Skeletal Radiology.* Baltimore, Williams & Wilkins, 1986.

CHAPTER 12

Muscle and Myofascial Pain Syndromes

MERIDEL I. GATTERMAN, M.A., D.C.
DONALD R. GOE, Ph.D., D.C.

The great majority of "pain patients" treated in pain centers by anaesthesiologists and psychiatrists, i.e., pharmacologically and psychologically, have undiagnosed problems of the motor system. Lewit (1)

The high prevalence of pain originating from muscles is not surprising since collectively, voluntary (skeletal) muscle constitutes the largest single tissue mass in the human body, accounting for 40% or more of body weight (2). What is surprising is how little emphasis is placed on the pathophysiology of muscles in both chiropractic and medical curricula. While the primary emphasis of chiropractic therapy is treatment by manipulation of joint dysfunction, concomitantly injured muscles, when left untreated, significantly prolong healing time and often result in unnecessary disability.

The residuals of muscle strain, whether due to repeated microtrauma or frank traumatic incidents, are characterized by tender areas readily palpable in the involved muscles. It is postulated that left untreated these localized tender points can progress to multiple areas of tenderness with systemic manifestations.

Typically, patients with widespread complaints of muscle pain, sleep disturbance, and mood swings have experienced major stressful life situations at the time of onset of their symptoms. They frequently report frightening but minor automobile or industrial accidents, or they have been helplessly involved in unsolvable domestic difficulties (3).

The consistent location of tender points at sites where mechanical stress in the muscles appears to be greatest (4, 5) implicates postural strain, possibly due to imbalance between agonist and antagonistic muscles. The most common sites of persistent tender points are the postural stabilizers (fixators) of the upper extremities (4, 5) and the rotator muscles of the hip and shoulders (5, 6).

With injury to the muscle, the pain-spasm-pain cycle is self-sustaining. The theory is that the entire symptom complex is an expression of reflex mechanisms, which once initiated, are self-sustaining by implication of closed, self-reexciting chains of internuncial neurons in the central nervous system (7). If the stimulation exceeds the threshold, a reflex cycle is set up whereby the sensation of pain may be referred to another area, with ultimate involvement of the autonomic nervous system (4).

LOCALIZED VERSUS SYSTEMIC MANIFESTATIONS OF MUSCLE PAIN

The term myofascial pain syndrome, popularized by Travell and Simons, (8) refers to pain originating from a specific muscle or muscle group. The widespread pain noted in multiple unrelated muscles and accompanied by systemic complaints is referred to as fibromyalgia (fibrositis) (9) (Table 12.1). Differentiation of what may at first appear to be two distinct clinical entities may be unnecessary, if one considers that unresolved myofascial pain can progress from a localized related group of muscles to involve multiple unrelated areas. Perhaps the chronic pain that results ultimately from the pain-spasm-pain cycle (8), through neurological channels, begins to affect more and more muscle areas, eventually involving also the autonomic nervous system.

This progression may account for the plethora of terms (8) used indiscriminately to describe muscle pain syndromes (Table 12.2), which may be stages (8) on a continuum of muscle dysfunction (Table 12.3). Adding to the controversy has been the paucity of objective findings necessary to characterize the various stages. Predisposing, precipitating, and

Table 12.1 Comparison of Myofascial Pain and Fibromyalgia Syndromes[a]

Characteristic	Myofascial Pain Syndrome	Primary Fibromyalgia Syndrome
Tenderness	Trigger points: belly and insertion	Multiple tender points
Pain	Referred pain	Generalized aching
Duration	Muscle specific—if untreated becomes chronic	Chronic—more than 3 months
Sex	Equal number of males and females	80% female
Prevalence	Common, 50% male and female	Uncommon, 4% primary, 11% secondary
Disturbed sleep pattern	Common secondary to discomfort due to position	Sleep disorder by definition greater than 80%
Treatment	Local muscle massage ice/heat, ultrasound, stretching exercises, ischemic compression, spray and stretch, nutritional support	Systemic light aerobic exercise, rest, decreased stress, psychologic support, nutritional support

[a]Modified from Simons DC: Fibrositis/fibromyalgia: a form of myofascial trigger points Am J Med 81:93–98, 1986.

Table 12.2 Terms Applied to Muscle Pain Syndromes

Fascitis	Myodysneuria
Fibromyalgia	Myesthesia
Fibrositis	Myofascial pain
Hypermyotonia	Myositis
Lumbago	Psychogenic rheumatism
Muscular rheumatism	Rheumatic myalgia
Myalgia	Rheumatic myopathy
Tension rheumatism	

perpetuating factors must be considered in the etiology of muscle pain syndromes (8) (Table 12.4).

Myofascial pain syndromes are characterized by hypersensitive trigger points described as hard, indurated nodules in the muscle, which refer pain in consistent patterns upon pressure (Table 12.5). Single or multiple trigger points with a twitch response and accompanying taut band are found with myofascial pain syndromes (8). Primary fibromyalgia patients present with multiple tender points in muscle and tendon insertions without the characteristic pattern of referral upon pressure. (Table 12.6). Skin-roll tenderness and cutaneous hyperemia are also found in these patients (10). Both trigger points and tender points are observed in some patients.

Confusing the issue is the observation that muscle pain is aggravated by psychological stress (10). This has led some to conclude that these muscle syndromes are primarily psychogenic (11). While the psychogenic component of muscle pain cannot be ignored, it is interesting to note that Sigmund Freud (12) treated muscle pain physiologically as well as psychologically, using massage and electrotherapy in addition to psychotherapy. While the psychological component no doubt is a factor in the perpetuation of muscle pain syndromes, it must not be assumed to be primary (8).

Chiropractic therapy has been reported to be among the most effective measures in the treatment of these muscle pain syndromes (13). Chiropractic care, along with life-style changes including stretching and light aerobic exercise, adequate rest, relaxation, and changes in attitude, can bring much relief to victims of myofascial pain and fibromyalgsia.

HISTORICAL OVERVIEW OF MUSCLE PAIN LITERATURE

German Literature

Prior to the 20th century, references to muscle pain syndromes appeared most extensively in the German literature (14, 15). As early as 1843, a German physician, Froriep, treated muscular rheumatism with electricity (15). He reportedly noted painful hard places in muscles that felt like tendinous cords or wide bands and referred to them as muskclschwiele (muscle callus) (14).

In 1876, Helleday described a myalgic condition characterized by nodules near the origin of muscles, which were tender on palpation. He noted that the rest of the pain of muscular rheumatism need not coincide with the location of palpable abnormalities. This phenomenon of "neurologic pain" spreading from nodules in rheumatic muscles was also re-

Table 12.3 Possible Causes of Muscle Syndromes

	Myofascial Pain Syndrome	Primary Fibromyalgia Syndrome
Characteristic history	Trauma or microtrauma	Chronic pain, delayed reaction to psychological stress
Clinical findings	Decreased ROM, trigger points, edema	Aching stiffness, fatigue, tenderpoints, sleep disorder, irritable bowel syndrome, headaches, joint pain
Management	Ice/heat ultrasound, ischemic compression, spray & stretch, active stretching exercises, nutritional support	Light aerobic activity, adequate rest & relaxation, active stretching exercises, stress reduction, psychological support, nutritional support

It has been postulated that myofascial pain in the presence of certain predisposing factors progresses to more and more sites, ultimately involving the autonomic nervous system. This progression places the patient's symptoms at a given time on a continuum, which frequently confounds the diagnostician.

Table 12.4 Factors Influencing Muscle Pain

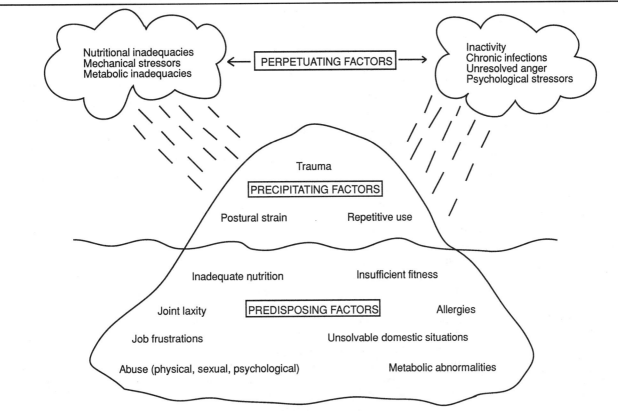

To fully comprehend the complexity of muscle pain syndromes, underlying predisposing and overlying perpetuating factors must be considered along with the precipitating factors that are more obvious like the tip of the iceberg.

Table 12.5 Terms Used to Describe Muscle Lesions

Muscle callus
Muskelharten
Myogelose
Receptor points
Sensitive deposits
Trigger points

Table 12.6 Comparison of Trigger Points and Tender Points[a]

	Trigger Points	Tender Points
Character-istic of	Myofascial pain	Primary fibromyalgia
Common sites	Belly and insertion of traumatized muscles or muscle groups	Prescribed locations in multiple areas
Referral pattern	Source of consistent referred pain	Localized tenderness without referral pattern

[a]Modified from Simons DG: Fibrositis/fibromyalgia: a form of myofascial trigger points. *Am J Med* 81: 93–98, 1986.

ported by German students of the Dutch masseur Mezger (15).

Building on these concepts, in 1912 Muller discussed three stages of muscular rheumatism, all exhibiting hypertonus as the primary clinical feature. He found that the acute stage was characterized by complaints of severe pain in the muscles, increased by pressure sensitivity, reflex spasm, swelling, impaired mobility, increased temperature, and involvement of multiple muscles. He noted that during the subacute phase, symptoms of pain, stiffness, and secondary spasm decreased, so that increased tension in the parts of the muscle primarily involved could be palpated. Further, in the chronic phase, residual signs included a variable combination of hypertonus, fiber hardenings, insertion nodules, and occasional swelling. He noted that generalized aching and painfulness were usually independent of palpable findings. He also reported that with pressure, some hardenings radiated pain to far-reaching areas, while others were even spontaneously painful. He noted that these hardenings were predictably found in specific locations in specific muscles.

Muller's unique contribution to the early German literature was the identification of insertion nodules, which he described as feeling like fine grains of sand up to pea-sized nodules. He found them hard like bone or crystal, immovable against bone, and very pressure sensitive. He also noted that during acute exacerbations the discrete, palpable hardenings were obscured by swelling and increased tonus. Muller described perpetuating factors including cold, momentary or sustained overexertion, psychic stress, poisons such as alcohol, and prolonged inactivity (15).

Schmidt, in 1914, elaborated on his earlier (1910) hypothesis that the pain associated with muscle hardenings is due to neuralgia of the sensory motor nerves. He was convinced that peripheral sensory nerve involvement was based on the pain sensitivity of vertebral structures to pressure. He demonstrated increased spinal fluid pressure in some patients, with a favorable response to epidural injection of local anesthetic in a number of patients with lumbago. He later implicated muscle spindles as responsible for the painfulness of the muscle hardenings, because of the anatomical location and known sensory function of spindles. He concluded that the fiber hardenings may be due to a functional phenomenon, since they felt to him like "a contraction of muscle bundle which one can easily produce by mechanical stimulation of the muscle substance." He also proposed that the toxic products of an infection progress centripetally via the terminals of sensory muscle nerves (14).

In 1917, Quinke compared the palpable muscular hardenings to the urticaria and acute edema observed in the skin, concluding that the frequent recurrence of circumscribed serous exudate finally leads to the development of connective tissue nodules, which might account for the inconsistent histological findings.

Other German authors disputed the nerve-mediated muscular-contraction theory after demonstrating that the muscle hardenings persisted in deep anesthesia and for a short time after death, the etiology possibly due to contracture. Other theories included decreased local circulation on a neurovascular basis producing a local stasis of the circulation, an allergic response involving histamine production, and an inflammatory response. A mechanism whereby a localized increase in reflex instability produces a sustained, localized, reflex muscle contraction, maintained by increased irritability of hypoxic muscle spindles was also proposed. Histological, biochemical, and serological studies of muscle tissue taken from patients with muscular rheumatism demonstrated fatty infiltration of the muscle cells (14).

English Literature

While the German literature focused on the muscles as the source of "muscular rheumatism" to explain those patients complaining of symptoms of myalgia and stiffness, the English literature focused on connective tissue as the site of origin of these widespread complaints (14, 15). This may have come about because rheumatism was defined in 1827 as "pain of a peculiar kind, usually attended with inflammatory action affecting the white fibrous textures belonging to muscles and joints such as tendons, aponeurosis, and ligaments; the synovial membranes of bursae and tendons; and nerves" (15).

Gowers, in 1904, introduced the term fibrositis to describe nonarticular rheumatism, while reasserting the idea that connective tissue was the site of rheumatism (15). Stockman reported in the same year that he had demonstrated nodules in muscle perimysium, beneath the skin, in subcutaneous fat, in fascia, and in the periosteum, which he considered to be an inflammatory hyperplasia of the connective tissue, causing chronic rheumatism (14). He reported the symptoms associated with these nodules to be "aching stiffness, a readiness to feel muscular fatigue, interference with free muscular movement, and very often a want of energy and vigour" (15, 16). He recommended a massage technique that must be continued until the nodule was completely resolved for permanent relief (14).

In 1915, Llewellyn and Jones (14) authored a book entitled *Fibrositis*, firmly entrenching the name and concept in the English language. They differentiated between articular fibrositis (chronic articular rheumatism or rheumatoid arthritis), myofibrositis (muscular rheumatism) and neurofibrositis (fibrositis of the nerve sheaths, associated with pain in the distribution of the nerve). They distinguished between acute and chronic stages of myofibrositis, defining the pathological process as an "inflammatory change in the interstitial fibrous tissue of a striated or voluntary muscle, the parenchymatous elements of which are only secondarily implicated."

Accordingly, acute symptoms of intense pain and markedly restricted function become chronic cases exhibiting annoying ache and eventually come to include stiffness and increased fatigue (14). The acute stage they found was characterized by hypertonus, swelling, and increased warmth of the involved muscles. They found that as the patient's condition becomes chronic the local hyperthermia disappears, and pressure-painful nodules may then appear. Controversy arose when subsequent researchers failed to find evidence of histological changes on biopsy (16–18). Elliot, in 1944, demonstrated EMG activity presenting evidence for a neurogenic mechanism (19). He postulated that sustained contraction of part of a muscle would lead to increased instability and pain sensitivity and eventually to pathological changes.

Kelly, in 1946, considered four features of fibrositis as evidence of reflex activity originating from the myalgic spot: widespread referred pain, deep hyperalgesia in that same area, edema of involved tissue, and stiffness or wasting of muscles (20). He reported success in 30–40% of cases, treating the involved muscles with procaine injection. He suggested that the development of myalgic lesions from the central connections of sensory neurons to other sensory and motor neurons arises from stimulation of either visceral or somatic tissues, by disease or injury, which is then transmitted in the CNS from the neurons directly affected to other sensory cells. From these cell bodies emanate antidromic impulses producing cutaneous or deep hyperalgesia and pain.

Good (21) considered nonarticular rheumatism to involve a dynamic pathology, with the disease consisting of disturbed circulation, with diminished blood flow leading to a relative hypoxia in the myalgic muscular areas. He concluded that "vasoconstriction appears reasonably and best to account for the triad of pain, disturbed muscular function, and paresthesia." He too recommended treatment of "myalgic spots" with procaine injection in addition to heat, deep massage, and a vegetarian diet.

American Literature

The terms trigger point and myofascial pain permeate the American literature that describes muscle pain syndromes. As early as 1936, Edeiken and Wolferth (22) used the term trigger zone to describe pain referred to the shoulder and down the left arm in response to pressure over the upper part of the left scapula, but they did not associate this referred pain pattern with muscles.

Steindler (23), in 1940, used the phrase trigger point to describe areas from which pain was referred. He described the treatment of chronic pain by injection of trigger points with procaine. In 1942 Travell, with coauthors Ringler and Herman (24), first reported on her many studies on trigger points. Since that time she has written extensively on this topic, publishing, with Simons in 1983, *Myofascial Pain and Dysfunction: The Trigger Point Manual* (8). In addition to procaine injections, medical treatment of trigger points has included stretching of the affected muscles, following topical spraying with vapocoolant. (8, 25)

Writing in the *Journal of the National Chiropractic Association* in 1957 (26), Nimmo discussed the concept that excessive contraction produced by mental tension, muscle strain, or other trauma, engages numerous receptors, producing a vicious cycle of noxious impulses. He developed a therapy in which pressure is applied to trigger points to interrupt the pain-spasm-pain cycle. Referred to by Travell and Simons (8) as ischemic compression, this type of therapy has been widely used by chiropractors in the treatment of trigger points.

MUSCLE CONTRACTION

In order to understand how muscle contraction results in the movement of bones and joints, it is important to understand the physical organization of skeletal muscle as well as its innervation. A typical skeletal muscle is made up of long muscle cells or fibers (some running the length of the muscle) that are arranged in bundles or fascicles bound together by connective-tissue perimysium. The fascicles are bound together with the tough epimysium that is continuous with the connective tissue attachments at the ends of the muscle (27).

Each muscle cell is composed of bundles of long myofibrils, 1000 to 2000 per cell. Myofibrils are linear arrangements of the contractile units of muscle,

the sarcomeres. In cross-section the sarcomeres can be seen to be made up of hexagonal arrays of two different kinds of long macromolecules or myofilaments. One kind is thick and heavy (myosin), and the other thin and light (actin). The interaction of the actin and myosin filaments is also the basis of the cross-striations characteristically seen in longitudinal sections viewed with the light microscope (2, 28).

Viewed longitudinally, each sarcomere is seen, in appropriately stained sections, to consist of alternating light and dark bands. The light or isotropic (I) bands contain only thin or actin filaments, while the dark or anisotropic (A) bands are regions where the thick myosin filaments are partially overlapped by interdigitating actin filaments. On closer inspection the A bands are seen to have a lighter center section where there is no actin-myosin overlap. This lighter region is known as the H region. A fine line, the M band, runs down the center of the H band. The actin filaments insert and run through the Z lines at each end of the sarcomere. The actin filaments, which are actually a long double helix, are arranged in a hexagonal array around each myosin filament. Along the actin filaments are receptors for the ATPase-containing myosin heads that are at the ends of the hinged, light portions of the myosin molecules.

Muscle contraction is thought to be caused by the hinged myosin arm making contact with the nearby actin receptor and pulling the actin filament toward the center of the sarcomere. Thus, shortening of the serially arranged sarcomeres results in shortening of the entire muscle (27).

The chemical events associated with muscle contraction center around the release of calcium from the sarcoplasmic reticulum in response to the electrical events of the muscle action potential. The sarcoplasmic reticulum is an extensive system of branching and anastomosing channels, filling most of the space between the myofibrils. The membrane of the sarcoplasmic reticulum is continuous with the outside cell membrane by means of the T-system, which is an invagination of the cell membrane.

An important feature of the sarcoplasmic reticulum is the presence of transverse channels, the terminal cysternae that are located at the level of the overlap of the A and I bands. The terminal cysternae store bound calcium, pending the arrival of an action potential. The release of calcium in response to an action potential results in the activation of the myosin-ATPase, interaction of the hinged portion of the myosin filaments with the actin filaments, and shortening of the muscle. The interaction of the calcium and the myosin ATPase is facilitated by another protein, troponin, which is located at intervals along a third filament, tropomyosin, intertwined in the actin helix. It is the free calcium liberated in response to the action potential that combines with the tropomyosin and thus affects the interaction of the actin and myosin and the shortening of the sarcomere (29).

There are two distinct types of muscle fibers or cells with respect to their action and composition, most muscles containing a mixture of the two. Type I (slow) fibers are so called because of their relatively slow twitch time. They tend to predominate in postural muscles such as the soleus. They are rich in mitochondria and oxidative enzymes but poor in phosphorylases. Type II (fast) fibers are characterized by fast twitch times, the best examples being the extraocular muscles and the muscles of the limbs, which produce large-scale movements.

The metabolic differences between the two types of fibers allow for the differences in function. Type I, slow fibers have a well-developed aerobic metabolism, with a rich supply of mitochondria concentrated in their thick Z bands. Type I fibers are thus capable of sustained action. Type II, fast fibers, on the other hand, are rich in glycolytic (anaerobic) enzymes (stored in thin Z bands) but are capable of only relatively short periods of sustained action. Another distinction (not invariably true) designates type I fibers as "red" fibers because of the rich blood supply required for their aerobic metabolism and type II fibers as "white" fibers because their anaerobic metabolism is relatively independent of a rich blood supply (27).

MUSCLE INNERVATION AND CONTROL OF MUSCLE LENGTH AND TENSION

The length and tension of an intact muscle at any moment is a function of two separate but interrelated nerve supplies. Anterior horn cells or lower motor neurons supply the bulk of the muscle mass. Each neuron supplies many muscle cells, and together they constitute a motor unit. The size of the motor unit is related to the function of the muscle; postural muscles such as the soleus have motor units with one or two thousand muscle cells supplied by a single nerve cell. The extraocular muscles have the smallest motor units, with an innervation ratio of less than one to ten (27).

A normal muscle at rest is electromyographically "silent," that is, no motor units are firing. Postural muscles under the influence of gravity must, however, maintain a degree of tension or contraction in order to maintain the stability of the body (30). This requires the cooperation of the lower motor or α motor neurons and a second, intrinsic level of muscle innervation, the muscle spindle system.

The spindle system provides information to the central nervous system about the length of a muscle at any given moment. In this regard it functions as a "myostat," which can assist the α motor neurons in maintaining a fixed muscle length for postural control or provide a smooth changing of muscle length (as in throwing a ball) (31).

Muscle spindles are fusiform structures, 4–7 mm long by 80–200 μ wide, that are located deep within the muscle mass. They are composed of 6–7 specialized muscle fibers (cells) of two different types. Running the length of the spindle and attached at either end to the inside of the connective tissue capsule are typically two nuclear-bag fibers, so named because the nuclei are collected in an expanded central region. Functionally, there are two types of bag fibers: slow and fast. The second fiber type, the nuclear-chain fibers (so called because the nuclei are arranged linearly in the central regions of the fibers), are shorter and thinner than the nuclear-bag fibers and are frequently attached to their polar ends.

The spindle functions, in general, to provide information to the central nervous system about the length and rate of change of length of the muscle in which it lies (32). These two kinds of information (static and dynamic) are supplied by two different kinds of sensory endings and their afferent processes. One type of ending, the annulospiral, or primary ending, wraps spirally around both the nuclear-bag and nuclear-chain fibers. The other, the flower-spray or secondary ending, is typically associated only with the nuclear-chain fibers (33).

In terms of their conduction velocities, the primary spindle afferents are classified as Ia, and the secondary endings as II. Both type Ia and type II afferents make monosynaptic excitatory synapses with homonymous α motor neurons (i.e., motor neurons supplying the muscle in which they reside).

The spindle with its intrafusal fibers is oriented parallel with the bulk of the muscle mass, the extrafusal fibers, so that when the muscle is stretched the spindle fibers are stretched, and when the muscle shortens the spindle fibers shorten.

It is possible to record separately from primary to secondary endings and to thus demonstrate the difference between dynamic and static responses. With a muscle at a given length, there is a characteristic rate of afferent discharge from both the primary and secondary fibers. When that muscle is lengthened at a constant rate to a new, longer length, two different kinds of response can be seen. While the muscle is being lengthened, a higher rate of firing occurs in the primary fiber until the new length is attained. The firing rate ceases to be as fast as it was during the lengthening (dynamic) phase, but it is maintained at a rate higher than that at the shorter length. On the other hand, the firing rate in the secondary fiber only gradually increases to a new, higher rate than at rest. In both cases the new, static length has new, higher rates of firing.

However, when the muscle is returned to its former shorter length, the response of the primary and secondary fibers is quite different. As soon as a muscle begins to shorten, the firing from the primary fiber ceases altogether until the length stabilizes, when it resumes its original firing rate. In the secondary fiber, decreasing length is signaled by a gradual decrease in firing rate, until the length is stabilized and the former firing rate is resumed (34).

Thus the principal functions of the primary endings are to give information about static length and about the rate of increasing muscle length. The secondary endings provide mainly information about length in general. It should be obvious from the above that there is an information gap or silent period in the output from the primary endings when a muscle is being shortened (as in contraction). This information gap is only slightly filled by the continuous firing from the secondary ending. It is mostly filled by activation of another system, the fusimotor or γ motor system.

These are motor fibers with cell bodies in the anterior horns, and endings on the polar ends of the intrafusal fibers, both nuclear-bag and nuclear-chain. When fusimotor activation causes contraction of the polar ends of the spindle fiber, traction is put on the central portions, where the sensory endings detect this change as they would if the entire muscle were being stretched. As a result, the information gap to the central nervous system is filled in, even while the muscle is being shortened (31).

There is evidence that some intrafusal innervation may come from slower-conducting A (or B) fibers whose cell bodies receive monosynaptic homonymous stimulation from primary and secondary spindle endings in the same way as do α motor neurons, and thus provide a positive feedback that also helps eliminate any information gap (35). Fusimotor neurons, however, receive their primary excitation from brainstem centers such as the vestibular nuclei and the cerebellum, which are concerned with maintaining appropriate tension in muscles.

Three different types of fusimotor fibers (and functions) have been described (32, 33): a dynamic or a static supply to nuclear-bag fibers, and a static supply to nuclear-chain fibers. Dynamic fusimotor activation provides for increased sensitivity of the stretch reflex, particularly during motion. Static nuclear-bag activation, on the other hand, results in an increased strength of extrafusal contraction at a given length of muscle, without changing the sensitivity of the stretch reflex.

The action of the static nuclear-chain activation is somewhat paradoxical in that it tends to increase the sensitivity of the stretch reflex while decreasing the sensitivity of the spindle to static change in length. This is thought to be important in enabling a muscle to support a heavy load, since a relatively small amount of lengthening would generate sufficient additional tension to support the load.

In summary, voluntary skeletal muscle activity is under the control of the motor cortex by way of the corticospinal projection to lower motor neurons. Lower motor neurons activate extrafusal muscle fibers that contain sensors, the spindles, whose afferent fibers send the spinal cord lower motor neurons information about the changes in both length and the rate of change of length of the muscle. The sensitivity of the spindle system to these changes is itself under the control of both positive and negative feedback from both segmental and suprasegmental systems. This feedback is accomplished primarily through the different fusimotor influences on the spindle fibers. Muscular control of posture, although the scale of the movements is much smaller, is based essentially on the same systems of activation and control. (36, 37)

MECHANISM OF MYOFASCIAL TRIGGER POINT DEVELOPMENT

Many factors interact to create myofascial trigger points (Table 12.7). Trigger points may develop in muscles that are either acutely or chronically strained. Particularly with acute strain, there is some degree of tissue damage. This may, on the cellular level, include disruption of some of the sarcoplasmic reticulum and release of some of the stored calcium. It also impairs the ability of the sarcoplasmic reticulum to remove calcium from the injury site. The availability of extra calcium (in the presence of normal amounts of ATP) to the myofibrils results in sustained contraction of the sarcomere and eventually in fatigue. This sustained local contraction produces the palpable taut band associated with myofascial trigger points.

The initial tissue damage may also result in the disruption of small blood vessels and the release of platelets, which in turn leak substances such as serotonin, which sensitizes nerve endings in the area. Connective tissue damage also results in the breakage of mast cells containing histamine, which can also sensitize and stimulate pain endings (38).

The sustained local (intramuscular) contraction has several consequences. It creates a region of uncontrolled metabolism that in turn can result in additional mast-cell liberation of histamine and the depletion of local ATP. Because the energy from splitting ATP is required to "recock" the contractile mechanism, its depletion results in a progressive failure of relaxation and eventually in contracture.

The sustained contractions have another important effect in reducing blood flow to the area, which is compounded by vasoconstriction from autonomic nerves that are activated because of trigger-point sensory-fiber input to the central nervous system. The resulting decrease in local blood supply results in the local accumulation of metabolites such as prostaglandins, which are also capable of sensitizing nerve endings. Thus a self-perpetuating local muscle condition is created, which is painful, resists stretching, and results in decreased range of motion and generalized disability.

PERCEPTION OF PAIN FROM MUSCLE

The perception of pain from muscles in general and myofascial trigger points in particular, must be understood from the perspective of how the central nervous system processes sensory information (39–44). The origin of pain may be perceived as being

Table 12.7 Trigger Point Genesis

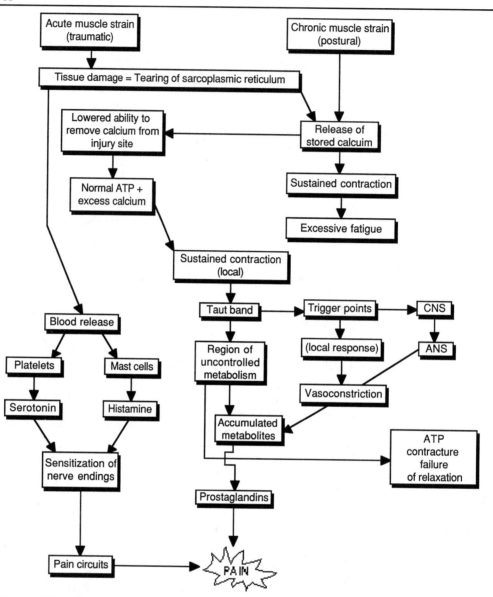

exogenous, that is, as arising from a specific sensory receptor or just from a free nerve ending. Pain may also be perceived as having an endogenous origin as in central pain or as with referred pain (pain that is displaced from its actual source to a distant site). An aspect of pain perception that has received increasing attention for the past two decades is pain modulation. It is now known that pain may be modulated at least four levels—the receptor, the spinal cord, the thalamus, and the sensory cortex (43, 44).

Sensory receptors subserving the function of pain (nociceptors) may be of two types, each with different characteristics and a variety of names (45). Epicritic receptors are responsible for localizing and discriminating pain. They are supplied by group III (A-δ) myelinated fibers that are fast conducting and, for the most part, are responsive to mechanical or thermal stimuli. Approximately one fourth of these fibers respond to stimuli that are potentially tissue damaging. Protopathic receptors, on the other hand, are slow-conducting, nonmyelinated group IV (C) fibers. Fifty percent of these supply the mechanoreceptors of hairy skin, while the other half are mechanical and/or thermal receptors, many being polymodal. Apparently none are purely chemical receptors.

The degree of pain perception for a given-strength stimulus depends first on the sensitivity of the receptor. Receptors may be sensitized by two different mechanisms, prior stimulation and a variety of chemical agents. The latter include histamine, prostaglandins, bradykinin, and serotonin (45). The results of their action locally may be not only sensitization of the pain receptors but also local inflammation and hyperirritability of myofascial trigger points.

Muscle receptors contain proprioceptors (muscle spindles and the Golgi tendon organs) and several different kinds of group III and group IV nerve fibers (46). There are no mechano- or thermoreceptors in muscle. Approximately half of all the sensory fibers from muscle fall into group II or IV. Some of the group III (A-δ) fibers are thought to be ergoreceptors or metaboreceptors. The type C fibers are those that respond to bradykinin, serotonin, histamine, prostaglandin E2, and injected potassium choloride. Stimulation of single group III or IV fibers in man results in a dull pain that is discrete but not sharp or itchy. Such stimulation also results in referral to other parts of the body, in addition to the muscle (47).

Modulation of Muscle Pain at the Spinal Cord Level

In the dorsal gray horn of the spinal cord, pain signals from the periphery are subject to a wide variety of processing and modulating mechanisms, depending initially on the fiber type carrying the signal. Anatomically, the dorsal horn is organized in six layers. Sensory root fibers enter the dorsal horn. They are separated into medial and lateral bundles. These are large, rapidly conducting fibers carrying primarily proprioceptive information. They collect medially and send collaterals to local interneurons before continuing on to make reflex connections in the ventral horn. Small, myelinated and unmyelinated fibers, many carrying pain signals, are collected in the lateral bundle. These fibers bend, ascend, or bifurcate, one branch making synaptic connection at the level of entry and the other ascending one or two segments before sending collaterals into the deeper layers of the dorsal horn. Second-order interneurons, which may be excitatory or inhibitory, may interconnect, via the tract of Lissauer, as many as five or six vertebral segments. Descending fiber tracts from the brainstem and higher centers can also provide inhibition or facilitation to interneurons receiving incoming pain signals from the periphery. This rich neuronal interplay at the dorsal horn level forms the anatomic basis for the gate-control theory of Melzack and Wall (48).

The two subdivisions of the spinothalamic tract transmit nociceptive information to the next relay center, the thalamus. Epicritic or fast pain is transmitted by the lateral (neo-) spinothalamic tract, while protopathic or slow pain travels in the ventral (paleo-) spinothalamic tract. The latter pathway is thought to give rise to the aversive responses of avoidance and inactivity to painful stimuli and is probably the basis for much of the suffering from chronic pain.

Modulation of Muscle Pain at the Subcortical Level

There are a number of structures concerned with the body's response to morphine, which, when stimulated appropriately, strongly inhibit the perception of pain by the release of neuromodulators known as enkephalins. Endorphin is one molecular fragment that has 48 times the analgesic effect of morphine. Acupuncture has been shown to result in the release of neuromodulators. Melzack and Wall (48) have suggested that the spinal gate in the dorsal gray horn may be "shut" either by a central biasing mechanism located in the reticular formation or by interruption of reverberatory circuits concerned with the memory of pain (44, 45, 48).

Modulation of Muscle Pain at the Cortical Level

Three kinds of responses to pain characterize the cortical level. Acute pain is interpreted as tissue threatening; sustained pain indicates the need for recuperative rest. When sustained pain becomes persistent, the patient is faced with chronic pain, a common situation with untreated myofascial trigger points.

The disruption of subcortical or cortical circuits involved with the memory of pain (mentioned in the section above) as a means of controlling pain, shows the importance of the individual's reaction to the painful experience. An example is the apparent lack of pain experienced by certain religious practitioners under circumstances that would normally result in severe pain.

Acute pain, even though severe, that diminished in the course of the natural healing process, does not present a psychological problem for the normal individual. However, chronic, persistent pain that seems inescapable or has no apparent explanation and which threatens the individual's present and future well-being, frequently results in depression, frustration, and further disability.

Such patients are all too frequently told that they "must learn to live with it." For such patients with myofascial pain dysfunction, Travell and Simons (8) have advised that "they must learn that the pain comes from muscles, not from nerve damage, and not from permanent arthritic changes in bones. Most important, they must know that it is responsive to treatment. This gives the pain new 'meaning' ... their lives take on new meaning and they are started on the road to recovery of function."(8).

Referred Pain

At least five mechanisms have been postulated to explain referred pain, not all of them mutually exclusive. (8, 49, 50)

Peripheral Branching of Axons

Extensive branching of sensory axons would be required to explain how a painful signal in one branch could be interpreted as having come from another. Each sensory fiber would also be required to have both visceral and somatic branches. This has not been demonstrated.

Convergence Facilitation

Convergence facilitation suggests that abnormal visceral afferent input to the cord raises the excitability of dorsal horn interneurons so that normal background sensory activity from the pain reference zone becomes interpreted as painful. If this were the case, application of local anesthetic to the reference zone should abolish the pain, which it does, but for longer than the existence of the anesthetic. This suggests an additional mechanism, perhaps interruption of a reverberating circuit in the central nervous system.

Convergence Projection

Convergence projection requires that both visceral (including muscle) and somatic (cutaneous) afferents converge on the same dorsal horn neuron. The cortex then could interpret a strong visceral input as coming from a corresponding skin locus. If this were the only mechanism involved, anesthetizing the reference skin area would have no effect on the perception of pain, which is not the case.

Reflex Constriction of the Vasa Nervorum

By this mechanism, vasoconstrictive ischemia of sensory fibers from the reference zone might cause pain to be perceived from that area.

Autonomic Nociceptive Feedback

This explanation proposes that autonomic neurons release nociceptive substances in the zone of referred pain, and thus it could be self-sustaining if the pain resulted in additional autonomic acitivity.

TRIGGER POINT DEVELOPMENT

Two phases have been proposed as contributing to the development of trigger points (8). It has been suggested that they begin as a neuromuscular dysfunction that, if prolonged, may result in a second phase with histologically demonstrable changes. Matching biopsy findings with clinical symptoms has been successful in a few instances (8). Three basic features characterize trigger points: hyperirritability, a region of increased metabolism and/or decreased circulation, and the presence of a palpable band.

Hyperirritability

Hyperirritability is characterized by (a) local tenderness to palpation, (b) spontaneous pain, referred tenderness, and referred autonomic phenomena, (c) local twitch responses, and (d) the typical, local twitch response to needling of the trigger point. An example of hyperirritability is the lowered EMG threshold due to the presence of a nearby trigger point (51).

Possible explanations for hyperirritability include (a) sensitization of muscle afferents by serotonin, histamine, kinins, and prostaglandins (supported by Awad's (38) demonstration of trigger points in biopsy specimens, with large numbers of platelets (containing serotonin) and mast cells (containing histamine)): (b) trigger points may be sensitized to pressure by mechano- or nociceptors (fast, group III or slow, group IV fibers); (c) afferent trigger point input to the CNS may be carried by more than one kind of nerve fiber; and (d) the afferents from trigger points that mediate different responses are not necessarily nociceptors.

Hypotheses to explain pain referral from trigger points include projection facilitation and projection convergence. Projection facilitation assumes that when afferent input from trigger points is superimposed upon the normal, neuronal-pool background activity from the referral area, signals are sent to the brain, which are interpreted as representing pain from the referral area. Projection convergence holds that different afferents from the trigger point and the referral area converge on the same ascending, dorsal horn cell, and the cortex misinterprets the information as a noxious stimulation of the referral area.

It has been suggested that the effectiveness of dry needling in reducing trigger point hyperirritability is due to mechanical disruption of sensory fibers. Substances causing hyperirritability may be washed out or dispersed by injections of saline or anesthetic or by the pumping action of alternate compression and release.

Increased Metabolism/Decreased Circulation

Evidence for this proposal comes largely from the observation of increased temperature at the trigger point. The increased metabolic demand for such substances as vitamins and hormones cannot be met by the decreased circulation. The presence of fine fat droplets and abnormal mitochondria in the region of trigger points in additional evidence of metabolic stress. Radioisotope studies have demonstrated a slowing of blood flow in the area of a trigger point, and needle thermocouple insertion into a trigger point shows an elevated temperature that subsides as sensitivity subsides. Furthermore, since stimulation of muscle nociceptors also activates γ-motor efferents, this activity could spill over to activate vasomotor sympathetic fibers and result in the observed ischemia in the area of trigger points.

Palpable Band

Although various explanations for this observation have been proposed (such as fibrous tissue deposition, myogelosis or gelling of muscle colloids, and muscle spasm), physiological contracture (failure of relaxation) appears to be the most plausible. Normal contraction is initiated by calcium release from the sarcoplasmic reticulum in response to an action potential, and it is terminated by the reuptake of calcium with resultant relaxation.

The interaction of actin and myosin and the subsequent splitting of ATP are interrupted by the reuptake of calcium. However, if the sarcoplasmic reticulum becomes damaged and free calcium remains, contraction will be maintained as long as the local energy supply holds out. When the ATP stores are depleted, relaxation can no longer be accomplished, and local contracture supervenes, resulting in a palpable band.

Dystrophic Changes

The development of demonstrable changes in muscles afflicted with trigger points may occur in some people in a relatively short time and not develop in others even after many years. This is apparently due to other contributing factors, and it may explain why some patients respond quickly to trigger point therapy and others respond slowly and incompletely.

Trigger Point Structure

Motor endplates are usually located close to the centers of muscle fibers. Sometimes trigger points are located close to motor endplate areas, and sometimes they are at some distance. Also, muscle spindles are generally located in the vicinity of motor endplates; however, muscle spindles have not been reported in biopsy specimens from trigger points, even when they have been specifically looked for in experimental, dog, trigger point studies. On the other hand, free nerve endings are widely dispersed throughout the connective tissue, between and around muscle fibers and in association with blood vessels (8). Sensitization of these nerve endings could explain the hyperirritability of trigger points.

MYOFASCIAL PAIN SYNDROMES

Myofascial pain is characterized by intense, deep muscular pain referred from hypersensitive trigger points located in the bellies of muscles and their tendinous attachments. This syndrome is most commonly found in the neck, back, and pelvis, including the postural stabilizers of the upper extremities and the rotator muscles of the hip and shoulder.

The trigger points are exquisitely tender to direct pressure or squeezing and are palpable as hard, indurated nodules in the muscle and/or fascia. The pain is frequently described as a deep ache like a toothache, which refers in constant patterns. It is this pain referral that characterizes myofascial trigger points and differentiates them from tender points that are sensitive to palpation and pressure, but which lack the classic referral pain pattern.

Multiple tender points in various muscle groups, without a pattern of referral, is characteristic of fibromyalgia, which appears to be the result of unsuccessfully treated myofascial pain syndromes in predisposed patients.

Clinical Features of Myofascial Pain

History

The patient exhibiting trigger points frequently gives a history of a traumatic incident producing muscle strain, such as lifting incidents on the job or a "whiplash" (flexion-extension) injury from a motor vehicle accident (52). Overuse of muscles, such as postural strain produced by static loading of the muscular stabilizers of the upper extremities, is also frequently reported in relatively sedentary workers (5, 52).

Myofascial pain syndromes are common among typists, CRT operators, and assembly line workers who repeatedly use the forearm muscles. Their postual muscles remain in a state of constant contraction in order to stabilize the neck and shoulder girdle. This type of static loading of the postural muscles produces overload fatigue and microtrauma to the muscle fibers, which is equally as devasting as frank trauma. Dysfunction of the deep transverse and intersegmental muscles is also exhibited by localized taut bands and trigger points. Eccentric contraction of the erector spinae, which occurs when lowering a heavy weight, is another common precipitating event.

Chilling from sleeping in a draft, exposure to air conditioning, or exposure to a sudden blast of cold air can produce self-sustaining torticollis from trigger points in the anterior strap muscles of the neck (Chapter 10). A history of acute infection, such as herpes simplex or herpes zoster, or immunization reactions has been noted (52, 53).

Symptoms

Myofascial pain referred from trigger points is usually dull and aching, varying in intensity from low-grade discomfort to severe and incapacitating torture (8). It may be intensified at rest or in motion. It is invariably increased by sharp, sudden motion such as occurs when the patient is startled or makes an unguarded movement.

Pressure on the trigger point produces referred pain. The pattern of pain referral does not follow segmental or neurological patterns, but the area where the pain is felt is consistent for trigger points in each individual muscle (21, 54). Pressure of the body on trigger points during recumbency frequently disrupts sleep (20). Myofascial stiffness is experienced following periods of inactivity, especially after a night's sleep or after sitting in one position for an extended period (20).

Muscle weakness is frequently reported, but true muscle weakness is not generally found. Rather, perceived weakness is thought to be due to a central inhibition that protects the muscle from a painful degree of contraction. Muscle strength then becomes unreliable, with objects dropping unexpectedly from the patient's grasp. This muscle "give-way" may be due to underlying joint dysfunction, which produces an arthrokinetic reflex. When a patient substitutes other muscles for the pain-producing one, atrophy and true weakness may occur without atrophy due to disease, but this is uncommon.

Signs

Pathognomonic of myofascial pain syndromes is the palpable trigger point that evokes the characteristic referred pain on compression (8, 20). Muscles in the immediate vicinity of a trigger point feel tense to palpation. When acute, the area over the trigger point may feel edematous and warm to the touch. Digital pressure may cause the patient to jump and cry out. This response is referred to as the "jump sign" (8).

Needle electromyography and a specific, reproducible snapping technique have been used to elicit and record the local twitch response (55, 56). A localized twitch response may be elicited when the trigger point is rolled under the fingers. The twitch may be vigorous enough to cause a perceptible jerk of the body part.

The increased tension of the taut bands will not permit the muscle to extend to its full range, restricting motion. Pain due to spasm blocks further lengthening of the muscle.

Dermographia (8) is frequently observed in areas overlying an active trigger point, particularly over the back and torso. Routine laboratory tests show no abnormalities or significant changes attributable to myofascial trigger points.

Diagnosis therefore depends on the doctor's skill at palpation and the correlation of the patient's history and complaints of pain radiation in the classic pattern of referral known to accompany myofascial pain.

Management

Myofascial pain may persist for decades, restricting range of motion and recurrently becoming active enough to cause attacks of referred pain without involving other muscles (8). In some cases, predisposing and perpetuating factors may prevail, and the patient falls victim to a generalized muscle pain syndrome involving multiple muscle groups, with widespread autonomic dysfunction and sleep disorders (fibrositis/fibromyalgia).

Treatment of myofascial trigger points is directed toward the disruption of reverberating neural circuits (56) responsible for the self-perpetuation of the pain-spasm-pain cycle (57). A number of techniques can be used to inactivate trigger points including needling, vapocoolant spray and stretch, injection of saline or anesthetic acupuncture (8, 53, 56–58), ultrasound, and ischemic compression.

Needle techniques employ one of the oldest methods of pain relief, by using hyperstimulation analgesia to interrupt or prevent recurrence of abnormal neural activity. Melzack (56) describes three major properties of hyperstimulation algesia: (a) a moderate to intense sensory input is applied to the body to alleviate pain; (b) the sensory input is sometimes applied to a site distant from the site of pain; and (c) the sensory input, which is usually of brief duration (varying from a few seconds to 20 or 30 minutes), may relieve chronic pain for days, weeks, and sometimes permanently.

Ischemic compression has been used by chiropractors for over 30 years in the treatment of myofascial pain syndromes (25). This mechanical treatment of myofascial trigger points consists of application of sustained pressure for a long enough time to inactivate the muscle spasm. Travell and Simons (8) termed this therapy ischemic compression because, on release of pressure, the skin is at first blanched and then shows reactive hyperemia. These changes correspond to circulatory changes in the underlying muscle, which is subjected to the same pressure.

Pressure can be applied with a thumb, finger, knuckle, or elbow depending on the size, depth, and thickness of the muscle being compressed. Moist hot-packs followed by ultrasound and light massage applied to the area of complaint helps to isolate the trigger point. Specific pressure can then be applied directly to the center trigger point to the patient's tolerance.

Care must be taken not to exceed the patient's tolerance, and if the patient tenses or pulls away, then a lighter pressure should be applied. If the pressure is too painful, the patient will respond with muscle tightening in the area (58).

Pressure is sustained for 10 to 20 seconds and gradually increased as the trigger point releases. A thumb or finger from the other hand may be used for reinforcement. Pressure is most effective when applied straight into the trigger point. The patient will generally be happy to confirm the exact site of pressure application, often with the statement that "it hurts good" or other indication that it is uncomfortable but on target. Mechanical devices can be used, but these do not give the necessary feedback as the trigger point releases.

Ischemic pressure therapy may have to be repeated every 2 to 3 days for several weeks, depending on the chronicity of the problem and the patient's response to treatment. Acute cases frequently respond with 3–4 treatments. Treatment time varies and may be extended in a patient with a long-standing history of pain and pain referral (58).

Nutritional supplementation and appropriate daily stretching exercises at home hasten recovery and prevent recurrence (58). Chilling and overexertion of the affected part should be avoided. Fixation of segmental joints of the spine and other areas, and mechanical stresses that perpetuate postural imbalance creating muscle stress, should also be corrected (see Chapter 11).

Stretch Techniques

A number of stretch techniques can be used effectively to inactivate trigger points. Travell and Simons (8) recommend the use of a vapocoolant spray along with passive stretching of the muscle. They emphasize that the "stretch is the action" while the "spray is the distraction." They state that gentle, persistent stretch without spray is more likely to inactivate trigger points than is spray without stretch. They recommend, however, that best results are obtained by spraying first and then stretching and spraying.

` Passive stretching without spraying will inactivate newly activated or moderately irritated trigger points (8). The patient is instructed to relax fully while the muscle is firmly and slowly stretched to the patient's tolerance, gradually restoring its full, normal length. Stretching is facilitated by moist heat applied over the reference zone prior to the stretch.

Proprioceptive neuromuscular relaxation (8) utilizes alternate contraction of agonist and antagonist muscle groups, which are resisted by a therapist. This technique keeps the muscles stretched isometrically at the limit of their range of motion. The alternating effort promotes a gradual lengthening of the affected muscles.

Lewit and Simons (59) describe a method utilizing passive stretch with lengthwise stabilization. The patient is instructed to exert minimal resistance to contract the affected muscle that has been stretched to the limit of its range. The patient holds this contraction for at least 10 seconds while the operator resists the isometric contraction. This is followed by gentle, passive stretching of the muscle when the patient has relaxed completely. This sequence is alternated until the muscle length no longer increases. They found that 94% of 244 patients treated by this method received immediate pain relief, with 63% reporting lasting pain relief.

Active resistance exercises for the involved muscles should not be implemented until trigger points have been inactivated and the affected muscle stretched. Low-impact aerobic activity provides the circulation necessary for a healthy musculoskeletal system without activating or exacerbating myofascial trigger points.

MYOFASCIAL PAIN SYNDROMES OF THE NECK, BACK, AND BUTTOCKS

A number of different muscle syndromes associated with neck, back, and buttock pain are commonly seen in chiropractic practice. Each involved muscle exhibits a characteristic pattern of pain and tenderness, which refers in a distribution specific for that muscle. Identification of these syndromes depends upon the location of the trigger points and the pattern of pain referred upon pressure.

Piriformis Syndrome

In spite of a number of articles discussing piriformis syndrome (60–73), it remains the most unrecognized cause of sciatica. Patients with this syndrome complain of pain and/or paresthesia in the distribution of the sciatic nerve (5, 60–75), which is commonly misdiagnosed as compression from nerve root lesions.

The piriformis muscle originates from the front of the sacrum, the gluteal surface of the ilium in the region of the posterior iliac spine, the capsule of the adjacent sacroiliac joint, and sometimes from the upper part of the pelvic surface of the sacrotuberous ligament. It passes out of the pelvis through the greater sciatic foramen attaching to the greater trochanter of the femur by a rounded tendon (27).

The sciatic nerve passes under the belly of the piriformis in more than 80% of the cases (Fig. 12.1A). It varies in relation to the muscle in the remainder, passing either through the belly of the muscle (Fig. 12.1B) or the nerve itself splits, with a portion passing through, as well as under, the muscle (Fig. 12.1-C&D).

Freiberg and Vinle (65) note that the piriformis muscle bridges over the sacroiliac joint, and a part of its origin is intimately bound up with the capsule of the joint and is therefore subject to reflex spasm from intraarticular irritation of the sacroiliac joint. The piriformis muscle is innervated by branches from the L5, S1, and S2 nerve roots. The piriformis rotates the extended thigh laterally and abducts the flexed thigh (27).

The two most common causes of piriformis syndrome are trauma to the sacroiliac joint producing a ligamentous sprain and hormonal changes such as occur in the female during the menstrual cycle, during pregnancy, or when taking estrogen replacement therapy or oral contraceptives. The hormonal factor probably accounts for the higher incidence in females (6:1) noted by Cailliet (63). The patient may also report a history of repeated sacroiliac manipulation of the ipsilateral sacroiliac joint or prolonged external rotation of the foot and leg, such as pressing the accelerator while driving.

Patients with piriformis syndrome complain of a deep, boring, ill-defined pain in the buttock, commonly radiating into the posterolateral thigh or calf, rarely to the foot (67, 68) (Fig. 12.2). They may also report a burning sensation in the hips over the greater trochanter, particularly at night, when they are unable to lie on the side.

Examination of the patient in the supine position reveals external rotation of the thigh on the affected side, known as the positive piriformis sign (Fig. 12.3). Internal rotation of the thigh is limited (64).

Figure 12.1. The sciatic nerve in relation to the piriformis muscle. **A,** The sciatic nerve passes under the belly of the piriformis muscle in 90% of cases. **B,** In the remainder it may pass through the belly of the muscle or **(C&D),** the nerve itself may be split by a portion of the muscle. This makes the sciatic nerve more vulnerable to irritation by trigger points. (Adapted from Beaton LE: The sciatic nerve and the piriformis muscle; their interrelation a possible cause of coccygodynia. *J Bone Joint Surg* 20:686–688, 1938.

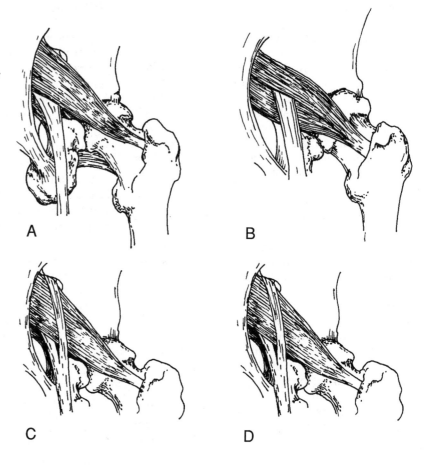

Trigger points are palpable in the belly of the muscle through the mass of the gluteus maximus muscle (64) and at the tendinous insertion at the greater trochanter (66) (Fig. 12.2). These trigger points are exquisitely tender. Deep pressure at the belly of the muscle produces radiation down the course of the sciatic nerve, while pressure at the tendinous insertion produces a localized burning sensation.

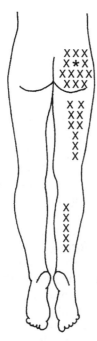

Figure 12.2. Piriformis syndrome. Trigger points (*) located near the belly and insertion of the piriformis muscle refer pain (×) in a characteristic pattern. (Adapted from Kirkaldy-Willis WH: *Managing Low Back Pain,* ed 2. New York, Churchill Livingstone, 1988, p 142.)

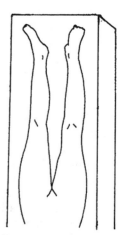

Figure 12.3. Positive piriformis sign. Examination of the patient in the supine position reveals external rotation of the thigh on the side of the piriformis syndrome.

Along with pressure therapy, hip or contralateral sacroiliac fixations should be manipulated; however, caution is advised against repeated non-specific pelvic manipulation, since this tends to perpetuate the condition. The use of a stabilizing trochanteric belt, preferably with an elastic bandage (Chapter 7), promotes stabilization of hypermobile sacroiliac joints. Stretching the involved muscle also prevents recurrence and enhances prompt resolution of the piriformis syndrome. To stretch the piriformis muscle, the knee on the affected side is tractioned slowly toward the opposite shoulder.

Gluteus Maximus Syndrome

The gluteus maximus muscle arises from the crest and posterior gluteal line of the ilium, from the aponeurosis of the erector spinae, from the lower dorsal surface of the sacrum and the side of the coccyx, from the sacrotuberous ligament, and from the gluteal aponeurosis. It runs obliquely and laterally, attaching to the iliotibial tract of the fascia lata, lateral to the greater trochanter.

The gluteus maximus is innervated by the inferior gluteal nerve, L5 and S1 and 2. Acting from above, it extends the flexed thigh, bringing it in line with the trunk. Fixed from below, it prevents flexion of the trunk of the supporting hip during bipedal gait. It assists in raising the trunk after stooping, by rotating the pelvis backward on the head of the femur. Its upper fibers are active in abduction of the thigh (27).

Trigger points in the gluteus maximus may evoke pain in practically any part of the buttocks, posterior thigh, and coccyx (76, 77) (Fig. 12.4). A trigger point in the lowest fibers refers pain deep in the coccyx. Examination of the patient reveals a slightly restricted straight-leg raise. Palpation reveals trigger points at the insertion and in the belly of the muscle, which reproduce and refer pain with sustained pressure on the tender spots.

Deep pressure is applied to the trigger points following physical therapy. The gluteus maximus can be actively or passively stretched by flexing the thigh on the abdomen (76).

Gluteus Medius Syndrome

The gluteus medius muscle arises above the upper part of the ilium, partly beneath the gluteus maximus. It runs downward and forward, attaching on the lateral surface of the greater trochanter. The gluteus medius is innervated by the superior gluteal nerve, L5 and S1. Acting from above, it abducts the thigh, and the anterior fibers rotate it medially. Acting from below, it tractions the pelvis on the side of the supporting leg, so that the unsupported contralateral side is raised slightly. If the pelvis sinks on the unsupported side when the patient stands on the opposite leg, it is known as the Trendelenberg sign and indicates gluteus medius dysfunction (27).

Gluteus medius trigger points refer pain medially over the sacrum, laterally along the iliac crest, and

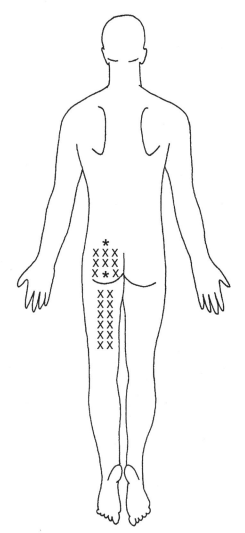

Figure 12.4. Gluteus maximus syndrome. Trigger points (*) in the upper and lower fibers of the gluteus maximus refer pain (×) into the ipsilateral buttock and posterior thigh. (Adapted from Kirkaldy-Willis WH: *Managing Low Back Pain*, ed 2. New York, Churchill Livingstone, 1988, p 142.)

occasionally downward to the midbuttock and the upper part of the thigh posteriorly (76, 77) (Fig. 12.5). Stretching the gluteus medius, along with physical therapy and pressure therapy, rapidly resolves this syndrome.

The middle fibers of the gluteus medius muscle can be passively stretched with the patient lying on the uninvolved side with the painful uppermost leg flexed to 90° at the hip, and with the knee of that leg resting on the surface of the treatment table. The thigh is then passively adducted further at the hip by pulling the pelvis backward while stretching the muscle fibers.

The anterior fibers of the gluteus medius can be passively stretched with the patient lying on the uninvolved side, close to the edge of the table. Standing behind the patient, the doctor lifts the affected thigh in extension, backward over the edge of

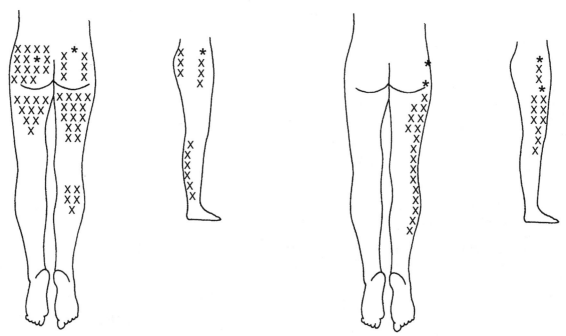

Figure 12.5. Gluteus medius and minimus syndromes. Trigger points (*) in the left gluteus medius refer pain (×) medially over the sacrum, laterally along the iliac crest, and occasionally downward to the midbuttock and the upper part of the posterior thigh. Trigger points (*) in the right posterior part of the gluteus minimus refer pain (×) down the lower part of the buttock, down the posterior thigh, and into the calf, skipping the knee. Trigger points (*) in the anterior part of the gluteus medius (lateral view) refer pain (×) into the buttock, lateral thigh, and leg, also skipping the knee. (Adapted from Simons DG: Muscle pain syndromes, part II. *Am J Phys Med* 55:15–42, 1976.)

Figure 12.6. Tensor fasciae latae syndrome. Trigger points (*) in the tensor fasciae latae refer pain (×) from the lateral pelvis down the lateral thigh and leg as far as the midcalf. (Adapted from Kirkaldy-Willis WH: *Managing Low Back Pain*, ed 2. New York, Churchill Livingstone, 1988, p 142.)

the table while adducting the thigh by lowering it toward the floor and crossing it behind the other thigh.

The posterior fibers of the gluteus medius are passively stretched with the patient lying on the uninvolved side, close to the edge of the table, facing the doctor. The thigh is lowered by crossing the painful uppermost leg in front of the other leg, to place the hip in slight flexion and full adduction (76).

Gluteus Minimus Syndrome

The gluteus minimus muscle attaches above to the ilium, beneath the gluteus medius. It is a fan-shaped muscle that converges to attach below to the greater trochanter. It is innervated by the superior gluteal nerve, L5 and S1. The gluteus minimus has the same action as the gluteus medius (26).

Trigger points in the posterior portion of the gluteus minimus refer pain downward to the lower part of the buttock, down the thigh posteriorly, and into the calf, skipping the knee (Fig. 12.6) (76). Trigger points in the anterior part of the gluteus minimus cause similar low-bottock pain, which projects to

the lateral thigh and leg as far as the lateral malleolus, also skipping the knee (Fig. 12.6).

Management includes pressure applied to the trigger points following physical therapy as well as stretching. The procedure for passively stretching the gluteus minimus is the same as that for stretching the gluteus medius. Like the piriformis muscle, trigger points in the gluteal muscles can cause "sciatica" (76), which is distinguished from sciatic neuritis by the absence of neurological deficit.

Tensor Fasciae Latae Syndrome

The tensor fasciae latae arises from the outer iliac crest, the anterior superior iliac spine and part of the notch below it, and from the deep surface of the fascia lata. It descends between and is attached to the two layers of the iliotibial tract of the fascia lata. It is innervated by the superior gluteal nerve, L4 and L5.

Through the iliotibial tract the tensor fascia latae extends the knee, with lateral rotation of the leg, and assists in abduction and medial rotation of the thigh. Acting from below it stabilizes the pelvis on the head of the femur (26).

Trigger points in the tensor fasciae latae refer pain from the lateral pelvis down the lateral thigh and leg as far as the midcalf (78) (Fig. 12.7).

In addition to deep pressure applied to the trigger points in the tensor fasciae latae, a stripping motion from the hip down the lateral thigh and leg passively stretches the muscle. The muscle can be ac-

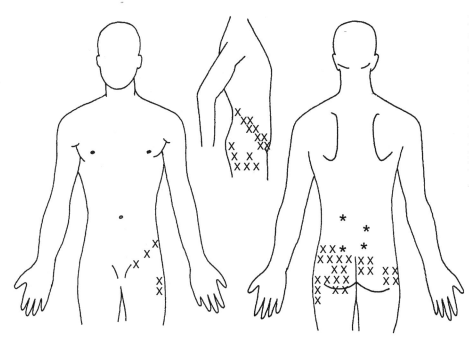

Figure 12.7. Quadratus lumborum syndrome. Trigger points (*) in the superficial lateral fibers of the left quadratus lumborum refer pain (×) to the abdomen and around the iliac crest. Trigger points (*) in the deeper diagonal fibers at the attachment on the right transverse processes refer pain (×) into the lower right buttock and sacroiliac region. (Adapted from Simons DG: Muscle pain syndromes, part II. *Am J Phys Med* 55:15–42, 1976.)

tively stretched by adduction of the hip with a straight leg.

Quadratus Lumborum

According to Simons (16), the quadratus lumborum is a frequently overlooked cause of low back pain of myofascial origin. Sola (79) attributes the high frequency of involvement to the fact that of all the lumbar muscles, the quadratus lumborum is the only one under active tension during walking, sitting, and lying. In particular, the slumped position as demonstrated in driving a car, accentuates stress in the attachment of the muscle.

The quadratus lumborum is an irregularly quadralateral muscle, with many of the fibers running nearly vertically, deep under the paraspinal muscles. These fibers connect above to the 12th rib and below to the posterior third of the iliac crest. In addition to the longitudinal fibers, four small tendons attach medially to the apices of the transverse processes of the upper four lumbar vertebrae (27). Some of the fibers are oriented diagonally downward to the iliac crest and upward to the 12th rib, forming a series of crisscrossing bundles. The quadratus lumborum is innervated by the ventral rami of the 12th thoracic and upper three or four lumbar spinal nerves (27).

The quadratus lumborum acts as a muscle of inspiration, by helping to steady the origin of the diaphragm, which attaches to the bodies of the upper lumbar vertebrae. Acting unilaterally, with the pelvis fixed, it flexes the vertebral column to the same side. Acting bilaterally, the quadratus lumborum extends the spine (27).

Acute strain of the quadratus lumborum muscle may result from a quick bending-and-twisting inci-

dent or from a fall in which the muscle is overstretched. Sustained or repetitive activities may also produce an overuse syndrome. Symptoms include pain on walking, when twisting, while stooping, when turning over in bed, in rising from a chair, when coughing or sneezing, and when climbing stairs. Pain at rest, especially at night, may be severe, and in the morning the patient may have extreme difficulty getting out of bed and may have to crawl on hands and knees to reach the bathroom (16). Because it assists respiratory function by anchoring the 12th rib for the pull of the diaphragm it frequently signals its distress with 12th rib pain in deep inspiration (80).

Examination reveals guarded movements when walking, lying down, or rising from a seated position. Postural evaluation shows a pelvic list to one side, when standing. Flexion and extension are limited, and lateral-bending away from the involved side is restricted, with exquisite spot tenderness in the involved muscle (16). Rapid stretching of the muscle by bending to the opposite side may exacerbate the symptoms (78).

Palpation of the quadratus lumborum is facilitated by positioning the patient on the examining table in a manner that separates the 12th rib from the iliac crest. Lying on the uninvolved side, the patient elevates the rib cage by reaching high overhead with the upper arm and grasping the edge of the examination table. The pelvis is drawn down by dropping the upper thigh and knee backward on the table. This results in tautening of the involved muscle, which lifts it nearer to the surface, making it more accessible to palpation.

The superficial portions of the muscle are palpated where they attach to the 12th rib and to the

Figure 12.8. Paraspinal muscle syndrome. Trigger points (*) in the midlevel of the right iliocostalis thoracis refer pain (×) in a roughly segmental pattern, anterolaterally. Trigger points (*) in the lower portion of the left iliocostalis thoracis refer pain (×) both caudally and cephalically. (Adapted from Simons DG: Muscle pain syndromes, part II. *Am J Phys Med* 55:15–42, 1976.)

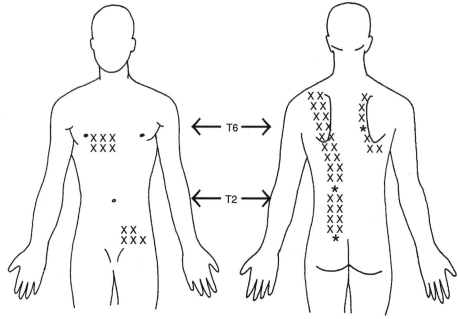

iliac crest. The deep portion of the muscle can be palpated with firm downward pressure toward the lumbar transverse process.

Trigger points located in the lateral, more superficial, longitudinal fibers of the quadratus lumborum refer pain downward, mainly over the iliac crest and the greater trochanter and occasionally anteriorly, to the lower abdomen and groin. When located in the medial deeper fibers, trigger points in the quadratus lumborum refer pain downward but more posteriorly to the sacroiliac joint and deep in the midbuttock (Fig. 12.8). This can be misdiagnosed as trochanteric bursitis or sacroiliac dysfunction (16). Bilateral involvement of the quadratus lumborum may lead to pain on both sides of the back, seen most frequently in females and often associated with symptoms of pregnancy.

Passive stretching of the quadratus lumborum can be achieved by two methods. With either position, the rib cage (12th rib) must be elevated while the pelvis is tilted to depress the iliac crest. The goal is to separate as far as possible the two regions of attachment of the muscle. With both positions the patient lies on the uninvolved side.

For the first position, the patient's back is to the doctor, close to the edge of the table, with the upper leg lowered behind the other leg. The patient then reaches overhead with the uppermost arm to grasp the edge of the table. The patient's uppermost lower extremity is tractioned in extension with adduction of the hips as tolerated. Maximal stretch of the quadratus lumborum requires that the thigh be fully adducted, to produce full tilt of the pelvis while the rib cage is elevated.

For the second position, the patient faces the doctor, again close to the edge of the table, and grasps

the end of the table to elevate the rib cage. The uppermost leg is then lowered in front of (rather than behind) the other leg. Pressure can then be applied to the leg, as tolerated, to help tilt the rim of the pelvis away from the rib cage. An assistant may help to elevate the ribs to improve the stretch (16).

Thoracolumbar Paraspinal Muscles

The thoracolumbar paraspinal muscles comprise three groups, the more superficial, longitudinally running sacrospinalis (erector spinae) group; the deeper, more diagonal group referred to as the transversospinalis group; and a less consistent group including the intersegmental muscles (interspinalis and intertransversarii). The thoracolumbar paraspinal muscles are a frequent source of referred back pain from both muscle spasm and specific trigger points (81).

The sacrospinalis (erector spinae) lie in the groove on the side of the vertebral column and comprise three groups, the iliocostalis, longissimus and spinalis. The most lateral group, the iliocostalis, attaches above the angles of the ribs. The intermediate erector spinae and the longissimus attach above the transverse processes of the thoracic and lumbar vertebra. Below, these two muscle groups attach to the posterior surface of the sacrum, the ilium, and the spines of the lumbar and 11th and 12th thoracic vertebrae, where they form a thick, fleshy mass that is readily palpable. The iliocostalis and longissimus are innervated by the dorsal rami of the spinal nerves. They both extend and laterally flex the spinal column. The most medial group, the spinalis, as the name suggests, attach to the spines of the upper and lower thoracic and upper lumbar vertebrae. The spinalis are innervated by the dorsal rami of the lower cervical and upper thoracic spinal nerves and act as extensors of the vertebral column (27).

Strain of the longitudinal muscles is common when the patient lifts a heavy object, facing forward. These muscles are most vulnerable to strain when they are eccentrically loaded. This occurs with contraction of muscle fibers while the muscle lengthens in a controlled manner. Repetitive bending and lifting can also lead to an overuse syndrome in which the patient may not notice a great deal of pain initially, with a gradual worsening within 2–3 days. As the muscle spasm increases the patient moves with the spine stiffened protectively.

When the superficial paraspinal muscles are involved, tense bands can be palpated against underlying structures. These bands exhibit exquisitely tender trigger points. To passively stretch the iliocostalis and longissimus paraspinal muscles the patient sits with the feet on the floor, leaning forward. The head is dropped with the arms hanging loosely between the legs. Forward pressure is then applied to the torso to further stretch the spine.

Trigger points in the thoracolumbar paraspinal muscles tend to refer pain caudally (16). Trigger points in the iliocostalis also refer pain anterolaterally to the lower chest and abdomen in a roughly segmental distribution and may refer pain upward through several spinal segments to the scapular region (Fig. 12.8). Referred pain from the iliocostalis and longissimus may refer down to the lower buttock, skipping several segments (Figs. 12.8, 12.9) (16).

The more deeply the transversospinalis muscles are located, the shorter and more diagonal they become. The multifidus attach to the maxillary processes in the lumbar region and the transverse processes in the thoracic region. They run diagonally upward, passing superficially from one vertebra to the third or fourth above, with the deepest fibers connecting contiguous vertebrae.

Deep to the multifidus are the rotatores muscles, which are most developed in the thoracic spine. In the lumbar region they are represented only by irregular bundles. The rotatores are small and somewhat quadrilateral in form. Each connects the transverse process of one vertebra to the lamina of the next vertebra above. Both the multifidus and rotatores are innervated by the dorsal rami of the spinal nerves.

The interspinalis are short, paired muscles between contiguous vertebrae, one on each side of the interspinous ligament. They are inconsistent and commonly found in the upper and lower thoracic region, being most developed in the lumbar region. They are innervated also by the dorsal rami of the spinal nerves.

The intertransversarii are small muscles joining the transverse processes of the upper and lower thoracic vertebrae. In the lumbar region they consist of 2 sets of muscles. The more medial intertransversarii medialis connects the accessory process of one

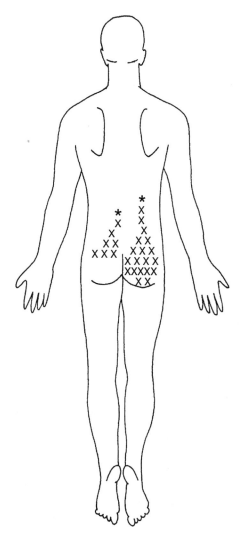

Figure 12.9. Paraspinal muscle syndrome. Trigger points (*) in the longissimus thoracis refer pain (×) caudally, sometimes as low as the buttocks (right side). Referred pain (×) from trigger points (*) in the iliocostalis lumborum also travels downward. (Adapted from Simons DG: Muscle pain syndromes, part II. *Am J Phys Med* 55:15–42, 1976.)

vertebra with the mamillary process of the next. The more lateral intertransversarii lateralis comprise dorsal and ventral parts. The dorsal part connects the accessory process of one vertebra to the transverse process of the succeeding vertebra. The ventral part connects the transverse processes of contiguous vertebrae.

The intertransversarii medialis lumborum and the thoracic intertransversarii are innervated by the dorsal rami of the spinal nerves. The intertransversarii lateralis are supplied by the ventral rami.

The deep, short muscles of the back serve as postural stabilizers. The short levers formed by the union of the vertebral motion segments would buckle during spinal movement without the bracing effect of these muscles. In this way they insure the efficient action of the long muscles (27).

Figure 12.10. Transversospinalis syndrome. Referred pain patterns (×) from corresponding trigger points (*) in the transversospinalis muscles (multifidus and rotators) are localized to the area around the trigger points and may refer anteriorly to the same level. (Adapted from Simons DG: Muscle pain syndromes, part II. *Am J Phys Med* 55:15–42, 1976.)

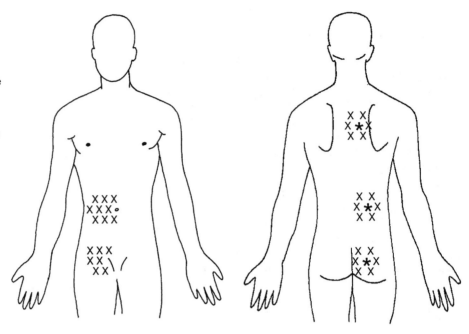

Patients with trigger points in the multifidus and rotatores muscles complain of deep pain and circumscribed tenderness adjacent to the spinous process at the level of the involved muscles. The vertebral spine is tender to tapping or firm pressure, and segmental motion may be restricted (referred tenderness).

Trigger points in the deep paraspinal muscles refer pain and tenderness to the midline from either side (Fig. 12.10). The patient's complaints are centered on the spinous process at the same level as the trigger point (14, 22). The deep paraspinal muscles cannot be actively stretched, but passive, deep compression of the trigger points brings effective relief of both local and referred pain with restoration of segmental motion (8).

Repeated manipulation of hypermobile vertebral joints that are restricted by hypertonic muscles rather than articular blockage brings only brief relief from pain and is not recommended (see "Hypermobility"). Patients with muscle fixation due to trigger points in the deep paraspinal muscle respond favorably to specific trigger point therapy to the involved muscle and should be treated accordingly. Injudicious repeated manipulation of these patients may perpetuate the patient's problem and create unnecessary dependence upon manipulation, without resolution of the problem.

Serratus Posterior Inferior Syndrome

The myofascial pain syndrome of the serratus posterior inferior muscle is seen less frequently than other muscle syndromes that produce back pain, but it is distressing when present (16). It responds well to trigger point therapy (16).

The serratus posterior inferior attaches above and laterally to the last four ribs. The fibers run obliquely and attach medially below to the spinous processes of the 11th and 12th thoracic and 1st and 2nd lumbar vertebrae. It is innervated by the ventral rami of the ninth, tenth, eleventh and twelfth thoracic spinal nerves (27).

The serratus posterior inferior depresses the ribs during forced expiration and assists in rotation of the spine at the thoracolumbar junction. Patients with trigger points in this muscle complain of pain over the lower ribs, often independent of spinal movement (Fig. 12.11). Flexion of the thoracolumbar spine is slightly restricted on examination (16). Patients with serratus posterior inferior muscle involvement often have disharmony between the respiratory muscles of the chest and abdomen (paradoxical breathing), but a deep breath is not painful, unlike intercostal muscle spasm and rib fixations (16).

Trigger points are found in the serratus posterior inferior over the lower ribs. Aching pain is referred in this region following trigger point therapy (ischemic compression). Passive stretching of the muscle may be achieved with the patient seated and leaning forward to achieve maximum flexion of the thoracic lumbar spine; the shoulder on the affected side is then rotated forward. Following a deep breath, the patient is further passively flexed and rotated to achieve maximum stretch of the serratus posterior inferior (16).

Rectus Abdominis Muscle

Trigger points in the rectus abdominis muscle refer pain in a distinctively horizontal pattern of low or mid back pain (Fig. 12.12). The rectus abdominis

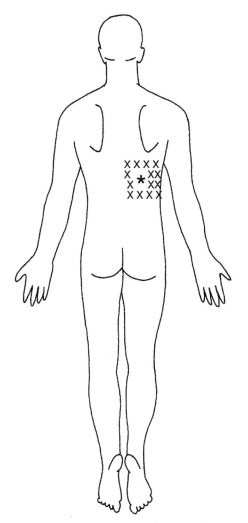

Figure 12.11. Serratus posterior inferior syndrome. Trigger points (*) in the serratus posterior inferior cause back pain (×) in a referral pattern in the lower thoracic and upper lumbar region. (Adapted from Simons DG: Muscle pain syndromes, part II. *Am J Phys Med* 55:15–42, 1976.)

attaches above to the fifth, sixth and seventh ribs anteriorly and below to the pubic bone. It is innervated by the ventral rami of the lower six or seven thoracic spinal nerves. The rectus abdominis is a strong flexor of the spine and also provides a compressive force on the abdominal viscera. It plays an important role in expiration with increased intraabdominal pressure (16).

Palpation reveals trigger points in terminal fibers of the rectus abdominis on one or both sides. The inhibition of contraction associated with trigger points in this muscle causes weakness of the abdominal wall, and the patient fails to "pull in" the protruded abdomen. Trigger points in the uppermost fibers are found in the angle between the midline and the rib cage at the level of and slightly below the tip of the xyphoid process. These trigger points refer pain horizontally across both sides of the back even when located on one side only (Fig. 12.12). Simi-

larly, trigger points in the lower fiber refer pain horizontally across the sacrum, iliac crests, and upper gluteal regions, whether located unilaterally or bilaterally (16). These can be located close to the symphysis pubis.

In addition to trigger point therapy, passive stretching of the rectus abdominis can be achieved by having the patient lie supine with the feet resting on a support below the level of the treatment table. This separates the pubis from rib cage, lengthening the abdominal muscles.

An active exercise program enhances recovery and prevents recurrence. Pelvic tilts with isometric contraction of the abdominal musculature strengthen the muscle initially. The patient can then proceed to reverse curl-ups. The lengthening contraction of the abdominal wall muscles during the controlled eccentric contraction of the reverse sit-up helps to restore the muscles to normal function. The patient can then proceed from 1 to 15 sit-ups in a series, with a pause and deep breathing between cycles (16).

Iliopsoas Syndrome

The psoas muscle arises from the bodies, intervertebral discs, and the transverse processes of the lumbar vertebrae. Along with the iliacus, it attaches below to the lesser trochanter on the medial aspect of the femur. The iliacus attaches above to the inner surface of the iliac bone. The psoas is innervated by the ventral rami of the lumbar nerves L1, 2, 3. The iliacus is innervated by branches of the femoral nerves L2 and 3.

Acting together from above, the psoas, assisted by the iliacus, flexes the thigh upon the pelvis. When the psoas and iliacus act bilaterally from below they contract powerfully to bend the trunk and pelvis forward against resistance, as in raising the trunk from the recumbent to the sitting posture (16). This action places a strong anterior pull on the lumbar spine, which increases with lumbar lordosis and intradiscal pressure, especially at L3, making full sit-ups contraindicated in patients with low back pain (82).

Patients with iliopsoas trigger points walk with a typical psoatic gait. They exhibit a stooped posture, with the hip flexed and the ipsilateral thigh externally rotated. Extension and rotation of the thigh is limited, as is extension of the spine. Palpation reveals trigger points immediately above the femoral attachment of the iliopsoas tendon, when pressure is applied deeply along the medial wall of the triangle toward the lesser trochanter. Trigger points can also be located by pressure applied to the iliacus against the iliac fossa just inside the brim of the pelvis behind the anterior superior iliac spine and by pressure applied medially, lateral to the rectus abdominis muscle, just below the level of the umbilicus (Fig. 12.13).

To passively stretch the iliopsoas muscle, the patient lies supine, with a rolled towel or small pillow

Figure 12.12. Rectus abdominis syndrome. Trigger points (*) in the rectus abdominis muscle refers pain (×) in a distinctly horizontal pattern across both sides of the back, whether located unilaterally or bilaterally. (Adapted from Simons DG: Muscle pain syndromes, part II. *Am J Phys Med* 55:15–42, 1976.)

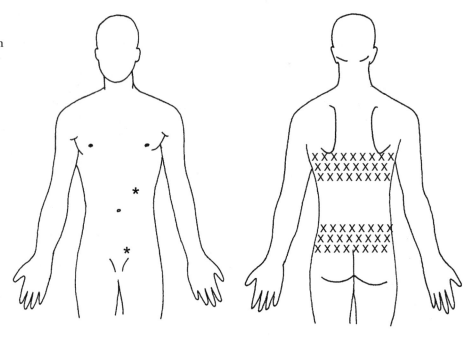

under the back and with the thigh on the involved side moderately abducted and extended over the side of the treatment table. The thigh can then be gradually extended and rotated internally (16).

Levator Scapulae

The levator scapulae is a common site of trigger points (4) that produce complaints of a stiff neck and restricted range of cervical motion (83). It is frequently strained in whiplash injuries and is the site of postural stress when the head is turned to one side for prolonged periods of time (8).

The levator scapulae is attached above by tendinous slips to the transverse process of the atlas and axis and the posterior tubercles of the transverse process of the third and fourth cervical vertebrae. It descends diagonally to attach below to the medial border of the scapula (27). It twists so that the C1 digitation is superficial to the others with the fibers vertical. The C4 digitation lies deepest and passes more diagonally to attach to the superior angle of the scapulae (8). Innervation is supplied directly by the third and fourth cervical spinal nerves and by the fifth cervical through the dorsal scapula nerve.

Figure 12.13. Iliopsoas syndrome. Pain referred (×) from trigger points (*) in the iliopsoas muscle forms a characteristic vertical pattern unilaterally along the lumbar spine, extending downward to the sacroiliac region, and over the front of the ipsilateral thigh. (Adapted from Simons DG: Muscle pain syndromes, part II. *Am J Phys Med* 55:15–42, 1976.)

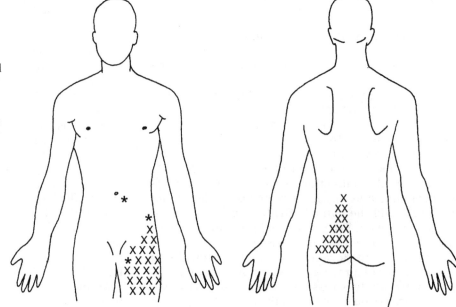

The levator scapulae acts in association with other muscles to stabilize the shoulder during movements of the upper extremity. When the cervical part of the spine is fixed, the levator scapulae acts with the trapezius to elevate the scapula or to sustain a weight carried on the shoulder. If the shoulder is fixed, the muscle inclines the neck to the same side. Both muscles acting together resist neck flexion. Acting with the rhomboid muscles and the latissimus dorsi, the levator scapulae rotates the glenoid fossa of the scapula downward, while pulling the inferior angles of the scapulae together. The levator scapulae, in conjunction with the upper trapezius and uppermost fibers of the serratus anterior, elevates the scapula, as when shrugging the shoulders (84).

Patients with trigger points in the levator scapulae complain of a "stiff neck." They frequently have been subjected to psychological stress, which produces the typical "weight of the world on my shoulders" posture (84) and a tense, hostile, repressive attitude. Occupations requiring the head and neck to be turned to one side for prolonged periods (such as typing or cradling the phone with the shoulders) can produce and perpetuate trigger points in the levator scapulae. Sleeping with the neck in a tilted position or in a cold draft can also precipitate this condition. Viral infections, especially oral herpes simplex, can activate trigger points in the levator scapulae, making it vulnerable to postural loads (8).

In addition to complaints of a stiff neck, patients complain of tension headaches and pain referred up the neck and into the shoulder posteriorly. Neck motion is moderately restricted, as the patient tends to look sideways by turning the eyes or body rather than the neck. The head may be tilted slightly to the involved side. If the patient's head is markedly tilted to one side (wry neck or torticollis), trigger points in the sternocleidomastoid muscle are more likely to be involved (Chapter 10).

Trigger points develop in the levator scapulae just cephalad to the attachment of the muscle to the superior angle of the scapula and at the angle of the neck where the muscle emerges from the upper fibers of the trapezius. To locate the trigger points, the patient is seated with the neck turned toward the opposite side to stretch and tighten the muscle and to lift it towards the palpating fingers. To locate the lower trigger point a stroking action back and forth across the muscle may be necessary. These trigger points are exquisitely tender to pressure and refer pain upward to the upper cervical region (8) (Fig. 12.14).

Repeated manipulation of the ipsilateral upper cervical vertebrae should be avoided. While manipulation provides temporary relief of symptoms (up to two hours), as with any muscular fixation, treatment is more effective when directed to the muscle rather than to the joints. In addition to pressure therapy, home stretching under a hot shower with the

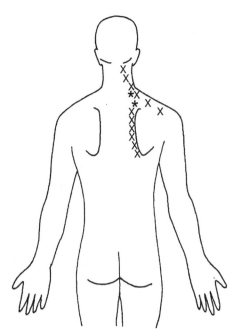

Figure 12.14. Levator scapulae syndrome. Trigger points (*) in the levator scapulae refer pain (×) up the neck, into the shoulder, and along the vertebral border of the scapula. (Adapted from Travell JG, Simons DG: *Myofascial Pain and Dysfunction: The Trigger Point Manual.* Baltimore, Williams & Wilkins, 1983.)

contralateral arm pulling the head down brings more effective relief. Ice packs offer palliative relief at times of acute exacerbations, allowing the patient to sleep better.

Trapezius Muscle

The trapezius muscle is a tripartite muscle with upper, middle, and lower fibers that often function independently. It is a flat, triangular muscle extending over the back of the neck and upper thorax. It is probably the muscle most often beleaguered by trigger points (4, 8), possibly because of its function as a stabilizer of the upper extremities. The frequent static loading of this muscle while the head is poked forward and the arms used repetitively out in front makes it vulnerable to chronic muscle pain due to overuse.

Anatomically the right and left trapezius muscles form a large trapezium from which it is named (27). It is attached to the medial one-third of the superior nuchal line of the occipital bone, the external occipital protuberance, the ligamentum nuchae, the seventh cervical and all the thoracic spinous processes, and the corresponding supraspinous ligaments. The superior fibers pass downward, attaching to the outer third of the clavicle. The middle fibers attach laterally to the acromion and superior border of the spine of the scapulae. The lower fibers proceed upward, attaching to the tubercle at the medial end of the spine of the scapula, just lateral to the lower attachment of the levator scapulae muscle.

The motor innervation of the trapezius muscle is supplied by the spinal accessory nerve (cranial nerve XI) arising from the ventral roots of the first five cervical segments, which ascend through the foramen magnum and exit the skull through the jugular foramen. This nerve joins a plexus beneath the trapezius with sensory (proprioceptive) fibers from spinal nerves (C 3, and 4).

The upper fibers act with the levator scapulae to elevate the scapulae and with it the point of the shoulder. Acting with the serratus anterior, the trapezius rotates the scapula in a forward direction, so that the arm can be raised above the head. Acting bilaterally, the upper fibers may extend the head and neck when the shoulder is fixed. The middle fibers abduct and retract the scapula (move it toward the midline). They also assist in rotating the glenoid fossa upward, allowing the arm to abduct, especially near the end of its full range. The lower fibers of the trapezius retract the scapula and rotate the glenoid fossa upward by depressing the vertebral border of the scapula. These fibers also assist in flexion and abduction of the arm.

Patients with trigger points in the upper fibers of the trapezius muscle complain of pain unilaterally upward along the posterolateral aspect of the neck to the mastoid process (Fig. 12.15). These trigger points are a common source of tension neckache and temporal headache on the ipsilateral side. Occasionally the pain may be referred to the angle of the jaw with a resultant misdiagnosis of cervical radiculopathy or atypical facial neuralgia (8). Trigger points in the upper fibers of the trapezius are found near the medial end of the spine of the scapula, just lateral to the attachment of the levator scapulae (Fig. 12.15).

Observation of the patient with trigger points in the upper trapezius often reveals a typical posture with bilateral shoulder elevation and a slight tilt of the neck toward the affected side. These patients may be observed to rub the trapezius muscle, and often they move the head in an attempt to stretch the muscle. Examination may reveal slight restriction of motion on contralateral lateral flexion, and flexion of the neck as well as abduction of the arm due to the restricted upward rotation of the scapula. These patients may also complain of pain on contralateral rotation at the extreme range of motion.

To locate and deactivate trigger points in the upper fibers of the trapezius, the patient is either supine or seated, with the ipsilateral ear drawn slightly toward the shoulder. A pincer grasp is then applied to the muscle mass that harbors the trigger point, lifting it off the underlying supraspinatus muscle. The muscle can then be rolled firmly between the thumb and fingers. These trigger points in the upper fibers of the trapezius often refer pain to the neck, occiput, and temple.

Trigger points in the middle fibers of the trapezius muscle produce a burning pain that is referred me-

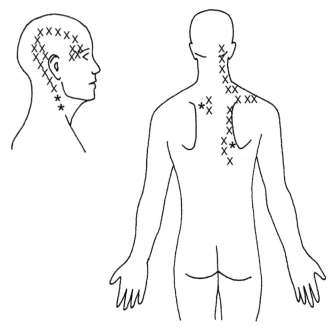

Figure 12.15. Trapezius syndrome. Trigger points (*) in the upper trapezius fibers (lateral view) characteristically refer pain (×) along the posterolateral aspect of the neck, behind the ear, and to the temple. Trigger points (*) in the middle trapezius refer pain (×) medially to the spinous processes and laterally to the top of the shoulder. Trigger points (*) in the lower fibers refer pain (×) mainly to the neck suprascapula and intrascapular region. (Adapted from Travell JG, Simons DG: *Myofasical Pain and Dysfunction: The Trigger Point Manual.* Baltimore, Williams & Wilkins, 1983.)

dially from the trigger points located near the upper border of the scapula. This pain may radiate upward as far as C7. Trigger points found near the acromion refer aching pain to the top of the shoulder or acromial process. The patient frequently gives a history of prolonged activity with the arm held up and forward, which creates an overuse syndrome with the middle fibers of the trapezius muscle attempting to counteract the unrelenting protraction of the scapulae. Trigger points from static loading of the middle fibers of the trapezius are commonly seen in drivers who grasp the top of the steering wheel, typists, CRT operators, and others who sustain a round-shouldered posture for prolonged periods. Often the antagonistic pectoral muscles become shortened, perpetuating the rounded shoulders.

Trigger points in the lateral lower trapezius fibers can refer pain downward along the vertebral border of the scapula. Those located more medially refer pain upward to the cervical region of the paraspinal muscles, the adjacent mastoid area, and the acromion (Fig. 12.15). The lower fibers are strained by prolonged bending and reaching forward while sitting.

To examine for trigger points in the middle and lower fibers of the trapezius, the patient is seated with the arms folded in front of the body to protract

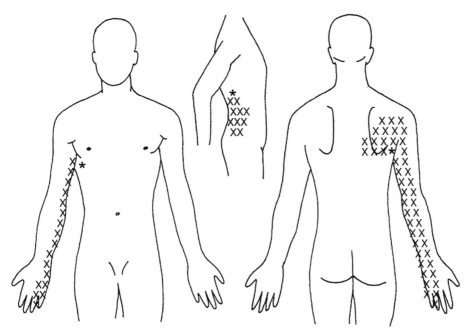

Figure 12.16. Latissimus dorsi syndrome. Trigger points (*) in the axillary portion of the latissimus dorsi refer pain (×) in the area of the back of the shoulder and down the medial arm and forearm. It may include the ulnar aspect of the hand, the ring, and the little fingers. Trigger points (*) in the fascial attachments of the latissimus dorsi (lateral view) refer pain (×) into the lumbosacral area. (Adapted from Travell JG, Simons DG: *Myofascial Pain and Dysfunction: The Trigger Point Manual.* Baltimore, Williams & Wilkins, 1983.)

the scapula and the trunk slightly flexed to place the muscle on stretch. The patient's head can then be tractioned to the contralateral side to add further stretch, while deep pressure is applied directly to the trigger points (8). The patient may apply ischemic compression at home by lying on a tennis ball that is positioned to press on tender spots (8).

Latissimus Dorsi

Trigger points in the latissimus dorsi refer pain into the midback region, which may be mistaken for intrathoracic disease (see Chapter 9). The latissimus dorsi is a large, flat, triangular muscle with fibers extending over the lumbar region and the lower half of the thorax, converging to a narrow tendinous attachment to the humerus.

Below, the muscle attaches to the sacrum and lumbar vertebrae via the lumbar aponeurosis, to the spinous processes of the lower six thoracic vertebrae, and to the superior border of the last three or four ribs. Above, the fibers converge and twist nearly 180° around the teres major muscle, merging with it to attach to the medial edge of the intertubercular groove of the humerus. Occasionally the nearly horizontal fibers attach to the tip of the scapula along with the teres major. The uppermost horizontal fibers of the latissimus dorsi attach distally on the humerus, while the lower, more vertical fibers attach proximally because of the way the muscle curves around the lower fibers of the teres major.

The latissimus dorsi is innervated by the thoracodorsal (long subscapular) nerve from the posterior cord of the brachial plexus, C6, 7, and 8. The primary actions of the latissimus dorsi is adduction, extension, and especially medial rotation of the humerus (26).

Patients with trigger points in the latissimus dorsi complain of a constant aching pain referred to the inferior angle of the scapula and the surrounding midthoracic region. This pain may also extend to the back of the shoulder and down the medial aspect of the arm, forearm, and hand, including the ring and little fingers (Fig. 12.16). Patients may indicate the origin of pain on the pain diagram as a circle centered on the inferior angle of the scapula (8). The pain is aggravated by reaching up and far out in front to handle an awkwardly large object or to pull something down (8).

The trigger points responsible for the pain are usually located in the axillary portion of the muscle, in the posterior axillary fold. A pincer palpation of the posterior axillary fold at approximately the midscapular level may be necessary to locate the source of pain and to inactivate the trigger points.

To examine the latissimus dorsi, the patient is supine, with the ipsilateral hand under the head and the arm abducted to approximately 90°. The examiner can then grasp the muscle along the free border of the axillary fold at the midscapular level. The muscle can then be lifted off the chest wall, and the firm bands and trigger points can be rolled between the fingers (9). The trigger points can then be inactivated by a pincer-like pressure, using the opposing fingers and thumb to apply the pressure.

Figure 12.17. Sternocleidomastoid syndrome. Trigger points (*) in the sternal division of the SCM may refer pain (×) to the vertex, to the occiput, across the cheek, over the eye to the throat and the sternum (view A). Trigger points (*) in the clavicular division refer pain (×) to the eye and face as well as the ipsilateral suboccipital region (view B). (Adapted from Travell JG, Simons DG: *Myofascial Pain and Dysfunction: The Trigger Point Manual*. Baltimore, Williams & Wilkins, 1983.)

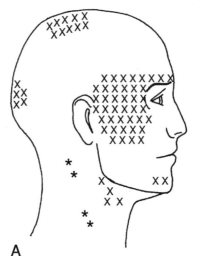

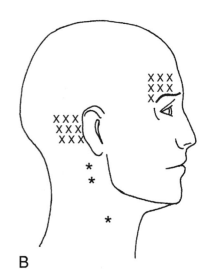

A

B

Sternocleidomastoid Muscle (SCM)

The sternocleidomastoid (SCM) muscle with the scalene muscles forms the anterior strap muscles that are a frequent site of muscle strain from "whiplash" injuries (Chapter 10). It is also the muscle involved in torticollis, commonly known as wryneck (Chapter 10).

Anatomically it is a complex muscle with two divisions, the sternal, which is more medial and superficial, and the clavicular, which lies lateral and deeper. Above, the muscle is attached by a short tendon into the lateral surface of the mastoid process and to the lateral half of the superior nuchal line of the occipital bone. Below, the medial or sternal head is attached to the manubrium sterni running obliquely upward, laterally, and backward. The lateral or clavicular head attaches below to the medial third of the superior border of the anterior surface of the clavicle. It passes almost vertically upward behind the sternal head and blends, with its deep surface forming a thick rounded belly (27).

The sternocleidomastoid is innervated by the accessory nerve, which arises within the spinal column from the ventral roots of the motor fibers of the upper five cervical segments. The motor nerve fibers ascend through the foramen magnum and then descend through the jugular foramen where they unite with sensory fibers from the anterior primary division of the second and sometimes third cervical nerves.

Acting unilaterally, the sternocleidomastoid muscle tilts the head toward the ipsilateral side while rotating the face to the contralateral side. Acting with the upper trapezius it laterally bends the neck, drawing the ear toward the ipsilateral shoulder. It acts along with the scalene and trapezius muscles to compensate for head tilt due to postural distortion. Acting together, the two muscles draw the chin forward, assisting the longi colli in neck flexion, checking hyperextension of the neck, and resisting forceful backward movement of the head. Acting with the trapezius, the two muscles stabilize the head during talking and chewing. If the head is fixed, they assist in elevating the thorax in forced inspiration. The two muscles are also active when the head is raised while the body is supine (27).

Trigger points in the SCM generate complaints of "soreness" of the neck and, most commonly, headaches (Fig. 12.17). These trigger points can be located with the patient seated or supine. The muscle is then slackened by laterally flexing the patient's head toward the shoulder on the symptomatic side and rotating the face slightly to the contralateral side. Trigger points can then be located by grasping the muscle between the thumb and fingers.

Pressure on the trigger points can be exerted by the pincer-like grasp rather than by direct pressure on the neck. The clavicular division of the SCM muscle can be stretched by extending the head and neck while rotating the face to the opposite side. To stretch the sternal division, the head is first rotated toward the side of complaint, and at full rotation, the chin is tipped downward toward the shoulder, elevating the occiput and mastoid to provide maximum stretch (8).

Scalene Muscles

Pain from trigger points in the scalene muscles can refer anteriorly, laterally, or posteriorly into the shoulders, chest, arm, and hand. This muscle group, along with the sternocleidomastoideus muscles, is frequently strained in whiplash-type injuries that produce painful trigger points (Chapter 10) (8, 52, 54, 85, 86).

The anterior scalene muscle attaches above to the anterior transverse processes of C3 through C6 and below to the inner border of the first rib. The medial scalene muscle attaches above to the posterior transverse processes of (usually) C2 through C7 (occasionally to only C4 and C5). This muscle starts diagonally and attaches below to the cephalad surface of

Figure 12.18. Scalene syndrome. Trigger points (*) in the scalene muscles refer pain (×) anteriorly to the chest, laterally to the upper extremity, and posteriorly to the medial scapular border and adjacent interscapular region. (Adapted from Travell JG, Simons DG: *Myofascial Pain and Dysfunction: The Trigger Point Manual.* Baltimore, Williams & Wilkins, 1983.)

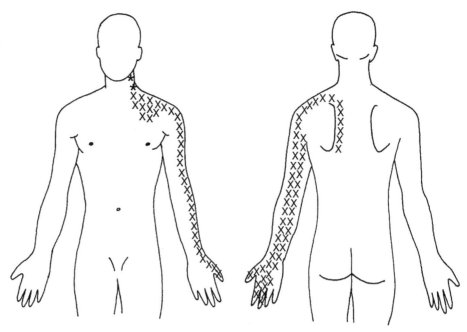

the first rib. The posterior scalene muscle attaches above to the posterior transverse processes of the lowest 2 or 3 cervical vertebrae and below to the lateral surface of the second and sometimes of the third rib. It lies deep to the levator scapulae muscle and posterior to the medial scalene muscle. Innervation of the scalene muscles is by motor branches of the anterior primary rami of the spinal nerves C2 through C3, corresponding to the segmental level of muscular attachment.

The action of the scalene muscles varies according to whether they are fixed from above or below. When fixed from above, the scalenes act as auxiliary muscles of inspiration. They help to support and elevate the upper rib cage when lifting, carrying, or pulling heavy objects. When fixed from below, the scalene muscles, acting unilaterally, laterally flex the cervical spine, moving the head obliquely forward and sideways. Acting bilaterally, the anterior scalene muscles assist neck flexion. The contralateral scalene muscles act as agonists, stabilizing the neck during lateral flexion.

Patients with a history of trauma to the neck should be examined for scalene muscle injury. Muscle strain of the scalene muscles frequently results from hyperextension (whiplash) injuries. If the head is turned during impact or is hit from the side, the injury will be unilateral. The characteristic pain pattern referred from trigger points in the scalene muscles extends over the deltoid area, down the front and back of the arm (over the biceps and triceps), and along the radial side of the forearm, thumb, and index finger (Fig. 12.18). When it occurs on the left side it may be mistaken for referred pain from the heart. Posteriorly, the pain may be referred over the

upper half of the vertebral border of the scapula and interscapular area (Fig. 12.18).

Entrapment of the brachial plexus between the anterior and middle scalene muscles refers pain down the ulnar side of the hand, with numbness due to sensory impairment. With swollen and taut scalene muscles, referred pain and entrapment pain may be present along with active trigger points. Motion palpation of the first rib will differentiate costovertebral fixation, which should be ruled out.

Examination will reveal restricted lateral bending of the neck to the contralateral side. Placing the ipsilateral forearm across the forehead while raising and pulling the forearm forward, lifts the clavicle off the underlying scalene muscles and brachial plexus, may relieve the pain (8), and may be used to differentiate cervical radiculopathy.

Trigger points in the anterior scalene are palpated beneath the posterior border of the clavicular division of the sternocleidomastoid muscle. Trigger points in the middle scalene can be palpated against the transverse processes of the cervical vertebrae, while those in the posterior scalene muscle are palpated medial to the levator scapulae which must be pushed aside. Pressure on the trigger points in the scalene muscles produces ischemic compression and brings rapid relief of the patient's symptoms.

Stretching to prevent recurrence can be performed by the patient at home. To stretch the anterior scalene muscle, the head and neck are tilted toward the opposite side, and the head is pressed in a posterolateral direction. To stretch the middle scalene muscle, head and neck are tilted toward the opposite side and pressed toward the contralateral shoulder. To stretch the posterior scalene muscle, the head and neck are not turned but are pressed in an antero-

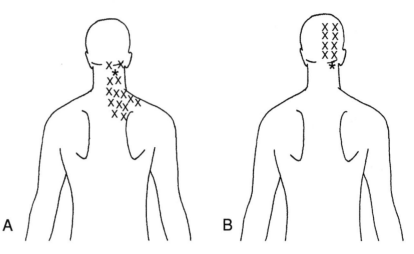

Figure 12.19. Posterior cervical muscle syndrome. Trigger points (*) in the posterior cervical muscles refer pain (×) upward to the suboccipital region and downward over the neck and upper part of the shoulder girdle (view A). If the greater occipital nerve is entrapped by trigger points in the posterior cervical region, pain is referred (×) over the occiput toward the vertex (view B). (Adapted from Travell JG, Simons DG: *Myofascial Pain and Dysfunction: The Trigger Point Manual.* Baltimore, Williams & Wilkins, 1983.)

lateral direction along the lines of the muscle fibers (8).

Posterior Cervical Muscles (Semispinalis Capitis, Semispinalis Cervicis, Multifidi, Rotatores)

Postural stress and trauma are key factors in the production of trigger points in the posterior cervical muscles. Patients with long, supple necks are more vulnerable to strain of these muscles than those with short, stocky necks, because of the greater leverage placed on the muscles (8). Trigger points found in the suboccipital region and face are common causes of pain in the upper posterior portion of the neck, back of the head, and face (87).

The semispinalis cervicis arises from a series of tendinous attachments to the transverse processes of the upper 5 or 6 thoracic vertebrae and inserts into the cervical spines from C2 to C5. The semispinalis capitis arises below from the transverse processes of the upper 6 or 7 thoracic and 7th cervical vertebrae and from the articular processes of the 4th, 5th and 6th cervical vertebrae. Above, it attaches to the occiput, between the superior and inferior nuchal lines.

The semispinalis extends the cervical spine and rotates the neck to the contralateral side. The semispinalis capitis extends the head and turns the face slightly toward the contralateral side.

The multifidus lie deep to the foregoing muscles, filling the groove at the side of the spines of the vertebrae. They arise from the articular processes of the lower four cervical vertebrae, passing obliquely upward and medially attaching to the spines C2 to C5. The most superficial pass from one vertebra to the 3rd or 4th above. The middle fasciculi attach from one vertebra to the 2nd or 3rd above. The deepest connect contiguous vertebrae.

Deep to the multifidus run the rotatores. They connect the transverse process of one vertebra to the lamina of the vertebra next above. They are irregular and variable in the cervical region. The semispinalis capitis and cervicis multifidi and rotatores are innervated by the dorsal rami of the spinal nerves. The multifidus and rotatores are thought to act as segmental stabilizers during spinal movement (Chapter 1).

The posterior cervical muscles are vulnerable to postural stress and trauma. Prolonged cervical extension or forced flexion can produce strain that activates trigger points in these muscles. Patients with trigger points in the posterior cervical muscles complain of pain in the neck, radiating upward to the suboccipital region and downward over the upper part of the shoulder girdle (Fig. 12.19). They frequently complain of tenderness over the back of the head and neck, and pressure from the weight of the head on the pillow may interfere with sleep. Range of motion of the neck is frequently restricted in all planes, especially head and neck flexion (8).

Prolonged activation of trigger points in the posterior cervical muscles may irritate or entrap the greater occipital nerve, producing numbness, tingling, and burning pain in the scalp over the ipsilateral scalp (occipital neuralgia). Ice effectively relieves the burning occipital pain, while heat tends to aggravate it (8). Patients with trigger points in the posterior cervical muscles often hold the shoulders high and restrict bobbing and nodding movements of the head. Significant restriction of flexion is often noted. If unilateral, the muscles on the side of the neck may be seen to stand out like a rope.

Cervical radiculopathy, which also produces hypertonic posterior cervical muscles, must be ruled out. While trigger points in these muscles do not produce limb signs as does cervical radiculopathy, concomitant trigger points in the shoulder girdle may confuse the diagnosis, since these patients complain of extremity pain and paresthesia. Axial (downward) pressure on the head with the cervical spine slightly extended (Spurling's test), which produces radicular pain, aids in the differential diagnosis (Chapter 10). Electrodiagnostic studies and enhanced imaging (CT, MRI, and myelography) are necessary for confirmation of the diagnosis of radiculopathy due to disc herniation.

Palpation of trigger points in posterior cervical muscles is facilitated by seating the patient with the head and neck flexed. Trigger points will be found in these muscles in a taut band. Some patients may find a side-lying or supine position more relaxing. Trigger points are usually found in the posterior cervical muscles a centimeter or two from the midline at C4 or C5, in the suboccipital region, or at the insertion of the semispinalis capitis or the occiput.

Stretching the muscles, along with pressure therapy, is helpful with the patient seated or in side-lying position. Patients positioned supine will respond faster if distraction of the head is employed along with pressure therapy. Travell and Simons (8) recommend a home stretching program performed by the patient seated on a stool under a hot shower. The patient is instructed to latch the fingers over the occiput, tractioning the head down and forward, passively stretching the posterior cervical muscles. It may be necessary for the head to be turned at various angles while this is repeated, to fully stretch the different lines of muscle fibers. Chronic postural strain on these muscles as they checkrein the weight of the head should be avoided, as should chilling the posterior muscles, since they are particularly vulnerable to cold.

Splenius Capitis and Splenius Cervicis Muscles

Patients with trigger points in the splenius capitis and splenius cervicis muscles complain of neck pain and deep, diffuse headaches, often involving the center of the head.

The splenius capitis attaches below to the lower half of the ligamentum nuchae muscles of the spine on the 7th cervical vertebra and the spines of the upper 3rd or 4th thoracic vertebrae. The muscle runs upward and laterally to attach to the mastoid process. It is innervated by the lateral branches of the dorsal rami of the middle cervical spinal nerves. The splenius cervicis attaches below to the spines of the 3rd to 6th thoracic vertebrae ascending laterally to attach to the transverse processes of the 2nd or 3rd cervical vertebrae. It is innervated by the lateral branches of the dorsal rami of the lower cervical spinal nerves.

The splenii, acting bilaterally, extend the head and neck. Acting unilaterally, they turn the face to the ipsilateral side (2). The patient with trigger points in the splenii muscles may give a history of prolonged postural stress or trauma. Activities that overload these muscles involve prolonged extension or rotation of the neck. Rear-end motor vehicle accidents in which the head and neck are rotated at the time of impact, frequently produce muscle strain with subsequent trigger points in these muscles.

Patients with trigger points in the splenius capitis complain primarily of pain referred to the vertex of the head on the ipsilateral side (Fig. 12.20). Trigger points in the splenius cervicis produce complaints of "stiff neck" and pain radiating up the neck into

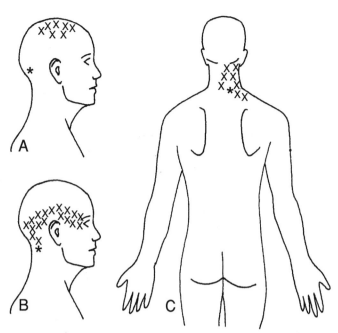

Figure 12.20. Splenius capitis and splenius cervicis syndromes. Trigger points (*) in the splenius capitis (view A) refer pain (×) to the vertex of the head on the ipsilateral side. Trigger points (*) in the upper splenius cervicis refer pain (×) to the orbit (view B). Pain is referred (×) to the angle of the neck from trigger points (*) in the lower splenius cervicis muscle (view C). (Adapted from Travell JG, Simons DG: *Myofascial Pain and Dysfunction: The Trigger Point Manual.* Baltimore, Williams & Wilkins, 1983.)

the head and eye (Fig. 12.20). Examination reveals restriction of motion on rotation of the head to the ipsilateral side, as well as neck flexion (8).

Trigger points in the splenius capitis are usually found in the belly of the muscles and at the insertion on the mastoid process. Trigger points in the splenius cervicis are palpable between the upper trapezius and the more lateral levator scapulae in the belly of the muscle and at the insertion of the muscle into the transverse processes.

To apply pressure to trigger points in the splenii muscles with the patient seated, the head and cervical spine are rotated and stretched away from the side of involvement. The patient may assist in stretching by grasping the back of the head and turning the face to the other side, pulling the head down in the direction of the face. This procedure may be used by the patient to stretch the muscles at home (8).

Suboccipital Muscles (Rectus Capitis Posterior Minor and Major, Obliquus Inferior and Superior)

Trigger points in the suboccipital muscles are a common source of "headaches" (86). The rectus capitis posterior minor arises from the posterior tubercle of the atlas and attaches into the medial part of the area between the inferior nuchal line and the foramen magnum. It extends the head at the atlantooccipital joint.

The rectus capitis posterior major starts with a pointed tendon from the spine of the axis and fans out, attaching to the lateral part of the inferior nuchal line of the suboccipital bone, lateral to the rectus capitis posterior minor. It extends the head and turns the face toward the ipsilateral side.

The obliquus capitis superior attach below to the transverse processes of the atlas, running almost vertically to insert above, between the superior and inferior nuchal lines of the occiput. It is narrow below and wide and expanded above. The obliquus capitis superior extends the head and laterally flexes it to the ipsilateral side.

The obliquus capitis inferior attaches medially and below to the spinous process and adjacent part of the lamina of the axis, running obliquely to fasten laterally and above to the transverse process of the atlas. This muscle turns the face towards the ipsilateral side. All of the suboccipital muscles are innervated by the dorsal ramus of the first spinal (suboccipital) nerve.

Patients with trigger points in the suboccipital muscles may give a history of cervical trauma (Chapter 10), maladjusted eye glasses, or postural strain from prolonged static loading with the head rocked forward or backward on top of the cervical spine. Patients with trigger points in the suboccipital muscles complain of headaches, usually unilateral, which extend forward from the occiput to the ipsilateral forehead and the eye (Fig. 12.21). If trigger points are found bilaterally, the headache involves both sides. The patient complains of deep-seated pain in the upper neck and can often locate an area of focal tenderness.

Examination reveals relatively minor restriction of motion on lateral flexion and rotation. Lower cervical motion may be noted sooner than normal during flexion and extension. Palpation locates trigger points within both the belly and upper attachment of the muscles. Pain referral on pressure is not always reproducible, but it may produce complaints of a deep "headache." To apply pressure on the trigger points, the head must be tilted on the neck to optimally stretch the involved muscle. To prevent recurrence, the patient should avoid chilling and prolonging postures that activate the trigger points.

Rhomboideus Major and Minor Muscles

Trigger points in the rhomboideus muscles are commonly found with patients exhibiting "round shoulders." The powerful pectoralis major muscles shorten and pull the shoulders forward in this characteristic posture that produces strain on the weaker, interscapular muscles. These patients are frequently unaware of the trigger points (latent trigger points) but often complain of superficial backache.

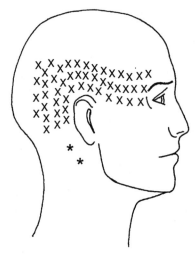

Figure 12.21. Suboccipital syndrome (tension headaches). Trigger points (*) in the suboccipital muscles refer pain (×) that radiates from the occiput to the orbit. (Adapted from Travell JG, Simons DG: *Myofascial Pain and Dysfunction: The Trigger Point Manual.* Baltimore, Williams & Wilkins, 1983.)

Anatomically, the rhomboideus major rises from the spines of the 2nd, 3rd, 4th, and 5th thoracic vertebrae and the supraspinous ligaments. It passes downward and laterally, attaching to the medial border of the scapula. The smaller and more cephalad rhomboideus minor arises from the lower part of the ligamentum nuchae and the spines of the 7th cervical and 1st thoracic vertebrae, attaching below to the medial border of the scapula at the end of the scapular spine. The rhomboids are innervated by the dorsal scapular nerve from the C4, 5 roots (2).

The primary action of the rhomboid muscles is retraction and rotation of the scapulae, turning the glenoid fossa downward. They serve as stabilizing muscles during abduction and to a lesser degree during flexion, fixing the scapulae firmly against the paraspinal soft tissue. (8).

Because of this stabilization function these muscles, along with the trapezius, are subject to overuse due to static loading when the upper extremities are used repetitively. Prolonged leaning forward and working in the round-shouldered position (as when writing, sewing, or working at a keyboard) activates trigger points in the rhomboid muscles. Patients with these trigger points complain of pain between the shoulders, along the vertebral border of the scapula. It may radiate upward over the scapula (Fig. 12.22). Examination typically reveals a round-shouldered posture.

The trigger points are readily palpated with the patient seated and the arms hanging forward to spread the scapulae apart. The trigger points are located in the firm "ropy bands" just medial to and along the vertebral border of the scapula (8). Ischemic compression is most effectively applied with the patient hunched forward with the weight of the

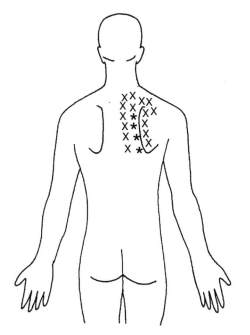

Figure 12.22. Rhomboid syndrome. Trigger points (*) in the rhomboid muscles refer pain (×) between the shoulders, along the vertebral border of the scapula radiating upward over the scapula. (Adapted from Travell JG, Simons DG: *Myofascial Pain and Dysfunction: The Trigger Point Manual.* Baltimore, Williams & Wilkins, 1983.)

arms pulling the shoulders forward. This protracts the scapulae and stretches the rhomboid muscles.

Travell and Simons (8) recommend teaching the patient to apply ischemic compression to the rhomboid trigger points by either lying on a tennis ball on the floor or lying on a large, thin book on a bed. The patient "presses out" the spot tenderness due to the trigger point by rolling the ball along the inner border of the scapula, holding it centered against the tender spot until the pain gradually fades, usually in 20 or 30 seconds.

Modification of the patient's work station to eliminate the round-shouldered posture prevents recurrence. The eyes should be focused straight ahead. A chair with adjustable height and lumbar support also improves seated posture. Patients with rounded shoulders should be encouraged to change position regularly and taught to roll the shoulder down and backwards, retracting the scapula. Stretches for pectoralis minor and major should be practiced frequently. A small hemipelvis that produces a functional scoliosis can be corrected by leveling the pelvis and straightening the spine with an appropriate lift (8).

Rotator Cuff Muscles (Subscapularis Supraspinatus, Infraspinatus and Teres Minor)

The rotator cuff muscles are discussed because the referred pain produced by trigger points in these muscles is commonly mistaken for cervical radiculopathy. Patients with trigger points in shoulder gir-

dle muscles are frequently subjected to much unnecessary treatment directed to the cervical spine and often end up branded malingerers, while still suffering from their original complaint when cervical radiculopathy is ruled out. These muscles may be strained in motor vehicle and lifting accidents when the body is torqued at the time of impact or rotated while lifting.

Anatomically, the supraspinatus attaches medially to the supraspinatus fossa of the scapula and laterally to the greater tubercle of the humerus. It is innervated by the suprascapular nerves (C4, 5, and 6). The supraspinatus muscle abducts the arm and pulls the head of the humerus into the glenoid fossa. This prevents downward displacement of the humerus when the arm is dependent.

Trigger points in the supraspinatus occur when the muscle is strained from carrying heavy objects with the arm hanging down or when lifted above shoulder height. Patients with trigger points in the supraspinatus complain of pain during abduction of the arm as well as a dull ache at rest. They may also complain of shoulder stiffness and sleep disturbances with nocturnal pain. Activities requiring the use of the arm overhead may be restricted. Some patients complain of a scraping crepitus or catch in the shoulder joint. This is thought to be due to interference with the normal glide of the head of the humerus in the glenoid fossa.

Examination reveals restriction of abduction of the arm. Palpation will reveal trigger points at the attachment of the tendon and through the trapezius muscle in the belly of the supraspinatus muscle. Pressure on the trigger points refers pain down the arm and often to the forearm or over the lateral epicondyle of the elbow (Fig. 12.23).

Frequently, ischemic compression alone does not resolve supraspinatus hypertonicity, and transverse friction massage across the fibers of the tendon is helpful (50). To stretch the supraspinatus, the forearm of the seated patient is placed behind the back at waist level or across the front of the chest with the patient grasping the elbow and actively stretching the muscle.

Trigger points in the infraspinatus muscle produce pain deep in the shoulder joint (Fig. 12.24). The infraspinatus attaches medially to the infraspinatus fossa of the scapula and laterally to the greater tubercle of the humerus. The infraspinatus is innervated by the suprascapular nerve through the upper trunk from spinal nerves C5 and C6.

The infraspinatus externally rotates the arms at the shoulder and assists in the stabilization of the head of the humerus in the glenoid fossa during upward movement of the arms. Muscle strain producing trigger points in the infraspinatus usually results from overload while reaching backward and upward. Abduction and restricted external rotation are due to pain.

Figure 12.23. Supraspinatus syndrome. Trigger points (*) in the left supraspinatus tendon refer pain (×) to the middeltoid region. Those trigger points (*) located in the belly of the muscle refer pain (×) around the shoulder and down the arm and forearm (right side). (Adapted from Travell JG, Simons DG: *Myofascial Pain and Dysfunction: The Trigger Point Manual.* Baltimore, Williams & Wilkins, 1983.)

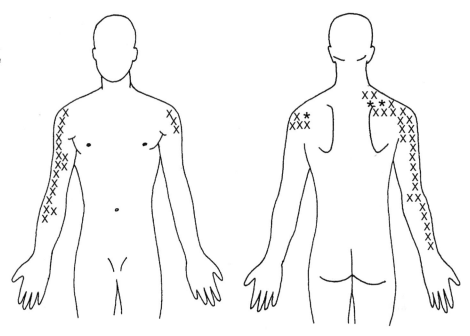

Trigger points in the infraspinatus muscle produce complaints that the patient cannot reach upward and back to pull down an automobile seat belt.

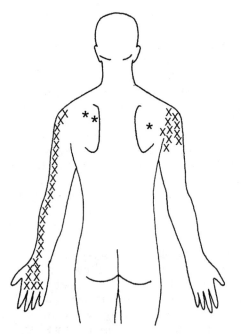

Figure 12.24. Infraspinatus and teres minor syndromes. Trigger points (*) in the left infraspinatus muscle refer pain (×) to the anterior deltoid region of the left shoulder, extending down the front and lateral aspect of the arm and forearm, occasionally including the radial half of the hand. Trigger points (*) in the right teres minor muscle refer pain (×) to the right posterior deltoid region (right side). (Adapted from Travell JG, Simons DG: *Myofascial Pain and Dysfunction: The Trigger Point Manual.* Baltimore, Williams & Wilkins, 1983.)

Sleep disturbances occur because lying on the involved shoulder produces referred pain due to compression and stimulation of the trigger points. Lying on the uninvolved side stretches the infraspinatus, also disturbing sleep. The patient is unable to internally rotate and adduct the arm at the shoulder. Complaints of shoulder fatigue are common.

Examination for trigger points is performed with the patient seated and the muscle stretched by bringing the hand and arm across the front of the chest. The patient may assist the stretch by grasping the elbow on the involved side and tractioning the shoulder, with the elbow close to the chest. Trigger points in the infraspinatus muscle are commonly found just caudal to the spine of the scapula and the midpoints about midmuscle along the vertebral border of the scapula and at the tendinous insertion of the humerus. Pressure is directed medially to inactivate the latter trigger point.

In addition to ischemic compression, regular home stretching under a hot shower directed on the involved muscle is beneficial. Travell and Simons (8) recommend home pressure therapy with the patient lying on a tennis ball under the trigger point, utilizing body weight to maintain increasing pressure for 1–2 minutes. They also recommend that a pillow be placed under the involved arm with the patient sleeping on the uninvolved shoulder. This relieves the pain-producing stretch that interferes with sleep.

The teres minor muscle is sometimes fused with the infraspinatus (2). The teres minor attaches medially to the dorsal surface of the scapula just below the infraspinatus and inserts laterally into the greater tubercle of the humerus. It is innervated by the axillary nerve through the posterior cord from

C5 and C6 spinal nerves. Like the infraspinatus, it externally rotates the arm at the shoulder and helps to stabilize the head of the humerus in the glenoid fossa during arm movement.

Trigger points in the teres minor rarely occur alone and are activated by the same overload stress that produces strain of the infraspinatus muscle (e.g., reaching out and behind the shoulder). These trigger points produce complaints of localized pain deep under the deltoid muscle in the belly of the teres minor. The patient is positioned as for examination of the infraspinatus and teres minor muscles. Trigger points are found in the belly of the muscle, with tenderness at the insertion into the humerus. Home stretching and corrective action for the teres minor are the same as those described for the infraspinatus.

The subscapularis forms the major part of the posterior wall of the axilla. It is a long, triangular muscle that arises from the inner surface of the scapula, filling the subscapular fossa from the vertebral border to the axillary border of the scapula. It converges laterally into a tendon that attaches to the lesser tubercle of the humerus and the front of the capsule of the shoulder joint. It is innervated by the upper and lower subscapular nerves: C5, 6, and 7. The actions of the subscapularis are primarily internal rotation and adduction of the arm at the shoulder. It also assists in the stabilization of the humerus in the glenoid fossa and thus assists in abduction of the arm.

Patients with trigger points in the subscapularis often have a history of trauma in which the body has been suspended by the ipsilateral upper extremity. In addition to sudden trauma, muscle strain due to overuse can produce trigger points in the subscapularis muscle. Subscapularis trigger points cause severe shoulder pain both at rest and in motion. The pain is concentrated in the posterior deltoid area and may extend medially over the scapula and down the posterior aspect of the arm (Fig. 12.25). It

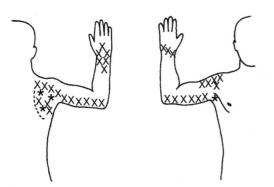

Figure 12.25. Subscapularis syndrome. Trigger points (*) in the subscapularis refer pain (×) to the posterior deltoid area, medially over the scapula, and down the posterior aspect of the arm, skipping to a band around the wrist. (Adapted from Travell JG, Simons DG: *Myofascial Pain and Dysfunction: The Trigger Point Manual.* Baltimore, Williams & Wilkins, 1983.)

commonly produces a strap-like distribution of referred pain around the wrist (8).

Examination reveals restriction of motion on abduction and internal rotation of the arm at the shoulder. Subscapularis myofascial pain syndromes are often diagnosed as "frozen shoulder" syndrome, which is a term that describes a number of conditions, including adhesive capsulitis and subacromial fibrosis. The clinical diagnosis of frozen shoulder does not identify the site of pathology and is not an accurate diagnosis.

Examination for trigger points in the subscapularis muscle is difficult and should be performed with the patient supine and the involved arm abducted away from the chest wall. In this position, trigger points can be palpated along the axillary border of the scapula.

Travell and Simons (8) warn that in patients with severe subscapularis involvement, deep tenderness in this muscle is usually so exquisite that they can tolerate only very light digital pressure on the trigger points. Patients should be watched carefully during ischemic compression of trigger points to insure that pressure is applied within the patient's tolerance. This is especially important when treating trigger points in the subscapularis muscle.

Home exercises can help to stretch this muscle. Rhythmic stabilization utilizing resisted abduction and external rotation at the shoulder to the limit of pain improves the range of motion of the subscapularis muscle.

FIBROMYALGIA (FIBROSITIS)

Much has been written about fibromyalgia (fibrositis), but there is still no general agreement among health professionals about this syndrome (87–100). Bennett (87) has stated that patients with fibrositis will not go away just because we disagree about its definition. Frequently the widespread and multiple complaints, recently labeled fibromyalgia, have been considered to be "all in the patients head" (11), and often they are not seriously considered when treating patients complaining of chronic muscle pain.

Although not a crippling disorder (87), fibromyalgia does cause widespread disability, primarily due to misdiagnosis and inappropriate therapy. Along with the multiple diagnostic terms used to describe this disorder (Table 12.2), there are numerous theories about the etiology, pathophysiology, and treatment of this common ailment. Adding to the confusion, there is not even a consensus on the criteria used to establish a diagnosis of fibromyalgia (90).

Clinical Characteristics of Fibromyalgia

Fibromyalgia is a chronic, noninflammatory, diffuse muscle pain disorder with constitutional manifestations suggesting a psychoneurophysiological mechanism of dysfunction. Patients typically com-

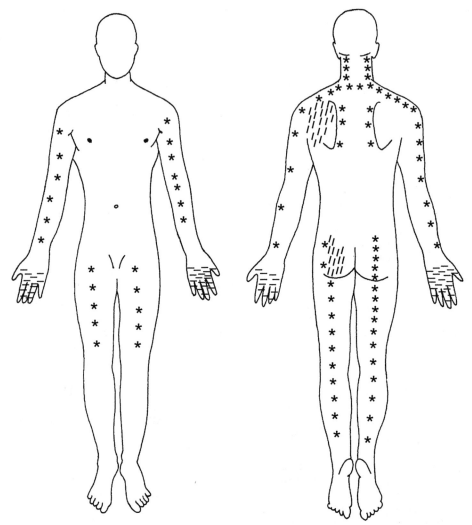

Figure 12.26. Fibromyalgia pain pattern. The typical pain drawing of patients with fibromyalgia is characterized by diffuse aching (*) in the back and in the upper and lower extremities, bilaterally. Areas of subjective numbness (---) in a glove distribution are commonly reported. Stabbing pain (///) is often noted when trigger points coexist with the tender points. The diffuse and bilateral nature of this pain pattern may be mistaken for hysteria or malingering (see Chapter 4).

plain of generalized aching and stiffness involving multiple muscle groups (Fig. 12.26) with well defined tender points in consistent locations (88). Unlike myofascial trigger points, these tender points are not always located in the muscle and do not refer pain in consistent patterns as do trigger points (90, 91).

This distinction is used to differentiate myofascial pain syndrome, characterized by referred pain from trigger points in a localized muscle group, from the more generalized fibromyalgia syndrome, which involves multiple muscle groups and nonreferring tender points. Differentiation becomes clouded when patients exhibit characteristics of both myofascial pain and fibromyalgia (91, 92). Myofascial pain may lead to fibromyalgia, with unresolved localized muscle pain ultimately involving multiple muscle groups (9) in addition to nervous system involvement. Masi and Yunas (93) suggest that establishing

scientific criteria for these muscle pain syndromes may be difficult because they are neighboring stages in a continuous biologic gradient of a single disorder. Clinically this pattern becomes more evident if a careful history is elicited.

Multiple host and environmental factors seem to contribute to the onset and course of fibromyalgia (93) (Table 12.8). Predisposing, precipitating, and perpetuating factors also appear to complicate the course of fibromyalgia. There is no doubt that psychological pressures affect the course of fibromyalgia syndrome (88). Whether these psychological factors are primary or secondary to the onset of muscle pain syndromes has not been determined (94). Unresolved resentment and anger from past abuse may be a predisposing factor that leads some patients with a localized muscle strain into the realm of systemic fibromyalgia. If this is so, the underlying

Table 12.8 Successful management of patients with primary fibromyalgia syndrome is dependent not only on interruption of the pain-spasm-pain cycle but also the relief of other factors feeding into the cycle.

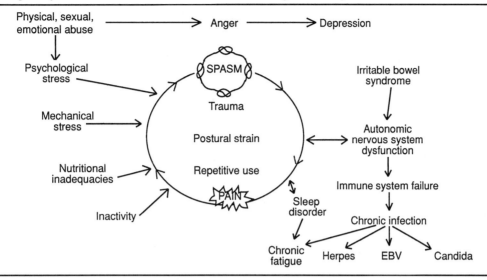

predisposition must then be dealt with, if a successful outcome is to be experiencd.

This emotional stress is not aways due to events prior to the accident. Trauma victims with chronic pain from misdiagnosis and/or inappropriate treatment can experience resentment and rage, which perpetuates and increases the pain-spasm-pain cycle. This may account for the spread of muscle pain from a localized muscle group to multiple tender points at the origin and insertion of the flight-or-fight muscles (6). The suppression of these hostile emotions then becomes the triggering factor responsible for autonomic nervous system dysfunction with subsequent sleep disorders and irritable bowel syndrome.

These seemingly unrelated complaints cause skeptics to question the fibromyalgia syndrome characterized by dysfunction of multiple systems. Lack of physician recognition may allow many of these patients ultimately to succumb to multiple chronic infections (88, 89, 100) (such as yeast, Epstein-Barr virus, and herpes simplex) as the immune system fails, due to chronic stress producing the chronic fatigue syndrome that has been linked to fibromyalgia (14, 88) (See Chapter 3).

Koch's postulates of disease etiology cannot be applied to these patients (93), for there does not appear to be a specific transferable agent that causes either fibromyalgia or chronic fatigue syndrome. Rather, the host's resistance is the deciding factor in the progression of this condition. When multiple environmental stresses overcome the host's resistance, chronic illness results (See Chapter 3).

Chronic muscle pain and exhaustion, with multiple somatic complaints, has often led to the diagnosis of hypochondriasis or hysteria in patients suffering from fibromyalgia syndrome. The uniform constellation of symptoms including tension headache, muscle aches, generalized stiffness, fatigue, and a high incidence of irritable bowel syndrome and sleep disorders in addition to tender points in consistent locations makes fibromyalgia a readily definable syndrome within the spectrum of muscle pain syndromes (94).

Pathomechanics of Fibromyalgia

Excessive mechanical stress on the postural stabilizers is one source of pain producing the pain-spasm-pain phenomena (6, 85). The prolonged static loading of the postural stabilizers produces a state of hypoxia, with a build-up of metabolites in the antigravity muscles. The shoulder girdle muscles (trapezius, rhomboid, and levator scapulae) are commonly affected.

Postural strain can also place additional stress on the lower cervical and lumbar spine musculature where the lordotic curvatures must be stabilized. Faulty sleeping posture as well as faulty upright posture can lead to painful muscle states. Sleeping prone places undue stress on both the cervical and lumbar spine, further accentuating the lordotic curves. Poor posture because of bad habits or occupational stress can produce microtrauma leading to a hyperalgesic state (6).

Constant pain can also produce prolonged muscle hypertonus, and patients with chronic pain are frequently unaware of how much their pain is suppressed. Some persons seem to be peculiarly prone to react to stress by hypertonicity of voluntary muscles, predisposing them to the development of profound discomfort (96). Kraft and coworkers (97) noted that certain patients appeared to be predisposed to fibrositis syndrome, reacting to stress situations as if their muscles were their shock organs. These patients developed the fibrositis syndrome following a variety of conditions, including minor

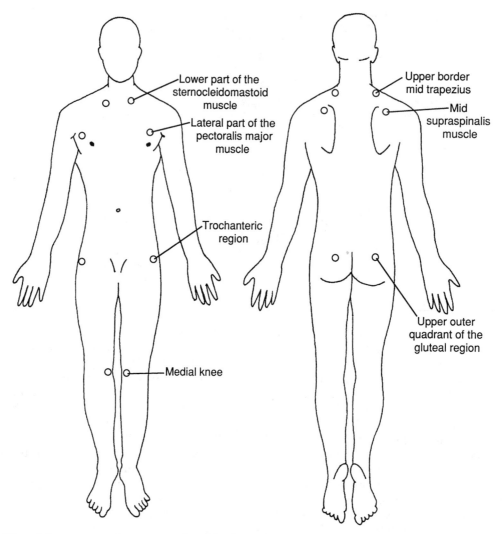

Figure 12.27. Sites of the seven most common pairs of tender points.

infections, psychologic or physical trauma, and fluid retention states.

Diagnostic Criteria for the Fibromyalgia Syndrome

The diagnosis of fibromyalgia should be based on consistent criteria. It should not be used as a "wastebasket" diagnosis for patients with generalized muscle aches and pains (88, 97). Criteria developed by Smythe (98) are widely used in the diagnosis of fibromyalgia. He suggests that diagnosis of fibromyalgia requires obligatory, major, and minor criteria.

Obligatory criteria that must be present include:

Subjective aching of more than 3 months duration;
Subjective stiffness of more than 3 months duration;
Point tenderness at multiple sites (Fig. 12.27);
Normal sedimentation rate, muscle enzyme levels, and sacroiliac radiographs, absent rheumatologic serologies.

Some, but not all, minor criteria must also be present (99). These include:

Chronic fatigue;
Sleep disorder;
Change in symptoms with anxiety/stress;
Change in symptoms with activity;
Change in symptoms with weather changes;
Headaches;
Irritable bowel syndrome;
Subjective swelling;
Nonradicular, nondermatomic numbness;
Dermographia.

Most contentious would seem to be the major criterion (tender points), with the number of tender points necessary to meet the major criterion varying from three to twelve. This seems to be nit-picking, since the number of tender points is probably a reflection of the degree of progression of the condition.

Psychogenic tension affects the flight-or-fight muscles, and due to such hostile emotions as chronic anxiety, resentment, or rage, can be a source of muscle pain. By a reflex mechanism, the pain is felt in a widespread area, so that pain and tenderness occur not only in the localized structures but also distally in various parts of the limbs. The pattern of referral does not follow known segmental patterns, but is consistent for individual muscles (91).

The location of tender points is frequently the site of increased mechanical stress at tendinous attachment to bone, as opposed to trigger points, which are commonly located in the belly of the muscle. This suggests involvement of the pacinian corpuscles and Golgi tendon organs as part of the neuropathological mechanism of the tender points, as opposed to muscle spindle involvement in the trigger points.

Cold and humid weather, abuse of muscles, and lack of adequate, restful sleep are known to potentiate this chronic syndrome (96). Unresolved pain from a state of localized hyperalgesia spreads by a reflex mechanism, producing a generalized aching and stiffness. In some individuals, physical stress from working long hours or performing strenuous, repetitive tasks is more important than anxiety or mental tension (100). Once a state of reflex hyperalgesia is established in the local and referred areas, other factors such as trauma, sleep disturbance, weather, and chronic tension states from mental stress can accentuate and perpetuate the symptoms.

History

A careful history of the duration of symptoms is necessary to determine the obligatory criteria for diagnosis of fibromyalgia (88). Subjective aching and stiffness of more than three months duration is a necessary component of the obligatory criteria (90). In addition, predisposing, precipitating, and perpetuating factors must be addressed.

Predisposing factors include prolonged psychological stress, such as emotional, physical, and sexual abuse. Women are more predisposed to fibromyalgia than men (70–90%), with an average age of onset between 34 and 55 years. Poor physical conditioning characterized as inadequate nutrition, rest, and exercise may also predispose individuals to this syndrome. Precipitating factors include chronic overuse, acute trauma, and environmental stressors such as cold, infectious agents, toxic substances, and excessive noise (89).

Perpetuating factors include repeated exposure to predisposing, precipitating factors, along with misdiagnosis and improper management. Historical symptoms easily distinguish patients with fibromyalgia but do not rule out those with similar conditions such as rheumatism, arthritis, osteoarthritis, and low back pain (87) (Table 12.9). The presence of criteria common to similar conditions does not pre-clude the diagnosis of fibromyalgia (87). Doctors do well to remember that patients have the right to have more than one thing wrong with them, including conditions with overlapping symptoms. Patients should not be denied appropriate treatment because of the physician's insistence on a mutually exclusive diagnosis. Other inflammatory or degenerative syndromes frequently mimic and coexist with fibromyalgia (89).

Symptoms of Fibromyalgia

The most common subjective complaints include an aching-type pain, stiffness, and overbearing fatigue. Location of the major complaint shifts from one muscle group to another, which can confound the diagnostician and eventually end in misdiagnosis and inappropriate treatment. In addition to a shifting in the site of pain, there is marked fluctuation in day-to-day severity. This causes some to discount the severity of the patient's complaints, pointing out that "the patient was fine yesterday, so why is he/she complaining today." A history of complete but transient remission of symptoms is an important clue to the diagnosis of fibromyalgia (fibrositis) (87).

Patients may also report a stabbing or "knife-like" pain, burning, and numbness. The complaints of numbness frequently fail to follow dermatomal patterns and are often inconsistent with sensory testing. Severe headaches (either tension or migraine), joint pain, and swelling are also frequent complaints (96). Joint laxity is not an uncommon finding in fibromyalgia patients and precludes routine manipulation.

Irritable Bowel Syndrome

Complaints of irritable bowel symptoms have been reported in over 50% of the patients with complaints of lower abdominal pain or distension, usually relieved by bowel movements (94). These patients often have characteristic small or thin stools, with or without mucus, and an absence of blood or weight loss. In many of these patients, the symptoms are made worse by increased emotional stress (96). Chronic *Candida* overgrowth in the GI tract may play a role in these complaints. Oral doses of nystatin with dietary restriction of concentrated sugars has brought relief from musculoskeletal complaints as well as relief of GI distress in some cases of fibromyalgia.

Sleep Disorder

Moldofsky and Scarisbrich (101) have described a disorder of nonrestorative sleep in fibromyalgia patients with specific neurochemical abnormalities and an alpha wave intrusion of delta sleep on sleep electroencephalogram recordings. They experimentally produced similar stage four sleep deprivation in normal subjects, with temporary appearance of musculoskeletal and mood symptoms characteristic of fibromyalgia patients.

Table 12.9 Differential Diagnosis of Common Disorders Exhibiting Muscle Pain

Condition	History & Symptoms	Diagnostic Indication	Therapy
Biomechanical disorders			
Degenerative joint disease (osteoarthritis)	Joint pain and stiffness after periods of rest; achiness at times of inclement weather; crepitation or joint motion with spasms of surrounding muscles.	Radiographic examination reveals narrowed joint space, subchondral sclerosis, subchondral cysts, and marginal osteophytes.	Swimming and stretching exercises, traction, weight reduction where indicated; treat secondary muscle spasm.
Bursitis/tendonitis	Localized pain and tenderness.	Decreased mobility of the affected part; pain on increased motion; localized edema and erythema when acute.	Rest of the part, cessation of aggravating activity, ice/heat therapy; moderately severe cases may require antiinflammatory medication.
Connective tissue disorders			
Rheumatoid arthritis	Morning stiffness, joint pain on motion, symmetrical joint swelling and subcutaneous nodules; weakness and atrophy of involved joints common, low-grade fever and lymphadenopathy may be present.	Positive agglutination test reveals rheumatoid factor elevated, mild anemia, elevated ESR and hypergammaglobulinemia often observed; radiographs reveal bony decalcification adjacent to involved joints; advanced disease shows joint deformities and subluxation due to erosion of cartilage and bone and destruction of supporting ligaments.	Rest, lightweight splints, especially at night; relieve muscle spasm and insure correct position; salicylates may provide relief from acute attacks.
Systemic lupus erythematosus	Fever, erythematous rash, polyarthralgia and arthritis, weakness, fatigability, and weight loss may be present.	Laboratory findings include mild normochromic and normocytic anemia, elevated ESR, LE cell reaction, and antinuclear antibodies.	Mild cases may spontaneously remiss; severe cases should be referred for corticosteroid therapy.
Polymyalgia rheumatica	Occurs in older individuals, most over 65; pain and stiffness in the proximal muscles, especially in the neck, back, shoulder, and pelvic girdles, marked in the morning; fever, anorexia, malaise, weight loss, and apathy may be present.	Greatly elevated ESR, increased fibrinogen and anemia	Refer for corticosteroid therapy; symptoms usually disappear rapidly with good prognosis.
Metabolic disorders			
Hypothyroidism	Muscle aching and mild weakness; pain and stiffness during rest and exacerbated by exposure to cold.	Decreased serum levels of thyroid hormones, elevated thyroid stimulating hormone, creatine phosphokinase.	Refer for thyroid hormone replacement.
Osteopenia/osteoporosis	Postmenopausal female and over 65 male; back pain, increased dorsal kyphosis.	Radiographs reveal thinning of the cortex and trabeculae of the vertebral body; concave endplates, "codfish" vertebrae.	Nutritional supplementation and increased activity; refer for hormone therapy if severe; rule out malabsorption.
Acromegaly	Coarse facial features, thick extremities and enlargement of the joints; myopathy and mild muscle weakness may be present.	Increased levels of plasma growth hormone and urinary hydroxyproline-containing peptide; radiographs reveal thickening of the soft tissues and widening of the joint space; enlarged bones, periosteal proliferation, thickened and widely spaced trabeculae.	Refer for surgical evaluation and hypophysectomy.
Hyperparathyroidism	Weakness and atrophy of muscles; bone pain and back pain.	Increased serum calcium and decreased serum phosphorus, elevation of alkaline phosphatase, increased urinary excretion of hydroxyprolin-containing peptides; radiographs reveal chondro-calcinosis; generalized skeletal demineralization.	Refer to an endocrinologist.

Note: Metabolic myopathy may also be caused by various factors including diabetes, chronic alcoholism, anemia, hypoglycemia, and nutritional inadequacies.

A similar nonrestorative sleep pattern has been demonstrated in patients with postaccident pain (102, 103) and depression (104–106). This suggests that chronic pain and depression may be related to neurochemical changes that affect sleep patterns. It has been noted that a decrease in serotonin produces an increased sensitivity to pain, suggesting that the serotoninergic system normally acts to inhibit the effects of painful stimuli (106). Moldofsky and Warsh (107) suggested that a metabolic disorder underlies both the physiologic sleep disturbances and symptoms characteristic of the fibrositis (fibromyalgia) syndrome.

Saskin, Moldofsky, and Lue (103) found sleep disorders (alpha EEG non-REM sleep anomaly) and a constellation of uniform complaints consisting of widespread musculoskeletal pain, localized areas of tenderness in specific anatomical regions, chronic fatigue, emotional distress, and nonrestorative sleep in nonphysically injured motor vehicle or work-related accident victims similar to patients with "fibrositis syndrome" (fibromyalgia).

Moldofsky and Warsh (107) observed an inverse relationship between plasma free tryptophan and pain severity in fibromyalgia patients, consistent with the hypothesis relating CNS serotonin metabolism and pain reactivity in animals. They also observed the influence of serotonin precursors and inhibitors on pain in humans.

Based on his studies, Moldofsky (104) has concluded that the chronic musculoskeletal pain and fatigue characteristic of fibromyalgia patients are associated with a physiologic arousal disorder within sleep. He states that in this nonrestorative sleep disorder, pain and mood symptoms may be mediated by psychologic distress. He cites nonphysically injurious industrial or automobile accidents, noxious environmental stimuli (e.g., noise), physiologic disturbance (e.g., sleep, related myoclonus, painful inflamed joints), and altered CNS metabolism (e.g., disordered brain serotoninergic functions) as agents influencing the fibromyalgia syndrome. He has reported that fibromyalgia patients describe light and/or restless sleep. They waken feeling unrefreshed, complaining of pains, stiffness, physical exhaustion, and lethargy. He noted that aspects of their sleep physiology are related to their pain and mood symptoms.

He found that patients with fibromyalgia typically reported an emotionally distressing event at the onset of their symptoms. Included were frightening but minor automobile or industrial accidents and unsolvable domestic difficulties. He suggests a self-perpetuating, vicious cycle of emotional distress, nonrestorative sleep, musculoskeletal pain, fatigue, and obsessional rumination about somatic symptoms.

He also observed that noise may have a negative influence on sleep, pain, and mood symptoms, and that sleep apnea may influence the musculoskeletal, fatigue, and mood symptoms (104). These mood changes were characterized as anger, irritability, anxiety, and sluggishness (3). Often, patients with fibromyalgia will complain that they are impatient and irritable with family members and coworkers, which increases tension, furthering the patient's muscle hypertonicity and pain-spasm-pain cycle. It is often difficult for people close to fibromyalgia patients to understand the marked fluctuation of symptoms and mood.

Physical Findings of Fibromyalgia

On physical examination, neurological findings and muscle strength are normal. Muscle and joint swelling with accompanying warmth and erythema are rare, but may be present when the symptoms are acute. Joint tenderness may be elicited by direct pressure.

The most definitive physical finding is localized, exaggerated tenderness (tender point) on pressure at specific periarticular, muscle, spinal, and muscle insertion sites. Patients may have from 4 to 40 of these tender points, with 8 to 12 the usual number (88). Pressure on the tender points commonly elicits a pain response with abrupt withdrawal of the palpated part. The locations of these tender points are remarkably consistent from patient to patient, and many patients are not aware of their presence (88). The use of a dolorimeter along with manual examination of tender points has demonstrated that a tender point examination can distinguish patients with fibromyalgia from normal controls (94).

Common sites of tender points in primary fibromyalgia are trapezius muscles, lateral and medial epicondyles of the elbows, attachments of the levator scapulae, pes anserine of the knees, posterior iliac crest, sternocleidomastoid muscles, spinal processes, paraspinal muscles, medial border of the scapulae, bicipital tendon area, suboccipital muscle insertion, costochondral junction, TMJ and sacroiliac joint areas, attachment of the pectoral muscles and greater trochanters, and the junction of the Achilles tendon and gastrocnemius muscle.

It is foolish to be dogmatic about the number of tender points required to substantiate a diagnosis of fibromyalgia, but most patients with well-defined fibromyalgia will respond significantly to at least seven of the tender points noted.

Interaction of Fibromyalgia and Psychologic Disturbance

The psychogenic component of fibromyalgia cannot be ignored, nor can it be considered the primary factor in the management of this disorder (108, 109). Polarization of treatment, based on lack of understanding of the etiology of fibromyalgia, does little good in the management of this complex problem and may even prove harmful.

While some researchers (94, 104, 110) did not demonstrate any difference in standard psychologic testing between patients with fibrositis (fibromyalgia) and control groups, others (110, 111) suggest an association of affective symptoms with fibromyalgia. It has not been established whether the affective symptoms noted were secondary to the pain and disability caused by fibromyalgia or were symptoms of a primary psychobiologic abnormality that causes both the affective and myofascial complaints (10).

Hudson et al. (111) observed that major depression had occurred at least one year before the development of fibromyalgia in 64% of the patients they studied. They contended that this could represent a preexisting condition or vulnerability. There certainly appears to be a predisposition in some patients for minor trauma or repeated microtrauma to develop into fibromyalgia. They (111) also noted that fibromyalgia does not appear to be related closely to hysterical or factitious illness. They found that patients suffering from fibromyalgia have specific chronic, stable, and stereotypical symptoms, in contrast to patients with factitious disorders, who often demonstrate vague, changeable, and bizarre symptoms. In spite of higher scores on the hysteria and hypochondriasis scales of the MMPI, profiles of patients with fibromyalgia indicate that fibromyalgia is not a simple affective disorder.

Goldenberg (88) contends that the MMPI was never intended to be used in chronic pain syndromes and that it is a poor scale for such application because of the nature of the questions. He states that elevation in the MMPI scale of hysteria, hypochondriasis, and depression will be present in any painful condition and does not constitute evidence that fibromyalgia patients are psychologically disturbed. Often, physicians who discuss the psychological component of fibromyalgia establish an adversarial barrier that magnifies any preexisting psychologic disturbance (112).

Many physicians share a common perception that patients with fibromyalgia exhibit characteristic personality traits (87, 113). Such patients have been described as perfectionistic, demanding of themselves and others, and often successful in their chosen areas of activity (87). Other psychological factors associated with muscle pain have been described, including tension, anxiety, type A behavior, emotional belief systems, and learned helplessness (114).

Anger and resentment, precipitated by abuse, may also play a role in the development of fibromyalgia. The heavy reliance of victims of abuse on somatization as a coping style may account for the higher incidence of fibromyalgia in females (80%). Within the last decade the abuse of females has become a problem of widespread interest. Despite attempts to expose this violent phenomenon, abuse often goes undetected because of taboo, its hidden nature, and a reluctance on the part of abused women to discuss their victimization. Even when directly asked about abuse, many women will not reveal the problem.

Psychologically, abused women use somatization and denial as their primary coping style, making their identification extremely difficult. Interestingly, socioeconomic differences are not significant between abused and nonabused groups; abuse occurs with low, middle, and high income people. Certainly, unresolved rage and resentment can cause the victim to tighten postural muscles, sustaining the flight-or-fight muscles in a state of chronic contraction. Such continuous, intense metabolic activity by muscles can produce substances that increase sensory nerve hypersensitivity (115).

Fibromyalgia Immune System Failure and Chronic Infection

Bennett (9, 89), has asked whether the fibromyalgia syndrome is a manifestation of persistent low-grade viral infection. Hudson et al. (111) noted that it is unclear to what extent fibromyalgia may represent an impairment in immune function. Chronic fatigue syndrome (Epstein-Barr virus infection), epidemic neuromyasthenia (116), epidemic myalgia, encephalomyelitis, and gastric intestinal yeast overgrowth are all characterized by muscle pain and fatigue. Clearly, the effects of chronic pain on the central and autonomic nervous system and the relationship to stress and immune system failure needs further study.

Sandman and Backstrom (114) discuss the function of the sympathetic nervous system in the preparation of the body for flight or fight. They note that after prolonged response to stress, such hormones as adrenalin, thyroxin, and the adrenocortical steroids do not always return to a normal level, and that the nervous system does not always differentiate between mental imagery and the actual threat of danger. Hence, an intense and often prolonged arousal response may occur inappropriately, with an autonomic nervous system imbalance upsetting the body's homeostasis. When the prolonged response becomes habituated, dysfunction occurs, and the condition may become debilitating with ultimate failure of the immune system. The role of the nervous system in immune system response is described in Chapter 3. Goldenberg (88) has concluded that a subset of patients may have fibromyalgia associated with classic immune-mediated symptoms.

Pathological Findings in Muscles

Yunas and coworkers (117, 118) have recently described muscle pathology in 12 well-defined cases of primary fibromyalgia syndrome. Studying muscle from an open biopsy of prominent tender points at the upper portion of the trapezius muscle, they noted the following changes:

1. Light microscope. Mildly scattered hyaline as well as split fibers in about 40% of patients.
2. Histochemistry. Type II fiber atrophy in 60% and a moth-eaten appearance of type I fibers in 40% of patients studied. Clusters of hyalinized fibers were sometimes seen.
3. Electron microscopy. Myofibrillar necrosis, with deposition of glycogen and mitochondria in all 12 patients.

While these findings were nonspecific, they do support the importance of further study of pathological muscle changes in patients with fibromyalgia syndrome. Opposition to recognition of fibromyalgia syndrome as a specific entity has long been based on the absence of specific pathological changes in patients suffering from this syndrome (11, 118, 119).

Management of Fibromyalgia

The management of patients with fibromyalgia is an art (6) as complex as the predisposing, precipitating, and perpetuating factors that produce this syndrome (Table 12.8). The key to management of fibromyalgia is a firm diagnosis, followed by assurance that the condition is benign, noncrippling, and may eventually remit (6). Patients must be encouraged to help themselves through positive environmental changes, and physicians must learn to accept the fact that they can do little to ameliorate these patients' conditions (87).

Patients must become better educated about fibromyalgia, and they must take responsibility for their own care (87). A necessary component in management is a change in attitude (114). Patients must be encouraged to remain active and to strive for a greater level of physical fitness. Most patients with fibromyalgia allow their muscles to become chronically unfit through disuse. Others may cause a flare-up of symptoms by pursuing a too-vigorous exercise program.

Gentle, progressive exercise can usually ease the symptoms of fibromyalgia; however, there is a fine line dividing the amount of exercise that is helpful and the amount that aggravates this condition. McCain (120) found that increased cardiovascular fitness significantly improved objective measurements of pain in 34 fibromyalgia patients who met Smythe's original criteria.

It is thought that exercise leads to significant alterations in opioid and nonopioid as well as neural and hormonal intrinsic pain-regulator systems that decrease pain sensitivity. McCain (120) cautioned, however, that strenuous exercise at sustained levels not only induces physiologic changes but also may be responsible for the development of a stress response that appears to perpetuate the fibromyalgia syndrome.

Bennett (9) noted that it may be relevant that the quality of stage four sleep has been linked to the amount of aerobic exercise performed by an individual. A combination of moderate aerobic and stretching exercises appears to prevent and alleviate the symptoms of temporary setbacks (121). Nonstraining exercises such as swimming have proven beneficial (6). Resistance exercises tend to aggravate fibromyalgia and, since the perceived muscle weakness and complaints of give-away are due to pain rather than to actual muscle weakness, strengthening exercises tend to be counterproductive. Postural dysfunction must be identified and corrected to relieve chronic muscle strain (6, 121).

Static loading of the antigravity muscles of the upper extremities is a common perpetuating factor in fibromyalgia, and an occupation change may be required if the cycle of pain-spasm-pain cannot be broken through relaxation and stretching of the involved muscles. A change from stressful occupations (physical, mental, or both) may be advisable (122) in addition to jobs requiring strenuous, repetitive muscular exertion (87).

The chiropractor treating fibromyalgia patients must encourage them to modify their life-style to maximize health. Palliative care can relieve the symptoms of temporary setbacks, but it does little to change the overall course of the condition. Heat, ultrasound, massage, and trigger point therapy, along with stretching exercises, reduce the muscle hypertonicity and can alleviate much of the patient's discomfort.

Manipulation of fixed joints is essential, however repeated manipulation of hypermobile joints tends to aggravate the overall condition. This is probably due to the joint laxity in some fibromyalgia patients. The reduction of reflex muscle spasm through manipulation may offer temporary relief, but it is counterproductive and contraindicated when joints are hypermobile. Passive therapy encourages the patient to seek help from outside sources, while the most beneficial therapy is a change of attitude and life-style with attention to goals, priorities, and pacing of activities. Fibromyalgia patients frequently describe the typical pattern of 1–2 hours of pain relief following manipulation, but a return of symptoms thereafter (See "Hypermobility," Chapter 8). This pattern, seen in the pain-spasm-pain cycle, can lead to both psychological and physical dependency on chiropractic manipulation.

Medication should play only a very minor role in the treatment of fibromyalgia (87). Painkilling (analgesic) drugs may be used occasionally to reduce the severity of musculoskeletal pain, but they should not be considered a major method of treatment (87). Because of the risk of dependency and intolerance to painkilling medication, these drugs are contraindicated for long-term use. While tricyclic antidepressants such as amitriptyline have been used in low dosages to treat the accompanying sleep disorder, they have been reported to be ineffective in relieving the tender point symptoms (121, 123).

Cognitive therapy can be effective in relieving the patient's depression as well as dealing directly with the patient's underlying anger. Changing the fibromyalgia patients' perspectives of themselves and their attitudes toward others can have a dramatic effect on them. These patients frequently think of themselves as helpless and hopeless. Their future becomes unrealistically bleak. They are often not only negative but also illogical.

Cognitive therapy works to change thought patterns and can help these patients to see more positive explanations for stressful situations. A well-trained cognitive therapist can help change the patient's "doomed-to-fail" attitude or help the patient deal with a difficult situation in specific, realistic terms. Patients must strive to reduce stressful factors that seem to exacerbate their symtoms, be these emotional or physical stressors.

Patients with fibromyalgia should not be allowed to use their condition as a scapegoat (87). Fibromyalgia is not a crippling disorder, and it must not be used as an excuse to evade irksome or unpleasant responsibilities (87). Family members and coworkers frequently become impatient with the fibromyalgia sufferer who exhibits an attitude of entitlement. Associates of fibromyalgia patients need to have a clear understanding of the condition and a willingness to encourage these patients to deal with their problem in a realistic manner.

Management of the fibromyalgia patient requires a good patient-physician relationship: patience, understanding, and firmness. It is both gratifying and demanding, for many of these patients have all but given up hope because of improper diagnosis and often years of seeking help to no avail.

Disability

There is no evidence to prove conclusively that any type of accident or job-related activity can cause or exacerbate the symptoms of fibromyalgia. Empirically, it appears that minor trauma can precipitate fibromyalgia; however, this has not been demonstrated by controlled studies. Clearly the stress of drawn-out legal proceedings can make the fibromyalgia symptoms worse, and such proceedings should be avoided (97). By focusing on what they are able to do (rather than bemoaning their disability), patients can lead a better quality life and recover faster.

Cathey and coworkers (124) have noted that patients with fibromyalgia (fibrositis) reported high levels of pain, mild disability, and moderate impairment of global health. They found also that work disability was limited and that most patients could work full work weeks, with only 6.3% of the patients studied describing themselves as disabled. They reported that their data suggest that fibromyalgia (fibrositis) is a painful and distressing disorder, but is not disabling. Generally, patients should be encouraged to be active and continue their employment (6).

Secondary Fibromyalgia (Fibrositis)

Fibromyalgia (fibrositis) is considered primary when there is no associated underlying disorder and secondary when it occurs in patients with underlying rheumatic or other organic disease (125). This distinction is necessary for scientific study, but primary fibromyalgia should be suspected by its own characteristic features and not diagnosed just by the absence of other recognizable conditions.

Symptoms of aching, stiffness, and tenderness of musculoskeletal tissues accompany many rheumatic diseases including rheumatoid arthritis, systemic lupus erythematosus, osteoarthritis, and subdeltoid bursitis (125). By careful application of the diagnostic criteria outlined by Smythe (95), primary fibromyalgia becomes a recognizable syndrome (fibromyalgia syndrome) and not just a diagnosis of exclusion.

Fibromyalgia syndrome may coexist with other conditions, such as osteoarthritis, and should be reported as such when the obligatory, major, and minor criteria have been met. Differential diagnosis of patients who have more than one condition is difficult at best. Because primary fibromyalgia is a poorly recognized condition, it is even more difficult to diagnose because there is no consistency in anatomic, serologic, or immunologic abnormalities (87).

Fibromyalgia and Chiropractic Therapy

Wolfe (13) found that 45.9% of patients with fibromyalgia who have received chiropractic care reported moderate to great improvement. Chiropractic scored among the most effective measures, with only rest providing more improvement. When treating fibromyalgia patients it is not appropriate to practice the art of medicine, as Voltaire has suggested, by keeping the patient entertained while the disease runs its inevitable course.

The course of fibromyalgia is frequently long, with characteristic remission. The most effective therapy is encouragement of life-style changes such as rest, relaxation, moderate stretching, and aerobic exercise (13) along with supportive chiropractic care. Patients with fibromyalgia improve dramatically when they take control of their life situation, rather than continuing in a state of learned helplessness (113).

While the psychologic factors influencing the course of fibromyalgia must be addressed, psychotherapy has not proven effective in this condition (108). Further study may find a neurochemical link explaining the autonomic nervous system involvement which can be pharmacologically mediated, but to date diagnostic reassurance, counseling, and moderate exercise, in addition to judicious use of chiropractic supportive therapy, helps the vast majority of patients suffering from fibromyalgia.

References

1. Lewit K: The muscular and articular factor in movement restriction. *Manual Med* 1:83–85, 1985.
2. Gray H: *Anatomy of the Human Body*, ed 29. Philadelphia, Lea & Febiger, 1973, pp 371, 510, 534, 539.
3. Moldofsky H, Scarisbrick P, England R, Smythe H: Musculo-skeletal symptoms and non-REM sleep disturbances in patients with "fibrositis syndrome" and healthy subjects. *Psychosom Med* 37:341–351, 1975.
4. Sola AE, Rodenburger ML, Gettys BB: Incidence of hypersensitive areas in posterior shoulder muscles. *Am J Phys Med* 34:585–590, 1955.
5. Good MG: Rheumatic myalgias. *The Practitioner* 146:167–174, 1941.
6. Yunas M, Masai AT, Calebro JJ, Miller K, Feigenbaum SL: Primary fibromyalgia (fibrositis): clinical study of 50 patients with matched normal controls. *Seminar on Arthritis and Rheumatism* 11:151–170, 1981.
7. Bonica JJ: Management of myofascial pain syndromes in general practice. *JAMA* 164:732–738, 1957.
8. Travell JG, Simons DG: *Myofascial Pain and Dysfunction: The Trigger Point Manual*. Baltimore, Williams & Wilkins, 1983, pp 2–4, 6–7, 12–13, 17–18, 27–28, 31, 36, 57, 64, 89, 103–164, 169, 183–184, 194, 210, 299, 310, 319, 334, 336–337, 359–360, 385, 393, 397, 410, 419, 426, 428–430, 648.
9. Bennett RM: Current issues concerning management of the fibrositis/fibromyalgia syndrome. *Am J Med* 81:15–18, 1986.
10. Salter RB: *Textbook of Disorders and Injuries of the Musculoskeletal System*. Baltimore, Williams & Wilkins, 1970, p 220.
11. Weinberger LM: Traumatic fibromyositis: a critical review of an enigmatic concept. *West J Med* 127:99–103, 1977.
12. Bruer J, Freud S: *Studies of Hysteria*. New York, Basic Books, 1957, pp 133–143.
13. Wolfe F: The clinical syndrome of fibrositis. *Am J Med* 81:81, 1986.
14. Simons DG: Muscle pain syndromes, part I. *Am J Phys Med* 54:289–311, 1975.
15. Reynolds MD: The development of the concept of fibrositis. *J Hist Med Allied Sci* 38:5–35, 1983.
16. Simons DG: Muscle pain syndromes, part II. *Am J Phys Med* 55:15–42, 1976.
17. Abel O, Siebert WJ, Earp R: Fibrositis. *J Min Med Assoc* 36:435–3437, 1939.
18. Collins DH: Fibrositis and infection. *Am Rheum Dis* 2:114–126, 1940.
19. Elliott FA: Tender muscles in sciatica, electromyographic studies. *Lancet* 1:47–49, 1944.
20. Kelly M: The nature of fibrositis. *Am Rheum Dis* 5:69–77, 1946.
21. Good MG: Objective diagnosis and curability of non-articular rheumatism. *Br J Phys Med* 14:1–7, 1951.
22. Edeiken J, Wolferth CC: Persistent pain in the shoulder region following myocardial infarction. *Am J Med Sci* 191:201–210, 1936.
23. Steindler A: The interpretation of sciatic radiation and the syndrome of low-back pain. *J Bone Joint Surg* 22:28–34, 1940.
24. Travell J, Ringler S, Herman M: Pain and disability of the shoulder and arm. *JAMA* 120:411–422, 1942.
25. Gorrell RL: Musculofascial pain. *JAMA* 142:557–561, 1950.
26. Nimmo RL: Receptors, effectors and tonus . . . a new approach. *J NCA*, 1957, 27:21–23, 60–64.
27. Warwick R, Williams PL: *Gray's Anatomy*, ed 35 (British). Philadelphia, WB Saunders, 1973, pp 432, 474, 475, 480, 505, 506, 511–513, 516, 534, 535, 562, 566–568.
28. Zierler KL: Mechanisms of muscle contraction and its energetics. In Mountevilla VB: *Medical Physiology*, ed 13. St. Louis, CV Mosby, 1978, p 78.
29. Needham DM: Biochemistry of muscles. In Bourne GH: *Biochemistry of Muscles*, ed 2. New York, Academic Press, 1973, p 377.
30. Basmasjian JV: *Muscles Alive*, ed 4. Baltimore, Williams & Wilkins, 1978, p 183.
31. Hunt C: Muscle stretch receptors, peripheral mechanisms and reflex function. *Symp Quant Biol* 17:113–121, 1952.
32. Boyd I: The response of fast and slow nuclear bag fibers and nuclear chain fibers in isolated cat muscle spindles to fusimotor stimulation and the effect of intrafusal contraction on the sensory endings. *J Exp Physiol* 61:203–254, 1976.
33. Boyd I: The nuclear-bag and nuclear-chain fiber system in muscle spindles of the cat. In Barker D: *Symposium on Muscle Receptors*, Hong Kong, Hong Kong University Press, 1962, pp 185–190.
34. Harvey RJ, Matthews PB: The response of differentiated muscle spindle endings in the cat's soleus to slow extension of the muscle. *J Physiol* 157:370, 1961.
35. Bessou P, Emonet-Denand F, Laposte Y: Occurrence of intrafusal muscle fibers innervation by branches of slow alpha-motor fibers in the cat. *Nature* 198:594–595, 1963.
36. Emonet-Denand F, Hunt CE, Laposte Y: How muscle spindles signal changes in muscle length. *NIPS (Nerves in Physiological Sciences)* 3:105–109, 1988.
37. Boyd I: The isolated mammalian muscle spindle. *Neuroscience* 258–265, 1980.
38. Awad EA: Interstitial myofibrositis: hypothesis of the mechanism. *Arch Phys Med* 54:440–453, 1973.
39. Bonica JJ: Neurophysiologic and pathologic aspects of acute and chronic pain. *Arch Surg* 112:750–761, 1977.
40. Ignelgic RJ, Atkinson JH: Pain and its modulation. Part 1—afferent mechanisms. *Neurosurgery* 6:377–583, 1980.
41. Ignelgic RJ, Atkinson JH: Pain and its modulation: Part 2—efferent mechanisms. *Neurosurgery* 6:584–590, 1980.
42. Wall PD, Melzack RJ. *Textbook of Pain*. New York, Churchill Livingstone, 1984, pp 1–16, 80–87.
43. Watkins LR, Mayer DJ: Organization of endogenous opiate and nonopiate pain control systems. *Science* 216:1185–1192, 1982.
44. Bishop B: *Pain: Its Physiology and Rationale for Management*. Washington D.C, American Physical Therapy Association, 1980, pp 1–25.
45. Dwarakanatz GK, Warfield CA: The pathophysiology of acute pain. *Hosp Pract* 64B-64R, 1986.
46. Henneman E: Peripheral mechanisms involved in the control of muscle. In Mountcastle VB: *Medical Physiology*, ed 13. St. Louis, CV Mosby, 1974, pp 617–635.
47. Brena SF: Nerve blocks and chronic pain states: basic considerations. *Postgrad Med* 78:62–71.
48. Melzack R, Wall PD: Pain mechanisms: a new theory. *Science* 150:971–979, 1965.
49. Ottoson D: *Physiology of the Nervous System* New York, Oxford University Press, 1983, pp 458–519.
50. Cyriax J: *Textbook of Orthopaedic Medicine*, vol 1. 1978, pp 30–34, 230.
51. Friction JR, Auvinen MD, Dyketra D, Schiffman E: Myofascial pain syndrome: electromyographic changes associated with local twitch response. *Arch Phys Med Rehabil* 66:314–317, 1985.
52. Sola AE, Kuitert JH: Myofascial trigger point pain in the neck and shoulder girdle. *Northwest Med* 54:980–984, 1955.
53. Simons DG, Travell JG: Myofascial origin of low back pain to principles of diagnosis and treatment. *Postgrad Med* 73:66–77, 1983.
54. Travell JG, Rinzler S: The myofascial genesis of pain. *Postgrad Med* 425–434, 1952.
55. Simons DG: Electrogenic nature of palpable bonds and "jump signs" associated with myofascial trigger points. In Boniler JJ, Albe-Fresard (eds): *Advances in Pain Research Therapy*. New York, Raven Press, 1:913–918, 1976.
56. Melczak R: Myofascial trigger points; relation to acupuncture and mechanism of pain. *Arch Phys Med Rehabil* 62:114–117, 1981.
57. Bonica JJ: Management of myofascial pain syndromes in general practice. *JAMA* June, 164–167, 1957.

58. Sandman KB: Myofascial pain syndromes: their mechanism, diagnosis and treatment. *J Manipulative Physiol Thera* 4:135–140, 1981.
59. Lewit K, Simons DG: Myofascial pain: relief by post-isometric relaxation. *Arch Phys Med Rehabil* 15:452–455, 1984.
60. Nakano KK: Sciatic nerve entrapment: the piriformis syndrome. *J Musculoskel Med* Feb:34–37, 1987.
61. Robinson DR: Piriformis syndrome in relation to sciatic pain. *Am J Surg* Mar:355–358, 1947.
62. Cailliet R: *Low Back Pain.* Philadelphia, FA Davis, 1968, p 124.
63. Cailliet R: *Soft Tissue Pain and Disability.* Philadelphia, FA Davis, 1963, p 124.
64. Maxwell TG: The piriformis muscle and its relation to the long legged sciatic syndrome. *J CCA* July:51–55, 1978.
65. Freiberg AH, Vinle TH: Sciatica and the sacroiliac joint. *J Bone Joint Surg* 16:126–136, 1934.
66. Retzlaff EW, Berry AH, Haight AS, Parente PA, Lechty HA, Turner DM, Yexbick AA, Labcevic JS, Devota JN: The piriformis muscle syndromes. *J Am Osteopath Assoc.* 73:55–63, 799–807, 1974.
67. Bernard N, Kirkaldy-Willis WH: Recognizing specific characteristics of nonspecific low back pain. *Clin Orthop* 217:266–280, 1987.
68. Corwin JM: Piriformis syndrome in the athlete. *ACA J Chiro* Jan:21–23, 1987.
69. TePoorten BA: The piriformis muscle. *J Am Osteopath Assoc* 69:78–88, 150–160, 1969.
70. Beaton LE: The sciatic nerve and the piriformis muscle: their interrelation a possible cause of coccygodynia. *J Bone Joint Surg* 20:686–688, 1938.
71. Good MG: Muscular sciatic. *Clinical Journal: A Record of Clinical Medicine and Surgery* 72:66–71, 1943.
72. Pace JB: Commonly overlooked pain syndromes responsive to simple therapy. *Postgrad Med* 58:107–113, 1975.
73. Ober FR: Back strain and sciatica. *JAMA* 104:1580–1583, 1935.
74. Yeoman W: The relation of arthritis of the sacroiliac joint to sciatica with an analysis of 100 cases. *Lancet* 2:1119–1122, 1928.
75. Singh Neel S, Singh Neel G: Piriformis Syndrome. *ACA J of Chiro* 20:32–35, 1986.
76. Simons DG, Travell JG: Myofascial origins of low back pain: 3. Pelvic and lower extremities. *Postgrad Med* 78:99–108, 1983.
77. Bernard TN, Kirkaldy-Willis WH: Recognizing specific characteristics of nonspecific low back pain. *Clin Orthop* 217:266–280, 1967.
78. Kirkaldy-Willis WH: *Managing Low Back Pain,* ed 2. New York, Churchill Livingstone, 1988, p 142.
79. Sola AE, Kuitert JH: Quadratus lumborum myofascitis. *Northwest Med* 53:1003–1005, 1954.
80. Sola AE: Myofascial trigger point therapy. *Medical Times* Jan:70–77, 1982.
81. Kellgren JH: Observation on referred pain arising from muscle. *Clin Sci* 3:175–190, 1938.
82. White AA, Panjabi MM: *Chemical Biomechanics of the Spine* Philadelphia, JB Lippincott, 1978, p 307.
83. Sola AE, Williams RL: Myofascial pain syndromes. *Neurology* 6:91–95, 1956.
84. Cailliet R: *Neck and Arm Pain.* Philadelphia, FA Davis, 1964, p 97.
85. Grice AS: Scalenus anticus syndrome: diagnosis and chiropractic adjustment procedure. *JCCA* March:15–19, 1977.
86. Berges PU: Myofascial pain syndromes. *Postgrad Med* 53:161–163, 1973.
87. Bennett KM: Fibrositis: does it exist and can it be treated? *J Musculoskeletal Med* June:52–72, 1984.
88. Goldenberg DL: Fibromyalgia syndrome: an emerging but controversial condition. *JAMA* 257:2782–2787, 1987.
89. Bennett KM: The fibrositis/fibromyalgia syndrome: current issues and perspectives. *Am J Med* 81:1–114, 1986.

90. Wolfe F: Workshop on criteria for diagnosing fibrositis/fibromyalgia. *Am J Med* 81:114–115, 1986.
91. Simons DG: Myofascial pain syndromes: where are we? where are we going? *Arch Phys Med Rehabil* 69:207–221, 1988.
92. Bennett KM: Fibromyalgia. *JAMA* 257:2802–2803, 1987.
93. Masi AT, Yunas MB: Concepts of illness in population applied to fibromyalgia syndromes. *Am J Med* 81:19–23.
94. Campbell SM, Clark S, Tindall EA, Forehand ME, Bennett RM: Clinical characteristics of fibrositis. *Arthritis Rheum* 26:817–824, 1983.
95. Smythe HA: Non-articular rheumatism and psychogenic musculoskeletal syndromes. In McCarty DJ: *Arthritis and Allied Conditions,* 9th ed. Philadelphia, Lea & Febiger, 1979, pp 881–891.
96. MacNab I: Acceleration injuries of the cervical spine. *J Bone Joint Surg* 46-A:1797–1799, 1964.
97. Kraft GH, Johnson EW, LaBon MM: The fibrositis syndrome. *Arch Phys Med Rehabil* 49:155–161, 1968.
98. Smythe HA: Fibrositis and other diffuse musculoskeletal syndromes. In Kelley WH, Havis JR, Ruddy S, et al. (eds): *Textbook of Rheumatology.* Philadelphia, WB Saunders, 1980, pp 485–493.
99. Wolfe F: Development of criteria for the diagnosis for fibrositis. *Am J Med* 81:99–104, 1986.
100. Bennett KM: Current issues concerning management of the fibrositis/fibromyalgia syndrome. *Am J Med* 81:15–18, 1986.
101. Moldofsky H, Scarisbrich P: Induction of neurasthenic musculoskeletal pain syndrome by selective sleep stage deprivation. *Psychosom Med* 28:35–44, 1976.
102. Modolfsky H, Tullis C, Lue FA, Quorce G, Davidson J: Sleep related myoclonus in rheumatic pain modulation disorder (fibrositis syndrome and in excessive daytime somnolence). *Psychosom Med* 46:145–151, 1984.
103. Saskin P, Moldofsky H, Lue FA: Sleep and post-traumatic rheumatic pain modulation disorder (fibrositis syndrome). *Psychosom Med* 48:319–323, 1986.
104. Moldofsky H: Sleep and musculoskeletal pain. *Am J Med* 81:85–89, 1986.
105. Withig R, Zourk FJ, Blumer D, et al.: Disturbed sleep in patients complaining of chronic pain. *J Nerv Ment Dis* 170:429–431, 1982.
106. Harvey JA, Schlosberg AJ, Yunger LM: Behavioral correlates of serotonin depletion. *Fed Proc* 34:1796–1801, 1975.
107. Moldofsky H, Warsh JJ: Plasma tryptophan and musculoskeletal pain in non-articular rheumatism ("fibrositis syndrome"). *Pain* 5:65–71, 1978.
108. Goldenberg DC: Psychologic studies in fibrositis. *Am J Med* 81:67–70, 1986.
109. Payne TC, Lewit F, Garron DC, Katz RS, Golden HE, Glickman PB, Vanderplate C: Fibrositis and psychologic disturbance. *Arthritis Rheum* 28:213–217, 1982.
110. Wolf F, Cathey MA, Kleinheked SM, Anon SP, Hoffman RG, Young DY, Hawley DJ: Psychological stature in primary fibrositis and fibrositis associated with rheumatoid arthritis. *J Rheumatol* 11:500–505, 1984.
111. Hudson JI, Hudson MS, Plines LF, Goldenberg DL, Pope HG: Fibromyalgia and major affective disorders: a controlled phenomenology and family history study. *Am J Psychiatry* 142:4, 1985.
112. Hadler NM: A critical reappraisal of the fibrositis concept. *Am J Med* 81:26–30, 1986.
113. Moskowitz RW: *Clinical Rheumatology: A Problem Oriented Approach,* ed 2. Philadelphia, Lea & Febiger, 1982, p 149.
114. Sandman KB, Backstrom CJ: Psychophysiological factors in myofascial pain. *JMPT* 7:237–241, 1984.
115. Haber JD, Roos C: Effects of spouse abuse and/or sexual abuse in the development and maintenance of chronic pain in women. In Fields H, Howard L: *World Congress on Pain: 4th Proceedings (Advances in Pain Research and Therapy).* New York, Raven Press, 1985, SER: 9:889–893.

116. Smythe H: Tender points: evolution of concepts of the fibrositis/fibromyalgia syndrome. *Am J Med* 82:2–6, 1986.
117. Yunas M, Kaylen-Raman UK, Kaylen-Raman K: Primary fibromyalgia syndrome and myofascial pain syndrome: clinical features and muscle pathology. *Arch Phys Med Rehabil* 69:451–454, 1988.
118. Yunas M, Kaylen-Raman UK, Kaylen-Raman K, Masi AT: Pathologic changes in muscles in primary fibromyalgia syndrome. *Am J Med* 81:38–42, 1986.
119. Bohr T: Painful questions about fibromyalgia. *JAMA* 258:1476, 1987.
120. McCain GA: Role of physical fitness training in the fibrositis/fibromyalgia syndrome. *Am J Med* 81:73–79, 1986.

121. Clark S: Workshop on managing fibrositis/fibromyalgia. *Am J Med* 81:110–112, 1986.
122. Yunas M, Masi AT, Calabro JJ, Indravaden KS: Primary fibromyalgia. *Am Fam Physician* May:115–121, 1982.
123. Carette S, McCain GA, Bell DA Fam AG: Evolution of amitriptyline in primary fibrositis. *Arthritis Rheum* 29:655–659, 1986.
124. Cathey MA, Wolfe F, Kleinhesel SM, Hawley DJ: Socioecomonic impact of fibrositis: a study of 81 patients with primary fibrositis. *Am J Med* 81:78–84, 1986.
125. Kahler Hench P: Secondary fibrositis. *Am J Med* 81:60–64, 1986.

CHAPTER 13

Adjunctive Procedures: Physiological Therapeutics

BONNIE L. McDOWELL, R.P.T., D.C.

Without question, the field of physiologic therapeutics has advanced because of both scientific and empirical findings of multiple minds seeking answers that have the potential of relieving pain and enhancing healing. (1)

Since the beginning of recorded history, man has used the natural forces of heat, light, sun, air, and water for the purpose of soothing and healing human disease. Tissue manipulation also has its roots in ancient history, though its exact origin cannot be traced. It seems only natural that these two forms of healing have in many cases been utilized concomitantly for maximum benefit to the patient.

Chiropractic physiological therapeutics, or physiotherapy, was defined by Stonebrink (personal communication, R.D. Stonebrink, Nov 28, 1986; 2) for the peer review procedures of the American Chiropractic Association (ACA) Council on Physiotherapy. His definition was later modified and published in the ACA Basic Chiropractic Procedural Manual: "Chiropractic physiotherapy is the therapeutic application of forces and substances that induce a physiologic response and that uses and/or allows the body's natural processes to return to a more normal state of health. It makes use of the therapeutic effects of:

- Soft tissue manipulation and massage; the latter including stroking, compression, percussion, touch, vibration, joint movements, and nerve compression.
- Mechanotherapy, including active and passive exercises; traction, either intermittent or sustained; and structural braces, shoe lifts, casts, or other supports.
- Hydrotherapy, in its traditional forms.

- Electrotherapy, when these procedures are in keeping with a physiologic therapeutic intent and reaction.
- Light, heat, cold, air, water, as natural forces which are the prerogatives of all people to be free to use.
- Nutritional planning, dietetics, and special food or nutritional supplementation" (3).

The first inclusion of physiological therapeutics into a chiropractic curriculum came in 1912 at the National College of Chiropractic. Otto J. Turek, business manager and director of the college, established the first Physiotherapy Center in the basement of the National College in 1927, under the guidance of Drs. John Howard, William Charles Schulze, and Arthur L. Forester. The center was equipped with colonic irrigation, steam baths, packs, massage, and needle-spray showers. Dr. Joseph Janse, who later became a president of the college, was one of the first interns to work at the Center. National College has remained in the forefront of the investigation and use of physiological therapeutics as an adjunct to chiropractic manipulation (4).

The use of physiological therapeutics has blossomed as the modalities have become researched, modernized, safer, and more effective. It is fortunate for chiropractic that we are not the only discipline taking advantage of these therapeutics. Physical therapists and medical doctors are also seeking state-of-the-art therapeutic equipment. We can all benefit from the knowledge gained by research and clinical use of the modalities.

A chiropractor might argue that the use of the modalities should be left to the physical therapists; that the chiropractor's purpose is to reduce the subluxation complex by means of the chiropractic adjustment. However, isn't it the chiropractor's purpose to restore health to the patient as quickly and effectively as possible? We should then employ whatever means are reasonable and necessary for achieving that purpose (5). Chiropractic manipulation is, however, generally the most effective chiropractic procedure (6) and remains the primary focus of treatment.

Malik and associates studied 333 cases for the effect of chiropractic manipulative adjustment alone compared to the combined treatment of chiropractic manipulative adjustment and physical therapy. He found that the recovery period in both male and female patients in the cervical and thoracic regions was dramatically shortened when the combined treatment was used rather than the adjustment alone (7).

The choice of physiological therapeutics can be a difficult one. Most modalities have a number of possible effects, and many modalities overlap in their repertoire of effects. Often there is no one "best" modality for the treatment of a particular phase of recovery for any given disease or condition. The doctor must then use clinical judgment in choosing the treatment modality or modalities that are best for the patient. There may be an element of trial-and-error. If a modality is used for a sufficient trial of treatments without the expected results, another may be tried. This process, however, should not continue endlessly. Discontinuation of the modalities or appropriate referral should be considered if results are not satisfactory.

Whether to use the adjunctive therapies before or after the adjustment is another decision that must be made by the doctor. Some feel that the adjustment "holds" better and the patient is able to relax more completely if the modality is given after manipulation, while others feel that the modality is important to prepare the tissues for the adjustment and that it allows the adjustment to occur more easily. Still others may use the simpler modalities (i.e., heat and cold) as home treatments and not use modalities in the office at all. Again, this appears to be left to the clinical judgment of the doctor. Each patient should be evaluated individually, and the treatment plan should be tailored to the patient's needs.

In any case, the physiological therapeutic procedures deserve high priority, as they support chiropractic manipulative treatment. Relief of symptoms, reversal of the disease process, and recovery time can all be enhanced by the appropriate use of these modalities.

CONDUCTIVE AND CONVECTIVE HEAT

Definitions

Conductive heat: transmission of heat from one body to another without evident movement of the conducting body.

Convective heat: transmission of heat in gases and liquids by circulation of heated particles.

Hydrotherapy: the application of water in any form, either internally or externally, in the treatment of disease.

Water temperatures:

Neutral: 94–97°F = 34.4–36.1°C
Tepid: 75–92°F = 23.9–33.3°C
Warm: 92–97°F = 33.3–36.1°C
Hot: 97–104°F = 36.1–40°C
Very Hot: above 104°F = above 40°C

Conversion factors for temperatures:

9/5 (temperature in °C) + 32 = temperature in °F
5/9 (temperature in °F − 32) = temperature in °C

Introduction

Heat is probably the oldest and most widely used of the physical modalities. Natural forms of heat—sun, sun-heated sand, and thermal waters—have been used therapeutically for as long as we can trace history. Stones heated by fire and animal bladders filled with hot water were placed against painful parts. Wounded soldiers in ancient Rome went to mineral springs for recuperation. The first artificial sources of heat were produced from the combustion of wood, coal, peat, oil, tallow, or alcohol. Electricity was not used for heat until the 1890s (8).

Even now, relatively simple forms of heat are used extensively to treat a wide variety of systemic and local conditions. Water is a common carrier for heat and has many advantages. It is inexpensive, readily accessible, can take many forms, and is able to conduct and absorb large quantities of heat.

Mechanism of Action

Vasodilation

At temperatures up to 42°C, there is vasodilation of the skin and superficial fascia, with an increase in blood flow of four to five times the resting level. This vasodilation is caused by histamine-like substances acting on the capillaries as well as a reflex action on the arterioles. Vasodilation continues as the temperature rises above 42°C, but burning becomes a danger.

Metabolism Increases

For every temperature rise of 1°C, there is a 13% increase in metabolism in the skin or muscle. Above 45°C, tissues become damaged irreversibly (9).

Collagen Extensibility Increases

At temperatures of 39 to 44°C, the viscous properties of collagen become more dominant, and tension relaxes (9).

Sensory Nerve Endings Are Stimulated

The sensation of heat is detected, but the effect of heat on nerve conduction is yet unproven (9).

Effects

Analgesia

Pain relief is probably due to the stimulation of sensory nerve endings, causing a counterirritant effect and a decrease in transmission by pain fibers (9).

Reduction of Muscle Spasm

This effect is probably also mediated by the stimulation of sensory nerve endings, causing decreased firing of secondary nerve endings, resulting in decreased muscle tone. Vasodilation causing a release of waste products from the muscle may also contribute.

Edema Reduction

Vasodilation increases capillary flow and the return of blood and lymph to the general circulation. However, heat may increase the trauma to the area and actually increase edema, especially in an acute inflammation.

Collagen Relaxes

Tendons and capsular ligaments increase their ability to extend with stretch.

Chronic Inflammation Decreases

Vasodilation increases the nutrient supply and white blood cells for the resolution of chronic inflammation (9, 10).

Indications

Subacute and chronic:

Neuromuscular, musculoskeletal conditions (e.g., myofascial pain syndromes, neuritis, neuralgia, sciatica);
Arthritic conditions: heat can effectively increase the extensibility of the joint capsule and decrease joint stiffness;
Sprains and strains;
Tendinitis, tenosynovitis;
Dysmenorrhea, amenorrhea;
Pelvic inflammatory disease;
Prostatitis (via sitz bath);
Benign prostatic hypertrophy (via sitz bath);
Hemorrhoids (via sitz bath);
Superficial abscesses, carbuncles, cellulitis, cystitis: heat localizes the inflammation and accelerates abscess formation (10);
Hematoma resolution: research results are not conclusive (10).

(Note: unfortunately the suffix -itis is misleading. While the term implies an active inflammatory process, conditions such as tendinitis may not be inflamed. Heat is appropriate in such conditions in the subacute and chronic stages.)

Contraindications

Insensitivity to heat (e.g., diabetics, postsurgical areas, drug-induced insensitivity, neurological deficit);
Heat sensitivity (e.g., multiple sclerosis);
Severe circulatory disturbances (e.g., peripheral vascular disease, arteriosclerosis, cardiac patient, varicose veins, aneurysm, hypertension, diabetes mellitus);
Tendency to hemorrhage (e.g., hemophilia);
Malignancy;
Advanced weakness;
Over a gravid uterus;
Active tuberculosis;
An encapsulated swelling in which rupture could cause damage;
An unreliable patient;
Severe edema.

Specific Methods of Application

Hydrocollator Packs

Hydrocollator packs or hot packs (Fig. 13.1) are probably the most commonly used form of heat. They are considered a form of conductive heat, as the heat is transmitted from the pack to the patient by heated water particles. The silica-gel pack covered with fabric is heated in a thermostatically controlled tank of water at a temperature of 130–170°F, and it delivers moist heat for approximately 30 min when removed from the water. The packs are available in a variety of shapes to conform to different body parts.

Approximately 6 layers of toweling are needed between the pack and the patient to avoid burning. More layers of toweling and extreme caution should be used if the patient lies on top of the pack, if the patient's heat sensitivity is in question, or if the pack feels too hot to the patient. Hot packs can burn, especially over bony prominences, so it is important to monitor the patient carefully and apply extra toweling as needed.

Hot Wet Compresses

Hot wet compresses may be used in place of hydrocollator packs as a form of moist heat. Towels are soaked in hot water and wrung out well before being placed against the patient's skin. The towels cool quickly, so they must be changed often or kept warm with a heating pad. The compress is left on for the usual 20 to 30 min for musculoskeletal conditions, but it may be left on for longer than an hour when treating infection. Hot wet compresses are conductive heat, as the compress lies directly against the skin.

Heating Pads, Hot Water Bottles

Dry heating pads do not have the ability to penetrate the skin that *moist heating pads* or hydrocollator packs do. Hot water bottles and some heating pads may be used with a wet towel to increase their penetration. More expensive moist heating pads are available that use a special cloth covering that draws moisture from the air. This type of moist heating pad is probably worth the investment in terms of ease of use and effectiveness if heat is indicated for a chronic, long-term condition.

Many lay people use heating pads or hot water bottles continuously for their soothing warmth. They should be taught that the physiological effects

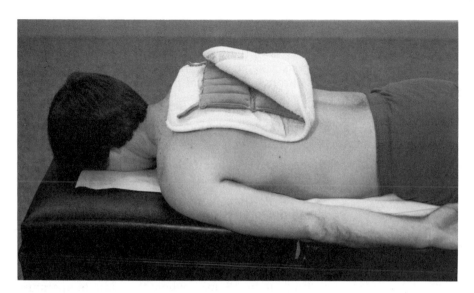

Figure 13.1. A hydrocollator or hot pack. A commercial hot-pack cover as shown here is equal to approximately four to five layers of toweling. Therefore, additional layers of toweling should be used to avoid burning the skin.

will be greatly enhanced by intermittent use (e.g., 20 minutes out of every hour or 20 minutes 3 to 4 times a day).

Extremity Baths

Warm water baths, a form of conductive heat, are useful for applying heat to hands, feet, elbows, etc. The temperature, usually 100–105°F, is easily controlled. The water may need to be changed or added to keep the temperature at the desired level. Medicinals, such as magnesium sulfate, can be added to the water for additional benefit, in this case, for the relief of edema.

Whirlpool Baths

Similar to warm water baths, *whirlpool baths* with their agitators have the additional advantage of a mechanical effect (i.e., the impact of water on the skin). Besides providing a pleasant form of heat for typical musculoskeletal conditions, whirlpools are also useful for increasing circulation and debriding dried or necrotic tissue from recently uncasted parts, burns, infected wounds, and decubitus ulcers. Whirlpools are a form of convective heat.

Fluidotherapy

Fluidotherapy is a dry whirlpool that uses circulating cellulose particles and enables the patient to tolerate higher temperature than are possible with water. An excellent discussion of fluidotherapy has been offered by Jaskoviak and Schafer (1).

Paraffin Baths

Paraffin baths (Fig. 13.2) are a mixture of 4 parts wax and 1 part mineral oil heated to a temperature of 125–130°F. The hand, foot, or elbow is dipped into the hot mixture 5 to 7 times, then quickly wrapped with wax paper or plastic, then a towel. Other body parts may be painted with paraffin and wrapped similarly.

Paraffin has the advantages of surrounding the small joints of the hands or feet, providing a consistent heat, and leaving the skin soft and pliable. Paraffin baths are particularly useful for chronic arthritic hands and Dupuytren's contractures. The paraffin bath is a form of conductive heat.

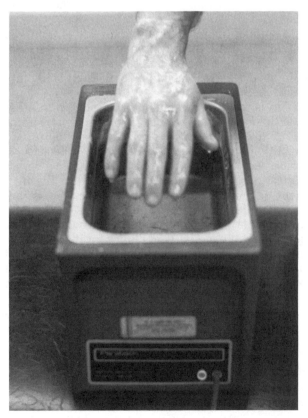

Figure 13.2. A paraffin bath. Illustrated here is a small, thermostatically controlled unit for limited office or home use.

Duration of Treatment

In general, the maximum beneficial effects of heat occur in the first 20 to 30 min. Beyond that time, blood flow plateaus and then declines, which may increase edema in the area. Therefore, 20 to 30 min is the standard time duration for heat treatments.

CRYOTHERAPY

Definitions

Cryotherapy: the therapeutic use of cold.

Hydrotherapy: the application of water in any form, either internally or externally, in the treatment of disease.

Water temperatures:

Neutral: 94–97°F = 34.4–36.1°C
Tepid: 75–92°F = 23.9–33.3°C
Cool: 65–75°F = 18.3–23.9°C
Cold: 40–65°F = 4.4–18.3°C
Very cold: below 40°F = below 4.4°C

Introduction

The use of ice externally for therapeutic purposes began in ancient times with Hippocrates and Celsius (11). In 1823, Scudamore used ice fragments for packing gouty joints, and in the next year Tanchou wrote a book on the therapeutic use of ice. About 1835, ice chips came into popular use for the treatment of wound inflammation. Artificial ice became commercially available in the United States about 1885 (8).

In spite of the relatively long history of the therapeutic use of ice, the physiological effects of ice and cold are still somewhat obscure. Some effects of cold have been assumed to exist without being fully researched.

The lack of research notwithstanding, cryotherapeutic modalities can have tremendous clinical value. Ice is inexpensive, readily available to both practitioner and patient, can be used in a variety of forms (see "Application"), has relatively few contraindications, and can be very effective in the treatment of musculoskeletal pain, edema, spasm, and inflammation, especially in the first 24–48 hrs after an injury (12). In many instances in which heat is considered the modality of choice for its "soothing" qualities, cooling would probably afford longer lasting and more complete results, and therefore should be considered more often. However, the choice of heat or cold is still under debate (13, 14).

The discussion of cold in this chapter will be limited to the external, local applications of cold.

Mechanism of Action

Blood Vessels Initially Constrict

The initial reaction of the blood vessels to cold results from the body's attempt to maintain its core temperature by constriction of the peripheral blood vessels. Lewis noted these actions:

Superficial vessels constrict; this is a direct and persistent action.

Vessels in the immediate area and consensual areas constrict transiently by reflex action through the central nervous system.

Systemically, blood vessels constrict through activation of the central nervous system as a result of cool venous blood returning to the core circulation from the cooled areas (15, 16).

Blood Vessels Dilate Intermittently

Lewis noted a "hunting reaction" in which vasoconstriction yielded to vasodilation as the tissue temperature dropped to 15°C or lower and continued to alternate between vasoconstriction and vasodilation as long as the cold was being applied (15, 17). Gucker described the vasodilation of this "hunting reaction" as occurring about every 30 min and lasting 10 to 15 min when the skin temperature dropped below 10°C (18). This intermittent vasodilation acts as a protective mechanism to guard the tissue against prolonged hypothermia, frostbite, and permanent tissue damage.

Skin Becomes Hyperemic

Cutaneous vessels dilate, causing a superficial reactive hyperemia (16), probably due to the release of histamines as a result of cellular damage (15).

Nerve Conduction Velocity Decreases

The frequency and velocity of both motor and sensory nerve impulses are decreased (19, 20), with small, myelinated fibers being most susceptible, then large, myelinated fibers, and finally unmyelinated fibers being least susceptible (21).

Muscle Tone Decreases

Cooling affects the muscle spindle by several mechanisms:

The rate of firing of spindle sensory fibers is directly decreased by the cooling of muscle spindles (22).

Muscle spindle activity decreases reflexly, possibly due to sympathetic influence on the muscle spindle (23).

Skin, Subcutaneous, and Intramuscular Temperatures Decrease

Maximum cooling occurs in the skin, with proportionately less cooling and more delayed cooling in the subcutaneous tissues and muscles. Reductions of muscle temperature of 1.2°C, measured approximately 4.3 cm below the skin, have been recorded within a 5-minute period by Wolf and Basmajian (24). Bierman and Friedlander studied temperature changes with a 2-hour application of ice to the human gastrocnemius muscle. They found that skin temperature dropped quickly and was maintained at approximately 6.1°C. Intramuscular temperatures, measured approximately 5 cm below the skin, took at least 30 min to show a significant drop and continued to drop to approximately 27°C (25).

Adipose tissue has a significant effect on cooling. A region covered by more than 2 cm of subcutaneous tissue shows significantly less cooling in a 10 min period than a region with less than 1 cm of subcutaneous fat (26).

Metabolism Decreases

Local reduction of metabolic rate has been demonstrated by the measurement of local oxygen uptake. Venous blood from cooled tissues is about 80% oxygen-saturated as opposed to 70% oxygen saturation of normal tissue (16).

Effects

Anesthesia

The patient will generally experience four phases of sensation within the initial 5 to 10 min of application of ice (12): cold, aching, burning, and numbness, easily remembered by the mnemonic C-A-B-N or "cabin." The patient may find the aching and/or burning phases to be reversed or nonexistent. When numbness has been achieved, there is a marked decrease in the conductivity of local nerve fibers and a resultant interruption of the pain-spasm-pain cycle. Treatment should cease at this point to avoid the "hunting reaction."

Analgesia

The mechanism of pain relief of musculoskeletal conditions is not clearly understood. Theories include:

Decreased nerve conduction velocity (20);
Stimulation of A-delta sensory fibers (for pain, temperature, and touch), activating descending "analgesia-producing systems" (27);
Bombardment of cold nerve impulses, causing an overload of the system and breakdown of the reflex arc (28).

Although these three theories of pain relief appear contradictory, none has been ruled out.

Reduction of Edema

A number of studies have been conducted to demonstrate the effect of cold on edema after an acute trauma. The results are inconclusive. Janssen and Waaler demonstrated that cooling blocks the release of histamine and therefore lessens vasodilation and the accumulation of exudates (29).

McMaster and Liddle found that cooling an acutely injured limb at 30°C for one hour produces less residual swelling than (a) no treatment, (b) cooling at 20°C for one hour, (c) cooling at 30°C for three sessions of one hour interspersed with one hour at room temperature, and (d) cooling at 20°C for three sessions as above (30).

However, Matsen and associates found that no cooling treatments lessened swelling, and in fact cooling of 5 to 15°C for 24 hours actually increased swelling (31). Likewise, Jezdinsky and associates showed that cold applied for 2, 5, 7, or 10 hours after injury had a tendency to increase swelling (32).

Further research is necessary to determine the optimum treatment regime for the reduction of posttraumatic edema. It is clear that cooling should be moderate and of short duration to avoid increased tissue damage and swelling.

Reduced Muscle Spasm

Muscle spasm or guarding is a protective mechanism of the body to avoid further trauma. Such a prolonged, involuntary, muscle contraction causes ischemia and the utilization of large quantities of nutrients, and further perpetuates the pain-spasm-pain cycle so commonly seen after injury. It appears that muscle spasm diminishes as pain is alleviated; therefore, the theories proposed to explain the analgesic effect of cooling can also apply to the reduction of muscle spasm by cooling (33). Mennell states that "the counterirritant application of cold plus muscle stretch reverses the pain mechanism of muscle spasm" (34).

Reduced Spasticity

Spasticity is "a pathological condition of the central nervous system characterized by hyperactivity of the stretch reflex in response to movement" (33). (The term spasticity is defined here so that it will not be confused with the term "spasm.")

It is generally agreed that cooling temporarily reduces stretch reflex activity, thereby reducing spasticity (23, 35–38), although several studies indicate that cooling initially increases spasticity (38, 39). As with other effects of cooling, the mechanism of action is merely theorized, not proven by research. Miglietta found an "immediate decrease in the mechanically induced stretch reflex response" which he explains as being "mediated through stimulation of cutaneous afferents and their secondary influence on the alpha and/or gamma motoneuron activity" (23). However, muscle spindle activity does not decrease until actual cooling of the muscles occurs (40, 41), indicating that spasticity is best reduced when cooling is prolonged long enough to cause an intramuscular drop in temperature (23).

Reduced Manual Dexterity

It has been postulated that increases in the viscosity of the fluids and tissues of the joints and tendons may account for the loss of dexterity with cooling at higher temperatures, while a loss of muscular power may have some effect on dexterity at lower temperatures (20).

Indications

Acute sprains and strains (42, 43);

Acute inflammatory processes: arthritis (33), bursitis, tendinitis (34), myositis, neuritis;

Acute trauma;

Acute and chronic muscle spasm;

Spasticity associated with neurological disorders (e.g., quadriplegia, paraplegia, hemiplegia, multiple sclerosis).

Contraindications

Weakened individuals such as geriatrics, infants, cachexics;

Individuals with psychological aversion to cold;

Hypersensitive individuals, secondary to (a) histamine release, (b) cold hemolysins and agglutinins, and (c) cryoglobulins. Symptoms of hypersensitivity may include urticaria (wheals), erythema, itching, Raynaud's phenomenon, ulceration, chills, gastrointestinal disturbances (44).

Circulatory disturbances (e.g., Raynaud's disease, thromboangiitis obliterans (Buerger's disease), peripheral vascular disease, high blood pressure, atherosclerosis, severe varicose veins, myocardial weakness).

Some rheumatoid conditions; cooling may increase joint stiffness.

Hypothermic individuals.

Application

General Considerations

Avoid generalized hypothermia by (a) keeping the room warm; (b) keeping the untreated parts of the body warm with blankets, heating pad, hot water bottle, etc.; (c) giving the patient a warm drink before and/or after the treatment; and (d) having the patient exercise before and/or after the treatment.

Healthy individuals will be able to tolerate and will respond more readily to drastic changes in temperature than will more debilitated individuals.

Specific Applications

The choice of cooling modalities will depend upon the size and contour of the area being treated, the degree of cooling desired, and availability of modalities. Major advantages of the cooling modalities over other physiotherapeutic modalities are their accessibility and low cost. Expensive cryotherapy units may be more convenient to use, but they do not afford superior results in any way.

Ice Packs or Cold Packs. Cold packs can take a number of forms, the simplest being a heavy plastic bag with ice cubes and water enclosed. These ice packs are readily available, can be made in any size, and will hold their cooling properties for a relatively long period of time. Refreezable gel packs are reusable and convenient for use in a clinical setting, but tend to lose their cooling properties somewhat more quickly than do ice packs (12, 45). Chemical-reaction packs are convenient for use where a refrigera-

tion unit is not available (e.g., on the football field), but they are more expensive than ice packs and only remain cold for 10 to 15 min and therefore are not effective for deep cooling (45). Bags of frozen vegetables and plastic bags frozen with a water/alcohol mixture are convenient for use at home.

Method

1. Inspect area to be treated.
2. Place warm wet towel against skin.
3. Place cold pack against towel and secure in place with a dry towel, strap, etc.

Duration. Because research has not determined the duration of treatment for maximum therapeutic effect, clinical judgment must be used. Treatment regimes generally include the use of a cold pack for 15 to 20 minutes, repeated between once an hour and once a day (13). This broad range suggests that further research would be most helpful.

Precautions

Do not place plastic directly against the skin.

Inspect skin often for signs of adverse reaction: pallor, cutis anserina (goose bumps), cyanosis, urticaria.

Monitor patient for hypothermia.

Ice Massage. Ice massage is a safe and effective method for cooling relatively small, superficial areas of the body. Once a treatment has been performed in the clinic without adverse reaction, it can be taught to a family member and performed safely at home without fear of tissue damage. The ice massage can be very effective at breaking the pain-spasm-pain cycle, probably due to both its cooling and its counterirritant effects. It should be considered in the treatment of both acute and chronic muscle spasm.

Method

1. Freeze water in a paper cup. A tongue depressor may be frozen into the cube to act as a handle. Individual ice cubes may be used, but larger pieces of ice are easier to handle.
2. Peel paper cup away. Hold ice in one hand with a towel. A rubber glove may be worn to further insulate the clinician's hand. A small towel is held in the other hand.
3. The ice is rubbed slowly and with moderate pressure (Fig. 13.3) on the affected area for several seconds, then the water is patted off with the towel in the other hand.
4. Warn the patient of possible discomfort, and monitor his sensation to the treatment. He will usually feel cold, aching, burning, and then numbness (mnemonic C-A-B-N, see "Effects").
5. When the patient reports that the area is numb, treatment is complete.

Duration. The treatment usually takes approximately 5 to 10 min.

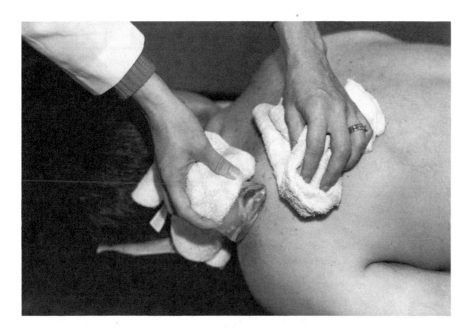

Figure 13.3. The application of ice for ice massage. The ice is rubbed on a small area, then the water is patted off with a small towel.

Precautions

Inspect skin for adverse reactions. If pallor persists for more than about 30 sec, the patient's circulatory status should be questioned, and treatment should cease. The part should be warmed gently; wrapping the patient and/or part in blankets is usually sufficient.

Avoid bony prominences.

Large areas should be divided into smaller areas and treated separately.

Cold Compresses. Cold compresses are useful for large areas of the body; however, they are difficult to keep cold.

Method

1. Dip turkish towels in cold or ice water and wring out.
2. Apply towels to the affected part.
3. Cover with plastic and dry towels.

Duration. Treatment time is similar to that for cold packs: 15–20 minutes, once an hour to once a day. Cold compresses can also be used for longer periods for treatment of fever.

Extremity Baths. Extremity baths can take the form of tubs or whirlpools. Treatment temperature is quite variable, depending upon water temperature and the amount of ice used. With smaller tubs, ice may need to be added to maintain a constant treatment temperature. Because very cold temperatures can be achieved with an extremity bath, the part should be closely monitored.

Vapor Coolant Sprays. Vapor coolant sprays will be discussed in Chapter 12, "Myofascial Pain."

CONTRAST HEAT AND COLD

Definitions

Contrast heat and cold: the alternating use of heat and cold in the form of water baths or packs.

Temperature ranges:

Heat: 95–110°F = 35.0–43.3°C
Cold: 50–80°F = 10.0–26.7°C

Actions

Since heat causes vasodilation and cold causes vasoconstriction, the contrast between heat and cold will cause intense stimulation of the blood vessels.

Effects

Stimulation of peripheral circulation
Edema reduction

Indications

Subacute and chronic

Postfracture;
Arthritic conditions;
Sprains and strains;
Neuromuscular, musculoskeletal conditions;
Contusions;
Edema;
Buerger's disease;
Chilblains.

Contraindications

Arterial insufficiency;
Advanced peripheral vascular disease;
Insensitivity to heat or cold;
Hypersensitivity to heat or cold.

Application

Contrast heat and cold may be applied in the form of extremity baths or hydrocollator packs and cold packs. All are described in "Specific Methods of Application" for "Conductive and Convective Heat" and "Cryotherapy."

Contrast applications should begin and end with heat. Five to seven total applications are given, with the heat applications lasting longer than the cold. For example, 3 min of heat is followed by 1 min of cold, or 5 min of heat is followed by 2 min of cold. Some authors suggest that the first application of heat should last up to 10 minutes.

LOW-VOLTAGE GALVANISM

Definitions

Low-voltage galvanism: a current of less than 50 mA which flows in one direction only.

Medical galvanism: the use of low-voltage galvanic current with water as the conducting medium to create chemical changes in the tissues.

Surgical galvanism: the use of low-voltage galvanic current for the surgical destruction of tissues.

Iontophoresis: the introduction of medicinal ions of soluble salts into the tissues using low-voltage galvanic current for therapeutic purposes.

Introduction

Galvani found in 1791 that the application of a direct current to a nerve and muscle could cause a twitch contraction. The electrical battery, which produced the first constant flow of galvanic current, was invented by Volta in 1800. Galvani's nephew Aldini first popularized the stimulating effect of the galvanic current. General galvanism (i.e., placing the positive electrode on the head and the negative electrode on the epigastrium or sacrum and running a low current) was originally used for insomnia and pain. The galvanic bath later became popular for its supposed ability to remove poisonous metallic ions and disease organisms from the body. It was therefore indicated for debility, nutritional deficiencies, and many disease processes. Localized galvanism was used for stimulation of cranial nerves for headaches, loss of smell, loss of vision, etc., for cardiorespiratory resuscitation, for cautery, and for fracture healing (46).

Low-voltage galvanism (LVG) was again popularized early in the 20th century for medical galvanism, surgical galvanism, and iontophoresis for the treatment of a wide variety of more local, superficial conditions. Recent studies are still demonstrating the benefits of LVG for the healing of fractures (47–50).

While LVG is still being utilized to some extent for a variety of effects, modern electronics have provided many more comfortable, more effective, and less dangerous modalities for treatment of the same conditions. LVG should only be administered with a

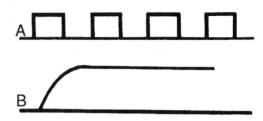

Figure 13.4. Low voltage galvanic current. **A,** *Interrupted.* The current may be interrupted manually or mechanically. A positive current is illustrated here. **B,** *Continuous.* The current is turned up to the desired level and remains at that level.

healthy respect for its ability to burn or damage tissue. If the desired effect can be accomplished with a safer modality, it is to the benefit of the patient that the safer modality be used.

Action

Interrupted LVG

When the LVG current is interrupted, either manually or mechanically (Fig. 13.4A), a twitch contraction of muscle fibers occurs at the "make" and the "break" of the current, with the "make" contraction usually being the stronger of the two. This LVG current is particularly useful for the stimulation of a denervated muscle, as an alternating current changes the direction of ion flow too quickly for stimulation of actual muscle fibers, and the pulsing direct current of high-voltage therapy is on for too short a time to stimulate muscle fiber.

Continuous LVG

Medical Galvanism. When a continuous LVG current is applied to the skin (Fig. 13.4B), chemical changes occur in the superficial tissues as a result of the interaction of sodium chloride (NaCl or table salt) and water (H_2O). At the cathode, or negative pole, the positively charged sodium ions from sodium chloride are attracted and combine with hydroxide ions from water to create sodium hydroxide (NaOH), a caustic soda, which tends to soften or liquify tissue. At the anode, or positive pole, the negatively charged chloride ions combine with hydrogen ions from water to create hydrochloric acid (HCl), which tends to harden or toughen tissue. The effects occurring at the two poles are summarized in Table 13.1.

Iontophoresis. When the solution of a soluble salt is placed under one of the galvanic electrodes, the polarity of the electrode will repel the ion of the same polarity, driving that ion away from the electrode and into the tissues. A number of different ions have been shown to be clinically useful in the treatment of various conditions, although sound physiological explanations for their actions are sometimes difficult to acquire. Some substances that have been used for their therapeutic effect are listed in Table 13.2.

Table 13.1 Effects of Low-Voltage Galvanism at the Positive and Negative Poles

Effects at the Positive Pole	Effects at the Negative Pole
Attracts oxygen	Attracts hydrogen
Attracts acids	Attracts alkalines
Dehydrates or hardens tissues	Liquefies or softens tissues
Vasoconstricts	Vasodilates
Causes ischemia	Creates hyperemia
Stops bleeding	Increases bleeding
More germicidal	Less germicidal
Sedating	Stimulating
Corrodes metals by oxidation	Does not corrode metal
Relieves pain in acute conditions by reduction of congestion	Relieves pain in chronic conditions by softening tissues and increasing circulation

Surgical Galvanism. LVG can be used for the surgical destruction of hair follicles, cysts, and hemorrhoids. The Keesey treatment, using negative LVG to reduce internal hemorrhoids, is the only form of surgical LVG used by the chiropractor.

Effects

Interrupted LVG

Twitch contraction of muscle.

Continuous LVG

Chemical changes that occur at the positive and negative electrodes (medical galvanism).
Therapeutic effects (e.g., fungicidal, antibacterial, analgesic) produced by various ions (iontophoresis).
Destruction of tissue (surgical galvanism).

Indications

Stimulation of denervated muscles (interrupted galvanism).
Stimulation of weak and/or atrophied muscles, when low-frequency alternating current is not effective (interrupted galvanism).
When the polar effects are desired (continous galvanism, see Table 13.1).
When medicinal ions are to be introduced into the tissues (iontophoresis, see Table 13.2).

Surgical galvanism (e.g., hair removal (positive pole), cyst removal (positive pole), hemorrhoids (negative pole)).

Contraindications

Malignancy;
Hemorrhage;
Infection;
Through the heart;
Through the brain;
Through the eye;
Where the polar effects are not desired;
Insensitivity;
Over recent scar tissue;
Over superficial metallic implants.

Application

1. Remove all metal from the treatment area.
2. Set all dials to zero.
3. Soak pads thoroughly.
4. Set the polarity desired at the active pad.
5. Place the smaller active pad over the area being treated. Place the larger dispersive pad on a large body part, preferably along the same fascial plane and close to the area being treated. Secure pads firmly with straps, weights, or body weight (Fig. 13.5A). A probe may be used instead of the active pad for stimulation of small muscles (Fig. 13.5B).
6. Set mode (if applicable):

Table 13.2 Some Common Substances Used for Iontophoresis

Substance	Ion Utilized	Polarity	Description
Copper sulfate	Copper	+	Fungicidal; used for fungus
Magnesium sulfate	Magnesium	+	Antiinflammatory, draws fluid "like a poultice"; used for adhesion, bursitis, edema, sprains
Mecholyl (acetyl-β-methyl choline chloride)	Choline	+	Vasoactive substance that stimulates parasympathetics and dilates peripheral vascular system at arteriole level
Methyl salicylate	Salicylate	−	Analgesic, antipyretic, antiarthritic; used for chronic neuritis, arthritis, boils, bursitis
Potassium iodide	Iodine	−	Antiinfective; used for adhesions, bursitis, Dupuytren's contracture, facial paralysis, sprains, calcific tendinitis, Pellegrini-Stieda disease
Silver nitrate	Silver	+	Caustic, fungicidal; used for fungus
Sodium Chloride	Chlorine	−	Mildly caustic, softens & loosens scars; used for bruises & scars
Sodium salicylate	Salicylate	−	See methyl salicylate
Zinc sulfate	Zinc	+	Caustic ion useful for its germicidal & astringent effects; used for sinusitis, otitis media, abscess

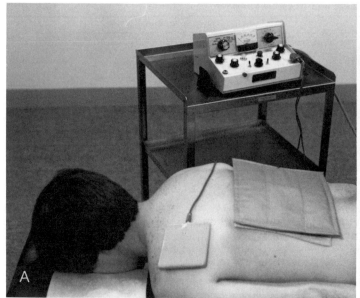

Figure 13.5. The application of low-voltage galvanism. **A,** A small, active pad is used with a larger, dispersive pad. (Securing straps are left out for the purposes of this illustration.) **B,** A probe may be used for stimulation of small muscles. A small pad may be used as the dispersive pad.

Continuous: for medical galvanism and iontophoresis.

Interrupted: for muscle stimulation.
7. Turn the rheostat up slowly to patient tolerance. Maximum current is 1 mA/cm² of active pad.
8. Treat for the desired time (see "Treatment Duration").
9. Turn rheostat to zero before removing pads.

Treatment Duration

For muscle stimulation: stimulate until muscle begins to fatigue. Treatment should be repeated several times a day for the maintenance of muscle tone.

For medical galvanism and iontophoresis: the first treatment should be no longer than 3 to 4 min. For subsequent treatments, increase time slowly up to a maximum of 10 minutes. Check carefully for signs of burning.

HIGH-VOLTAGE THERAPY

Definition

High-voltage therapy: a unidirectional, pulsed current of up to 500 V force and average current of 1.0–1.5 mA. The wave form most commonly used is a twin-peaked pulse with a quick rise to peak and a slower decay (Fig. 13.6). Pulse duration is generally between 20 and 200 microsec (51).

Introduction

High-voltage therapy (HVT) was developed in the 1970s and has since come into popular clinical use.

The traditional term "high-voltage galvanism" is somewhat misleading, as clinicians tend to confuse and/or equate the effects of HVT with low-voltage galvanism (LVG). Because HVT utilizes a pulsed monophasic current of short duration, high peak voltage, and long interpulse interval, the chemical effects of LVG simply do not occur to any great extent (52), making medical galvanism and iontophoresis impossible. For this reason the author has chosen to use the term "high-voltage therapy" rather than "high-voltage galvanism."

Manufacturers of the HVT equipment offer guidelines for the choice of polarity in particular situations, but research has not yet substantiated these guidelines. Polarity appears relatively unimportant in many circumstances.

In contrast to LVG, HVT offers a more comfortable current that is safer to use and more universal in its application. Because of its high peak current, low average current, and short pulse duration, penetration is deeper, with less sensory disturbance and less heat production (51).

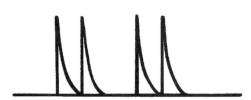

Figure 13.6. High-voltage current is a twin-peaked, monophasic current with a quick rise and slower decay.

Mechanism of Action

Sensory Nerve Stimulation

Because of the short pulse duration, large, myelinated, alpha sensory fibers are stimulated with minimum stimulation of small, C-type pain fibers (51, 53).

Motor Nerve Stimulation

As intensity is increased beyond initial sensory stimulation, motor nerve fibers are stimulated. Superficial, small muscles are stimulated easily, but a high peak current is required to stimulate deeper, larger muscles. In fact, full contraction of the largest muscles cannot always be achieved, even with maximum tolerable intensity.

Because of the short pulse duration, HVT is not able to stimulate muscle fibers directly, and therefore is not useful for the stimulation of denervated muscles.

Effects

Analgesia

Theories for the pain-relief effect of HVT include the following:

Endogenous discharge of opiate substances occurs with somatic stimulation. Low-frequency stimulation (2–5 pulses per second) appears to stimulate endorphins for the relief of chronic pain, whereas higher frequency stimulation (50–120 pps) apparently stimulates serotonin and other nonendorphin analgesics for acute pain relief (51, 54, 55).

Direct blocking of action potential propagation has been demonstrated in the laboratory but not clinically (56).

The classic gate-control theory of pain postulates that stimulation of the larger, myelinated, sensory fibers will inhibit the conduction of the smaller, unmyelinated, pain fibers (56).

Edema Absorption

Both acute and chronic nonsystemic edema can be well controlled with the application of HVT. With chronic edema, the electrical stimulation of muscle contraction assists the pumping action of the muscles, aiding lymphatic absorption of exudates. With acute edema, where muscle contraction may produce increased inflammation, sensory stimulation has been shown to be adequate for edema reduction. It is postulated that creation of an electrical potential field in the tissues may enhance lymphatic absorption (56).

Muscle Contraction

Intermittent HVT, in conjunction with voluntary muscle contraction, enhances muscle reeducation in cases of disuse atrophy, whether the atrophy results from an orthopaedic cause or from a central nervous system lesion (57). The combination of HVT and voluntary contraction increases muscle strength more effectively than voluntary contraction alone (58).

HVT can also be used to fatigue muscles for the relief of pain and muscle spasm. Alon states that continuous stimulation at a high pulse rate (100–200 pps) will decrease muscle contraction to 20–30% of its maximum within a 2 to 3 minute period (56). Rosenblueth and Luco (as cited by Wakim) found that stimulation at 60 pps progressively reduced muscle tension until it ceased completely after about an hour (59).

Tissue Regeneration

Healing of dermal and subdermal ulcers can be hastened by the application of HVT (60–62). The change in the electrical charge of the wound by HVT appears to enhance the healing process. Katzberg has demonstrated artifical induction of reorientation of the fibrin network with weak galvanic currents (63). Improved microcirculation and the bactericidal effect of HVT may also contribute to the healing process.

It is not clear whether positive or negative polarity is more beneficial, but it does appear that a monophasic current must be used rather than a biphasic one (56, 64). One author suggests alternating the polarity each week of treatment (62). Also suggested is using the negative pole initially and the positive pole after bacterial growth has been arrested.

Increased Peripheral Circulation

Although HVT does not affect the peripheral blood flow of normal individuals (65), it does improve impaired circulation in such disease processes as Volkmann's ischemia, reflex sympathetic dystrophy, venous insufficiency, and peripheral arterial occlusive disease. The theories supporting this effect include:

Direct sympathetic activation;
Somatic sympathetic reflex;
Discharge of neuropeptides such as ACTH and endorphins (at a pulse rate of 2 pps) which cause vasodilation of the microcirculation;
Muscle pumping enhancing venous return (at pulse rates of less than 10 pps);
Muscle metabolites produced by muscle contraction stimulating blood supply to remove metabolites (56).

Indications

Acute and Chronic

Musculoskeletal conditions, soft tissue injuries;
Neurogenic conditions: neuritis, radiculitis, neuralgia, sciatica;
Arthritic conditions;
Nonsystemic edema;
Muscle spasm;
Muscle reeducation;

Open wounds: ulcer, burns, decubiti;
Peripheral circulatory disturbances: Volkmann's ischemia, reflex sympathetic dystrophy, venous insufficiency, peripheral arterial occlusive disease;
Trigger point therapy.

Contraindications

Malignancy;
Patient with a pacemaker;
Pregnancy.

Application

1. Inspect part and remove metal from treatment area.
2. Set all intensity controls to zero.
3. Soak pads thoroughly.
4. Set the polarity desired at the active pad or pads. Remember that all treating pads are of the same polarity and the dispersive pad is of the opposite polarity.
5. Set the pulse rate desired:
   Low pulse rate (2–5 pps), sensory stimulation only, for long-lasting analgesia,
   High pulse rate (80–120 pps), sensory stimulation only, for immediate analgesia (51),
   Middle pulse rate (40–60 pps), sensory and muscle stimulation, for tetany without fatigue,
   High pulse rate (80–120 pps), sensory and muscle stimulation, for tetany with fatigue;
6. Choose continuous or alternating current:
   Continuous: all treating pads operate continuously; for edema reduction, pain control, or tissue regeneration.
   Alternating: current alternates between two or four treating pads; for muscle fatigue or re-education.
7. Choose the appropriate number of active pads (one or two on some units, one to four on others) and apply firmly to the part being treated. The dispersive pad should be larger than the treating pads and should be placed firmly on a muscular part of the body (preferably the back or thigh). For superficial treatments, it should be placed as close to the treating area as possible and a long the same fascial plane (Fig 13.7). For deeper treatments, it should be placed farther away and/or on the opposite side of the body.
8. Turn timer on to the desired time period, usually 5–20 minutes.
9. Turn intensity up gradually to patient tolerance or until the desired effect is achieved within patient tolerance. For acute pain, the intensity should not be higher than the minimal sensory level. Turn the intensity down before moving pads or changing polarity or pulse rate.

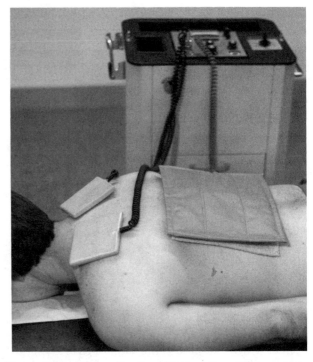

Figure 13.7. The application of high-voltage therapy. One to four active pads may be used. Illustrated here are two small active pads and a large dispersive pad. (Securing straps have been left off for the purposes of this illustration.)

10. If applicable, adjust the balance control so that the stimulation at the treating pads feels balanced to the patient.
11. At the end of treatment, return the intensity to zero and remove pads.

If treating trigger points, acupuncture points, or motor points, use the procedure above except use a probe instead of active pads. Turn the intensity to the level of mild sensory stimulation and probe the area to locate the exact point to be stimulated. Continue to increase the intensity until the desired effect is achieved. Trigger points will usually become less painful in 15–30 sec. Motor points are stimulated in an interrupted manner until fatigue is noticeable.

LOW FREQUENCY ALTERNATING CURRENTS

Definitions

Hertz (Hz): cycles per second.
Low frequency alternating current: a current in which the direction of electron flow changes at a rate between 1 and 2000 Hz.
Sine wave: a low frequency alternating current that takes the shape of a sine curve.
Faradic current: a low frequency alternating current with 2 unequal phases.

Introduction

The use of electrical stimulation dates back to 2750 BC, when the current from electric fish was used to treat a variety of ailments including headaches. The first alternating current was introduced by DuBois-Reymond in 1848 in the form of the induction coil stimulator. Unlike galvanic current, the faradic current produced by the induction coil was able to cause tetany of an innervated muscle and stimulate a wide variety of excitable tissues. Interest in this new current led to treatment of many forms of disease, with either general faradism (i.e., full-body treatment) or local faradism.

While the faradic current had many beneficial stimulating effects, it could also cause undesirable side effects such as hysteria, nervous exhaustion, paralysis, and even death (46). When the dangers of faradism were realized, its popularity waned, although faradism continued to be used for respiratory resuscitation. The newer low frequency alternating currents (LFACs), developed since World War II, have become popular because of their increase in patient comfort and the continued need for electrical stimulation of atrophied muscle, especially for patients with central nervous system lesions (66).

Mechanism of Action

Action Potential

The normal resting membrane potential is between 70 and 100 mV. Excitation of a nerve by electrical stimulation is caused by a rapid change in the membrane potential of the nerve. Electrical stimulation causes a momentarily increased permeability to sodium, which lowers the membrane potential of the cell to 25 to 50 mV for about 1 msec. Adequate intensity and duration of stimulation are necessary for the creation of the action potential. The action potential continues along the nerve fiber as a result of increased permeability of neighboring regions to sodium ions until the resting potential is reestablished by the sodium pump.

Factors that determine whether the current is sufficient to create an action potential include:

Impedance of the tissue: Bone and fat have higher impedance than do muscle and blood, requiring greater current flow.

Size and placement of electrodes: Small, closely spaced electrodes require less current than larger, more widely spaced electrodes. However, the farther apart the electrodes, the deeper the stimulation.

Current intensity: As the intensity is increased, smaller diameter and deeper nerve fibers are stimulated.

Pulse width: The wider the pulse ("on time"), the stronger the muscle contraction. Wider pulse widths are necessary to cause full contraction of large muscle groups such as gluteals and quadriceps.

Pulse rise time: A slow rise time allows accommodation, and if it is too slow, no excitation will occur.

Pulse rate: Slow pulse rates allow repolarization of the membrane between each stimulus, thus creating a twitch contraction. Higher pulse rates (usually 30–50 Hz) cause summation of contractions and tetany of the muscle. As the pulse rate is increased from the tetany level, the muscle will fatigue more quickly (67).

Waveform: Devices that generate many waveforms have been developed by different manufacturers, often under the assumption that the new waveform will prove superior to the others. To date, no single waveform has been shown to be more effective than the others if the aforementioned factors have been considered. Common waveforms (Fig. 13.8) include:
   1. Sine wave: a smooth, symmetrical current
   2. Faradic: a sharply rising, asymmetrical current
   3. Square wave: a symmetrical current with abrupt rise and abrupt fall. Some of the newer units being developed use the square wave because the pulse width can be varied, thus allowing for maximal contraction of large muscle groups.
   4. Burst modulation: Some newer units use a medium-frequency current that significantly reduces skin resistance, and they burst the pulses at a low frequency to cause the desired nerve excitation.

Effects

Contraction of innervated muscle, by stimulation of the nerve that innervates that muscle. It has been shown that electrical stimulation (with or without isometric exercises) increases muscle strength more than no electrical stimulation or exercise (68, 69) (Selkowitz DM: Thesis, SUNY at Buffalo).

Contraction of smooth muscle.

Pain relief. The mechanism of pain relief is not fully understood. Possible theories include stimulation of large, myelinated sensory fibers or the release of endorphins and enkephalins (see "TENS: Mechanism of Action").

Edema reduction. This effect probably occurs as a result of the creation of an electrical field in the lymphatic system and the pumping action of the muscles.

Indications

Stimulation of weak and/or atrophied muscles;
Stimulation of smooth muscle;
Treatment of hysterical paralysis;
Treatment of upper motor neuron lesions in which the lower motor neuron is intact;

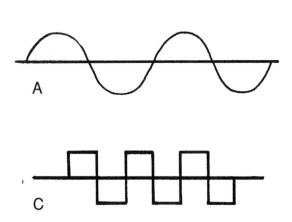

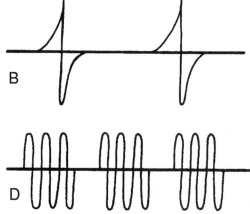

Figure 13.8. Low frequency alternating currents. **A,** Sine wave. **B,** Faradic current (may vary in its appearance). **C,** Square wave. **D,** Burst modulated.

Pain;
Swelling, nonsystemic.

Contraindications

Through the brain;
Through the heart;
Through the eye;
Over bony prominences;
Where muscle contraction is not desired; (e.g., in some cases of fracture, dislocation, osteoporosis, rickets, osteomalacia, Pott's disease);
Skin lesions;
Infection;
Thrombosis;
Active tuberculosis;
Malignancy;
Insensitive area;
Unreliable patient;
Superficial metal.

Application

1. Remove all metal from the treatment area.
2. Set all dials to zero.
3. Soak pads thoroughly and place firmly on treating parts; use straps, hot packs, cold packs, or the patient's weight. Two or four pads may be used. If unequal-sized pads are used, the smaller pad will produce a greater effect. A probe may be used for specific stimulation of motor points (consult a motor point chart for the approximate location of motor points).
4. Set mode (if applicable) to:
   a. Pulse: if a gentle treatment is desired, to avoid further trauma or to disperse fluid (Fig. 13.9A).
   b. Surge: if a series of muscle contractions is desired (e.g., for muscle reeducation) (Fig. 13.9B).
   c. Tetanize: if a tetanic contraction is desired to fatigue the muscle (e.g., for a muscle spasm or muscle tension) (Fig. 14.9C).

5. Choose the pulse width, "on ramp" time, and/or "off ramp" time (if applicable). A wider pulse width is less comfortable but allows for contraction of larger muscle groups. A slower on or off ramp time allows for slower, more comfortable contraction or relaxation of the muscle.
6. Turn the timer on (see "Treatment Duration").
7. Increase the intensity slowly to patient tolerance or until the desired muscle contraction is achieved.
8. After treatment, return all dials to zero and remove pads.

Treatment Duration

Treatment time depends on the effect desired and the integrity of the muscle being stimulated. If reeducation of a weak muscle is desired, the muscle should only be exercised until fatigue begins. The muscle should not be exercised to complete fatigue. However, if electrical stimulation is being used to

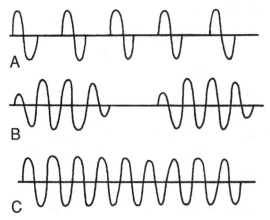

Figure 13.9. Modes possible on many low frequency alternating current units. **A,** Pulse: causes a twitch contraction. **B,** Surge: causes full contraction and relaxation. **C,** Tetanize: Causes a tetanic contraction without relaxation.

fatigue a muscle in spasm, treatment time should be adequate to insure fatigue, usually 10–20 min.

Time on and time off are also factors to be considered. Dr. Kots of the Soviet Union has suggested the following times:

To increase circulation: 2 sec on, 2 sec off;
To reduce spasm and pain: 12 sec on, 8 sec off;
For strength, endurance, and velocity: 10 sec on, 50 sec off.

(Lecture notes, Y.M. Kots, Canadian-Soviet Exchange Symposium on Electrostimulation of Skeletal Muscles, Concordia University, December 6–15, 1977.)

TRANSCUTANEOUS ELECTRICAL NERVE STIMULATION

Introduction

Transcutaneous electrical nerve stimulation (TENS) for the relief of chronic pain was first described in the first century AD when Scribonius Largus applied electrical torpedo fish to the head of a patient suffering from headaches, utilizing the electrical current generated by the fish. Electrical stimulation reached its peak popularity in the 19th century when manually operated stimulators were reported to treat many forms of disease. Overzealous claims for its abilities led to its wane in popularity (70). Interest was renewed in 1965 when Melzack and Wall published their "gate-control theory" that proposed an explanation for the use of electrical stimulation for the relief of pain (71).

Since 1965, the gate-control theory has been disputed, and new theories for the mechanism of pain have been suggested. However, the utilization of electrical stimulation has not diminished but rather has increased as a result of increased clinical effectiveness. In fact, where TENS was originally used almost exclusively for the relief of chronic pain, its efficacy is now being explored for the relief of acute pain. Many health practitioners are finding TENS to be an effective, safe, noninvasive, and cost-effective method of treating acute, chronic, and psychogenic pain of innumerable origins (72).

Technically, the term TENS should apply to any form of electrical stimulation that is applied via surface electrodes. However, the term is generally reserved for the small portable stimulators that can be conveniently attached to the belt or clothing and used for various time periods for the relief of pain (Fig. 13.10).

Mechanism of Action

In spite of the abundance of research being devoted to the mechanism of pain, no single theory prevails. Until pain is understood, the relief of pain remains equally unclear. Therefore, the mechanism of action of TENS can only be explained in terms of current theories of the mechanism of pain.

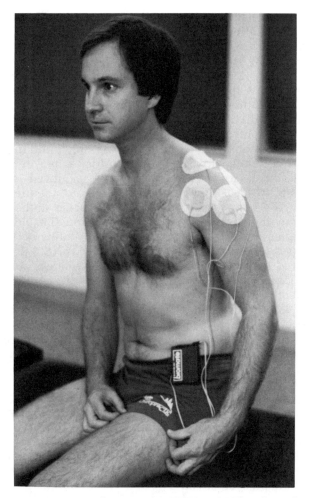

Figure 13.10. Application of a TENS unit. The electrodes here are attached with round adhesive patches. The unit is clipped to the waistband.

Melzack and Wall's gate-control theory, while not perfect, has not been replaced in the 20 years since its origin. According to this theory, activity in large, myelinated sensory nerve fibers stimulates interneuronal activity of the substantia gelatinosa of the dorsal horn of the spinal cord, causing presynaptic inhibitory effects on the small nociceptive (pain) fibers. Therefore, electrical stimulation of the large sensory fibers in effect "closes the gate" to the small pain fibers, blocking the perception of pain in the brain. Wall and Sweet showed that electrical stimulation of large sensory fibers did indeed elevate the pain threshold. However, subsequent research has shown that stimulation of large sensory fibers does not result in presynaptic effects of polarity opposite that of stimulation of small pain fibers, thus refuting the basic premises of Melzack and Wall's theory (73).

Livingston, in 1943, and Melzack, in 1973, proposed that prolonged pathological pain may cause self-exciting neuron chains or loops that act as a memory-like process and that brief intense stimulation with TENS can interrupt that process, relieving pain and allowing more normal neural activity long after the stimulation has ceased (74, 75).

In 1973, Andersson and associates found that low frequency (2 Hz) electrical stimulation of acupuncture points increased the pain threshold in volunteers by 2 to 4 times (76). Hypothesizing that acupuncture-like TENS causes the endogenous release of endorphins (which are morphine-like, pain-relieving substances), Sjolund and Eriksson found that injections of naloxone hydrochloride, a morphine antagonist, reversed the analgesia achieved by TENS, whereas the injection of saline did not affect the TENS analgesia (77). Later, the same authors found that acupuncture-like stimulation (i.e., low frequency (2 Hz), high-intensity pulse trains of 18 pulses per train at 70 Hz, termed "low TENS") produced endorphin-mediated analgesia, whereas conventional TENS (termed "high TENS") did not (78). Therefore, it is suggested that TENS, at least "low TENS," produces endogenous endorphins for pain relief (79).

O'Brien and associates could find no evidence that TENS, at either 2 Hz or 80 Hz, altered the experimental pain threshold or plasma β-endorphin levels (80). This group and others imply that the effect of TENS may be largely placebo (81, 82).

To summarize, the analgesic action of TENS may be mediated by: (a) stimulation of large sensory fibers (the gate-control theory), (b) interruption of a self-perpetuating, memory-like loop or chain of neural activity, (c) release of endogenous endorphins, or (d) the placebo effect.

Effect

In brief, the primary effect of TENS is the relief of pain. The degree of effectiveness of TENS is still under debate. While some studies show significant analgesia from TENS (83), others indicate that TENS may have no greater effect than the placebo effect (80, 84). It is generally agreed, however, that because of its safe and noninvasive nature, TENS should be utilized before more invasive and potentially harmful methods of pain relief are considered.

Indications

Chronic Pain

Pain relief has been demonstrated in patients with rheumatoid arthritis (85, 86), chronic low back pain syndrome, chronic cervical syndrome, postherpetic neuralgia, and other chronic pain conditions (87–90). Success rates vary from the approximately 30% expected from a placebo treatment to as high as 75% (88, 91–94).

It is difficult to predict who will respond favorably to TENS. One study found no significant correlation between the success rate with TENS and preexisting physical or social factors except that the success rate was higher for retired patients than for those unemployed or holding blue-collar jobs. TENS

appears to be slightly less successful in patients with pain of greater than 1 year duration, patients with a history of multiple surgeries, those using tranquilizers, and those not working because of pain (95).

One should keep in mind that the use of TENS may result in obliteration of the pain signals that normally warn patients when they are overstressing the injured area. TENS should not be used by patients who will ignore other cues of overwork and will cause further injury to themselves. Patient education is critical in this situation.

Postoperative, Obstetric, and Other Acute Pain

TENS is now being utilized to shorten rehabilitation time, reduce pain medication needs, and hasten mobilization time postoperatively and after an acute injury. Success rates reported are as variable as those for chronic pain (96–100). One study of postoperative patients reports similar pain relief with functional and sham TENS, while both groups showed superior relief to the drug-administered group (96). Another study reported 80% of the postoperative patients reported pain reduction (97). Use of TENS during delivery had an 88% rate of moderate to very good pain relief in one study (98).

Intractable Pain

TENS can provide adequate relief of pain secondary to malignancy. One study reported an initial 65% success rate, which declined to 33% within 3 months, indicating that long-term relief is less likely than short-term relief. Results were best with trunk and extremity pain and worst with pelvic and perineal pain (101). Success rates are high enough to warrant trial of TENS for intractable pain.

Rehabilitation

The use of TENS for the reduction of pain during rehabilitation can increase performance and shorten hospital stay time (102). In at least one case, TENS allowed reversal of a Sudeck's atrophy by controlling pain, thereby allowing weight acceptance on the involved extremity (103). Care must be taken to not allow the TENS to obliterate pain to the extent that the patient loses protective cues and overstresses the part being rehabilitated. Use of TENS prior to and after exercise may alleviate this potential hazard.

Contraindications

Cardiac pacemaker;
Carotid nerve stimulation;
Laryngeal stimulation (may occlude airway);
During pregnancy (91, 104).

Application

Units Available

TENS units are being manufactured with a variety of features and waveforms. Knowledge of several

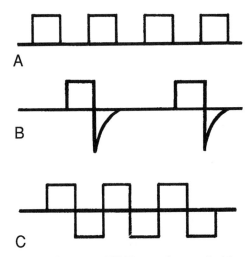

Figure 13.11. Common TENS waveforms. **A**, Monophasic rectangular. **B**, Modified rectangular asymmetrical biphasic. **C**, Symmetrical biphasic rectangular.

different TENS units is necessary before an intelligent choice can be made.

Common waveforms include the monophasic rectangular, modified rectangular asymmetrical biphasic, and symmetrical biphasic rectangular types (Fig. 13.11). Because the most effective waveform has not yet been established, comparison of pain relief with several units of different waveforms is appropriate (104).

Maximum amplitude is an important feature of a TENS unit. In a study of eight different TENS units, maximum amplitudes ranged from 30 to 120 mA (105). The lower maximum amplitudes may not be adequate for the strong stimulation that some clinicians feel is necessary for prolonged pain relief (105).

Minimum and maximum frequencies are also important to note. Units generally range from about 10–100 Hz with wide variation on either end. Most clinicians find good pain relief with a high frequency, low intensity stimulation of approximately 80–100 Hz, termed "high TENS" (106). However, Eriksson and associates found that 30% of the patients in a study of 123 patients had to use "low TENS" to achieve useful analgesia (i.e., a low frequency, high intensity stimulation delivered in pulse trains of about 8 70 Hz pulses per train and 1 to 4 trains per sec) (107). Mannheimer and Carlsson found no significant difference between the analgesic effect of low TENS and high TENS (85). The capability for low TENS is not available on all TENS units.

Pulse widths generally range from 10 to 350 microsec, again with wide variation. The most desirable pulse width demonstrates the widest separation of amplitudes between sensory detection threshold and initial motor response. Of the pulse widths tested thus far, the shortest pulse width, 10 microsec, has the widest separation. However, shorter pulse widths have not been tested (105).

Other features of TENS units to be considered include size, number of channels and leads available, ease of operation, and method of recharging (i.e., disposable batteries, rechargable batteries, or rechargable unit). One should be leery of inexpensive TENS units that are limited in their capabilities. Some TENS units are even considered "disposable" (i.e., they are not rechargable in any manner).

Electrode Choice and Placement

Many varieties of electrodes have been developed for use with TENS. The most popular electrodes are a soft, carbonized, silicone rubber and are applied with a thin layer of electrode gel and tape.

The most significant complication of TENS is local skin rashes produced by the conduction gel or tape. Several other electrodes have been developed to reduce this complaint, including the karaya pad, which comes from the karaya gum tree. The karaya pad is moistened and placed between the skin and electrode, eliminating the need for gel or tape. The pad is reusable, but still less cost-effective than gel and tape (91).

Electrode placement is one of the most critical factors for the success of TENS, yet guidelines for electrode placement are vague (108). Suggestions include:

Directly over or around the painful site;
Over trigger points;
Over acupuncture points;
Within a specific dermatome;
At the site of the corresponding nerve root;
Along the pathway of a peripheral nerve.

One author suggests attaching one electrode to the patient and having the other in the clinician's hand. The clinician then uses an index finger and a mild current to locate the pathway of the nerve (109).

A small area may be adequately treated with a single-channel, dual-lead unit, whereas most conditions will respond more effectively with a dual-channel, four-lead unit. With a dual-channel unit, placement of at least one electrode contralaterally and/or crossing channels may prove more effective (87, 110).

In any case, several electrode placements should be tried before TENS is abandoned as being ineffective.

Treatment Duration

There is no contraindication to 24 hour use of "high TENS." "Low TENS," however, should be used only 30–40 min at a time, as "low TENS" causes muscle contraction and may cause soreness if used for longer periods (111). Electrodes should be removed every day or two to clean the skin and inspect the area.

In cases of acute and chronic pain, dependency on TENS may become a problem. Encourage patients to use the TENS as little as is needed for adequate pain relief and to decrease "on" time as they are able. Keeping a daily log of "on" time and relief time may help them keep track of these factors so that they may be systematically "weaned" from the unit. They may work toward using the unit for only short periods of time in the morning and evening or abandoning it completely. The problem of dependency is less critical for patients with intractable pain (e.g., secondary to malignancy).

General Considerations

It cannot be overemphasized that patient education and cooperation are essential for the success of TENS. Patients must have a complete understanding of the purpose and operation of TENS, as well as the confidence that the unit will help them. This of course necessitates complete understanding and confidence on the part of the clinician. If the clinician does not have that knowledge and confidence, referral to a TENS specialist would be prudent.

MICROAMPERAGE NEURAL STIMULATION

Definition

Microamperage neural stimulation: electrical stimulation, either biphasic or monophasic, with peak pulse current to 1000 microamps.

Introduction

Microamperage neural stimulation (MNS) is among the newest and least well researched modalities in physiotherapy. The current is being utilized by a variety of techniques for analgesia and tissue healing. The techniques include stimulation of acupuncture points, auricular points, Golgi tendon organs, and more generalized stimulation of tissue in need of repair. Discussion here will be limited to the use of MNS for tissue repair. The use of MNS for the stimulation of acupuncture points will be discussed in the section on meridian therapy.

Mechanism of Action

Enhancement of Tissue Repair

It appears that stimulation of damaged tissue with small amounts of electrical current can have a significant healing effect on the tissue. When nucleated red blood cells are involved in bone repair, they lose their normal elliptical shape and become more spherical (i.e., more embryonic-like) in a process termed "dedifferentiation" (112). Further experimentation has shown that stimulation of cells with various direct or alternating currents produces these morphological changes in the cells and that the cells exhibit increased RNA and protein synthesis immediately after stimulation (113, 114), initiating the repair process. Clinically, it appears that currents in the range of 10–1000 microamps are adequate to stimulate this dedifferentiation and healing process.

Effects

Analgesia (115);
Antiinflammatory;
Tissue healing.

Indications

Pain;
Tissue healing, including decubitus ulcers.

Several microamperage stimulators are being used for the treatment of acute and chronic sports injuries because of their analgesic, antiinflammatory, and healing properties (116).

Contraindications

Demand-type cardiac pacemakers;
Over the carotid sinus;
Over the eyeball or eyelid;
Safety and effectiveness of MNS has not been established in pregnancy; avoid the stimulation of any area that might affect the pregnancy.

Application

Pads and/or probes may be used, depending upon the area being treated and the degree of treatment specificity desired.

Two or four pads may be placed around the lesion and stimulated for a desired length of time, usually 10–60 minutes, as an unattended treatment. If four pads are used on two different frequency settings, the two sets of pads may be crisscrossed to create a sort of interferential treatment. For example, if a 0.3 Hz current is crossed with a 0.9 Hz current, the tissues will receive treatment at those frequencies, as well as at their difference and their summation (i.e., 0.6 Hz and 1.2 Hz).

Two probes may be utilized as an attended treatment to increase the specificity of treatment area. Points are chosen on either side of the lesion and stimulated for approximately 30 sec. Adjacent points are then stimulated until the lesion has been circumscribed. Acute conditions should be stimulated in a counterclockwise direction and/or away from the midline, while chronic conditions should be stimulated in a clockwise direction and/or toward the midline (Fig. 13.12) (Seminar notes, Wing's Electro-point Systems). A longitudinal muscle or treatment area should be stimulated in a similar fashion along the length of the muscle.

Another treatment option is placing a single pad on the patient near the lesion and a second pad on the hand or arm of the clinician. In this manner, the clinician completes the electrical circuit, and the clinician's hand becomes the second treatment pad during palpation or massage of the affected area.

Treating frequencies and intensities will not be suggested here as the optimum parameters have yet to be established.

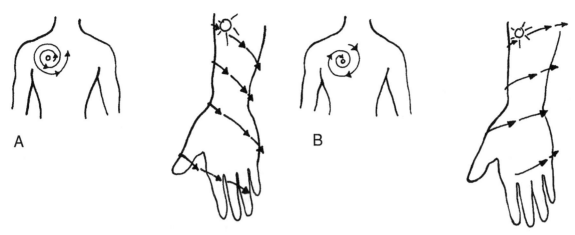

Figure 13.12. Treatment patterns with microamperage neural stimulation. **A**, For *acute conditions*, treatment is performed in a counter-clockwise and proximal-to-distal manner. **B**, For *chronic conditions*, treatment is performed in a clockwise and distal-to-proximal manner.

MERIDIAN THERAPY

Definitions

Acupuncture: the treatment of disease by the insertion of fine needles into specific points (i.e., acupuncture points), from Latin *acu* meaning needles and *punctura* meaning to pierce or puncture.

Electroacupuncture: the treatment of the acupuncture points using an electrical current as the stimulus.

Meridians: the 12 channels of energy of the body, according to Chinese medicine. Stimulation of any acupuncture point along the meridian will change the energy of that meridian.

Introduction

Acupuncture has been successfully practiced in China for thousands of years for the treatment of a great variety of symptoms and disease processes. According to Chinese medicine, acupuncture is used to affect the "Chi," or life force, of the human body. Stimulation of the acupuncture points can strengthen or weaken the meridians, thereby balancing the energy of the meridians and allowing energy to flow optimally.

The 14th century Europeans coined the term "acupuncture." However, a number of techniques have been used historically to stimulate acupuncture points including pressure, heat, moxa, steel bars, and of course needles. Therefore, the term "meridian therapy" (MT) probably more accurately describes the discipline that we have come to know as acupuncture.

In 1953, Dr. Yoshio Nakatani developed a sensitive ohmmeter that could be used to detect acupuncture points on the skin's surface. This discovery has altered many clinicians' practice of MT. Acupuncture points can now be located precisely with the aid of electronics and stimulated electrically with the same probe.

A variety of techniques based on MT remain in use today. Several are summarized here. A more complete discussion of the theory and practice of MT has been presented by Jaskoviak and Schafer (1).

In the United States, the Food and Drug Administration (FDA) regulates the manufacturing of all medical devices. Medical devices for electroacupuncture have not been shown to be safe and effective and therefore are not approved for that use (117). It is important to check any individual device for the particular uses that have been approved by the FDA (conversation with Dave Chesney, supervisor, Food and Drug Administration, Portland, OR, July 30, 1986).

Mechanism of Action

Electronic Stimulation of Acupuncture Points

Clinicians are finding that many acupuncture points can be located and stimulated by electrical currents, including microamperage and milliamperage currents. Acupuncture points show increased electrical conductivity (118) and can therefore be located by the stimulator in the "search" mode. Once the point has been located, it can be stimulated by small amounts of either an alternating or a direct current.

Research done by Matsumoto and Hayes showed that the skin resistance of certain acupuncture points changed significantly after vagotomy in a rabbit, but that electrical stimulation minimized those changes and the resultant gastrointestinal dysfunction (119). Studies indicate that the analgesia produced by acupuncture point stimulation is much greater when small, nonmyelinated C-fibers are stimulated with brief, intense stimulation than when larger, myelinated A-fibers alone are stimulated (120, 121). This technique, referred to as "hyperstimulation analgesia," may possibly be explained by a central biasing mechanism in which input from the body projects to widespread parts of the spinal cord and brain, causing inhibition of pain transmission (75, 122).

Stimulation of Acupuncture Points by Other Means

Acupuncture points may be stimulated by any technique that is fairly specific and causes an adequate stimulus. Techniques commonly used include finger pressure, tapping with a probe, needles, and needles with an electrical current coursing through them.

Effects

The effects of MT can be quite varied, depending on its use by the clinician. Possibilities include:

Analgesia (115);
Anesthesia;
Antiinflammatory action;
Relief of disease symptoms;
Balancing of meridians, thereby balancing body energy;
Tissue healing.

Indications

A World Health Organization Interregional Seminar on Acupuncture, Moxibustion and Acupuncture Anaesthesia held in 1979 in Peking drew up a provisional list of diseases that lend themselves to acupuncture treatment.

This list is based on clinical experience, and not necessarily on controlled clinical research. The inclusion of specific diseases is not meant to indicate the extent of acupuncture's efficacy in treating the following conditions.

Upper respiratory tract
Acute sinusitis
Acute rhinitis
Common cold
Acute tonsillitis
Respiratory system
Acute bronchitis
Broncial asthma (most effective in children and in patients without complicating diseases)
Disorders of the eye
Acute conjunctivitis
Central retinitis
Myopia (in children)
Cataract (without complications)
Disorders of the mouth
Toothache
Postextraction pain
Gingivitis
Acute and chronic pharyngitis
Gastrointestinal disorders
Spasms of esophagus and cardia
Hiccough
Gastroptosis
Acute and chronic gastritis
Gastric hyperacidity

Chronic duodenal ulcer (pain relief)
Acute duodenal ulcer (without complications)
Acute and chronic colitis
Acute bacillary dysentery
Constipation
Diarrhea
Paralytic ileus
Neurological and musculoskeletal disorders
Headaches
Migraine
Trigeminal neuralgia
Facial palsy (early stage, i.e., within 3 to 6 months)
Pareses following a stroke
Peripheral neuropathies
Sequelae of poliomyelitis (early stage, i.e., within 6 months)
Ménière's disease
Neurogenic bladder dysfunction
Nocturnal enuresis
Intercostal neuralgia
Cervicobrachial syndrome
"Frozen shoulder"
"Tennis elbow"
Sciatica
Low back pain
Osteoarthritis (123)

Contraindications

Pregnancy (123);
Pacemaker patients (123);
Skin infections (123);
Tumor sites (123);
Through the heart;
Through the brain.

Application

Because of the variety of equipment being used and effects desired, techniques of application vary greatly.

Local Stimulation

A specific area of the body may be treated simply by palpating the area for unusually tender points and applying pressure to those points. Similar "hot spots" may also be located electronically and treated with either pressure or electrical stimulation.

"Cookbook" Stimulation of Acupuncture Points

Many books and charts contain listings of points that have been shown to be effective for the treatment of particular diseases or symptoms of diseases. The points are located by probe with the stimulator in the "search" mode (with the patient holding the ground electrode), then stimulated for approximately 30 seconds with electrical current (Fig. 13.13). Three to six points are generally stimulated in a treatment session. This technique may include stimulation of auricular points.

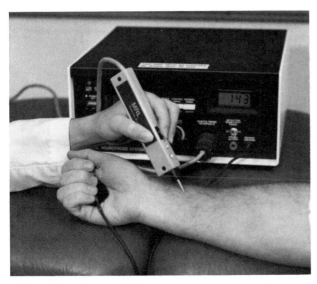

Figure 13.13. Stimulation of an acupuncture point with microamperage neural stimulation. The doctor locates the point with the probe. The patient holds the ground electrode.

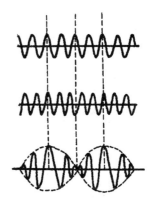

Figure 13.14. Interference of a 4000 Hz current and a 4100 Hz current to create a beat frequency of 100 Hz.

Balancing Meridians

The electrical conductivity of a particular point, the test point, on each meridian is determined with the probe and compared for right-to-left symmetry and for balance with the other meridians. Depending upon the readings, other points (such as tonification or sedation points) are then stimulated to balance the energy in the meridians. Two such systems for balancing meridians are called Akabane and Ryodoraku. (Seminar notes, Wing's Electro-point Systems, (124)) Further study of this method of treatment would be necessary for a complete understanding.

Other MT Points

Specific points associated with the meridians can be used to create specific effects. These points include source, alarm, associated, master, and miracle points. Again, more extensive study would be necessary for the proper use of these points.

MEDIUM-FREQUENCY CURRENT: INTERFERENTIAL THERAPY

Definitions

Interference: the mutual action of waves of any kind (water, sound, heat, or light) upon each other, by which the vibrations and their effects are increased, diminished, or neutralized.

Medium-frequency alternating current: an electrical current in the range of 1000 to 10,000 Hz.

Frequency-difference interferential current therapy: electrical stimulation with two intersecting medium-frequency alternating currents that differ in frequency by 0–100 or 0–200 Hz.

Amplitude-summation interferential current therapy: electrical stimulation that utilizes two medium-frequency currents that are identical in frequency but differ in amplitude.

Introduction

Dr. Hans Nemec of Austria originally developed frequency-difference interferential current therapy (FDICT) in the late 1940s to overcome the skin resistance created by the introduction of low-frequency currents through the skin. By increasing the frequency of the current, skin resistance was dramatically reduced (e.g., skin resistance at 50 Hz = 3200 ohms, whereas skin resistance at 4000 Hz = 41.6 ohms (125)). Two medium-frequency currents differing by 0–100 Hz were crossed, allowing the interfering frequency of 0–100 Hz to provide deeper and more specific treatment stimulation than the conventional low-frequency currents, with less sensory stimulation (126).

Unfortunately, Dr. Nemec's invention was not readily accepted in the United States, perhaps because of the simultaneous advent of powerful anti-inflammatory drugs (127) and perhaps because of the popularity of the low- and high-voltage galvanic units (personal communication, Juergen F. Kopf, Nemectron Medical, Inc. Dec 8, 1986). The use of interferential therapy continued in Europe for many years but has only recently become popular in the United States.

A second type of interferential therapy has recently been developed. Amplitude-summation interferential current therapy (ASICT), as the name implies, relies on the summation of the amplitudes of two intersecting, medium-frequency currents rather than on the difference between their frequencies.

Mechanism of Action

FDICT utilizes two medium-frequency alternating currents that differ in frequency by 0–100 Hz (or 0–200 Hz, depending on the particular piece of equipment). For example, one circuit is set at 4000 Hz, while the other oscillates between 4000 and 4100 Hz. When the two circuits are allowed to cross or

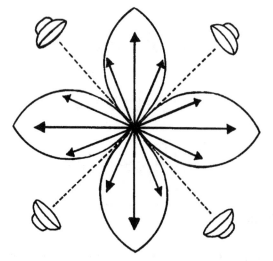

Figure 13.15. Cloverleaf pattern of treatment with frequency-difference interferential current.

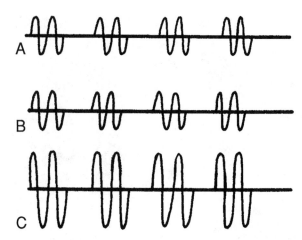

Figure 13.17. Interference of two burst modulated currents (**A** and **B**) to create an amplitude-summation interferential current (**C**).

interfere with each other, a beat frequency is created (Fig. 13.14). This beat frequency of 0–100 Hz acts as a low-frequency alternating current, which is capable of stimulating nervous tissue. Because of the nature of interfering electromagnetic currents, stimulation occurs in a cloverleaf pattern around the electrodes (Fig. 13.15). If a more generalized treatment is desired, the rotating vector is utilized, which causes the cloverleaf pattern to rotate within the tissues (Fig. 13.16).

ASICT utilizes two medium-frequency alternating currents that are "burst modulated" to 0–100 Hz (i.e., are allowed to fire in sets of 0–100 bursts per sec). The interference of these two circuits allows the summation of the amplitudes of the circuits (Fig. 13.17), creating a low-frequency, alternating current treatment that is maximal at 45° to the out-of-phase electrodes (Fig. 13.18). Because the circuits are

premodulated, the tissues immediately beneath the electrodes are stimulated at the medium-frequency rate, allowing more superficial treatment than provided by FDICT (128). Some clinicians will argue that this superficial treatment is actually a disadvantage, as the superficial stimulation will cause the patient to reach tolerance at a lower amperage and therefore will not allow as great a deep treatment. A rotating vector is optional, as with FDICT, to allow a more generalized treatment area (128) (Fig. 13.19).

Both FDICT and ASICT allow for a continuous, medium-frequency current (not burst modulated) to be utilized for constant depolarization of nerves, re-

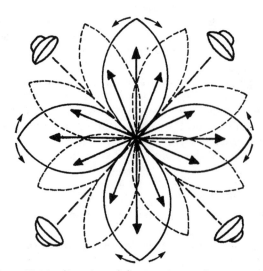

Figure 13.16. Rotation of the interferential current, creating a more generalized treatment area.

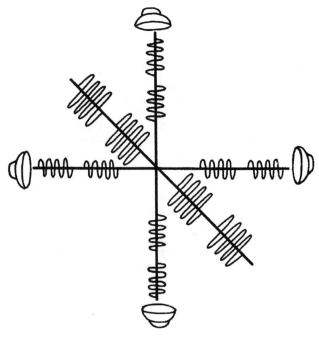

Figure 13.18. Treatment pattern of amplitude summation interferential current.

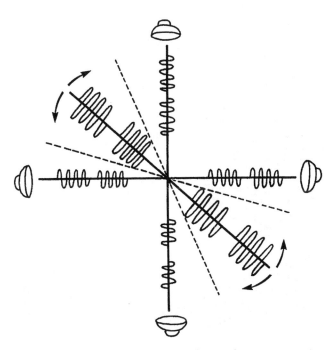

Figure 13.19. Rotation of the interferential current, creating a more generalized treatment area.

sulting in Wedenski inhibition and a rapid nerve-blocking effect (128).

Whichever the mechanism, the action is the stimulation of nervous tissue. According to their strength-duration curves, each nerve type has an optimum frequency at which maximum response will occur. Some examples are:

0–5	Sympathetic nerves;
10–150	Parasympathetic nerves;
10–50	Motor nerves;
90–110	Sensory nerves;
130	Nociceptive system (nerve fibers for pain);
0–10	Smooth muscle (129).

Effects

Analgesia

Treatment in the 90–100 Hz range is recommended for the analgesic effect. One source states that constant stimulation at 130 Hz is optimal, if available (129). Presumably this frequency allows for stimulation of C-type pain fibers, which can produce a longer-lasting analgesia than stimulation of the larger, A-type sensory fibers (111, 112). Although research has not substantiated optimal treatment frequencies for analgesia, it is logical to assume that guidelines similar to those for HVT could be used: high-frequency stimulation (50–120 Hz) for rapid analgesia and low-frequency stimulation (2–5 Hz) for longer-lasting analgesia (see "High Voltage Therapy: Analgesia Effect").

Muscle Contraction

The 10–50 Hz treatment frequency is suggested for maximal muscle contraction (129). Muscle rehabilitation is only possible if the unit is equipped with on/off capabilities and is optimal if on/off times as well as pulse width times are variable.

Reduction of Bruising and Swelling

Treatment in the 10–150 Hz range stimulates parasympathetic nerves, which increases blood flow to the treatment area. Muscle contraction in the lower-frequency ranges (10–50 Hz) also assists in the dispersion of excess fluids. The 0–5 Hz range should be avoided, if possible, to minimize stimulation of sympathetic nerves (129).

Because stimulation ooccurs with no appreciable heat production, both acute and chronic conditions can be treated.

Promotion of Healing

Although accelerated healing has been noted clinically, the reason for this is undetermined. Increased circulation as well as improved electrical "charge" of the damaged cells are possible explanations.

One study showed that in 150 subjects with mandibular fractures treated with interferential current, there were no nonunions, compared to 2% nonunions in 150 control subjects with mandibular fractures (127). Another study of 812 patients with fractures showed that interferential current had a favorable effect on delayed callus formation and Sudeck's atrophy (130). The healing effect has been shown to be better than those of microwave diathermy and ultrasound (131).

Indications

Neuromusculoskeletal conditions: to relieve pain and/or swelling and/or bruising, acute and chronic;
Muscle stimulation: to relieve muscle spasm, prevent atrophy, or provide muscle reeducation;
Postherpetic neuralgia, after skin lesions have healed;
Arthritic conditions;
Intervertebral disc lesions;
Incontinence secondary to weakened muscles (132);
Asthma: to relax the smooth muscle of the lungs;
Circulatory disorders: intermittent claudication, lymphedema, Sudeck's atrophy (133);
Migraine headaches;
Fracture and dislocation healing (130, 131).

Contraindications

Thrombosis;
Pacemaker patients;
Cardiac conditions: current should not go through the heart or stellate ganglion;
Bacterial infections, unless there is open drainage;
Malignancy;

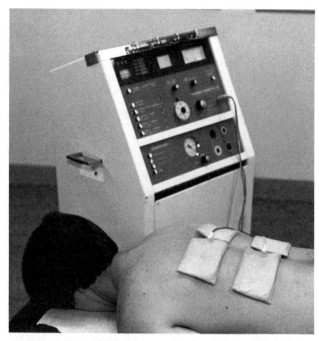

Figure 13.20. Interferential therapy. Application of plate electrodes. The four electrodes must be placed so that the two circuits intersect.

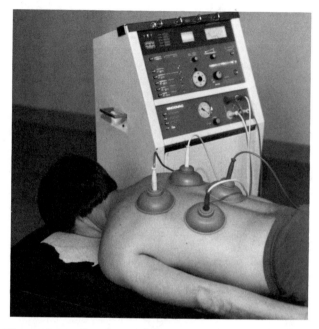

Figure 13.21. Interferential therapy. Application of vacuum electrodes. The vacuum electrodes are easily applied or rearranged.

Within 20 feet of an operating, short-wave diathermy machine.

Application

1. Apply electrodes as symmetrically as possible, with the treatment area at the intersection of the two circuits.
   a. For plate electrodes: dampen sponge covers and apply electrodes firmly with straps, sandbags, etc. All four plates may be the same size, or each circuit may have one large and one small plate (Fig. 13.20).
   b. For vacuum electrodes: dampen the sponges, squeeze them out until almost dry, then place in cups. Arrange cups on the top of the unit and turn the vacuum on. Wait for suction to begin and adjust suction to a moderate range (more suction is required for smaller cups). Place the electrodes on the skin in pairs. Reduce suction to the minimum amount needed to keep the cups from falling off. Keep cups as round as possible. All four cups may be the same size, or each circuit may have one large and one small cup (Fig. 13.21). (This description applies only to units with the more common negative vacuum system.)
   c. Mixing electrodes: each circuit may have one cup electrode and one plate electrode. Cup sizes must be equal, plate sizes must be equal but cups and plates may be of different sizes.
   d. A single combined electrode may be used for small, localized areas of treatment (Fig. 13.22).
2. Choose treatment range:
   90–100 Hz for analgesia
   10–50 Hz for muscle contraction
    0–100 Hz for full range treatment
   Treatment range may have to be altered, depending on the equipment being used.
3. Choose the rotating vector mode if a more generalized treatment is desired.
4. Turn the intensity up slowly until patient reports a strong but comfortable prickling sensation. If a muscle contraction is desired, the in-

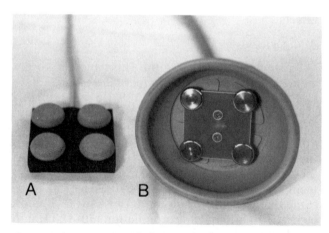

Figure 13.22. Combined electrode for interferential current is used for small superficial areas. **A,** Electrode used without vacuum. **B,** Electrode used with vacuum.

tensity should be increased to the desired level if it is within the patient's tolerance.

5. The current should be felt at the site of the lesion. If it is not, the electrodes should be rearranged. The vacuum electrodes can be easily relocated by lifting up on the collars of the electrodes.

6. Treatment time is generally 10–15 minutes, with a maximum of 20 minutes at normal intensity. In some acute cases, only a low intensity will be tolerated, in which case treatment time may be increased.

7. At the end of treatment, turn the intensity down to zero. Vacuum electrodes should be removed before the vacuum is turned off to keep them from falling off (129).

DIATHERMY

Definitions

Shortwave diathermy: the production of therapeutic heat using high-frequency, alternating, electromagnetic waves in the frequency range of 10 to 100 MHz. The primary frequency utilized is 27.12 MHz.

Microwave diathermy: the production of therapeutic heat using high-frequency, alternating, electromagnetic waves in the range of 100 to 10,000 MHz. The primary frequency utilized is 2456 MHz.

Introduction

Clinical application of high-frequency electromagnetic waves began in the early 1900s for the cauterization of malignant and other tissues (8). This form of diathermy, later designated long-wave diathermy, proved to cause unfilterable static in nearby and remote radio stations. In the 1930s, the Federal Communications Commission (FCC) was given the authority to regulate the frequency and power of diathermy. The FCC proceeded to ban long wave diathermy and designate 27.12 MHz as the primary frequency for the newer shortwave diathermy (SWD). In the late 1940s, microwave diathermy (MWD) was assigned a frequency of 2456 MHz and came into clinical use. SWD and MWD both remain in use today (66).

Both SWD and MWD have declined in popularity in recent years because they can be dangerous and difficult to use. Subcutaneous burns can occur with concentration of heat in those tissues. Conversely, if the correct type of diathermy, electrode type (134), or electrode placement are not utilized, the diathermy will be ineffective. Also, the advent of ultrasound has given clinicians a safer, easier, and less time-consuming method of creating heat deep in the tissues (66, 135).

However, several indications for the use of diathermy cannot be adequately treated by any other modality to date. Infectious conditions of the lungs such as pneumonia, bronchitis, and bronchiectasis, as well as inflammatory conditions such as chronic pelvic inflammatory disease, benign prostatic hypertrophy, osteomyelitis, and prostatitis can respond very well to diathermy. And there are no doubt other situations in which the deep heat of diathermy is more effective than ultrasound or other methods of heat. Therefore, while diathermy has somewhat limited use, it should not be abandoned.

Mechanism of Action

General Mechanism of Action

Production of an Electrical or Electrostatic Field. The electrical field is created by the high-frequency alternating current being applied to the two condenser plates or electrodes. The patient's tissues and the space between the electrodes and the skin act as the condenser, or capacitor, and are thus able to store the electrical energy created between the electrodes (Fig. 13.23A). Because the current is rapidly alternating, free ions in the tissues alternate back and forth, creating a vibration. This vibration causes friction between ions and thus produces heat. Polar molecules (such as water) will change direction rapidly, and therefore they produce more heat than nonpolar molecules (such as fat).

Production of an Electromagnetic Field. The electromagnetic field is created around the thick, insulated cable through which the current flows (Fig. 13.23B). The cable completes the circuit from the machine and therefore does not require a patient for completion of the circuit. The cable is coiled in close proximity to the patient's tissues so that the eddy currents created around the cable cause friction in the superficial tissues and the production of heat.

Mechanisms of Action Specific to Electrode Types

Diathermy can be administered through a variety of electrodes, each with its own advantages and disadvantages. Therefore, the mechanisms of action will be discussed in terms of the different electrode types.

SWD Air-Spaced Electrodes (Fig. 13.24). Air-spaced electrodes contain rigid metal plates in electrically insulated housing. The patient's tissues act as the condenser between the two plates and are necessary for the completion of the circuit. The depth of heat penetration is proportional to the distance of the metal plate from the skin, that is, the farther the plate is placed from the skin (within the limit of approximately 3 cm), the deeper will be the penetration. Also, the deeper the penetration, the less will be the sensation of warmth to the patient and vice-versa. Air-spaced electrodes are useful for treating large areas where direct contact of the electrode is not desired.

SWD Pad Electrodes (Fig. 13.25). Pad electrodes consist of a flexible metal plate covered with rubber insulating material. Two pads and the patient's tissues are required for completion of the circuit. The spacing needed between the pads and the skin can

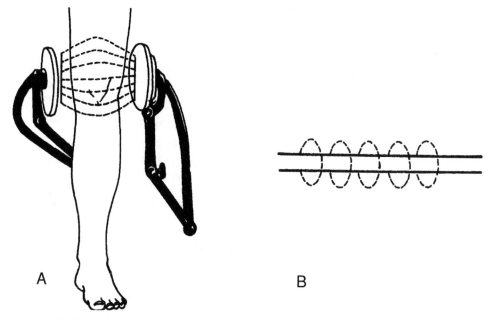

Figure 13.23. **A,** Electrostatic field created by diathermy. **B,** Electromagnetic field created by diathermy.

be provided by felt pads, layers of toweling, or rubber "knobs" that are sometimes fabricated into the pads. Uniform contact throughout the electrode surface is required for deep penetration. Because uniform contact is difficult to achieve, the older pads have been considered ineffective and have even been banned by the American Medical Association (66). Pad electrodes are useful for treating large, flat areas that can tolerate electrode contact.

SWD Drum or Induction-Coil Electrodes (Fig. 13.26). The drum or induction-coil electrode can take several forms. It consists of one or more monoplanar coils of thick copper wire embedded in a housing. A single coil takes the form of a drum and can be used for relatively small, flat areas. Two or three coils can be hinged together in a "butterfly" fashion so that the electrode can be bent to conform to body contours.

In either case, the patient's tissues are not necessary for completion of the circuit. Consequently, the patient's tissues lie more within the electromagnetic field than in the electrical field, so that polar tissues will be heated to a greater extent than nonpolar tissues. Although the area that can be treated is smaller

Figure 13.24. Shortwave diathermy air-spaced electrodes. Both electrodes are needed to complete the circuit.

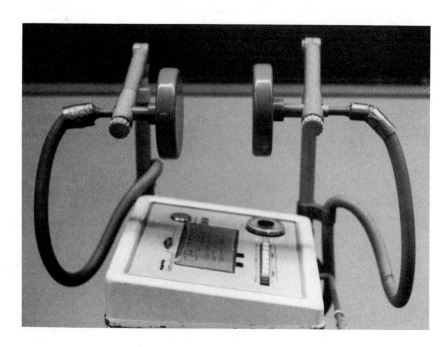

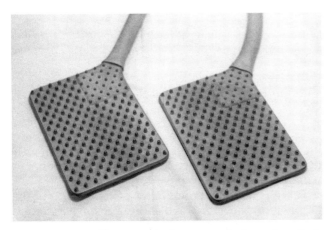

Figure 13.25. Shortwave diathermy pad electrodes. Both electrodes are needed to complete the circuit.

than with air-spaced or pad electrodes, penetration is deeper, with less danger of burning the subcutaneous tissues.

SWD Cable Electrodes. Cable electrodes are rarely used. They are appropriate only for use on extremities. They consist of a long copper cable that is insulated with flexible rubber. The cable is carefully wound around the extremity with adequate spacing

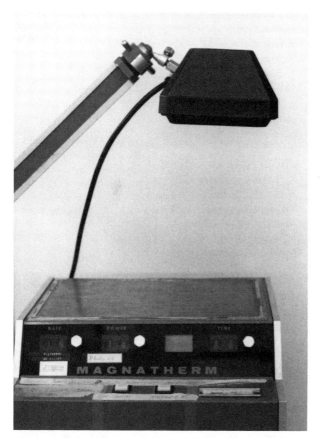

Figure 13.26. Shortwave diathermy drum electrode. A single electrode may be used. Two electrodes are used to increase the area of treatment.

(approximately 1 cm), with towels between the cable and the skin. As with the drum electrode, the patient is not needed to complete the circuit, and the patient's tissues lie more within the electromagnetic field than the electrical field.

MWD Directors (Fig. 13.27). Because the MWD wavelength is shorter than the SWD wavelength, the energy can be directed toward the skin from a greater distance (up to 15 cm) without significant loss of energy. The farther the director is placed from the skin, the greater will be the area treated, but more power will be needed for equally deep heating. The energy must be directed perpendicular to a flat, even surface. MWD energy causes oscillation in polar molecules and therefore heats polar tissues more than nonpolar tissues. In an area of little fat, MWD energy can penetrate as deeply as 5 cm. However, in a fatty area, penetration is limited markedly.

MWD directors take a variety of forms. Most are tent-shaped (Fig. 13.27A) or hemispheric (Fig. 13.27B). With the tent-shaped and some of the hemispheric directors, maximum heating occurs in the center of the treating area, with less heating toward the periphery. Other hemispheric directors are constructed so that approximately 50% of the maximum heating occurs in the center of the treating field, with maximum heating occurring in a donut-shaped ring around the center, allowing placement of the director at the center of a joint without concern for too much heating effect within the joint. A MWD director may be placed 2 to 15 cm from the skin; the farther from the skin, the larger will be the treatment area and the more power will be needed. MWD units are most useful for treating relatively small areas with minimal fat.

Effects

Continuous SWD or MWD

The effects of diathermy can be attributed primarily to the production of heat and consequent increased blood supply. They include:

Decreased pain;
Decreased muscle spasm;
Decreased inflammation;
Increased healing;
Decreased infection;
Increased extensibility of fibrous tissue (9).

Pulsed Diathermy

Pulsed SWD has existed almost as long as the more common continuous SWD. Theoretically, pulsing the energy allows dissipation of the heat, leaving only the nonthermal effect (i.e., the "electromagnetic" effect). Therefore, many conditions (such as acute inflammatory processes) can be treated with pulsed SWD that would be contraindicated for continuous SWD. Although many cases have been cited indicating that pulsed electromagnetic fields

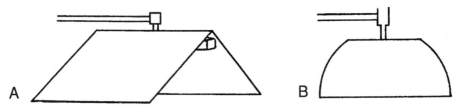

Figure 13.27. Microwave diathermy directors. **A,** Tent-shaped. **B,** Hemispheric.

(PEMFs) have improved the healing of nonunion fractures, congenital pseudarthrosis, failed fusions, peripheral nerve regeneration, and various soft tissue injuries (136–146), other studies have shown no significant changes in bone growth (147, 148). Waveform characteristics may play a significant role in the success or failure of PEMFs (140), or the conservative management of the nonunion fractures studied may account for much of the success attributed to PEMFs (149).

Because of overexuberant claims made by the manufacturer of one PEMF unit, the Food and Drug Administration has removed it from the market and banned its use. Another remains on the market, but no claims are made for any effects other than the thermal effects.

Indications

Diathermy is used for the production of heat in deep and superficial structures. Indications include subacute and chronic:

Bursitis;
Tendinitis, tenosynovitis;
Neuromuscular, musculoskeletal disorders;
Sprains and strains;
Fractures with closed reduction, after callus formation has begun;
Arthritic conditions;
Pelvic inflammatory disease;
Wound healing;
Pneumonia;
Bronchitis, bronchiectasis;
Benign prostatic hypertrophy;
Osteomyelitis;
Prostatitis;
Amenorrhea, dysmenorrhea;
Pleuritis;
Hematoma (150);
Abscess.

Precautions

Diathermy is probably one of the most potentially dangerous modalities in use today, and it should be administered only with knowledge and respect. Contraindications to diathermy are numerous and should be heeded. Diathermy has the ability to heat subcutaneous tissue dramatically with little sensation to the patient; therefore, it is possible to pro-

duce subcutaneous burns without the clinician's or patient's awareness (66).

There is also the potential of overexposure of the clinician to the shortwave and microwave radiation (151). The United Kingdom has suggested limits on exposure to microwave radiation and their National Radiation Protection Board and others have determined from their studies that there is no hazard to the operator or patient with the use of normal correct procedures (152, 153). A Canadian study agrees but concludes that overexposure may occur if the operator stands within one-half meter of the applicators or cables of a SWD unit (154).

Contraindications

Acute inflammatory processes;
Metal implant;
Wet dressing;
Plaster cast;
Peripheral vascular disease;
Over a gravid uterus;
Profuse menstruation;
Malignancy;
Desensitized skin;
Hematemesis, hemoptysis;
Over epiphyseal centers;
Varicosities;
Advanced osteoporosis;
Occlusive arterial disease;
Moderate or severe edema;
Within the same room as a cardiac pacemaker patient;
Tuberculous joints;
Unreliable patient;
Severe cardiac conditions;
Severe hypertension;
Through the brain.

Application

1. Do not use a treatment table with metal parts.
2. Remove all metal from the patient.
3. Preheat the unit.
4. Inspect the part to be treated and place a towel over it.
5. Place electrodes.
   SWD pads: place against the skin with a towel in-between. Leave as much space between the pads as possible.

SWD air-spaced electrodes: place 1–3 cm from the skin, following the contours of the body as much as possible.

SWD drum or induction coil electrodes: place electrode as close to the skin as possible without touching it. Follow the contours of the body as much as possible.

MWD director: place 2–15 cm from the skin with the beam of energy perpendicular to the skin. The greater the distance from the skin, the greater the treatment area and the higher the dosage required.

6. Make sure cables are not crossing or touching patient or metal.
7. Turn dosage on to the desired level. Superficial and subacute conditions should be treated on low power. Dosage levels are
   25% power: nondetectable warmth; for the treatment of subacute and inflammatory conditions;
   50% power: barely detectable heat; for more chronic inflammatory conditions;
   75% power: comfortable warmth; for the treatment of soft tissue and articular conditions of a chronic nature;
   100% power: maximum tolerable warmth; rarely used.
8. Monitor patient carefully; decrease dosage if patient feels too warm or if profuse sweating occurs.
9. Treat for desired length of time:
   5–10 min for subacute conditions;
   15–20 min for chronic conditions.

ULTRASOUND

Definition

Ultrasound: Sound waves vibrating at frequencies above those that the human ear can hear. Therapeutic ultrasound is that which is used for therapeutic (rather than diagnostic) purposes and is usually produced at 1 megacycle or 1 million cycles per sec.

Introduction

Ultrasound (US) was first researched in Europe, especially Germany, and was brought to the United States in the early 1950s. Since that time, the use of ultrasound has grown, and it remains a very popular modality today.

US has replaced diathermy for many types of conditions because it is less time-consuming and penetrates tissues well. US is safe to use over metal implants (155), there is less danger of burning, it takes only 5–10 min, and it is capable of penetrating approximately 5 cm into the tissues.

Mechanism of Action

US is produced by a high-frequency alternating current being applied to a crystal made of quartz or a synthetic (i.e., barium titanate or lead zirconate). The current causes the crystal to bend, first in one direction and then the other, as the current alternates. This deformation of the crystal creates what is called *piezoelectric energy.* This vibratory energy is transferred to a metal plate, usually nickel-plated brass, and then to the patient's tissues. The crystal and metal plate are housed in the *transducer* or *sound head* of the unit.

Physical Properties

Because US is part of the acoustic spectrum rather than the electromagnetic spectrum, its physical properties differ from those of other physiotherapy modalities.

It is not transmitted through a vacuum.
It is transmitted poorly through gases.
It is transmitted best through gas-free liquids and high-density solids.

Absorption

The absorption of ultrasonic energy is dependent upon a number of factors, including:
Acoustic Impedance of the Tissues. Energy is absorbed at tissue interfaces (i.e., places where the acoustic impedance of the two media are different). Reflection of the acoustic energy occurs at these tissue interfaces and increases as the difference of the acoustic impedance of the two media increases according to the formula

$$x = \frac{Z_1 - Z_2}{Z_1 + Z_2},$$

where x is the intensity of reflection coefficient, and Z_1 and Z_2 are characteristic impedances (9).
Density of the Tissues. The denser the tissues, the greater the transmittance, hence the less the absorption.
Protein, Fat, and Water in Tissues. Proteins are the major absorbers of US (66, 156). Muscle absorbs twice as much US as fat does. The hemoglobin of blood absorbs US. Absorption by fluids depends upon their viscosity and heat conduction. The absorption in water is very low (9).

Actions of US on Human Tissue

Continuous US

Thermal. The friction caused by the vibration of the molecules within the patient's tissues will produce heat. Because US is easily transmitted by skin and fat, the heat can be directed to the deeper muscle layers where it is needed. Heat will be greater at tissue interfaces, where increased reflection occurs.
Mechanical. The tissues alternately compress and expand because of the pressure of the sound waves. This action causes a micromassaging effect that will loosen the microscopic cell structures, break down complex molecules, and accelerate diffusion across cell membranes. The effects of the micromassage are difficult to separate from the thermal effects, because micromassaging will also cause

friction among cells, which contributes to the thermal effect.

At high intensities, usually beyond reasonable therapeutic range, cavitation may occur. During the expansion stage, gas-filled cavities may form which then collapse during compression, causing mechanical destruction (9). Cavitation should be avoided.

Chemical. US has the effect of increasing chemical reactions. In vitro, hyaluronic and chondroitin sulfuric acids become significantly less viscous when exposed to US, assisting in the repair of connective tissue after injury (66, 157). Again this effect is difficult to separate completely from the thermal effect.

Pulsed US

Most units are able to administer pulsed US. The energy is on for a short period of time, then off, alternating so that the "on time" or duty cycle is approximately 5–50% of the total time. The "off time" allows the tissues to disperse the heat created, thereby minimizing or eliminating the thermal effect. With the 5% duty cycle, there is virtually no heating, whereas with the 50% duty cycle, some heating occurs. Pulsing US is advantageous when the thermal effect may be detrimental (e.g., when treating acute conditions or when the stationary method is used for treating small areas).

Phonophoresis

Sound waves can apparently be used to drive large, complex molecules into the tissues, although this has not been proven. Preparations containing menthol, eucalyptus, herbs, etc. can supposedly be phonophoresed.

Advantages of phonophoresis over iontophoresis are:

US is safer to use than LVG;
Complex molecules can be phonophoresed in their entirety and need not be broken down into their ionic components;
Substances can be driven deeper into the tissues.

Effects

Tissue temperature rise. The degree of tissue temperature rise depends on the previously mentioned absorption factors (see "Mechanism of Action"). With the normal operating frequency of 1 megacycle, approximately one-half of the ultrasound energy will penetrate 5 cm into soft tissue (66).
Decreased nerve conduction velocity between 0.5 and 1.5 W/cm^2 (but increased above 2.0 and 0.5 W/cm^2). This effect is transient, lasting approximately 30 min (66).
Increased circulation. This is mainly due to the thermal effect.
Increased tendon extensibility.
Reduced adhesion formation.
Decreased pain.
Increased wound healing.
Muscle relaxation.
Inhibition of sympathetic nervous system.

Note: no antiinflammatory effect has been documented (158).

Indications

Neuromuscular, musculoskeletal disorders;
Sprains and strains;
Adhesive capsulitis;
Arthritic conditions—acute and chronic;
Bursitis;
Tendinitis, including calcific tendinitis;
Neuromas;
Scars;
Dupuytren's contracture;
Acute herpes zoster radiculitis (159);
Plantar warts;
Hematoma;
Pain secondary to sympathetic dysfunction;
Minimum to moderate swelling;
Wound healing, surgical (160) or otherwise. However, one study showed an adverse effect on the early repair process on flexor tendon repairs in rabbits (161);
Adhesions;
Peyronie's disease (162).

Precautions

Overheating of the cutaneous tissues may occur if too much gel is used, not enough gel is used, the intensity is too high, the transducer is moved too slowly, or the transducer surface is not kept parallel to the skin surface.

Overheating of the periosteum may occur if the transducer is held too close to the bone, the intensity is too high, or the transducer is moved too slowly. Reflected heat is absorbed and not allowed to dissipate because of the periosteum's poor blood supply. The patient will complain of a deep, gnawing pain. If the US is turned down or removed quickly, no permanent damage will occur.

Contraindications

Epiphyses of growing bones;
Over reproductive organs;
Over a gravid uterus;
Over the heart;
Over the eye;
Over anesthetic areas;
Over the lower cervical sympathetic ganglia;
Over ischemic areas;
Directly over the spinal column or brain;
Over a fracture (until well healed);
Near an acute infection;
Patients having deep x-ray therapy or radium isotopes;
Deep vein thrombosis;
Arterial disease;
Hemophilia;

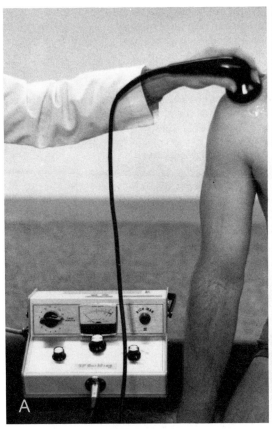

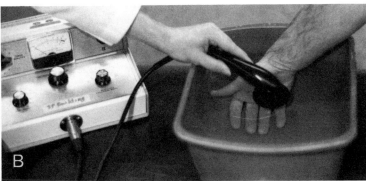

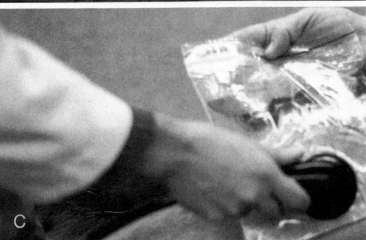

Figure 13.28. Application of ultrasound. **A,** *Direct contact method.* Adequate coupling medium is necessary for proper conduction of the ultrasound energy. The transducer should always remain in contact with the skin while the unit is on. **B,** *Immersion method.* The transducer is held close to the skin under the water. **C,** *Fluid-filled bag method.* The bag acts as the coupling medium over uneven or inaccessible areas. Gel must be used on both sides of the bag.

Tuberculosis of the lungs or bone;
Malignancy;
Over the thoracic region of a patient with a pacemaker (66).

Application

General Application

1. Apply coupling medium to the part being treated and place the transducer against the coupling medium. The unit should never be turned on without coupling medium because the crystal may overheat.
2. Keep the transducer moving slowly.
3. Turn the intensity up to the desired level (see "Dosage" below).
4. Avoid bony prominences and keep the transducer as parallel to the skin as possible.
5. The patient may get a mild sense of warmth. If the patient gets too hot or uncomfortable, the wattage should be reduced to a tolerable level.
6. Treat for the desired time (see "Duration" below).
7. Return the intensity to zero before removing the transducer from skin.

Specific Methods of Application

1. Direct contact (Fig. 13.28A)
   a. Most common method.
   b. Use an adequate layer of thixotropic gel between the transducer and the skin. Glycerol is acceptable, but mineral oil or massage lotion should not be used (66).
2. Immersion method (Fig. 13.28B)
   a. Good for treating hands, wrists, feet, elbows (i.e., any area that can be comfortably immersed in water).
   b. Place the transducer and the treating part in a container of water. Metal containers are not contraindicated.
   c. Keep the transducer within 1 cm of skin without contacting it; keep the transducer moving slowly.
3. Stationary method
   a. Good for treating small, localized areas such as small muscle spasms, hematomas, trigger points, or acupuncture points.
   b. Use a low intensity (0.2 W/cm^2) for 2–3 min, or pulsed US.
   c. Be careful to avoid a periosteal reaction.

4. Fluid-filled bag method (Fig. 13.28C)
   a. Good for difficult-to-reach and/or bony areas, such as the anterior knee, clavicle, etc.
   b. Fill a finger cot, rubber glove, or plastic bag with coupling gel, glycerol, or degased water.
   c. Fix the cot or glove over the transducer. Apply coupling gel to the outside of the bag and place it against the patient's skin, or tie off the cot or glove. Apply coupling gel to two sides of the bag. Place one side against the patient and place the transducer against the other side.
5. Neurotrophic method
   a. Good for a problem involving an extremity.
   b. Prior to using US on the injured part, treat the corresponding nerve root.

Dosage

With gel: Acute: 0.5–1.5 W/cm^2
         Chronic: 1.0–2.0 W/cm^2
Under water: Acute: 1.0–2.0 W/cm^2
         Chronic: 1.5–2.5 W/cm^2

Duration

Acute: 3–4 min
Chronic: 5–10 min

PHOTOTHERAPY

Definitions

Phototherapy: the use of light rays for therapeutic purposes.

Ultraviolet therapy: the use of the ultraviolet portion of the light spectrum, between approximately 1800 and 4000 angstroms wavelength.

Infrared therapy: the use of the infrared portion of the light spectrum, between approximately 7000 and 30,000 angstroms wavelength.

Introduction

In the early 1900s, ultraviolet (UV) was being used in the treatment of extrapulmonary tuberculosis and rickets. When it was discovered in 1924 that food could be irradiated with artificial light, rather than the patient, with the same beneficial effect on vitamin D conversion, UV lamps lost their popularity. Manufacturers of the UV equipment, to avoid wasting their electrical parts and skilled workers, converted their lamps to infrared (IR), selling the IR lamps to clinicians as a source of heat not available in the home. While it is difficult to relate the phototherapies directly to spine-related disorders, the topic is included here for the sake of completeness of the physiological therapeutics.

Neither UV nor IR is very popular today, although both have a place in the clinician's armamentarium of modalities. UV is useful in the symptomatic treatment of psoriasis and other skin disorders, as well as in the irradiation of superficial bacterial infections. IR is a good source of superficial heat with which it is not necessary to touch the patient's skin or disturb the patient in any way.

Both UV and IR, being sources of light, follow the physical laws of light.

Inverse Square Law

The *inverse square law* states that the intensity of radiation from any source of light varies inversely with the square of the distance from the source. For example, dividing the distance from the lamp to the patient by *two* increases the intensity of the rays *fourfold.* When changing lamp distance, the new time may be calculated by

$$\frac{(\text{New distance})^2}{(\text{Old distance})^2} \times \text{Old time} = \text{New time}.$$

Lambert's Cosine Law

Lambert's cosine law states that the patient receives maximum radiation at right angles to the center of the area being treated. Radiation loss becomes significant at about 30° from the central ray.

Ultraviolet

Mechanism of Action

UV light is categorized as UVA, UVB or UVC, each with its own properties.

UVA and UVB

Erythema. UV light destroys cells in the prickle cell layer of the skin, causing the release of a histamine-like substance.

Pigmentation. Cell destruction also releases tyrosine, which causes the migration of melanin from the deeper skin layers.

UVB

Stimulation of Calcium and Phosphorus Metabolism. UV light activates cholesterol and ergosterol to convert provitamin D to vitamin D$_3$.

UVC

Germicidal. UV light causes dimerization of thymine, which suppresses the synthesis of DNA in bacteria.

Penetration of ultraviolet is minimal, 90% is absorbed in the first 0.1 mm of the skin. Almost any substance (cloth, glass, paper, etc.) will block the penetration of ultraviolet and may be used as draping.

Effects

The effects of ultraviolet depend upon the particular lamp used.

Hot Quartz Lamps. Hot quartz lamps emit a combination of 2537, 2800, and 2900–3200 Å wavelength. They produce a strong erythema effect with delayed onset and short duration, strong pigmentation, excellent stimulation of calcium and phosphorus metabolism, and good germicidal effects.

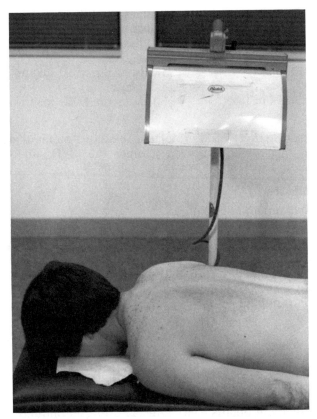

Figure 13.29. Hot quartz ultraviolet is used for the treatment of psoriasis.

Cold Quartz Lamps. Cold quartz lamps emit ultraviolet light at 2537 Å only. They produce a moderate erythema with early onset and short duration, poor pigmentation, negligible calcium and phosphorus metabolism, and excellent germicidal effects.

Indications

Psoriasis;
Indolent ulcers;
Rickets;
Infantile tetany or spasmophilia;
Infected ulcers and wounds;
Mild degrees of calcium and phosphorus deficiency in children;
Osteomalacia in pregnant or nursing women;
Acne;
Seborrheic dermatitis;
Pityriasis rosea;
Anemia;
Extrapulmonary tuberculosis (bones, joints, skin—if non-progressive and no fever);
Lupus vulgaris;
Erysipelas;
Impetigo;
As generalized tonic.

Contraindications

Active and progressive tuberculosis;
Advanced heart disease with failure of compensation;
Advanced arteriosclerosis;
Renal or hepatic insufficiency;
Hyperthyroidism;
Diabetes mellitus;
Generalized dermatitis (e.g., measles, chicken pox);
Porphyrias;
Pellagra;
Lupus erythematosus;
Sarcoidosis;
Xeroderma pigmentosum;
Skin malignancies and/or precancerous lesions.

Application

Hot Quartz (Fig. 13.29).

1. Preheat lamp about 5 min.
2. Protect the eyes of doctor and patient with goggles.
3. Place lamp at a distance of 18–30 inches from the skin (keeping the cosine law and the inverse square law in mind).
4. Do a sleeve test if the patient's minimal erythemal dose (MED) is not known (see "Dosage").
5. Drape the patient carefully.
6. Expose the skin for the proper length of time. Four exposures will generally be required for full-body exposure.
7. Increase exposure time each treatment, so that the exposure time continues to cause minimal erythema.

Cold Quartz Lamp (Fig. 13.30A). Application is the same as with the hot quartz lamp except the lamp need not be preheated. Lamp-to-skin distance may have to be decreased. (Cold quartz is more germicidal than hot quartz, but it is not as effective at treating psoriasis.)

Cold Quartz Spot Lamp or Orifical Lamp (Fig. 13.30B).

1. Protect the eyes of doctor and patient with goggles.
2. Turn unit on (preheating is not necessary).
3. Place lamp about one-half inch from treatment area.
4. Expose area for 5 sec for the first treatment; increase 5 sec each treatment.

Dosage

For general body exposures, a minimal erythemal dose (MED) is desired. An MED is the amount of UV that in 4 to 6 hr will produce a minimal erythema on the volar surface of the forearm.

The MED is determined by the sleeve test, or patch test. The entire body is draped except for five

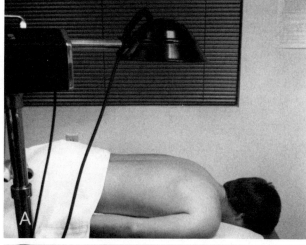

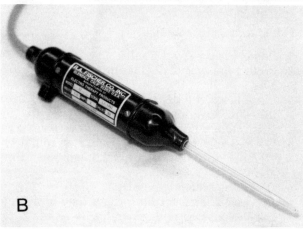

Figure 13.30. Cold quartz ultraviolet. **A**, Lamp used for treating large areas. **B**, Orificial lamp used for treating bacterial infections of the throat and ears.

patches on the anterior forearm, which are progressively opened or closed to expose each patch for a different period of time. The least amount of time needed to produce an erythema is the MED. The MED may vary tremendously from one machine to the next, depending upon the strength and age of the UV tube. A time period as short as 15 sec may produce the MED.

Because the skin builds up a tolerance to UV, treatment time must be increased each treatment to maintain the MED, unless a number of days has elapsed between treatments.

Different parts of the body have different tolerances for UV. Compared to the MED of the forearm, the following parts can tolerate these dosages:

Face	Same as MED for forearm
Chest	1.5 times the MED for the forearm
Thigh	1.5 times the MED for the forearm
Mucous membranes	1.5 times the MED for the forearm
Back	2 times the MED for the forearm
Back of hands	4 times the MED for the forearm
Palms	15 times the MED for the forearm
Soles of feet	20 times the MED for the forearm

Because there is no protective skin layer on an ulcer or open wound, up to 10 times the MED can be given. Be careful to drape all normal skin.

Infrared

Mechanism of Action

Superficial heating is the main action of IR. Nonluminous heaters emit near IR rays in the range of 20,000–30,000 Å wavelength; penetration is limited to 1 mm. Luminous heaters emit far IR in the range of 2,000–15,000 Å; heat of this type penetrates to 10 mm.

Effects

Analgesia;
Reduction of muscle spasm;
Reduction of edema;
Decreased chronic inflammation.

(For more details, see "Effects" under "Conductive and Convective Heat.")

Indications

See "Conductive and Convective Heat."

Contraindications

See "Conductive and Convective Heat."

Application

1. Remove all metal from the treatment area.
2. Inspect the part to be treated and drape appropriately.
3. Preheat unit if it takes longer than 5 minutes to heat.
4. Protect the patient's eyes.
5. Place the lamp 2 to 3 feet from the patient, with the light beam perpendicular to the area of treatment.
6. Tell the patient to expect a mild sense of warmth. If the patient feels too warm or if the skin feels too warm to the clinician, pull the lamp farther away from the patient.
7. Treatment time of 20 minutes is standard.

BIOFEEDBACK

Definitions

Biofeedback: a process in which information about an aspect of bodily functioning is displayed to the patient via an auditory or visual signal (163).

Galvanic skin response: changes in the skin conductance of the hand, caused by activity of the sweat glands (163).

Introduction

Interest in biofeedback began in 1938 with B. F. Skinner and O. Hobart Mowrer. Unfortunately their results were not favorable, and biofeedback was forgotten until the 1960s when E. Kimmell and F. Hill got some promising results with galvanic skin response (164). Other early methods of biofeedback attempted the voluntary control of autonomic functions such as heart rate and blood pressure. Since then, applications have been expanded to include work with muscle training, relaxation, and posture control. These latter applications are more relevant to today's chiropractor. Biofeedback techniques appear to be gaining in popularity as their effectiveness is being shown, and carryover to nontherapy activities is at least postulated (163).

Mechanism of Action

By giving the patient an immediate and on-going display of a specific biological function that was formerly "silent," the patient can make continual, voluntary changes in that function and gain voluntary control over it. The display is a visual or auditory signal that may occur when a particular threshold is reached or may be variable in proportion to the function being measured.

Effects

Depending upon the bodily function being measured, the effects may include:

Control of heart rate;
Control of blood pressure;
Control of skin temperature;
Improved skill (i.e., control of specific muscle action and/or proprioception);
Reduced tension.

Indications

High blood pressure;
Stress and tension;
Muscle reeducation (e.g., after disuse or cerebral vascular accident);
Muscle tension (e.g., tension headaches);
Migraine headaches; the difference in temperature between the temple and the hand is minimized, thus shunting blood from the head region to the peripheral circulation (164);
Postural faults.

Contraindications

None known.

Application

Specific application depends upon the machinery used and the function being monitored. Training sessions range from 10 to 30 minutes duration, occurring somewhere between daily and weekly. Significant changes are usually noted in only a few sessions (164).

SPINAL TRACTION

Definitions

Spinal traction: the application of a drawing or pulling force along the long axis of the spine in order to (a) stretch soft tissues, (b) separate joint surfaces, or (c) separate bony fragments.

Distraction: a form of dislocation in which joint surfaces have been separated without rupture of the binding ligaments and without displacement.

Inversion: turning upside-down or other reversal of the normal relation of a part.

Introduction

As early as 400 BC, Hippocrates witnessed the application of spinal traction in the form of inversion—a man was tied by his legs to a ladder and then inverted. Since then, traction has taken many forms and remains a useful adjunct to the chiropractic adjustment, both in the office and as a home treatment.

For the purposes of this book, discussion of traction will be limited to the application of traction to the spine for the purpose of stretching soft tissues or separating joint surfaces. Chiropractors would probably not have an occasion to use traction for separating bony fragments.

Types of Traction

Static Traction

Static traction is used for several minutes to several hours at a time for the purpose of immobilizing a part and allowing soft tissue to relax.

In the clinic or hospital setting, a cervical or lumbar harness is attached to a rope, and a small amount of weight is suspended over a pulley. For lumbar traction, either the bed is "gatched" (i.e., head elevated and knees flexed) or a counterharness is used to stabilize the upper body.

For home use, a cervical traction unit uses pulleys with a water bags or weights (patient is in the sitting position) (Fig. 13.31A), springs (patient is supine) (Fig. 13.31B), or pulleys with a locking mechanism (patient is supine) (Fig. 13.31C). Home lumbar traction is most conveniently and effectively performed with a "90/90" traction unit (Fig. 13.32), originally devised by Cottrell (165), which utilizes a frame that rests on the bed, a pelvic harness, a pulley attached to the frame, and a locking mechanism. The patient pulls on the rope, which flexes the pelvis and tractions the lumbar spine. The rope is locked into position when the desired amount of traction is achieved.

Intermittent Mechanical Traction

Intermittent mechanical traction (Fig. 13.33A, B) utilizes a mechanical traction device that alternately applies traction and allows relaxation for a time period of several minutes to one-half hour. This allows intermittent stretch of soft tissues, joint separation,

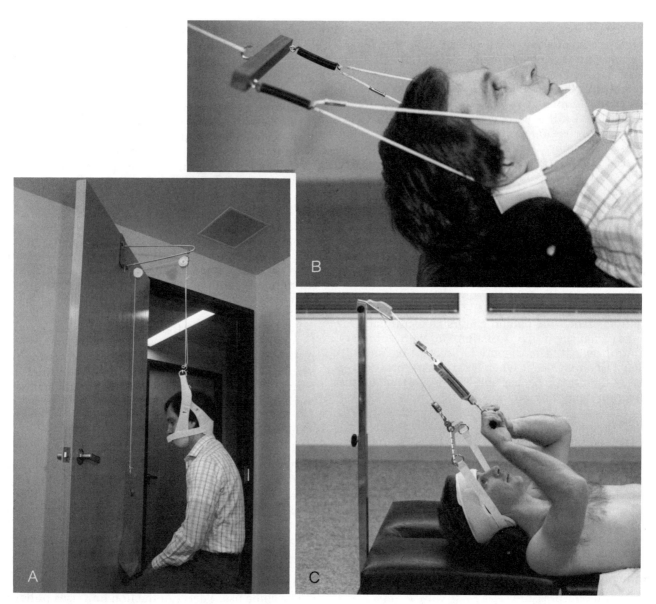

Figure 13.31. Home cervical traction. **A,** Traction with weights. The patient is easily able to control the bag of water or sand. **B,** Traction with springs. This unit can be screwed into the wall or attached to a piece of heavy furniture. The patient pulls away from the unit, placing tension on the springs. **C,** Traction with pulleys. The patient is able to control the amount of traction and read the poundage on the scale.

and imbibition of the disc, which can be beneficial for the treatment of soft tissue injuries, joint fixation, nerve root compression, degenerative disc disease, or an acute or chronic herniated disc. For lumbar traction, counterstabilization via a thoracic harness is necessary. A split table or table with rollers is also advantageous to reduce friction.

Manual Traction

Manual traction is traction applied manually by the doctor. The amount of traction applied may vary tremendously, depending upon the patient's condition, the part of the spine being tractioned, and the strength of the doctor. Belts, towels, or harnesses

may be used to increase the mechanical advantage of the doctor and leave the hands free for palpation of the affected area.

Positional Traction

Positional traction (Fig. 13.34) involves placing the patient in a particular position to increase motion in a specific direction at a specific segment of the spine. Pillows, blocks, and sandbags may be used to accentuate the position and increase traction.

Inversion

Inversion therapy may be achieved by a variety of inversion apparatuses. Basically, the patient is se-

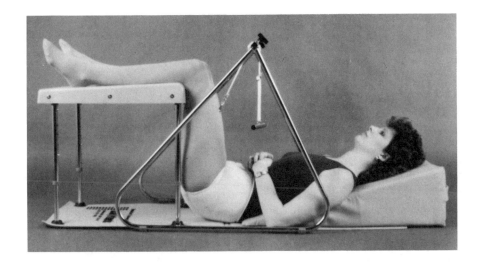

Figure 13.32. "90/90" Traction. The hips and knees are placed at 90°. The belt pulls the pelvis into flexion while it tractions. (Photo courtesy of Lossing Orthopedic.)

cured by the ankles or thighs and allowed to invert to some degree, up to 90°. The weight of the upper body is affected by gravity and allows traction of the spine, especially of the lumbar segments. Unfortu-

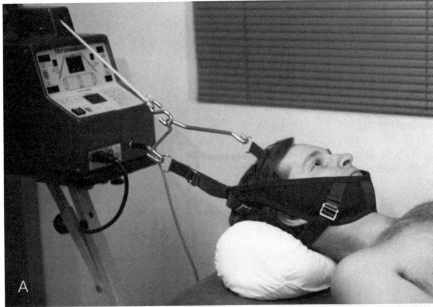

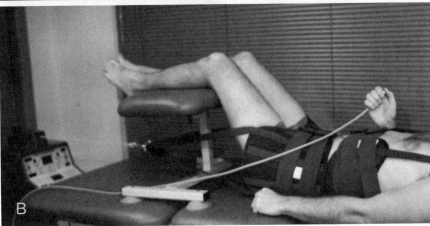

Figure 13.33. Intermittent traction. **A,** Intermittent cervical traction. The rope angle of pull is approximately 30° from horizontal. **B,** Intermittent lumbar traction. The rope angle of pull is approximately horizontal. A counterharness is used for stabilization.

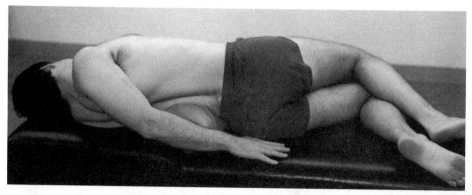

Figure 13.34. Positional traction of the lumbar spine. Traction is accomplished by rotating and sidebending at the spinal level desired.

nately, each type of inversion apparatus has its unique disadvantages, making the choice of a unit somewhat difficult.

The *standard inversion table* (Fig. 13.35), in which the body is suspended by ankle cuffs, does allow controllable, variable degrees of inversion, but it may cause or aggravate ankle, knee, or hip joint dysfunction. In addition, with the legs in full extension, the lumbar spine is placed in some degree of lumbar lordosis by the passive pull of the vertebral portion of the psoas muscles, placing an unnecessary load on the lumbar spine during traction (166).

The apparatus that utilizes a *thigh and behind-the-knee inversion* (Fig. 13.36) has the advantages of placing the hips and knees in flexion (thus decreasing the load on the lumbar spine) and of applying no pull to the joints of the lower extremities. However, there is no variable degree of inversion; it is all-or-nothing. Also, many of the units are not large enough to accommodate a tall person.

The *mechanical chair-type inversion unit* combines the advantage of the flexed hip and knee positioning with variable degrees of inversion. Disadvantages include possible discomfort across the thigh belt and difficulty with patient control of the degree of inversion.

The *electric chair-type inversion unit* appears to combine the greatest advantages of inversion; hips and knees are in a flexed position, and the degree of inversion is infinitely variable and controllable. However, the cost is quite high, and discomfort across the thigh belt is possible.

An inexpensive alternative to inversion is *inversion boots* (Fig. 13.37). This system utilizes specifically designed ankle boots with hooks that are secured over a chin-up bar, usually placed in a doorway. While the cost and the utilization of a small space are desirable, the boots unfortunately allow inversion with extended hips and knees. They place stress on the joints of the lower extremities and allow no variation in inversion (i.e., they provide all-or-nothing inversion). In addition, the system may be difficult for the patient to get in and out of and

may be dangerous if the chin-up bar is not secured properly.

In spite of the disadvantages of each type of inversion, all are viable means of achieving inversion when chosen carefully and when patient education is adequate.

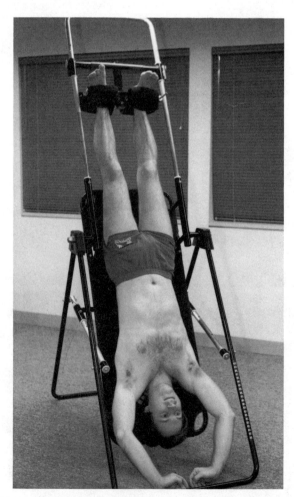

Figure 13.35. Standard inversion table allows varying degrees of inversion and a comfortable pumping action.

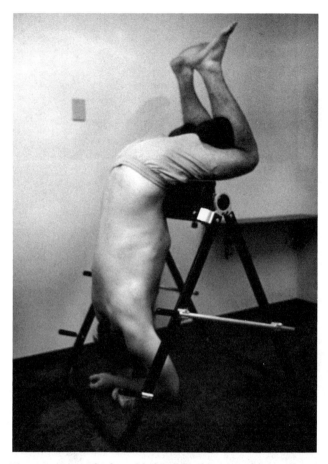

Figure 13.36. Thigh and behind-the-knee inversion reduces the lumbar lordosis while it tractions.

Flexion-Distraction

Flexion-distraction (Fig. 13.38) is achieved with a specialized table on which the patient is placed in a prone position with the ankles strapped to the caudal end of the table. The table is then unlocked, so

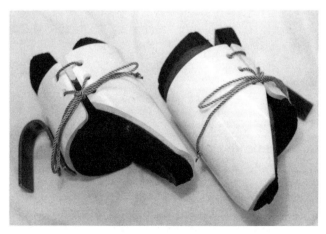

Figure 13.37. Inversion boots are placed around the ankles and hooked to a chin-up bar to provide an inexpensive form of traction.

that the lower half of the table is allowed to flex. By placing cephalad and anterior pressure on the vertebra above the motion segment being treated, very specific distraction is applied to the motion segment involved. Many tables can also rotate and/or sidebend their lower half, allowing even more specifically therapeutic distraction to the segment. Traction is applied in an intermittent fashion, creating a pumping effect.

Flexion-distraction can be a very effective method for the treatment of acute and chronic intervertebral disc protrusion (medial and lateral), facet syndrome, spondylolisthesis, retrolisthesis, discogenic spondyloarthrosis, anterior or posterior innominate, and sacrum inferiority (167).

Results from a similar type of treatment, autotraction, have been reported by Gertrude Lind. With autotraction, traction is generated by the patient's arms pulling against a fixed pelvic belt in a variety of positions. Lind reported good results in 1 week in 16 of 20 patients with confirmed disc lesions awaiting surgery. She further reported satisfactory results in 929 of 1023 patients with low back pain and/or sciatica (168).

Cox, using the flexion-distraction technique, found in 43 cases of medial disc protrusion that 34 responded to this treatment; in 57 cases of lateral disc protrusion, 55 responded to his treatment, alleviating the need for surgery (167).

Effects

Suction. A subatmospheric pressure is created when two vertebrae are pulled part, causing a centripetal force on the disc.

Distraction. The distance between the articular surfaces increases with sufficient traction. Studies have shown that traction of 10 lbs for the atlantooccipital and atlantoaxial joints (169), 20–50 lbs for the remainder of the cervical spine (170–172), and 80–200 lbs for the lumbar spine are needed for measurable joint separation (173).

Ligamentous tautening. The anterior and posterior longitudinal ligaments are stretched, causing further centripetal force on the disc.

Relaxation of the musculature. Cyriax reported EMG silence 3 minutes after continuous traction (174), while Nosse reported maximum EMG activity reduction in a minimum of 70 sec with inversion of healthy male subjects (175).

Widening of the intervertebral foramen.

Straightening of the spinal curves.

Indications

Intervertebral disc protrusion, medial and lateral;
Facet syndrome;
Nerve root compression;
Spondylolisthesis;
Retrolisthesis;
Discogenic spondyloarthrosis;

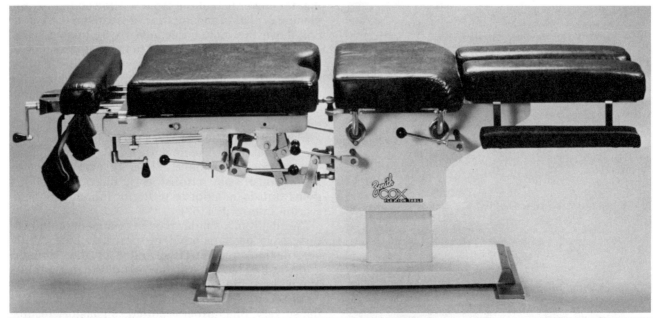

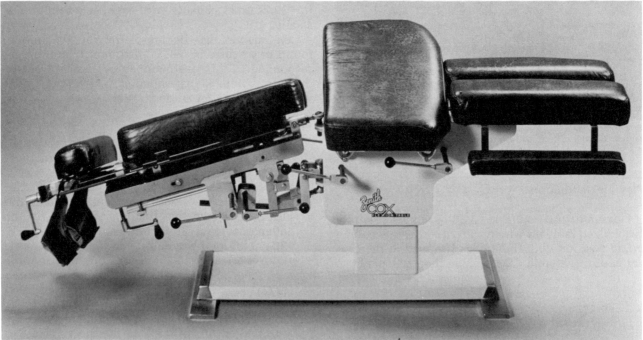

Figure 13.38. Flexion-distraction of the lumbar spine allows traction and flexion with or without rotation and sidebend at a specific level of the spine. (Photo courtesy of Williams Manufacturing.)

Anterior or posterior innominate;
Sacrum inferiority;
Early scoliosis;
Muscular spasm.

Indications specific to inversion:

Visceroptosis;
Organ prolapse;
Uterine anteversion;
Varicosities;

Pulmonary congestion.

Contraindications

Structural disease secondary to tumor or infection;
Vascular compromise—severe hypertension, atherosclerosis, phlebitis, angina, history of stroke or transient ischemic attack;
Acute sprains, strains, and other musculoskeletal inflammatory processes;
Pregnancy.

Osteoporosis and other bone-weakening conditions;

Claustrophobia;foContraindications specific to inversion:

Hiatal hernia;
Ankle, knee, or hip joint dysfunction (some units);
Anatomical short leg (some units);
Middle ear disease, motion sickness, dizziness, vertigo.

Application

Application of traction is unique, depending upon the specific traction unit being used. However, some generalities can be made for cervical and lumbar traction.

Cervical Traction

Maximum separation of the cervical vertebrae occurs when the cervical spine is flexed to 25 to 30°, except for the atlantooccipital and atlantoaxial joints, which should be tractioned with a 0° angle of pull (176).

The patient should feel more pull on the posterior aspect of the occiput than on the mandible. Changing the angle of pull, changing strap tension, or removing dentures may be helpful. A unique cervical traction attachment is available which eliminates traction on the mandible altogether.

Research has shown that supine traction is superior to sitting traction (177, 178).

Lumbar Traction

1. In the supine position, the hips and knees should be flexed sufficiently to minimize the lumbar lordosis.
2. Rope angle should be approximately 0°.
3. A counterharness is necessary to stabilize the upper body. Usually a thoracic harness is used.
4. Some method of reducing friction is desirable. A split table or table with rollers is commonly used.
5. Thoracic and lumbar belts must fit snugly. Placing the belt directly against the skin may help reduce slippage.

MASSAGE

Definition

Massage: "certain manipulations of the soft tissues of the body; these manipulations are most effectively performed with the hands, and are administered for the purpose of producing effects on the nervous and muscular systems and the local and general circulation of the blood and lymph" (179).

Introduction

Massage was first described in 2696 BC by Hwang Ti. Hippocrates was the first to advocate massage in a centripetal direction, presumably based on clinical observation, as the circulation of the blood was not to be discovered by Harvey for another 2000 years (179). The Greeks and Romans continued the practice of massage until the fall of the Roman Empire. The art of massage was nearly lost during the Middle Ages (180), but was again revived in the 16th century by a French physician Ambroïse Paré (181). In the latter 19th century, Metzzer of Holland and Ling of Sweden helped to formulate a scientific system of massage. World War I and World War II were partially responsible for the increased use of massage in the United States (180).

Today massage remains a useful treatment for many conditions, although its popularity waxes and wanes. There is no doubt that the laying on of the hands can have tremendous physical as well as psychological benefits and can be used not only for the treatment of disease but also for the maintenance of overall well-being.

Effects

Removal of dry skin and opening of sweat and sebaceous glands;
Mechanically assisting the flow of blood and lymph to increase circulation and reduce edema;
Maintenance of muscle flexibility and viability;
Breaking up scar tissue, adhesions, and fibrosis;
Sedation;
Stimulation;
Mobilization of lung secretions.

Indications

Muscle spasm;
Local edema;
Myofascial pain syndrome. (see Chapter 12);
Adhesions, scar tissue;
Following cast removal or other immobilization;
Tendinitis, tenosynovitis;
Lung congestion;
Joint contracture.

Contraindications

Acute circulatory disturbances (e.g., phlebitis or lymphangitis);
Acute inflammation;
Malignancy;
Edema secondary to heart decompensation, kidney disease, embolus, obstruction of lymph channels, thrombus;
Skin conditions such as acne, eczema, furuncles, ulcerations, acute burns, wounds;
Communicable disease;
Hyperesthesia of the skin.

Specific Methods of Application

Effleurage

Effleurage consists of a stroking motion. Superficial effleurage creates a reflex increase in circulation, while deeper effleurage creates a reflex as well as a mechanical increase in circulation. Strokes should parallel the direction of the muscle fibers and should be heavier in the centripetal direction (i.e., toward the heart). Massage should begin with light pressure, progress to heavier pressure as tolerated, and terminate with light pressure.

Petrissage

Petrissage consists of a kneading or rolling motion. It has the effect of mechanically milking the muscles. The motion is performed either between the thumb and fingers or chiefly with the palm. Pressure can vary from light to heavy. Strokes are either in a centripetal direction or transverse to the muscle fibers (179).

Rolfing

Rolfing is a deep massage that strives to separate the fascia between muscles. It is believed that gravity will have a more beneficial effect on posture when the muscles are free to move more independently on each other.

Friction Massage

Friction massage is used to break up superficial and/or deep adhesions of muscle or other soft tissue. No lotion is used. The fingers or thumb are placed on the skin and not allowed to slide on the skin. Small circular or linear strokes are used to loosen the tissue beneath the skin.

Transverse Friction Massage

Transverse friction massage is a specific type of friction massage that is used to treat tendinitis or tenosynovitis. Friction massage is performed perpendicular to the tendon sheath, causing the tendon to separate from the sheath and slide through it more easily.

Tapotement

Tapotement includes tapping, slapping, cupping, and hacking motions. It is useful for increasing circulation to an area and for postural drainage to increase the release of abnormal secretions from the lungs.

Pneumatic Massage

Pneumatic massage utilizes a machine that provides intermittent air pressure. The air is injected into a sleeve that is placed on an extremity. Pneumatic massage is useful for the reduction of extremity edema.

ORTHOTICS

Definitions

Orthotics: the field of knowledge relating to orthoses and their use.

Orthosis: an orthopaedic appliance or apparatus used to support, align, prevent, or correct deformities or to improve the function of movable parts of the body.

Mechanism of Action

Orthoses act to immobilize or stabilize a joint or joints. Orthoses with minimal support (e.g., elastic or cloth), may serve to merely keep the area warm or remind the patient to be cautious of the injured part. More rigid orthoses with plastic or metal stays are needed to provide adequate joint immobilization or stabilization. Orthoses may also be used to stimulate skin sensory receptors that facilitate motor nerves to increase muscle tone and strength in cases of muscle imbalance.

Effects

Allows relaxation of muscle, joint, ligament, or other soft tissue.
Stabilizes a joint to allow more functional motion of more distal joints.
Facilitates muscle tone.

Indications

Acute soft tissue injury;
Joint instability;
Muscular imbalance.

Contraindications

None known.

Application

The orthosis should be tailored and fit to the patient so the maximum support occurs where it is needed, and adjacent areas are not unnecessarily restricted.
The orthosis should be applied firmly without compromise of circulation.
The patient should be able to don the orthosis independently, unless a suitable assistant has been instructed in its application.
In the case of acute soft tissue injury, patients should be instructed to gradually decrease the use of the orthosis as they are able. Excessive use of an orthosis may lead to atrophy of the muscle, increased fibrosis formation, contracture, vascular stress, and/or an increased dependence on that orthosis.

ASSISTIVE DEVICES FOR WALKING

Introduction

There are a variety of assistive devices available to decrease weight bearing on one or both lower extremities or to merely assist with balance. An assistive device can increase a patient's self-confidence and/or independence tremendously. It is important that the proper assistive device be chosen, that it be properly fit, and that the patient be educated as to its use.

Types of Assistive Devices

Crutches

Uses. Crutches are used to decrease or remove weightbearing of one lower extremity or to add support when both lower extremities are weak.

Fitting.

1. Crutch tips are placed about 9 inches in front of the patient's feet and 9 inches out to the side.
2. The patient stands erect with shoulders relaxed.
3. Two or three fingers should fit between the axilla and the axillary pad.
4. With the patient's arms at the side, the handgrips should be positioned at wrist level, allowing a 30° elbow bend when the handgrips are held.

Gaits.

Four-Point Gait. Used when both legs are weak. Right crutch is advanced first, then left foot, then left crutch, then right foot.

Two-Point Gait. Used when both legs are weak and a faster gait is desired.

Right crutch and left foot are advanced at the same time, then left crutch and right foot are advanced together.

Three-Point Gait. Used when decreased weight is desired on one leg. Weight-bearing status may be:

a. Weightbearing to tolerance: the patient is allowed to take as much weight as is comfortable.
b. Partial weightbearing: 5–95% weightbearing on th affected leg.
c. Toe touch: for balance only.
d. Nonweightbearing: affected leg is held off the ground entirely.

Crutches are advanced first, then the affected leg, then the normal leg.

Swing-to Gait. Used when both legs are very weak. Legs are usually braced to keep knees in extension.

Crutches are advanced first, then both legs are swung to the crutches.

Swing-through Gait. Used when the patient described in the swing-to-gait gets stronger and wants to move faster.

Crutches are advanced first, then both legs are swung past the crutches.

Walker

Uses. A walker is used in place of crutches for an older less stable patient. Walkers stand up by themselves and are often easier to use around the house.

Fitting. The patient stands erect with shoulders relaxed. With the patient's arms to the side, handgrips should come to the patient's wrist, allowing a 30° elbow bend when the handgrips are held.

Gait. See three point crutch gait.

Accessories. A folding walker is good for storing or carrying in the car. Wheels on the front legs eliminate the need to lift the walker. Most patients prefer wheels.

Cane

Use. A cane is used for balance, not for weightbearing.

Fitting. See fitting of a walker.

Gait. The cane is carried on the side contralateral to the leg being supported and is advanced before or with the affected leg (i.e., cane, then the affected leg, then the normal leg).

Quad Cane

A cane with four small legs on the bottom.

Uses. A quad cane is used when more support than offered by a straight cane is needed and/or when it is desirable for the cane to be able to stand by itelf.

Fitting. See fitting for walker.

Gait. See gait for a cane. A quad cane requires more space and is a little more awkward to use than a straight cane.

APPROPRIATE PHYSIOLOGICAL THERAPEUTICS FOR DIFFERENT STAGES OF TISSUE REPAIR

Introduction

When a tissue is injured, via either frank direct trauma or microtrauma, that tissue will generally go through recognized stages of pathophysiological changes. Each tissue will have its own timetable for progressing through the stages, so tissues in a single area may be in different stages of change, though one stage usually predominates.

It is important to coordinate the doctor's choice of physiological therapeutics with the correct stage of tissue repair in order to stop and/or reverse the process and allow the tissues to resume a more normal physiological function. Treating a patient for a stage through which the tissues have passed is futile, while treating for a stage that has not yet been reached may prove to be injurious and detrimental to the patient's recovery.

Stages of Tissue Repair and the Appropriate Therapeutics

Stage of Hyperemia or Active Congestion

Rest: to reduce further damage;
Immobilization: a splint or brace may be appropriate;
Elevation: to reduce edema;
Ice packs: to vasoconstrict;
High-voltage therapy: at subcontraction level, to reduce edema and relieve pain;
Interferential current: at subcontraction level, to reduce edema and relieve pain;
TENS or microamperage current: to relieve pain;
Low-voltage galvanism: positive, to vasoconstrict and harden tissues;

Ultrasound: pulsed, for its micromassage effect without heat;

Iontophoresis: for various effects (e.g., with magnesium sulfate, to reduce edema).

Stage of Passive Congestion

Contrast heat and cold: for a pumping action of the blood vessels;

Gentle, active range of motion: to maintain mobility;

Light effleurage: to reduce edema;

Gentle manipulation and/or manual traction: to maintain mobility;

High-voltage therapy: at subcontraction or mild contraction level, to relieve pain and reduce edema;

Interferential current: at subcontraction or mild contraction level, to relieve pain and reduce edema;

Sine wave: gentle surging or pulsing, to reduce edema;

Microamperage current: to relieve pain;

Ultrasound: pulsed, for its micromassage effect;

Low-voltage galvanism: alternating positive and negative, for the pumping action of the blood vessels.

Stage of Consolidation and/or Formation of Fibrinous Coagulate

Superficial moist heat: (e.g., hot packs), for vasodilation;

Moderate active exercise: to free coagulate and early adhesions, maintain muscle tone and joint mobility;

Moderate effleurage: to free coagulates and early adhesions;

High-voltage therapy: at contraction level, to increase circulation and maintain muscle tone;

Interferential current: at contraction level, to increase circulation and maintain muscle tone;

Microamperage current: to relieve pain and other symptoms;

Ultrasound: continuous, for vasodilation, softening of ground substance;

Sine wave: surging or pulsating, to maintain muscle tone;

Low-voltage galvanism: (negative), to vasodilate.

Stage of Fibroblastic Activity and Fibrosis

Deep heat: (e.g., diathermy), to vasodilate;

Petrissage or friction massage: to break down fibrous adhesions;

Vigorous active and/or resistive exercise: to maintain or increase muscle and joint viability, break down adhesions, increase elasticity;

Vigorous manipulation: to increase joint mobility, break down adhesions;

Intermittent mechanical traction: to increase joint mobility, break down adhesions;

High-voltage therapy at strong but comfortable contraction level, to vasodilate and increase muscle tone, may tetanize muscle to relieve spasm;

Interferential current: at strong but comfortable contraction level, to vasodilate and increase muscle tone;

Microamperage current: to relieve symptoms;

Ultrasound: continuous, to vasodilate and soften tissues;

Sine wave: surging or tetanizing, to maintain muscle tone or relieve muscle spasm;

Low-voltage galvanism: negative, to vasodilate;

Iontophoresis: (e.g., potassium iodide to antisclerose).

This section was adapted from R. D. Stonebrink, Synopsis of Physiotherapeutic Procedures in Relation to Disease Processes, Peer Review Procedures of the ACA Council on Physiotherapy.

References

1. Jaskoviak PA, Schafer RC: *Applied Physiotherapy.* Arlington, Associated Chiropractic Academic Press, 1986, pp VII, 87–118, 152–161.
2. Brandstetter C: Physiotherapy council report. *ACA J Chiro* 12:27–28, 1975.
3. Schafer RC (ed): *American Chiropractic Association Basic Procedural Manual,* ed 3. Des Moines, Associated Chiropractic Academic Press, 1980, pp X-1, X-2.
4. Ransom JF: The origins of chiropractic physiological therapeutics: Howard, Forester and Schulze. *Chiro Hist* 4(1):47–52, 1984.
5. Ramby, D: The use of physical therapy in chiropractic. *Digest Chiro Econ* 23(2):36–37, 1980.
6. Nwuga VCB: Relative therapeutic efficacy of vertebral manipulation and conventional treatment in back pain management. *Am J Phys Med* 61(6):273–278, 1982.
7. Malik DD, Slack JM, Brooks S, Wald L: Effectiveness of chiropractic adjustment and physical therapy to treat spinal subluxation. *ACA J Chiro,* 20(6):63–69, 1983.
8. Licht S: History of therapeutic heat and cold. In Lehmann JF (ed): *Therapeutic Heat and Cold,* ed 3. Baltimore, Williams & Wilkins, 1982, pp 5–7, 28–30.
9. Wadsworth H, Chanmugam APP: *Electrophysical Agents in Physiotherapy,* ed 2. Marrickville, NSW (Australia), Science Press, 1983, pp 23–24, 73, 113–115, 117.
10. Lehmann JF, deLateur BJ: Therapeutic heat. In Lehmann JF (ed): *Therapeutic Heat and Cold,* ed 3. Baltimore, Williams & Wilkins, 1982, pp 414–420.
11. Bierman W: Therapeutic use of cold. *JAMA* 157(14): 1189–1192, 1955.
12. Hocutt JE: Cryotherapy. *Am Fam Physician* 23(3):141–144, 1981.
13. Tepperman PS, Devlin M: Therapeutic heat and cold: a practitioner's guide. *Postgrad Med* 73(1):69–76, 1983.
14. Landen BR: Heat or cold for the relief of low back pain? *Phys Ther* 47(12):1126–1128, 1967.
15. Lewis T: Observations on some normal and injurious effects of cold upon skin and underlying tissues: I. Reactions to cold, and injury of normal skin. *Br Med J* 2:795–797, 1941.
16. Coulter JS: Physical therapy: heat and cold. In Glasser OV (ed): *Medical Physics,* ed 2. Chicago, Year Book, 1944, pp 1043–1054.
17. Lewis T: Observations upon the reactions of the vessels of the human skin to cold. *Heart* 15:177–208, 1930.

18. Gucker T: The use of heat and cold in orthopedics. In Licht S (ed): *Therapeutic Heat and Cold*, ed 2. Baltimore, Waverly Press, 1965, pp 399–400.

19. Zankel HT: Effect of physical agents on motor conduction velocity of the ulnar nerve. *Arch Phys Med* 47(12):787–792, 1966.

20. Fox, RH: Local cooling in man. *Br Med Bull* 17(1):14–18, 1961.

21. Douglas WW, Malcolm JL: The effect of localized cooling on conduction in cat nerves. *J Physiol* 130:53–71, 1955.

22. Eldred E, Lindsley DF, Buchwald JS: The effect of cooling on mammalian muscle spindles. *Exp Neurol* 2:144–157, 1960.

23. Miglietta O: Action of cold on spasticity. *Am J Phys Med* 52(4):198–205, 1973.

24. Wolf SL, Basmajian JV: Intramuscular temperatures changes deep to localized cutaneous cold stimulation. *Phys Ther* 53:1284–1288, 1973.

25. Bierman W, Friedlander M: The penetrative effect of cold. *Arch Phys Ther* 21:585–592, 1940.

26. Lehmann JF, deLateur BJ: Cryotherapy. In Lehmann JF (ed): *Therapeutic Heat and Cold*, ed 3. Baltimore, Williams & Wilkins, 1982, p 591.

27. Melzack R, Jeans ME, Stratford JG, Monks RC: Ice massage and transcutaneous electrical stimulation: comparison of treatment for low back pain. *Pain* 9(2):209–217, 1980.

28. Ellis M: The relief of pain by cooling of the skin. *Br Med J* 1:250–252, 1961.

29. Janssen CW, Waaler E: Body temperature, antibody formation and inflammatory response. *Acta Pathol Microbiol Immunol Scand* 69:557–566, 1967.

30. McMaster WC, Liddle S: Cryotherapy influence on posttraumatic limb edema. *Clin Orthop* 150:283–287, 1980.

31. Matsen FA III, Questad K, Matsen AL: The effect of local cooling on postfracture swelling. *Clin Orthop* 109:201–206, 1975.

32. Jezdinsky J, Marek J, Ochonsky P: Effects of local cold and heat therapy on traumatic oedema of the rat hind paw. *Acta Univ Olomuc Fac Med* 66:185–201, 1973.

33. Olson JE, Stravino VD: A review of cryotherapy. *Phys Ther* 52(8):840–853, 1972.

34. Mennell JM: The therapeutic use of cold. *J Am Osteopath Assoc* 74:1146–1158, 1975.

35. Levine MG, Kabat H, Knott M, Voss DE: Relaxation of spasticity by physiological technics. *Arch Phys Med* 35:214–223, 1954.

36. Knutsson E: Topical cryotherapy in spasticity. *Scand J Rehabil Med* 2:159–163, 1970.

37. Petajan JH, Watts N: Effects of cooling on the triceps surae reflex. *Am J Phys Med* 41:240–251, 1962.

38. Hartviksen K: Ice therapy in spasticity. *Acta Neurol Scand* [suppl3] 38:79–84, 1962.

39. Viel E: Treatment of spasticity by exposure to cold. *Phys Ther Rev* 39(9):598–599, 1959.

40. Lippold OCJ, Nicholls JG, Redfearn JWT: A study of the afferent discharge produced by cooling a mammalian muscle spindle. *J Physiol* 153:218–231, 1960.

41. Ottoson D: The effects of temperature on the isolated muscle spindle. *J Physiol* 180:636–648, 1965.

42. Hocutt JE, Jaffe R, Rylander CR, Beebe JK: Cryotherapy in ankle sprains. *Am J Sports Med* 10(5):316–319, 1982.

43. Basur RL, Shephard E, Mouzas GL: A cooling method in the treatment of ankle sprains. *Practitioner* 216:708–711, 1976.

44. Lehmann JF, deLateur BJ: Cryotherapy. In Lehmann JF (ed): *Therapeutic Heat and Cold*, ed 3. Baltimore, Williams & Wilkins, 1982, pp 594–596.

45. McMaster WC, Liddle S, Waugh TR: Laboratory evaluation of various cold therapy modalities. *Am J Sports Med* 6(5):291–294, 1978.

46. Geddes LA: A short history of the electrical stimulation of excitable tissue including electrotherapeutic application. *Physiologist* 27(suppl):s1-s47, 1984.

47. Brighton CT, Black J, Friedenberg ZB, Esterhai JL, Day LJ, Connolly JF: A multicenter study of the treatment of non-union with constant direct current. *J Bone Joint Surg* (AM) 63A(5):2–13, 1981.

48. Brighton CT: Current concepts review: the treatment of non-unions with electricity. *J Bone Joint Surg* (AM) 63A:847–851, 1981.

49. Steinberg ME, Brighton CT, Steinberg DR, Tooze SE, Hayken GD: Treatment of avascular necrosis of the femoral head by a combination of bone grafting, decompression, and electrical stimulation. *Clin Orthop* 186:137–153, 1984.

50. Paterson DC, Carter RF, Tilbury RF, Ludbrook J, Savage JP: The effects of varying current levels of electrical stimulation. *Clin Orthop* 169:303–312, 1982.

51. Quirion-deGirardi C, Seaborne D: *High Voltage Galvanic Stimulation (HVGS)*. Montreal, University of Montreal, 1983, pp 1–58.

52. Newton RA, Karselis TC: Skin pH following high voltage pulsed galvanic stimulation. *Phys Ther* 63(10):1593–1596, 1983.

53. Howson DC: Peripheral neural excitability: implications for transcutaneous electrical nerve stimulation. *Phys Ther* 58(12):1467–1473, 1978.

54. Andersson SA: Pain Control by Sensory Stimulation. In Bonica JJ, (ed): *Advances in Pain Research and Therapy*. New York, Raven Press, 1979, vol 3, pp 569–585.

55. Cheng RSS, Pomeranz B: Electroacupuncture analgesia could be mediated by at least two pain-relieving mechanisms: endorphin and non-endorphin systems. *Life Sci* 25(23):1957–1962, 1979.

56. Alon G: *High Voltage Stimulation (High Voltage Pulsating Direct Current): A Monograph*. Hixson, Tennessee, Chattanooga Corporation, 1984, pp 1–18.

57. Baker LL, Yeh C, Wilson D, Waters RL: Electrical stimulation of wrist and fingers for hemiplegic patients. *Phys Ther* 59:1495–1499, 1979.

58. Eriksson E, Haggmark T: Comparison of isometric muscle training and electrical stimulation supplementing isometric muscle training in the recovery after major knee ligament surgery. *Am J Sports Med* 7(3):169–171, 1979.

59. Wakim KG: Influence of frequency of electrical stimulation on circulation. *Arch Phys Med Rehabil* 34:291–295, 1953.

60. Thurman BF, Christian EL: Response of a serious circulatory lesion to electrical stimulation. *Phys Ther* 51(10):1107–1110, 1971.

61. Akers TK, Gabrielson AL: The effect of high voltage galvanic stimulation on the rate of healing of decubitus ulcers. *Biomed Sci Instrum* 20:99–100, 1984.

62. Harrington EL: The use of high voltage galvanic stimulation for wound healing in a long-term care setting. *Phys Ther Forum* 5(30):1–4, 1986.

63. Katzberg AA: The induction of cellular orientation by low-level electrical currents. In Liboff AR, Rinaldi RA (eds): Electrically mediated growth mechanisms in living systems. *Ann NY Acad Sci* 238:445–450, 1974.

64. Harrington DB, Meyer R, Klein RM: Effects of small amounts of electric current at the cellular level. In Liboff AR, Rinaldi RA (eds): Electrically mediated growth mechanisms in living systems. *Ann NY Acad Sci* 238:300–306, 1974.

65. Alon G, Bainbridge J, Croson G, Genendlis R, Hurlon D, Meany J, Simon M, Smith AR Jr: High-voltage pulsed direct current effects on peripheral blood flow. *Phys Ther* 61(5):734, 1981.

66. Griffin JE, Karselis TC: *Physical Agents for Physical Therapists*. Springfield, IL, Charles C Thomas, 1982, p 37, 177–182, 280, 287–288, 294, 308.

67. Davis RV: Clinical electrical muscle stimulation. *Am Chiro* May/June, p 48, 1982.

68. Laughman RK, Youdas JW, Garrett TR, Chao EYS: Strength changes in the normal quadriceps femoris muscle as a result of electrical stimulation. *Phys Ther* 63(4):494–499, 1983.

69. Currier DP, Mann R: Muscular strength development by electrical stimulation in healthy individuals. *Phys Ther* 63(16):915–921, 1983.

70. Miles J: Electrical stimulation for the relief of pain. *Ann R Coll Surg Engl* 66(2):108–112, 1984.

71. Melzack R, Wall PD: Pain mechanisms: a new theory. *Science* 150:971–979, 1965.

72. Paxton SL: Clinical uses of TENS: a survey of physical therapists. *Phys Ther* 60(1):38–44, 1980.

73. Kerr FWL: Pain: a central inhibitory balance theory. *Mayo Clin Proc* 50:685–690, 1975.

74. Lenhart JP: Transcutaneous electrical nerve stimulation (TENS): a review. *Digest Chiro Econ* 26(4):59–62, 1984.

75. Melzack R: *The Puzzle of Pain.* New York, Basic Books, 1973, pp 142–143, 183–190.

76. Andersson SA, Ericson T, Holmgren E, Lindgvist G: Electro-acupuncture: effect on pain threshold measured with electrical stimulation of teeth. *Brain Res* 63:393–396, 1973.

77. Sjolund B, Eriksson M: Electro-acupuncture and endogenous morphines. *Lancet* 2:1085, 1976.

78. Sjolund BH, Eriksson MBE: The influence of naloxone on analgesia produced by peripheral conditioning stimulation. *Brain Res* 173:295–301, 1979.

79. Salar G, Job I, Mingrino S, Bosio A, Trabucchi M: Effect of transcutaneous electrotherapy on CSF β-endorphin content in patients without pain problems. *Pain* 10(2):169–172, 1981.

80. O'Brien WJ, Rutan FM, Sanborn C, Omer GE: Effect of transcutaneous electrical nerve stimulation on human blood β-endorphin levels. *Phys Ther* 64(19):1367–1374, 1984.

81. Langley GB, Sheppeard H, Johnson M, Wigley RD: The analgesic effects of transcutaneous electrical nerve stimulation and placebo in chronic pain patients: a double-blind non-crossover comparison. *Rheumatol Int* 4(3):119–123, 1984.

82. Strassburg HM, Krainick JU, Thoden U: Influence of transcutaneous nerve stimulation (TNS) on acute pain. *J Neurol* 217:1–10, 1977.

83. Melzack R, Vetere P, Finch L: Transcutaneous electrical nerve stimulation for low back pain. A comparison of TENS and massage for pain and range of motion. *Phys Ther* 63(4):489–493, 1983.

84. Lewis D, Lewis B, Sturrock RD: Transcutaneous electrical nerve stimulation in osteoarthrosis: a therapeutic alternative? *Ann Rheum Dis* 43(1):47–49, 1984.

85. Mannheimer C, Carlsson C: The analgesic effect of transcutaneous electrical nerve stimulation (TNS) in patients with rheumatoid arthritis: a comparative study of different pulse patterns. *Pain* 6:329–334, 1979.

86. Abelson K, Langley GB, Sheppeard H, Vlieg M, Wigley RD: Transcutaneous electrical nerve stimulation in rheumatoid arthritis. *NZ Med J* 96(727):156–158, 1983.

87. Moore DE, Blacker HM: How effective is TENS for chronic pain? *Am J Nurs* 83(8):1175–1177, 1983.

88. Roberts CW: Transcutaneous nerve stimulation: an outline of the theory and application. *Bull Eur Chiro Union* 28(3):40–44, 1980.

89. Loeser JD, Black RG, Christman A: Relief of pain by transcutaneous stimulation. *J Neurosurg* 42:308–314, 1975.

90. Lundeberg T: The pain suppressive effect of vibratory stimulation and transcutaneous electrical nerve stimulation (TENS) as compared to aspirin. *Brain Res* 294(2):201–209, 1984.

91. Stamp JM: A review of transcutaneous electrical nerve stimulation (TENS). *J Med Eng Technol* 6(3):99–103, 1982.

92. Fried T, Johnson R, McCracken W: Transcutaneous electrical nerve stimulation: its role in the control of chronic pain. *Arch Phys Med Rehabil* 65:228–231, 1984.

93. Thorsteinsson G, Stonnington HH, Stillwell GK, Elveback LR: Transcutaneous electrical stimulation: a double-blind trial of its efficacy for pain. *Arch Phys Med Rehabil* 58:8–13, 1977.

94. Stonnington HH, Stillwell GK, Ebersold MJ, Thorsteinsson G, Laws ER: Transcutaneous electrical stimulation for chronic pain relief: a pilot study. *Minn Med* 59:681–683, 1976.

95. Reynolds AC, Abram SE, Anderson RA, Vasudevan SV, Lynch NT: Chronic pain therapy with transcutaneous electrical nerve stimulation: predictive value of questionnaires. *Arch Phys Med Rehabil* 64(7):311–313, 1983.

96. Taylor AG, West BA, Simon B, Skelton J, Rowlingson JC: How effective is TENS for acute pain? *Am J Nurs* 83(8):1171–1174, 1983.

97. Hymes AC, Raab DE, Yonehiro EG, Nelson GD, Printy AL: Acute pain control by electrostimulation: a preliminary report. *Adv Neurol* 4:761–767, 1974.

98. Augustinsson LE, Bohlin P, Bundsen P, Carlsson CA, Forssman L, Sjoberg P, Tyreman NO: Pain relief during delivery by transcutaneous electrical nerve stimulation. *Pain* 4:59–65, 1977.

99. Rooney SM, Jain S, Goldiner PL: Effect of transcutaneous nerve stimulation on postoperative pain after thoracotomy. *Anesth Analg* 62(11):1010–1012, 1983.

100. Cotter DJ: Overview of transcutaneous electrical nerve stimulation for treatment of acute postoperative pain. *Med Instrum* 17(14):289–292, 1983.

101. Avellanosa AM, West CR: Experience with transcutaneous electrical nerve stimulation for relief of intractable pain in cancer patients. *J Med* 13(3):203–213, 1982.

102. Smith MJ, Hutchins RC, Hehenberger D: Transcutaneous neural stimulation use in postoperative knee rehabilitation. *Am J Sports Med* 11(2):75–82, 1983.

103. Bodenheim R, Bennett JH: Reversal of a Sudeck's atrophy by the adjunctive use of transcutaneous electrical nerve stimulation: a case report. *Phys Ther* 63(8):1287–1288, 1983.

104. Lampe GN: Introduction to the use of transcutaneous electrical nerve stimulation devices. *Phys Ther* 58(12):1450–1454, 1978.

105. Howson DC: Peripheral neural excitability: implications for transcutaneous electrical nerve stimulation. *Phys Ther* 58(12):1467–1473, 1978.

106. Andersson SA, Hansson G, Holmgren E, Renberg O: Evaluation of the pain suppressive effect of different frequencies of peripheral electrical stimulation in chronic pain conditions. *Acta Orthop Scand* 47:149–157, 1976.

107. Eriksson MBE, Sjolund BH, Nielzen S: Long term results of peripheral conditioning stimulation as an analgesic measure in chronic pain. *Pain* 6:335–347, 1979.

108. Wolf SL, Gersh MR, Rao VR: Examination of electrode placements and stimulating parameters in treating chronic pain with conventional transcutaneous electrical nerve stimulation (TENS). *Pain* 11:37–47, 1981.

109. Berlant SR: Method of determining optimal stimulation sites for transcutaneous electrical nerve stimulation. *Phys Ther* 64(6): 924–928, 1984.

110. Mannheimer JS: Electrode placements for transcutaneous electrical nerve stimulation. *Phys Ther* 58(12):1455–1462, 1978.

111. Finneran J: The important parameters for effective TENS usage. *Phys Ther Forum* 5(17):1–3, 1986.

112. Becker RO, Murray DG: The electrical control system regulating fracture healing in amphibians. *Clin Orthop* 73:169–198, 1970.

113. Harrington DB, Becker RO: Electrical stimulation of RNA and protein synthesis in the frog erythrocyte. *Exp Cell Res* 76:95–98, 1973.

114. Pilla AA: Electrochemical information transfer at living cell membranes. *Ann NY Acad Sci* 238:149–170, 1974.

115. Szczudlik A, Lypka A: Plasma immunoreactive β-endorphin and enkephalin concentration in healthy subjects before and after electroacupuncture. *Acupunct Electrother Res* 8:127–137, 1983.

116. Mladenoff E: Sports chiropractic: acupuncture treatment of shin splints. *Am Chiro* May/June, p 42, 1982.

117. Food and Drug Administration: *Compliance Policy Guides* #7124.11, Mar 1, 1983, Rockville, MD, Food and Drug Administration.

118. Roppel RM, Mitchell F Jr: Skin points of anomalously low electric resistance: current-voltage characteristics and relationships to peripheral stimulation therapies. *J Am Osteopath Assoc* 74:877–878, 1975.
119. Matsumoto T, Hayes MF Jr: Acupuncture, electric phenomenon of the skin, and postvagotomy gastrointestinal atony. *Am J Surg* 125:176–180, 1973.
120. Fox EJ, Melzack R: Transcutaneous electrical stimulation and acupuncture: comparison of treatment for low-back pain. *Pain* 2:141–148, 1976.
121. Melzack R: Prolonged relief of pain by brief, intense transcutaneous somatic stimulation. ·*Pain* 1(14):357–373, 1975.
122. Melzack R: Phantom limb pain: implications for treatment of pathologic pain. *Anesthesiology* 35(4):409–419, 1971.
123. Bannerman RH: Acupuncture: the WHO view. *World Health* 28:24–29, 1979.
124. Veglia MP: "High tech" acupuncture: a new look at the old Ryodoraku therapy and its role in today's technology. *Am Chiro* Mar/Apr, p 6–8, 1984.
125. Willie, CD: Interferential therapy. *Physiotherapy* 55(12):503–505, 1969.
126. Ganne JM: Interferential therapy. *Aust J Physiother* 22(3):101–110, 1976.
127. Ganne JM, Speculand B, Mayne LH, Goss AN: Interferential therapy to promote union of mandibular fractures. *Aust NZ J Surg* 49(1):81-83, 1979.
128. Couch RT: *Omnistim. Interferential current therapy: theory, rationale, and clinical applications,* (brochure). Topeka, Kansas, Physio Technology, 1985, pp 1–11.
129. Savage B: *Interferential Therapy.* Boston, Faber and Faber, 1984, pp 17, 53, 58, 61.
130. Nikolova L: Physiotherapeutische rehabilitation bei knochenbruchkomplikationen. *Munch Med Wochenschr* 111(11):592–599, 1969.
131. Nikolova-Troeva L: Interferenzstromtherapie bei distorsionen, kontusionen und luxationen der gelenke. *Munch Med Wochenschr* 109(11):579–582, 1967.
132. McQuire WA: Electrotherapy and exercises for stress incontinence and urinary frequency. *Physiotherapy* 61(10):305–307, 1975.
133. Schoeler H: Physical block of the sympathetic chain. *Technik in der Medizin* 1:16–18, 1972.
134. Lehmann JF, McDougall JA, Guy AW, Warren CG, Esselman PC: Heating patterns produced by shortwave diathermy applicators in tissue substitute models. *Arch Phys Med Rehabil* 64(12):575–577, 1983.
135. Jones RJ (program director): Diagnostic and therapeutic technology assessment. Diathermy. *JAMA* 250(4):540, 1983.
136. Kahanovitz N, Arnoczky SP, Hulse D, Shires PK: The effect of postoperative electromagnetic pulsing on canine posterior spinal fusions. *Spine* 9(3):273–279, 1984.
137. Binder A, Parr G, Hazleman B, Fitton-Jackson S: Pulsed electromagnetic field therapy of persistent rotator cuff tendinitis: a double-blind controlled assessment. *Lancet* 1(8379):695–698, 1984.
138. Bassett CAL: The development and application of pulsed electromagnetic fields (PEMFs) for ununited fractures and arthrodeses. *Orthop Clin North Am* 15(1):61–87, 1984.
139. Barclay V, Collier RJ, Jones A: Treatment of various hand injuries by pulsed electromagnetic energy (Diapulse). *Physiotherapy* 69(6):186–188, 1983.
140. Bassett CAL, Valdes MG, Hernandez E: Modification of fracture repair with selected pulsing electromagnetic fields. *J Bone Joint Surg (AM)* 64A(6):888–895, 1982.
141. Sutcliffe ML, Goldberg AAJ: The treatment of congenital pseudarthrosis of the tibia with pulsing electromagnetic fields: a survey of 52 cases. *Clin Orthop* 166:45–57, 1982.
142. Raji ARM, Bowden REM: Effects of high-peak pulsed electromagnetic field on the degeneration and regeneration of the common peroneal nerve in rats. *J Bone Joint Surg (Br)* 65B(14):478–492, 1983.
143. Bassett CAL, Mitchell SN, Schink NM: Treatment of therapeutically resistant non-unions with bone grafts and pulsing electromagnetic fields. *J Bone Joint Surg (AM)* 64A(8):1214–1220, 1982.
144. Botwin CA: A noninvasive treatment utilizing pulsating electromagnetic fields for promoting healing of nonunited fractures, failed fusions, and congenital pseudarthrosis. *J Am Osteopath Assoc* 82(10):779–781, 1983.
145. Ito H, Bassett CAL: Effect of weak, pulsing electromagnetic fields on neural regeneration in the rat. *Clin Orthop* 181:283–290, 1983.
146. Raji AM: An experimental study of the effects of pulsed electromagnetic filed (Diapulse) on the nerve repair. *J Hand Surg (Br)* 9B(2):105–112, 1984.
147. Enzler MA, Sumner-Smith G, Waelchli-Suter C, Perren SM: Treatment of nonuniting osteotomies with pulsating electromagnetic fields. *Clin Orthop* 187:272–276, 1984.
148. Smith RL, Nagel DA: Effects of pulsing electromagnetic fields on bone growth and articular cartilage. *Clin Orthop* 181:277–282, 1983.
149. Barker AT, Dixon RA, Sharrard WJW, Sutcliffe ML: Pulsed magnetic field therapy for tibial non-union. interim results of a double-blind trial. *Lancet* 1(8384):994–996, 1984.
150. Lehmann JF, Dundore DE, Esselman PC, Nelp WB: Microwave diathermy: effects on experimental muscle hematoma resolution. *Arch Phys Med Rehab* 64(3):127–129, 1983.
151. Lau RWM: Some observations on stray magnetic fields and power outputs from short-wave diathermy equipment. *Health Phys* 46(4):939–943, 1984.
152. Microwave diathermy: safety in normal use. *Physiotherapy* 67(4):108–109, 1981.
153. Moseley H, Davison M: Exposure of physiotherapists to microwave radiation during microwave diathermy treatment. *Clin Phys Physiol Meas* 2(3):217–221, 1981.
154. Stuchly MA, Repacholi MH, Lecuyer DW, Mann RD: Exposure to the operator and patient during short wave diathermy treatments. *Health Phys* 42(3):341–366, 1982.
155. Skoubo-Kristensen E, Sommer J: Ultrasound influence on internal fixation with a rigid plate in dogs. *Arch Phys Med Rehabil* 63(8):371–373, 1982.
156. Piersol GM, Schwan HP, Pennell RB, Carstensen EL: Mechanism of absorption of ultrasonic energy in blood. *Arch Phys Med Rehabil* 33:327, 1952.
157. El'Piner IE: *Ultrasound: Its Physical, Chemical and Biological Effects.* New York, Consultants Bureau, 1964, pp 154–156.
158. Goddard DH, Revell PA, Cason J, Gallagher S, Currey HLF: Ultrasound has no anti-inflammatory effect. *Ann Rheum Dis* 42(5):582–584, 1983.
159. Jones RJ: Treatment of acute herpes zoster using ultrasonic therapy: report on a series of twelve patients. *Physiotherapy* 70(3):94–96, 1984.
160. Ferguson HN: Ultrasound in the treatment of surgical wounds. *Physiotherapy* 67(2):43, 1981.
161. Roberts M, Rutherford JH, Harris D: The effect of ultrasound on flexor tendon repairs in the rabbit. *Hand* 14(1):17–20, 1982.
162. Miller HC, Ardizzone J: Peyronie disease treated with ultrasound and hydrocortisone. *Urology* 21(6):584–585, 1983.
163. Caudrey DJ, Seeger BR: Biofeedback devices as an adjunct to physiotherapy. *Physiotherapy* 67(12):371–376, 1981.
164. Public information office of UC Irvine College of Medicine: Biofeedback: part of the controversial. *The Bulletin.* Irvine, UC Irvine College of Medicine, Jan 2, 1975, pp 12–14.
165. Cottrell GW: New, conservative, and exceptionally effective treatment for low back pain. *Compr Ther* 11(11):59–65, 1985.
166. Meschino JP: The role of spinal inverted traction in chiropractic practice. *J Chiro* 18(2):63–68, 1984.
167. Cox JM: *Low Back Pain,* ed 3. Ft Wayne, JM Cox, 1980, pp 8–11, 79–184.
168. Lind G: *Auto Traction Therapy,* 1974.
169. Daugherty R, Erhard R: Segmentalized cervical traction. *Proceedings Intl Fed of Orthopaedic Manipulative Therapists,* Vail, B Kent, 1977, pp 189–195.

170. Colachis SC, Strohm BR: Cervical traction: relationship of traction time to varied tractive force with constant angle of pull. *Arch Phy Med Rehabil* 46:812–819, 1965.

171. Judovich BD: Herniated cervical disc: a new form of traction therapy. *Am J Surg* 84:646–656, 1952.

172. Jackson R: *The Cervical Syndrome*. Springfield, IL, Charles C Thomas, 1958, pp 284–286.

173. Lawson G, Godfrey C: A report on studies of spinal traction. *Med Serv J Can* 12:762, 1958.

174. Cyriax J: Diagnosis of soft tissue lesions. In *Textbook of Orthopaedic Medicine*, ed 6. London, Bailliere Tindall, vol 1, p 316.

175. Nosse LJ: Inverted spinal traction. *Arch Phys Med Rehabil* 59:367–370, 1978.

176. Lawson G, Godfrey C: A report on studies of spinal traction. *Med Serv J, Canada* 12:762–767, 1958.

177. Harris PR: Cervical traction: review of literature and treatment guidelines. *Phys Ther* 57(8);910–914, 1977.

178. Deets D, Hands KL, Hopp SS: Cervical traction: a comparison of sitting and supine positions. *Phys Ther* 57(3):255–261, 1977.

179. Beard G, Wood EC: *Massage: Principles and Technique*. Philadelphia, WB Saunders, 1964, pp 6, 8.

180. Nichols F: *Theory and Practice of Body Massage*. New York, Milady Publishing, 1982, pp 5–7.

181. Lidell L: *The Book of Massage*. New York, Simon & Schuster, 1984, p 12.

Suggested Readings

Beideman RP: Seeking the rational alternative: (the National College of Chiropractic, 1906–1982). *Chiro Hist* 3(1):17–22, 1983.

Cox JM: Unilateral distraction in scoliosis, subluxation and disc protrusion. *Digest Chiro Econ* 24(3):46–49, 1981.

Downey JA: Physiological effects of heat and cold. *Phys Ther* 44(8):713–717, 1964.

Haines J: A survey of recent developments in cold therapy. *Physiotherapy* 53:222–229, 1967.

Lundberg T: Electrical stimulation for the relief of pain. *Physiotherapy* 70(3):98–100, 1984.

McMaster WC: A literary review on ice therapy in injuries. *Am J Sports Med* 5(3):124–126, 1977.

Meschino JP: The treatment of low back pain by combined inverted spinal traction and chiropractic manipulation. *J Chiro* 21(2);68–72, 1984.

Moor FB, Peterson SC, Manwell EM, Noble MF, Meunch G: *Manual of Hydrotherapy and Massage*. Mountain View, CA, Pacific Press, 1964, pp 129–160.

Parrish MC, Loskot CA: Therapeutic effectiveness of cold (cryotherapy) on circulation, edema, musculoskeletal pain, and spasticity. In Coyle BA (ed): *Proceedings: Conference on Current Topics in Chiropractic: Reviews of the Literature*. Sunnyvale, CA, Palmer College of Chiropractic-West, 1983, pp C1-1–C1-12.

CHAPTER 14

Visceral Disorders Related to the Spine

MICHAEL R. WILES B.S.,M.Ed., D.C., F.C.C.S.(C)

Every organ and muscle in the body is dependent, more or less, upon the spinal nerves. Risadore, 1842

Disease of every organ or portion of the body may, and very frequently do, arise from defect in the nerve centers rather than in the organ itself. D. D. Palmer, 1910

Pathology is function gone wrong. Boyd

Chiropractors have traditionally treated patients with the general goal of restoring and/or enhancing the natural healing process. This is accomplished by "removing interferences from the nervous system" by correcting subluxations. In the infancy of the profession, much of the practice of chiropractic depended upon adherence to an underlying philosophy as a firm foundation of clinical decision making. Chiropractors tended to differ, over the years, on the degree to which clinical decision making should depend upon matters of philosophy. This in turn contributed to the classic schism of "straights and mixers."

Recently, however, the scientific advancements in this field by Korr, Denslow, Sato, Koizumi, and many others (described in Chapter 3) have added support to the original model of chiropractic. Although the contemporary model is far more sophisticated than that envisioned by D. D. Palmer, the fact remains that chiropractic seems to influence the natural functioning of the body (homeostasis) through normalizing the tone of the autonomic nervous system. Subluxations are associated with segmental facilitation, and this phenomenon, in turn, involves hyperactive sympathetic neuromeres, segmental sympatheticotonia, and finally tissue and cell pathophysiology. From Denslow's historic studies in the early 1940s to the contemporary work of Swenson and Sato, all related research has tended to support this model of chiropractic, itself a variant of D. D. Palmer's concept of "life as a function of tone."

This current model supports the notion of preventive chiropractic care through lasting correction of subluxations. In cases of postural deterioration or induced asymmetry, subluxation correction may involve a long term process whereby the central neurological patterning of the original subluxation requires long-term correction. In fact, a recent study by Patterson and Steinmetz (1) demonstrated that a 30 to 35 minute stimulation of spinal muscle resulted in segmental reflex activity for up to 72 hours. This central neural patterning was called a "neural scar." This neural scar probably produces recurrent subluxations in some individuals and requires repeated manipulative therapy for lasting correction.

This model of chiropractic also supports the role of chiropractic care not only in musculoskeletal conditions but in all patient situations involving subluxations, notwithstanding contraindications to manipulation. Thus a patient with low back pain would naturally benefit from manipulation; a patient with peptic ulcer and related subluxations in the midthoracic region or upper cervical region would also benefit from manipulation, although if actual visceral pathology has occurred, other forms of therapy would probably be required as well. We are primarily concerned with the state of health (physiology) prior to pathology. Gastrointestinal disorders are discussed in detail later in this chapter; however, suffice it to say that midthoracic subluxations are definitely associated with peptic ulcer disease. Whether this is cause or effect can only be determined by individual case assessment. The concern of the modern chiropractor (in this example) is the patient with a well-established midthoracic subluxation, without either musculoskeletal or visceral symptoms. It is this author's opinion that such a subluxation is disruptive to normal homeostatic behavior at that neuromere and will eventually lead to pathophysiology and pathology. It definitely should be corrected by manipulation.

We are left with the simple conclusion that the main therapeutic target of chiropractors, the subluxation, exists in both symptomatic and asymptomatic patients. Whether these patients are suffering with tennis elbow, low back pain, peptic ulcer, multiple sclerosis, or nothing, is, in a sense, irrelevant to the primary therapeutic goal of subluxation correction. Naturally, in symptomatic patients, if the subluxation is thought to be the origin of symptoms (e.g., pain), then initial care should be patient-oriented to provide the earliest alleviation of suffering. However, the chiropractor should not forget that the ultimate goal is a healthier patient with fewer, if any, subluxations.

Obviously, subluxations are more likely to be found in patients with symptoms. The most common presenting complaints in chiropractic offices are musculoskeletal problems. Subluxations, however, can occur anywhere in the spine and need not only be related to musculoskeletal problems. For example, well-defined patterns of thoracic subluxations have been associated with peptic ulcer disease. These may cause midback pain, tenderness on palpation only, or no symptoms at all. In any case, they are still treatable lesions in the chiropractic office.

Subluxations need not cause musculoskeletal symptoms or any symptoms at all. They are, however, just as important to treat by manipulation, whether symptomatic or not. Only by their reduction can the doctor be assured that segmental sympatheticotonia (and its pathophysiologic effect) is relieved. In symptomatic patients, initial care is specifically directed to the area of complaint to alleviate suffering before proceeding with the (often) longer task of subluxation correction. Manipulative care and adjunctive therapy for musculoskeletal conditions are discussed throughout this book. For conditions relating to the viscera, the physician must answer three questions.

1. Are the visceral symptoms related segmentally to the observed subluxation? If not, the patient still requires chiropractic care for any subluxation found on examination, but should be referred to practitioners who deal specifically with the presenting pathology or pathophysiology. An example is a patient with severe dysmenorrhea who is found to have subluxations of T1, T4, and T5. These levels are unlikely to be related to pelvic symptoms, and this patient would be referred for allopathic consideration, as well as being treated chiropractically for the asymptomatic subluxations.

2. Are the segmentally related visceral symptoms due to visceral pathology? If so, then the patient should be referred for allopathic consideration as well as treated vigorously, by chiropractic, in order to relieve segmental reflexes of sympatheticotonia. An example is a patient with T6–8 subluxations, presenting with what appears to be cholecystitis. Medical referral is necessary, along with aggressive manipulative care of affected vertebral levels. If no visceral pathology is found and visceral symptoms are considered to be physiological or functional in nature, then an aggressive course of chiropractic care may be initiated. An example is a patient with severe dysmenorrhea who has been examined for pelvic pathology (with negative results) and who is found to have subluxations of L1–2 and L4–5. Naturally, clinical judgement must be used in order to rule out visceral pathology. In cases of doubt, referral is in order.

3. Is manipulative care contraindicated? This topic is covered elsewhere and is of great relevance when treating patients with visceral disorders. For example, manipulation may be indicated for thoracic subluxations in the otherwise healthy spine of a patient with pancreatitis, but relatively contraindicated due to the clinical condition of the patient. Note, however, that this is a very individualized clinical decision of the chiropractor and that neither febrile illness, visceral disease, or debilitation are necessarily contraindications to manipulative therapy. Daiber (2) in *Osteopathic Medicine* says that patients who are hospitalized with acute glomerulonephritis require manipulative care as much as medication, and they should be given adjustments around the clock, every four hours, even being awakened at night for treatment.

An important distinction must be made between treating visceral disease and treating patients *with* visceral disease. Chiropractors, as has been said, have the therapeutic goal of subluxation correction. This in turn normalizes neurologic function and promotes the healing process. Subluxations are found in patients with and without visceral disease. For example, a patient may present for a check-up and subluxations of T7–9 may be found. These will naturally be treated. Another patient may present with diabetes mellitus and on examination, T7–9 subluxations may be found. These will also be treated, albeit more aggressively because of the potential segmental relationship with the pancreas. The chiropractor in this case is *not* treating diabetes. He is treating a patient with diabetes.

Of course, in such a case the chiropractor is concerned primarily with subluxation correction and will not interfere with a patient's medication regimen, since unlike the chiropractor, the allopath *does* treat the diabetes (as well as the patient with diabetes). This point must be clear, since misconception will otherwise occur when manipulation is discussed in relation to specific visceral disorders.

To summarize with one more example: a patient presents with neck pain, who also happens to have lung cancer. On examination, subluxations are found at C5–6 and T5–6. He complains of gastrointestinal symptoms of heartburn and esophagitis since undergoing radiation treatment. First, are the symptoms related segmentally to the subluxations? In the cervical area, yes, but the thoracic subluxations are asymptomatic. Second, are related visceral symptoms due to visceral pathology? Yes, esophagitis in this case is due to radiation exposure. This patient will be under the primary care of an oncologist. Third, are there any contraindications to manipulation? This requires careful clinical and radiographic evaluation. Neoplasm of the vertebrae or related structures is a contraindication to manipulation. However, this patient may have cancer limited to the lung. If so, such a patient should not be denied care simply because he has cancer (which does not involve the spine). The care of this patient would therefore be the primary care of oncologist for cancer and esophagitis, secondary care of chiropractor for neck pain and cervical subluxations (assuming no local contraindications), and asymptomatic thoracic subluxations (assuming no local contraindications). This latter treatment may have a beneficial healing effect on the postradiation esophagitis. Such a patient can, and should be treated chiropractically. The chiropractor is *not* treating cancer, but a patient with cancer who happens to have other problems as well. The proper understanding of this principle is crucial for any chiropractor seeking to help patients other than musculoskeletal ones.

A full discussion of chiropractic care for patients with visceral disease would require a separate textbook. In order to give the reader some idea of specific issues and data in this area, the gastrointestinal, cardiovascular, and respiratory systems were chosen, and the physiology, pathophysiology, and pathology of these systems are discussed from a chiropractic viewpoint. This is intended to give the reader a clear illustration of the relationship between subluxations and visceral pathophysiology. The reader is advised, however, that this summary is not exhaustive and is representative only of the kind of documentation available supporting manipulative care of patients with visceral disease. Hopefully as the profession expands its activities, more interest will be given to this aspect of chiropractic, and more literature (e.g., texts) will become available.

GASTROINTESTINAL SYSTEM

The gastrointestinal system is tremendously influenced by the autonomic nervous system. It is not surprising, therefore, that subluxations have been shown to have a strong segmental relationship in cases of visceral pathophysiology and pathology, and manipulative therapy has both a demonstrated and a theoretical role. This system is generally considered diagnostically and therapeutically from the standpoint of its anatomical divisions.

For example, gastrointestinal diagnosis and therapy is based, generally, upon disorders of the mouth, esophagus, stomach, small intestine, large intestine, and rectum. Chiropractic applications in gastrointestinal disorders have sometimes been classified according to these divisions. For example, Solheim's text (3) outlines chiropractic care of major gastrointestinal problems in a "cookbook" fashion (look up the disease and read the "recipe"). The modern chiropractic approach, however, recognizes "functional" divisions to be of greater relevance than the structural divisions of the gastrointestinal system. The entire system, really, is just a long tube with storage, absorption, and expulsive functions.

It is necessary, before discussing the chiropractic role in gastrointestinal health and disease, to review briefly the function and control of the gastrointestinal system. In general, the parasympathetic nervous system prepares the gut for digestion and mediates the processes of digestion and motility. Parasympathetic function, therefore, increases gastric and intestinal motility, increases acid production, and relaxes the anal sphincter (4). Under parasympathetic function, the gall bladder contracts, thereby facilitating digestion.

The sympathetic nervous system generally inhibits the digestive function. The effects of sympathetic activity are inhibition of motility and peristalsis, inhibition of gastrointestinal secretions (acid and mucous gland secretion), vasoconstriction, and constriction of sphincters (pyloric and anal). The gall bladder relaxes under sympathetic stimulation. Stimulation of sympathetic nerves at physiological frequencies produces "drastic and sustained blanching of colonic mucosa" (5). Furthermore, sustained sympathetic stimulation causes an initial neurogenic constriction, followed by a decline to a new steady state of *moderately increased resistance* (5). Thus, theoretically at least, there is good reason to suspect the subluxation as an etiologic factor in gastrointestinal pathophysiology (since the subluxation is known to cause facilitation of lateral horn cells and resultant sympatheticotonia).

Neurologically, we can divide the gastrointestinal system into a proximal section (vagus) and a distal portion (pelvic parasympathetic). Although pelvic autonomics may overlap with vagal autonomics, the vagus nerve is reasonably consistent in its colonic innervation. The proximal portion has functions that are primarily related to storage and absorption. The principal parasympathetic innervation is the vagus nerve (absorptive function). In the proximal colon, some pelvic autonomics overlap the vagal innervation; their function (pelvic PNS) is primarily expulsive. The sympathetic nervous system, in the proximal gastrointestinal portion, can be said to have an "anti-absorptive" effect (vasoconstriction). The distal gastrointestinal portion (last 2/3 of colon) is innervated by pelvic parasympathetic nerves (expulsive function) and lumbar sympathetic nerves (antiexpulsive function).

Table 14.1 Subluxations and Peptic Ulcers[a]

Finding	Ulcer Patients (N = 79) %	Controls (N = 36) %
T5–6 subluxation	68.4	27.8
Sacroiliac subluxation	87.4	44.4
Occ-C1 subluxation	58.2	41.7
Normal thoracic spine	11.4	63.8

[a]From Lewit K, Rychlikova E: Reflex and vertebrogenic disturbances in peptic ulcer. In Lewit K, Gutman G (eds): *Rehabilitacia: Proceedings of the IV Congress, Prague*. International Federation of Manual Medicine, 1975.

Functionally, the gastrointestinal system is under parasympathetic control. The sympathetics seem to have a moderating, antiparasympathetic effect that quickly and simply inhibits digestive function under conditions of sympathetic activation ("stress"). Since the subluxation can affect the sympathetic nervous system, it is reasonable to implicate this lesion in gastrointestinal pathophysiology. Basic science research suggests this contention. Sato and coworkers have demonstrated that pinching the abdominal skin of cats causes decreased motility of the stomach via the sympathetic nerves (a somatoautonomic reflex) (6). Pinching the skin of the head, tail, legs, and paws results in increased gastric motility. This was felt to occur via vagal and pelvic parasympathetic nerves. Kametani et al. (7) have similar results and concluded that "efferent activity of the vagus was responsible for the gastric motility facilitation." Jansson (8) demonstrated an inhibitory sympathetic effect even in spinal cats, suggesting a local, spinal reflex was responsible for somatoautonomic gastric inhibition. Furthermore, he demonstrated that afferent stimulation of group III muscle afferents was mainly responsible for gastric inhibition (sympathetic stimulation), and he concluded that "stimulation of somatic afferent 'pain fibers' seems to produce similar adrenergic activity."

Recently, Swenson (9) has demonstrated that "suboccipital muscles are capable of participating in somatovisceral reflexes in α-choralose anesthestized rats." This effect is presumably via the efferent effect of the vagus nerve. Studies of these phenomena in humans are scarce. There is a lot of Russian literature on gastric motility measurements (a good indicator of autonomic function) in relation to various gastrointestinal disorders and as a prognostic indicator in following surgical cases. Wiles published a short report demonstrating a relationship between upper cervical manipulation and changes in gastric motility as measured by the electrogastrogram (10).

Literature pertaining to the clinical application of manipulative therapy in gastrointestinal disorders is usually general, without specific guidelines for diagnosis or therapy. Harakal and Burns (11) wrote that biliary and digestive dysfunction were "amenable to modification toward health by treatment of the related somatic dysfunction." Their model was simple: subluxations produce visceral dysfunction that leads to pathology via abnormal autonomics. Lewit and Rychlikova (12) published results of a survey of adolescents with peptic ulcers (Table 14.1). They concluded that there is a "characteristic (subluxation) pattern in peptic ulcer patients."

Banner published an interesting paper relating spinal palpation, thermography, and x-ray findings in duodenal ulcer patients (13). Although he failed to demonstrate any major relationship, his study did reveal one fact: all 30 patients were chosen because of clinical suggestion of duodenal ulcer; only 17 had radiographic evidence of ulceration, but all 30 had midthoracic subluxations. Given the scientific rationale of chiropractic and the abundance of evidence linking subluxations with sympatheticotonia and sympathetic dysfunction with patholophysiology and disease, this is not surprising.

Although Banner failed to show a relationship between ulcers and thoracic x-rays, Kamieth (14) did relate x-ray findings of spatial infringement in the intervertebral foramen from T6–9 in 90 of 100 ulcer patients. His work is interesting, also, since it was abstracted in the *Journal of the American Medical Association* as far back as 1958. He concluded that "morphologic changes seem to be less important than functional-dynamic changes," and "processes in the vertebral column seemed to play a part in 90 of the 100 patients with peptic ulcers."

More recently, Nicholas studied palpatory findings in a sample of hospital patients (15) that included 42 patients with gastrointestinal disease. In this group of patients, T7–12 subluxations predominated, with the most common levels being T5–6 (left), T8 (left), T7–9 (right).

There are two theories regarding the role of manipulative therapy in treating patients with peptic ulcer disease (16). Since the gastric acid levels in patients with gastric ulcer are either normal or low, it is envisioned that sympatheticotonia from subluxations of the midthoracic spine facilitates gastric neuromeres and causes diminished secretion of both acid and protective mucus (17). Basic science studies support this theory, demonstrating that the SNS plays an important role in the protective mechanisms of the gastric mucosa (18) and that increased sympathetic activity is involved in the pathogenesis of gastric ulcer (19). Besides sympatheticotonia (associated with thoracic spine subluxations), parasympatheticotonia associated with vagal facilitation and upper cervical subluxations has been suggested as an etiologic factor. The beneficial effects of vagotomy are well-known and support this view. Also, there is some clinical evidence (3, 10, 12, 16) and basic science evidence (9) linking the upper cervical spine to gastric function.

Regardless of which mechanism is occurring, it is quite likely that the upper gastrointestinal system is very sensitive to autonomic dysfunction. Therefore, subluxations of either the upper cervical or midthoracic segments could disturb normal autonomic activity and result in pathophysiology leading to ulceration. Combined subluxations of both areas would undoubtedly be a pathogenic influence on gastric function.

Describing a comprehensive approach to ulcer disease, with reference to both cervical (PNS) and thoracic (SNS) involvement, Robuck (20) and Magoun (21) both mentioned the etiologic significance of the midthoracic spine as did Lewit (12) and Kamieth (14). Indeed Magoun states that (subluxations) "at the 5th or the 5th and 6th thoracic supply the missing link in present-day medical etiology of peptic ulcer" (21). Robuck's approach to ulcer treatment included manipulative therapy, psychotherapy, medication, rest, and diet. The specific spinal involvement mentioned was 7th thoracic, 3rd to 5th cervical, and suboccipital triangle. Finally, the role of manipulative therapy in ulcer disease is so scientifically plausible and reasonable, and clinically demonstrable, that Dr. William Strong, an osteopathic internist, wrote (in Hoag's text), "manipulative therapy can play a major role in the management of the ulcer problem, both specifically and supportively, and it should be a routine and continuing feature of the emergency, maintenance, and follow-up care of the patient" (22).

The lower gastrointestinal tract has been related empirically to results from chiropractic care for constipation and functional colon disease. Strong (22), describes the value of manipulative therapy for colitis by saying that "manipulative therapy of the lumbar spine and pelvis with the aim of normalizing abnormal irritation to the pelvic parasympathetics is probably the *most important* area of treatment." He goes on to describe the need for regular preventive manipulative care to prevent the reestablishment of chronic subluxation patterns. "Manipulative therapy", he says, "should be continued on a regular basis." In a general review of the topic, Smeyne relates "stress" to diseases of the colon (23) and emphasizes the therapeutic need for removing stressors when treating colon disease. Such a model is very compatible with the chiropractic view of subluxations as a source of colonic dysfunction. Going further, English (24) not only describes the role of somatic dysfunction as an etiologic component of colon disease, but also proposes specific levels of involvement based on his clinical experience. He lists the following areas of spinal involvement: stomach (T5–9), small intestine (T5–9, especially T8–9), and colon (T10–12, especially T11–12).

Masterton has written a very good paper on irritable bowel syndrome (25) which includes neurology, diagnosis, and treatment. She states that "the irritable bowel syndrome probably accounts for at least one half of all gastrointestinal complaints." Levels of spinal involvement are given very specifically (e.g., T4–8 subluxations "can cause venous congestion of the small bowel, and gas; T6–8 lesions will produce disturbed splanchnic secretion, atonic bowel, and diarrhea; T10–12 lesions can produce an atonic bowel, gas, decreased peristalsis, and constipation"). Indeed, the role of chiropractic care in patients with colon disease is very clear, considering the data presented by Dr. Masterton, and definitely should be a major part of the care of such patients.

On the same topic, Strong (22) states that "manipulative treatment directed to the pelvic parasympathetic nerves is extremely useful in helping to restore and control normal function of the colon" (in irritable bowel syndrome). Constipation has been reported to be successfully treated by manipulation. Strong (22) reports success through manipulation for both atonic and spastic constipation. The treatment program should consist of a variety of components including "careful attention to the lumbar spine and pelvis, a bland diet, sufficient rest, adequate fluid intake, and appropriate manipulative therapy." Such a program is said to "quickly resolve" the (constipation) problem. Dr. Overton wrote a classic paper on the topic of constipation in 1956 (26). His program likewise consisted of multiple components (including electrotherapy). He described the levels of T10 to L3 as being most important for adjustive procedures.

Finally, disorders of both the liver and the gallbladder have been described in relation to manipulative therapy. Probably the best-known clinical entities of these organs in chiropractic practices are postcholecystectomy syndrome, and chronic right thoracic subluxations associated with latent or active gallbladder disease.

Sympathetic innervation to the gallbladder produces relaxation and diminished emptying. Clearly, then, sympatheticotonia from subluxations could produce decreased emptying leading to stasis, irritation, inflammation, and stones. This is precisely what Strong proposed (22): "musculoskeletal disturbances, therefore, in the area of T6 to L1 are considered capable of impairing circulation or increasing ischemia in the gallbladder and ducts." Lewit (27) described good results in cases of gallbladder colic treated by manipulation to "fixed segments" and local massage. His findings suggested that "attacks can usually be controlled and results compare favorably with the administration of a good antispasmodic agent."

Studies of liver disease and manipulative therapy are less common. However, Cole's study (28) reveals fascinating experimental results: almost identical histological liver changes were produced by direct injection of chemical irritants (into the liver), injection of irritants into the paraspinal muscles of the T6 level, and experimental induction of a subluxation at T6. Strong proposes a significant prophylactic role for manipulative therapy in liver disease (22). He states (with respect to infective disorders such as amebiasis), "managing the autonomic nervous system *by means of manipulative therapy* directed chiefly to the cervical and mid-thoracic areas should be the best method of preventing the breakdown in parenchymal liver defense that permits invasion in the first place." He goes on to describe manipulative therapy as playing an important role in the care of patients with many liver diseases, especially hepatitis ("manipulative therapy should be applied as often as may seem necessary") and cirrhosis ("manipulative therapy directed to T5–T10 should assist in establishing improved vascular control to the liver").

Clearly, the role of chiropractic care in treating patients with disorders of the gastrointestinal tract is a strong one, supported by basic science and clinical science literature. Perhaps one of the greatest frustrations in practice is the urgent need for both public education about such roles for chiropractic care, and professional education such that other primary care physicians (mostly allopathic) can properly understand and utilize the services of chiropractors in the care of patients with gastrointestinal disease. The role of subluxations in disturbing innervation and producing pathophysiology should not be taken lightly. All the evidence points to a very potent tool in the form of properly utilized manipulative diagnosis and treatment. The chiropractic profession should utilize these skills to their maximum benefit for the well-being of mankind.

CARDIOVASCULAR SYSTEM

The cardiovascular system is another system immensely influenced by the autonomic nervous system. Therefore, it is also not surprising that much has been written describing the effects of manipulative therapy on cardiovascular physiology and diseases. One can get another perspective on the topic by looking at chiropractic as a therapy that affects the input to the nervous system (by correcting subluxations) thereby diminishing abnormal levels of output from the nervous system. This "output" can only represent muscle activity and glandular secretion, since these are the only targets of motor innervation. Muscle activity can be divided into that of skeletal muscle (and cardiac muscle) and smooth muscle. Since the entire cardiovascular system is smooth muscle (except the heart), it follows that this system is under considerable influence from somatic sensory irritations (subluxations).

The chiropractic approach to disorders of this system is no different than that to disorders of any other system. First, the chiropractor must appropriately diagnose the patient and, if necessary, make appropriate referrals. Next, the chiropractic evaluation will determine if subluxations are incidental to the patient's chief complaint or directly related to it. In either case, if subluxations are diagnosed, then the patient is treated chiropractically. If the subluxations are considered to be related to the visceral disease or presenting complaint, then vigorous treatment including other methods of natural hygiene, such as diet and exercise, are in order.

The osteopathic profession functions similarly, and a recent paper by Rogers (29) describes this approach. Rogers, a cardiologist, feels that the context of care is important and that care should be both comprehensive and consistent with philosophical principles. In a carefully worded statement, he says, "if, in fact, (manipulative therapy) exerts its effects on visceral function through the autonomic nervous system, there is a theoretic reason to believe that manipulation may be of some short or long term benefit in patients with heart disease." No doubt every chiropractor would agree with such a prudent statement, and it is on this reasonable basis that we should evaluate the literature in this area.

A number of studies have described palpatory findings and subluxations in relation to heart disease. While classical orthopaedics described a "flat upper thoracic spine" in relation to heart disease, as early as 1961, chiropractors and osteopaths were describing "somatic components to heart disease," and "vertebrogenic syndromes." The "flat thoracic spine" or "straight back syndrome" was described in several papers (30–32) as an accompaniment to heart murmurs, pulmonary problems, and other forms of cardiopulmonary disease. Although no connection to thoracic autonomics was mentioned, chiropractors would likely relate the flat upper dorsals to subluxations and anticipate some segmentally related pathophysiology. In an earlier chiropractic review (33), Egli describes the thoracic portion of the spine as a significant contributor to thoracic and chest complaints.

From the manipulative therapy standpoint, palpatory diagnosis offers another important clue to the nature of heart disease. Three separate papers, written more or less a decade apart describe the somatic component of heart disease and demonstrate the timeless quality of this approach. Koch, for example, in 1961 (34) described the somatic component to heart disease. His numerous observations included: upper thoracic subluxations are common in heart patients; these subluxations appeared months or years before the cardiac symptoms; previous thoracic trauma was recalled by many patients; organic heart disease followed "functional heart disease"; marked subjective and objective improvement followed manipulative therapy; no cardiac deaths occurred during the spinal corrective program (150 cases).

These findings "say it all" and clearly support the role of chiropractic in treating patients with heart disease. More recently, Tilley described the same phenomenon (35). He concluded with a philosophical invitation to practitioners to utilize their manipulative skills in the treatment of all patients with heart disease, whether acute, chronic, or emergency. Finally, in a much more sophisticated analysis, Beal (36), on 108 patients, found upper thoracic subluxations commonly associated with heart disease, and demonstrated that spinal palpation alone was 76%

accurate in "indicating the presence of cardiac disease." Furthermore, he accumulated specific data from 21 studies demonstrating the presence of T1–4 subluxations in cases of heart disease.

A few studies have been done on the physiological effects of manipulation on the cardiovascular system (37–39). However, like other studies of manipulation on "normal" populations, they failed to show any major consistent effects. Blood pressure changes were seen with adjustment to the upper cervical and upper thoracic spine, but we must view such studies with caution because (a) their populations were physiologically normal and (b) chiropractic, as an art, is much more than the physical act of manipulation.

An interesting and related study (40) relates head-up tilt to hypertension. A 25° head-up inclination was related to increased blood pressure and urinary catecholamines. No specific mechanisms were postulated, but chiropractors may tend to relate this to the commonly seen head-up posture of a slumped, hyperlordotic posture with hyperextended upper cervical region. Such postures involve many chronic subluxations and therefore could be related to increased autonomic tone and essential hypertension.

Numerous studies have demonstrated a beneficial effect of manipulation on hypertensive patients. Theoretically there is a major role for chiropractic in these cases. The primary problem in essential hypertension is peripheral vascular resistance. Since this physiological parameter is directly linked to autonomic tone, it follows that subluxations (especially at multiple sites, which would cumulatively affect the visceral motor output of the nervous system) are likely a major component of primary hypertension.

In an unpublished study of 241 chiropractors, Wiles and Diakow (personal communication) found that 98% of chiropractors treat hypertensives and that their approach to this problem was generally consistent, including manipulation, nutrition, and exercise. Among the published reports of specific palpatory findings of subluxations in hypertensive patients, the most extensive series is by Dr. W. Johnston and colleagues. Initially, Johnston studied electrodermographic findings in hypertensive patients (41). This small study of 20 patients and 20 controls demonstrated that there were differences between these groups in sympathetic patterns of the skin. Later, he went on to study palpation findings in hypertensive patients. In 1979 (42), a study demonstrated that hypertensive patients were significantly differentiated from normotensive patients by the number of subluxations and the degree of agreement on those subluxations by multiple examiners. Finally, a major paper in 1982 (43) demonstrated similar findings. His study group was divided into two subgroups: those with "unstable" somatic findings (low agreement on subluxations by three doctors) and those with "stable" somatic findings (high

agreement). In the low agreement group, 22.2% were hypertensive, but in the "stable" or high-agreement group, 52.7% were hypertensive. It was concluded that stable, consistent somatic findings do exist in hypertensive patients.

The nonpharmacologic treatment of hypertension is an important topic of national interest. Since this problem is so common and potentially dangerous, and since compliance with drug treatment is low (not to mention the potential risk), all non-drug methods deserve serious consideration. While techniques of relaxation, stress control, and biofeedback are well known (44), manipulative therapy may well offer these patients an effective method of hypertension control.

These sentiments are echoed by Baldwin, an osteopathic internal medicine specialist, who writes,

> Imbalance at the peripheral vascular level would mean increased sympathetic tonicity and continuous pathologic vasoconstriction. This is the rationale underlying surgical treatment by sympathectomy which has now been replaced almost entirely by potent ganglion-blocking drugs. From the osteopathic viewpoint, such treatment is not only a poorly directed means of correcting autonomic imbalance, compared with the natural means afforded by manipulative therapy, but it also opens the way to a great many iatrogenic ailments stemming from the widespread and powerful effects of the drugs themselves (45).

He goes on to describe the benefits of manipulation and concludes, "with regard to treatment, manipulation of the musculoskeletal system is a far better means of correcting or modifying the pressure levels than are most of the hypotensive drugs," and finally, "in the procedures mentioned (manipulation), the . . . physician has at his command the most natural, direct, and comprehensive means of dealing with practically all the complexities of hypertension."

Numerous general publications on this topic can be found. Goodheart (46) and Hood (47) have described general manipulative techniques as well as other methods of natural hygiene. Hood found that manipulation alone was not as effective as it was in combination with efforts to control diet, exercise, and sleep habits. Welberry published a much more detailed chiropractic approach (48) in which he outlined the specific dietary and manipulative programs of 136 cases. Manipulation generally lasted for four weeks at three times per week and good (but not specific) results were recorded.

Some specific techniques of chiropractic (such as Basic (49), Goodheart (46) and Gonstead (47)) have also been shown to be effective in treating hypertensive patients. This author, however, cautions readers using such an approach. The goal in treating *patients with hypertension* (not hypertension itself) is to reduce somatic sources of irritation to the nervous system (primarily subluxations). Using this approach, treatment should not be given which treats the symptoms only, and techniques should therefore be utilized with an ultimate goal of autonomic normalization, not just pressure regulation.

There are a number of osteopathic papers on the treatment of patients with hypertension, by manipulation. Northup (50) published a general paper outlining his care of a "long series" of hypertensives over a 30-year period. He boldly stated, "after more than 30 years of practice, I know of no other modality that will as effectively maintain blood pressure at a safe level as appropriate osteopathic manipulative treatment." Northup gives very specific advice including the direction of therapy to the upper cervical area and the lower thoracic area. This latter region is considered important because of its relationship with the kidneys, and later research has supported this relationship by demonstrating changes in aldosterone levels following manipulation. In an older review, the work of Wilson (51) is described, including a detailed approach for treating hypertension. He proposes that the objectives of treatment are the restoration of physiologic motion of the occiput, C7–T2, and T10–12.

Many other papers outline the manipulative treatment of hypertension and the physiologic effects of manipulative therapy on blood pressure (52–59). Blood (in 1964) described the role of gentle, low-velocity manipulation in treating these patients. This is a common theme throughout this literature and reflects the concept of attempting to lower efferent sympathetic tone by manipulative therapy. Stimulative procedures would only increase peripheral vascular tone and hypertension. A similar paper by Norris (53) described the mechanisms by which such treatment might affect the body. He concluded that the therapeutic goal was "normalizing" or "balancing" the autonomic nervous system via manipulative therapy. Miller (54) again described the dangers of stimulating the autonomic nervous system by vigorous adjustments or rapid adjustment of chronic lesions and postural patterns. He also advocated cranial techniques, cervical (particularly occipital) manipulation, and general attention to the thoracic spine and thoracolumbar area (renal involvement). All of the aforementioned approaches are consistent with the concept of manipulation reducing sympatheticotonia. Too much physical stimulation during this process could conceivably stimulate the sympathetic nervous system, leading to augmentation of hypertension.

In the late 1960s Celander and coworkers (55, 56) studied the effect of manipulation on autonomic tone, as evidenced by blood pressure changes. They found that manipulation caused a decrease in plasma fibrinogen which they felt indicated a fibrinolytic change favoring the parasympathetic nervous system. This later work (56) provided evidence of this effect *and* decreased blood pressure in 86% of hypertensives studied. In a related study of cardiovascular physiology, Kolman et al. (57) demon-

strated a reduction in blood pressure following manipulative therapy. They were unable to explain this observation, but postulated a "compensatory vasodilation in the viscera with a net increase in visceral blood flow and associated blood pressure and respiratory rate decrease."

In a more recent brief review of the topic (58), Stiles also mentions the concepts of subluxation being associated with facilitation and the resultant sympatheticotonia. He specifically mentions the "upper dorsal and cervical areas" as playing a role in increasing the peripheral resistance "in a significant portion of the body." He also mentions the thoracolumbar region and its relation to the efferent supply to the kidneys and adrenal glands. His conclusion is bold, "it is also thought that specifically designed manipulative care for the somatic dysfunction of the patient will also help to delay the onset of secondary visceral problems such as stroke and renal and myocardial decompensatory changes."

Two studies of manipulation and hypertension have shown that under certain circumstances there may be no changes in blood pressure following manipulation. Mannino (59) studied the effects of Chapman's reflexes (a neurolymphatic reflex procedure) on blood pressure. He found that although a significant reduction in serum aldosterone was observed, no statistically significant changes in blood pressure were observed.

Morgan et al. (60) performed a detailed, 18-week, controlled study of the effect of manipulation on hypertension. Their results failed to demonstrate that either manipulation or a sham manipulation could reduce or control elevated systemic blood pressure in the study population. However, even the authors make careful conclusions (in light of the abundant nonexperimental clinical literature supporting this effect of manipulation) and comment that future studies best be directed at studying manipulative procedures that are reportedly effective in lowering blood pressure. In their study, the authors utilized a specific manipulation-mobilization technique that did not involve specific directional thrusts. Moreover, patients reaching higher than 150 systolic or 110 diastolic were discharged from the study. Many clinical reports suggest that manipulative care is effective above these levels. Nonetheless this study is one of the only attempts at a controlled experimental analysis of this phenomenon.

The contemporary chiropractic approach to the treatment of hypertensives has been described (61). In this small survey of 17 chiropractors, the authors were able to describe the general approach to care, which included manipulation (88% of chiropractors)—specifically to upper cervical (60%), lower cervical (13%), upper thoracic (33%), lower thoracic (27%), lumbar (13%); nutritional therapy (82% of chiropractors); exercise (35% of chiropractors); soft tissue massage (18% of chiropractors); and psychotherapy (35% of chiropractors). A more recent and larger study (as yet unpublished) by these same authors (Wiles and Diakow, personal communication), surveying 241 chiropractors yielded similar results: manipulation (83.8%)—upper cervical (40.1%), lower cervical (19.8%), upper thoracic (36.6%), lower thoracic (13.9%), lumbar (3.5%); nutrition (74.3%); exercise (49.4%); soft tissue massage (15.8%); and psychotherapy (5.5%).

Clearly, there is agreement among chiropractors about the type of natural health approach to be taken when treating hypertensive patients. This approach is reviewed in a recent paper by Crawford et al. (62) in which hypertension is described as "a prime condition warranting specialized care that includes proper education during the formative years, modification of dietary habits in conjunction with daily exercise regimes, and regular spinal maintenance, all of which are covered by modern chiropractic clinical practice."

The theoretical and empirical data all support a role for manipulative therapy in decreasing total peripheral resistance and reducing hypertension.

Manipulative therapy has also been described in relation to coronary artery disease, as well as other types of heart disease. The classic work of Dr. Louisa Burns during the 1940s demonstrated the detailed cardiopathology of midthoracic subluxations in small animals (63). She found that T3–4 lesions produced, initially, a staccato pulse and an irregular pulse, followed by myocardial congestion and hemorrhage. This led to loss of contractile force and myocardial fibrosis. Similar changes in humans would likely result in coronary heart disease.

Around this same time, Travell and Rinzler were recording and discussing the somatic component of cardiac disease. Their work (64) focused on "trigger points" and the relationship between somatic afferent activity and converging visceral afferent activity. They also described how somatic afferent discharges originating in "trigger points" could spatially summate with subliminal visceral afferent activity, resulting in the sensation of cardiac pain. Their work clearly shows how therapy directed toward somatic structures can affect sensation from visceral disease. The chiropractic significance of such work lies in the fact that subluxations are also a potent subliminal (or nociceptive) influence on neuromeric activity and likely have the same summative effects as trigger points.

Foreman and Ohata (65) did, in fact, demonstrate that coronary occlusion did result in facilitation of 53% of the thoracic spinal neurons receiving viscerosomatic input from the heart. Clearly, the overlap and interaction of somatic and visceral afferents is a significant determinant of the impact of subluxations on symptomatic forms of heart disease.

The effect of sympathetic stimulation by subluxations is probably a more important pathophysiologic phenomenon to chiropractors. Raab demonstrated a "cardiotoxic" effect of sustained adrenergic stimulation to heart muscle (66). He reported "prolonged electrical stimulation of the norepinephrine discharging cardiac sympathetic nerves has been found to elicit electrocardiographic signs of hypoxic myocardial damage and subendothelial hemorrhages and necrosis." In other words, sympatheticotonia produces a histologic result identical to that of myocardial infarction. No direct evidence has been published linking subluxations to such damage in humans, however Burns' work on animals did relate these two phenomena, and the published clinical observations do lend further support to the existence of vertebrogenic cardiac pathophysiology and pathology.

In a detailed description of 30 years' experience in treating coronary disease, Wilson's classic paper (67) of 1949 gives clear practical advice for practitioners of spinal manipulation. The doctor is given four objectives: extend T1–3, adjust T3 and the related left rib, raise the sternum, and raise the diaphragm. Supportive patient activities are also described including rest, relaxation, proper diet and posture, and exercise.

Kletzel described a favorable response to manipulation, in conjunction with dietary and exercise advice, in the management of 21 patients with atherosclerosis (68). No other literature could be found on this topic from 1963 to 1972 when Johnson described the importance of manipulation in the management of a series of six patients with heart disease (69). He is specific in his observations and reports a clear relationship between T2 (and related ribs) and heart disease.

Rychlikova also specifically described a vertebral pattern in myocardial disease (70). In his study of 260 patients, he demonstrated the relationship between midthoracic subluxation (specifically T4–6) and anginal pain. Patients having myocardial infarction without prominent anginal pain had subluxation patterns similar to healthy controls; however, those with significant cardiac pain appeared to have a high prevalence of T4–6 subluxation.

Other published works have provided either general advice and comments regarding thoracic subluxations and heart disease (71) or more specific observations and recommendations regarding the care of such patients (71–73). Miller, an osteopathic internist, describes the importance of C7-T5 subluxations in disturbing cardiovascular autonomics, leading to coronary disease (72). He goes on to describe the importance of manipulative therapy in the care of patients with angina or myocardial infarction. Although the chiropractic physician will readily acknowledge that manipulative therapy has only a limited role in life-threatening cardiac accidents, Miller does go on to say, "the presence of an acute myocardial infarction does not contraindicate the use of osteopathic manipulative therapy. The areas treated include the cervical and upper dorsal spine. Treatment is directed to the paraspinal musculature to reduce spasm and local vasomotor changes." Miller quotes the classic work of Richmond (73) who demonstrated electrocardiographic changes of lessening of the RT segment and an absence of previously noted T-wave changes in patients with angina who were treated with manipulation.

It would appear that the evidence supporting the relationship of subluxations, manipulative therapy, and cardiac disease is clear. Chiropractic physicians should be providing this type of care to heart patients in both the ambulatory and hospital setting. Given the abundance of evidence, patients should be given the benefit of manipulative procedures as a matter of routine care and not just in specialized centers such as osteopathic hospitals.

Greenman has in fact described this need for manipulative care of hospitalized heart patients (74). He feels that the relationship between coronary heart disease and subluxations is so clear that the *specific* type of vertebral dysfunction can be described. Lesions from T1–5 are mentioned, especially those producing restriction in extension, left lateral flexion and right rotation. By old "static" listing systems this would approximate T1–5(pr), or T1–5(left). Greenman feels that the somatic reflection of chest pain is a helpful diagnostic tool in acute emergencies. Left-sided lesions tend to more strongly reflect heart disease (according to Greenman) as opposed to right thoracic lesions which he feels more likely reflect acute pulmonary disease (such as embolism).

In a very detailed and recent article, Rogers and Rogers (75), two osteopathic cardiologists, have described the role of manipulation in coronary heart disease. Their model is the same as described in this text: vertebral lesions (subluxations) produce segmental sympatheticotonia that has adverse effects on target tissues, in this case, the heart and coronary vessels. They conclude, "osteopathic manipulative therapy has been demonstrated to be of significant value in some patients with coronary insufficiency." Their final statement is an echo of previously mentioned sentiments: "it is logical to assume that manipulative treatment, by normalizing the action of the autonomic nervous system, might influence both cellular metabolism and the vasomotor dynamics of the coronary arteries."

Further evidence, supporting the above-mentioned model, comes from the radiographic and palpation studies of Cox et al (76, 77). Subluxations of the upper and midthoracic spine have repeatedly been mentioned as a cofactor in cardiac pathophysiology. Since spinal dysfunction is not a static process but one in which slowly progressive degenerative changes are observed ("subluxation degeneration"), it is reasonable to assume that cardiac disease might be correlated with radiographically demonstrable thoracic degenerative disease.

Cox describes this relationship in a review of 92 patients undergoing coronary arteriography for sus-

Table 14.2 Thoracic Lipping and Coronary Stenosis[a]

| | | Thoracic Osteophytosis | |
		Present (N = 34)	Absent (N = 58)
Coronary stenosis	Present (N = 72)	31	41
	Absent (N = 20)	3	17

[a]N = 92, P = 0.02.

pected coronary atherosclerosis (77). Seventy-two of these patients had angiographic evidence of coronary stenosis, and of these, 31 (or 43%) had thoracic osteophytic lipping (defined in this study as lipping of at least 5 mm, in at least 1 thoracic segment). The x-rays were reviewed by a radiologist who was unaware of the patient's clinical status, ruling out subjective bias. In the 20 patients without angiographic evidence of coronary stenosis, only 3 had thoracic lipping (Table 14.2). The authors concluded that "the presence of thoracic osteophytosis is a specific predictor of coronary atherosclerosis."

In a related study of spinal palpation in 97 coronary patients, Cox was able to demonstrate a "high correlation between coronary atherosclerosis and abnormalities of range of motion and soft tissue texture in the fourth thoracic vertebral segment" (76). Agreeing with Greenman that spinal palpation may be a valuable diagnostic aid in heart disease, the authors state that in their study,

the predictive accuracy of the palpatory findings was not affected by the presence or absence of a history of myocardial infarction or of typical angina pectoris. Therefore, it appears that a musculoskeletal examination with emphasis on the presence or absence of soft tissue and range of motion abnormalities of T4, will add to the ability of the examiner to diagnose coronary atherosclerosis in patients in whom the diagnosis is not obvious.

These palpatory phenomena are also described by Frymann (78) in a very practical paper that includes detailed technique for restoring rib, cranial, and vertebral mobility in cardiac patients. She also mentions further literature describing manipulative benefits to cardiac patients (79, 80), and quotes the great osteopathic cardiologist, Dr. Sam Robuck (81), who stated that "during the period of emergency and many times after the period of emergency, the difference in success and failure may be determined by a timely and efficiently applied osteopathic manipulative therapy."

Finally, manipulative therapy has been discussed in regards to the treatment of other types of heart problems, including arrhythmias and congestive heart failure (82–84). Howell and Kappler detailed a case report in which manipulative therapy was shown to significantly alter the subjective status of a patient with advanced cardiopulmonary disease, as well as significantly improve the arterial oxygen level (82).

Thomas more specifically outlines the manipulative approach to patients with congestive heart failure (84) and gives clear practical instruction on techniques that have been found to be helpful in treating such patients in the hospital environment. He goes on to say, "for many years, osteopathic physicians have reported clinical improvement in patients with congestive heart failure following certain manipulative procedures for mobilizing areas of restricted motion that are associated with observed changes in tissues." These changes, he suggests, occur most frequently on the left side at T3-T5, which is in general agreement with all other published reports of subluxations in patients with heart disease.

Arrhythmias, particularly sinus bradycardia and sinus tachycardia are logically related to subluxations, in that they represent abnormal heart rhythm via autonomic dysfunction. Dr. William Baldwin agrees (83) and states that although drug therapy can be used to control arrhythmias, "a more natural approach is to remove or modify those disturbing influences within the central nervous system which affect the autonomic neural pathways." Manipulative therapy is proposed by Dr. Baldwin as a way of accomplishing this objective. Tachycardia is proposed as being related to subluxations of C7-T5 (naturally, however, only after thyroid hyperfunction or other underlying diseases have been ruled out), and he suggests that "recurrent episodes of tachycardia suggest the presence of a chronic type of (vertebral) lesion." As predicted, sinus bradycardia, which is logically related to parasympatheticotonia and associated upper cervical subluxations, is described by Baldwin as related most frequently to lesions of C1–3.

The role of manipulative therapy in treating patients with cardiovascular disease is clear and has been described in detail by numerous authors from medical, osteopathic, and chiropractic backgrounds. Perhaps more important is the preventive role of care that is directed at maintaining a subluxation-free spine. Stary (85), writing of the status of manipulative therapy in Czechoslovakia, suggests that his data indicate that more than half of the population suffers from vertebrogenic disease during their lives. He also proposes that "active prevention is important as subclinical disorders of the vertebral column are reversible." A statement in a recent textbook emphasizes the need for a preventive approach: "In the majority of patients with coronary heart disease, the initial presentation will be a myocardial infarction and/or sudden death, rather than angina pectoris" (86). There is no doubt that the chiropractic profession has an extremely valuable therapy in this regard, which must be appropriately utilized for the public's benefit in both ambulatory and hospital settings.

RESPIRATORY SYSTEM

This system presents a classic example of the chiropractic concept of "double-diagnosis"—that is, the analysis of the patient from the standpoint of (a) "classical diagnosis" (i.e., nomenclature describing the primary pathologic phenomenon, such as "pneumonia" or "atalectasis") and (b) the diagnosis of the structural lesion associated with, or occurring as an adaptation to the classical diagnosis. For example, a patient may be described (medically) as having pneumonia; chiropractically, the patient may be described, using double-diagnosis, as having pneumonia in assocation with subluxations of T1–2 and myofascitis of the trapezius, rhomboid, and pectoralis major muscles.

Much has been written of the associated musculoskeletal findings in respiratory disease. Such phenomena are well recognized, and their treatment constitutes an important part of the care of patients with respiratory disease. Not as well researched or understood is the role of subluxations of the thoracic neuromeres in producing pathophysiology in the respiratory tract. Such considerations are primary to the chiropractic care of patients with respiratory disease.

The chiropractic approach to patients with respiratory disease includes three dimensions of care. The first is chiropractic care of related subluxations (in order to correct segmental sympatheticotonia and its disruptive influence on respiratory physiology). Second is the treatment of secondary or related somatic disturbances (such as intercostal muscle spasm and strain of the muscles of forced expiration). Third is the provision by referral for any necessary medical care (as dictated by patient needs and the classical diagnosis—for example, antibiotics in cases of pneumococcal pneumonia).

Lewit (87) recently synthesized this chiropractic approach with the statement, "the mobilization of the ribs and of blocked segments of the thoracic spine" (i.e., correction of subluxations) "and training of correct breathing patterns" (i.e., secondary, related somatic disturbances) "will thus be the logical treatment for patients with respiratory disease, particularly those with obstructive respiratory disease." Lewit has described the mechanics of respiration in detail (88), especially the relationship of faulty respiration and posture. He feels that the presence of somatic disturbances in cases of faulty respiration is so frequent, that faulty respiratory patterns (in particular, exaggerated lifting of the thorax in inspiration) should be sought in patients with chronic cervical syndromes.

This general relationship between respiration and somatic dysfunction has also been described in relation to physical performance, by Bergsmann and Eder (89). Their study of 100 patients demonstrated that circulatory and respiratory parameters showed improvement during work activities, following normalization of the thoracic spine and ribs. They concluded that "respiration and circulation can be improved by releasing the (thoracic) arthrogenic malfunction by manual medicine, which results in an increase in physical performance."

Osteopathic physicians, like chiropractic physicians, have long described an approach to the treatment of respiratory disease compatible with the aforementioned model. Citing specific clinical procedures and goals, Miller described this approach (90) and stressed the role of osteopathic health care in maintaining health rather than in treating disease. He states that physicians "must depend on the inherent ability of the body to help maintain its health." Consistent with the model, he describes the treatment of pneumonia, which includes antibiotics, manipulative therapy, and supportive measures. He emphasizes manipulative care, stating, "(manipulative therapy), called supportive therapy by many, should be primary therapy. Osteopathic manipulative therapy improves venous and lymphatic return, normalizes rib cage and diaphragmatic motions, aids in expectoration and makes the patient more comfortable."

Further evidence of respiratory system improvement in function, following manipulative therapy is given by Hviid (91) and Murphy (92), who described (respectively) the effect of manipulation on vital capacity and arterial oxygen saturation. Three medical professions: chiropractic, osteopathic, and allopathic have recognized the importance of manipulative therapy in respiratory disease and its treatment. Our approach, as chiropractic physicians, recognizes the need and importance of allopathic care as circumstances dictate. However, we cannot lose sight of the great role manipulative care has to play by both normalizing the autonomic innervation of the lungs and correcting the somatic disturbances of faulty respiration.

Let us first look at the interaction between the respiratory tract and the neuromusculoskeletal system in terms of the effects of sustained sympatheticotonia and somatic adaptation to respiratory disease. Droste et al. (93) described the effect of prolonged sympathetic stimulation on the lungs as reduced compliance and altered alveolar surface tension. Through a series of studies, they determined that these effects were independent of circulatory phenomena. Quite probably, an autonomic "pulmonary-toxic" effect may occur as a direct result of autonomic dysfunction on lung parenchyma (similar to the cardiotoxic effect described by Raab). Chiropractic theory postulates such an effect and the previous evidence of Louisa Burns (studying the effects of subluxations on the lungs of small animals) and the more recent work of Droste (for example) supports this concept.

Somatic involvement in respiratory disease can be viewed from the perspective of somatic adaptation to respiratory disease. In fact, Hoag (94) said "the chief aim of manipulative therapy is to aid the musculoskeletal system to respond to the pathophysiologic changes (of lung disease)." Dr. Hoag, a specialist in rehabilitation medicine, also says that "involvement of the musculoskeletal system in chronic lung disease is direct as well as subtle and complex." Somatic involvement in lung disease can be a secondary phenomenon, whereby local and general reflex mechanisms may result in restricted thoracic mobility via rib or thoracic subluxations. Somatic involvement can also be somatogenic, or primary, related to the (indirect) "pulmonary-toxic" phenomenon described above, or related to a more direct respiratory embarassment caused by hypoventilation from musculoskeletal dysfunction (95).

Any approach to somatic involvement in respiratory disease must also consider whether the respiratory dysfunction is obstructive or restrictive. Obstructive lung diseases, caused by the trapping of air in alveolar dead space, result in hyperinflated lungs and musculoskeletal demand upon expiratory muscles. Therefore in such disorders as asthma (acute obstructive) and emphysema (chronic obstructive), the related musculoskeletal dysfunction will involve the abdominal muscles, intercostals, quadratus lumborum, and iliocostalis lumborum. Restrictive lung diseases, caused by restriction of air flow into the lungs, result in musculoskeletal demand upon the muscles of forced inspiration. Thus, in such disorders as pneumonia (acute restrictive) and scoliosis or pulmonary fibrosis (chronic restrictive), the related musculoskeletal dysfunction will involve the diaphragm, scaleni, sternocleidomastoids, trapezii, serrati anticus and posticus, pectorales, latissimus dorsi and the spinal extensor muscles.

Four approaches to chiropractic care of patients with respiratory disease can be summarized: (a) correction of subluxations involved in producing reflex respiratory dysfunction via the autonomic nervous system (this primarily involves the pulmonary neuromeres, T1-T6); (b) correction of musculoskeletal dysfunction directly associated with respiratory disease. This may be primary (somatogenic) or secondary (viscerogenic) and may involve the muscles of expiration or inspiration (or both). Naturally there may also be related (or interrelated) subluxations. For example, trapezius hypertonicity may cause reflex C3–4 subluxations or may be caused by such subluxations; (c) Correction of respiratory or musculoskeletal dysfunction that may directly or indirectly impair vital processes such as respiratory circulation and lymphatic circulation. Much has been written about lymphatic involvement, especially by the osteopaths (90, 96–98), and a number of techniques such as Chapman's reflexes and the thoracic pump have been described; (d) Provision of any nonmanipulative aid necessary for such patients. This may be allopathic (i.e., pharmacologic) or not, depending on the presence of life-threatening circumstances, and may involve hygienic measures (such as hydration) as well as nutritional measures.

These topics are beyond the scope of this presentation.

Asthma is probably the most commonly discussed respiratory complaint with regards to clinical applications of manipulative therapy. Pneumonia, chronic obstructive lung disease, and acute upper respiratory disease have also been described in this regard. These four problems will be briefly discussed as illustrative of the chiropractic approach.

Asthma

Hoag (94) states that "asthma is second only to the common cold as a classic symbol of medical frustration." This statement contrasts clearly with "the place and importance of spinal manipulative therapy in bronchial asthma can no longer be denied or taken lightly." Kunert quoted by Beyeler (99) states that this form of therapy often leads to astonishing results, pushing the pharmacological treatment into the background (Further, Lewit says "the mobilization of the ribs and of blocked segments of the thoracic spine . . . will thus be the logical treatment for patients with respiratory disorders" (87).

If manipulation is this important in the treatment of asthma, it can play a major role. It remains for the chiropractic profession to fully define and document this treatment. There are recent reports of research in this area (100–102) as well as calls for research into the relationship of respiratory disease and the response to manipulation (103).

Asthma is generally considered to arise from spastic obstruction to airflow due to bronchospasm. This can be extrinsic in origin (e.g., pollution) or intrinsic (e.g., neurogenic swelling due to fear). In any event, neurogenic spasm of smooth muscle or allergic swelling of mucous membranes accounts for the majority of cases and the most severe cases.

Manipulative therapists (in particular, osteopaths) have long considered midthoracic and/or rib subluxations to be causative factors (via reflex relationships) of neurogenic bronchospasm. Modern concepts of neuropathogenesis do not fully rationalize a midthoracic origin, since sympatheticotonia of the respiratory neuromeres would tend to reduce bronchospasm, not cause it.

The classic argument has always been that subluxations can also reduce the efferent discharge activity, although most evidence suggests segmental facilitation to be the most likely effect of a subluxation. The most plausible theory related to the "reduced neural output" concept is Korr's idea that long-term sympatheticotonia can be deleterious not only to target tissues but also to the efferent nerves themselves. A trophic involutionary effect can be seen whereby the clinical picture can resemble a trophic disturbance rather than facilitation and hypertonus.

Thus, the clinical picture of asthma appears to be neurologically related to trophic disturbance of the respiratory sympathetic neuromeres (T2–7), reflecting sympathetic depletion, or to facilitation of the respiratory parasympathetic neuromere (the vagus nerve, related to the C1 segment by proximity, with respect to somatoautonomic reflex mechanisms) resulting in parasympatheticotonia. There is evidence supporting both concepts. Of course asthmatic symptoms can also be secondarily vertebrogenic (i.e., as a component of vertebral disease in which respiratory disease is simulated). A condition has been described in which dorsal spine radiculitis simulates asthma (104).

Beyeler takes a rather broad approach, suggesting that both mechanisms may be at work in the rather complex etiology of asthma. He says, "we have to assume that in the genesis of the asthmatic attack, the influence of the vagus and reflexes from spinal centres play the predominant role" (99). Beryl Swan, M.D., presented a case of chronic asthma very significantly reduced by upper cervical manipulation only, in the *Medical Journal of Australia* (105), and others have given general coverage to the idea of upper cervical subluxations being related to asthma (97, 106), but more documentation is required for this mechanism to be supported.

Literature supporting a thoracic origin of vertebrogenic asthma is more abundant. Lewit suggests that mobilization of blocked segments of the thoracic spine is the "logical treatment of patients with respiratory disease" (87). As mentioned above, Beyeler assumes a thoracic origin (99), and mention of subluxations of the thoracic spine in asthma (particularly T2–7) can be found in other reports (90, 96, 97, 101, 106–111).

An interesting idea was put forward by O'Donovan, an allergist (108). He speculates that minor scoliosis due to a short leg could stimulate local thoracic neuromeres (not a new idea now, but O'Donovan proposed this in 1951) thereby causing them over a period of time to "burn out," resulting in depletion of sympathetic catecholamines. The resulting autonomic imbalance causes asthma, in O'Donovan's view. His treatment consisted of heel lifts applied to the short leg (determined by upright pelvic x-rays) and manipulation. (Indeed he states, "I treat the scoliosis by inserting a solid heel lift into the shoe of the short side . . . the patient is then treated by manipulation which aims at restoring the spine to its normal position. After a few weeks a vast improvement is noticed in children in the first decade of life.") In a review paper on this topic (107) he summarized three cases where asthmatic cure was achieved using only a heel lift. O'Donovan further supported his theory by adding the observation that many asthmatics are hypotensive. This finding would logically follow in cases of sympathetic depletion or underactivity. There have been other studies of the effect of posture on asthma (112), but only O'Donovan's specifically suggests scoliosis as a cause of sympathetic disturbance.

Table 14.3 Summary of Treatment Modalities Used for Bronchial Asthma Patients[a, b]

Adjustment	94.6%
Nutrition	61.8%
Soft tissue	
Manipulation	44.4%
Exercise	31.1%
Psychotherapy	27 %
Electrotherapy	20.8%
(Do not treat patients with asthma)	3.7%

[a]From Wiles M, Diakow P: (unpublished, personal communication).
[b]N = 241.

Table 14.4 Summary of Spinal Regions Adjusted in Patients with Bronchial Asthma[a, b]

Upper C (C0-C2)	36.4%
Lower C (C3-C7)	21.5%
Upper T (T1-T6)	58.8%
Lower T (T7-T12)	29.8%
Upper L (L1-L3)	2.6%
Upper L (L4-L5)	0.4%
S/I	1.8%
Ribs	13.2%
Nonspecific	50.4%
Other	2.6%

[a]From Wiles M, Diakow P: (unpublished, personal communication).
[b]N = 228.

Table 14.5 Nutritional Therapy in Bronchial Asthma[a, b]

Vitamin and mineral supplements	
Vitamin A	16.8%
Vitamin B	9.4%
Vitamin C	29.5%
Vitamin D	4.7%
Vitamin E	7.4%
Panthothenic acid	2.0%
Multiple vitamins	6.7%
Calcium	6.0%
Magnesium	0.7%
Other supplements and dietary advice	
Herbals	6.7%
Glandulary	5.4%
General advice	33.6%
Remove food triggers	43.6%
No sugar	9.4%
No caffeine	6.0%
No salt	0.7%
No smoking	8.7%
Other	6.7%

[a]From Wiles M, Diakow P: (unpublished, personal communication).
[b]N=149.

Table 14.6 Soft Tissue Therapy in Bronchial Asthma[a, b]

Cervical muscles	3.7%
Thoracic pump	43.0%
Upper Thoracic	32.7%
Lower Thoracic	2.8%
Intercostal muscles	17.8%
Diaphragm	15.0%
Psoas muscle	2.8%
"Sinus massage"	3.7%
Nonspecific soft-tissue therapy	17.8%

[a]From Wiles M, Diakow P: (unpublished, personal communication).
[b]N = 107.

Table 14.7 Electrotherapy in Bronchial Asthma[a, b]

Low volt	32%
Short wave diathermy	34%
Diapulse	20%
Interferential therapy	18%
Ultrasound	10%
Acupuncture	8%
Percussion therapy	12%
Other	18%

[a]From Wiles M, Diakow P: (unpublished, personal communication).
[b]N = 50.

Table 14.8 Exercise in Bronchial Asthma[a]

Breathing exercise	58.7%
General activity	40.0%
Other	33.3%

[a]N = 75.

Table 14.9 Psychotherapy in Bronchial Asthma[a, b]

General counseling and relaxation therapy	52.3%
Identification of environmental and emotional trigger	49.2%
Other	7.7%

[a]From Wiles M, Diakow P: (unpublished, personal communication).
[b]N = 65.

Wilson, in discussing the osteopathic approach to asthma, gave his opinion of the time required to restore thoracic mechanics to normal in cases of asthma (106). He stated that patients should be treated once per week for about one year in order to achieve optimal results in asthmatic cases. Wiles and Diakow (unpublished) surveyed 241 chiropractors about their approach to the care of patients with asthma. Only 3.7% did not treat asthmatic patients. Of those who did treat them, 94.6% adjusted the spine, 61.8% used nutrition, 44.4% used soft tissue techniques, 31.1% used exercise, 27% used hypno-sis and/or counseling, and 20.8% used electrotherapy. The details of this treatment are given in Tables 14.3 to 14.9.

Clearly, since asthma is such a significant problem for so many patients (and a "symbol of medical frustration") and since manipulative therapy has been utilized with success for many years in these cases, we can only hope that there will be renewed interest in fully defining and demonstrating a role for chiropractic care of asthmatic patients.

Pneumonia

In terms of its pathophysiological mechanism, pneumonia is generally considered an opportunistic infection. There are numerous inherent defense mechanisms protecting the warm, moist, pulmonary environment from infection. These include the epiglottal reflex, mucous-covered ciliated epithelia, cough reflex, macrophages, lymphatic drainage, and antibodies (90). These mechanisms are present in everybody, yet in susceptible individuals they individually or collectively fail, bringing about clinical evidence of pulmonary infection. Among the more common factors leading to this susceptibility are decreased rib cage motion and decreased diaphragmatic excursion. These lead, in turn, to fascial congestion and poor venous and lymphatic return. The result is a major disturbance in the normal homeostatic processes protecting the lungs, thereby providing an environment for opportunistic infections.

Subluxations in the upper to midthoracic spine will tend to diminish respiratory excursion (giving rise to a restrictive type of pulmonary embarrassment and decreased compliance). This initiates the aforementioned cascade of events and disturbs normal vasomotor events in the pulmonary neuromeres. The result is trophic disturbance along the pulmonary neuromeres, as well as a more direct embarrassment of pulmonary physiology.

This sequence of events has long been recognized (90, 94, 98, 113, 114), and from this follows a logical and rational role for manipulative therapy in treating patients with pneumonia, consistent with the chiropractic strategy in respiratory disease.

1. Correction of subluxations causing vasomotor disturbances in the pulmonary neuromeres (T1–6);
2. Correction of somatic dysfunction (i.e., thoracic and rib problems directly causing decreased respiratory excursion (primary), or somatic problems that exist as a result of lung disease, such a rib fixation due to restricted movement in pleurisy (secondary));
3. Correction of direct somatogenic respiratory embarrassment (such as diaphragmatic excursion limitation or rib subluxations causing decreased thoracic cage compliance);
4. Provision of nonmanipulative aid such as natural hygiene methods and allopathy.

Several detailed discussions of this approach to pneumonia have been published (90, 94, 98, 114). In addition to thoracic and rib manipulative procedures, cranial and sacral procedures have been recommended because of the proposed relationship between cranial-sacral movement patterns and CSF movement (and hence generalized resistance and well-being). Thoracic pump procedures have been recommended to enhance lymphatic flow in the thoracic cage.

The manipulative approach seems so logical that it may be a frustration to chiropractors that it is not utilized more in the treatment of patients with pneumonia. Indeed, Miller (90) states: "(Manipulative) therapy, called supportive therapy by many, should be primary therapy. Manipulative therapy improves venous and lymphatic return, normalized rib cage and diaphragmatic options, aids in expectoration and makes the patient more comfortable. As supportive as well as primary therapy, it acts by improving arterial supply and venous return so that

the delivery and detoxification of medication will be at a maximum." Acuteness of symptoms is not a contraindication to treatment, although any treatment must be given with care and discretion to acutely ill patients. In fact, specific advice has been published about dealing with hospitalized patients (97, 98). This advice suggests treatment in the sitting or side-posture if necessary, and encourages soft-tissue techniques as a prelude and accompaniment to regular manipulative therapy. Wilson suggests two treatments per day are sufficient for hospitalized patients.

Pneumonia, as a common opportunistic infection, is a good example of disease secondary to decreased resistance as a consequence of structural dysfunction. It offers a tremendous opportunity to chiropractors to demonstrate their role in general health care by aiding such patients in achieving a more rapid and effective resolution to their disease.

Chronic Obstructive Pulmonary Disease

Manipulative therapy is considered to be extremely effective in assisting patients with chronic obstructive pulmonary disease (COPD). Indeed, the 1975 NINCDS conference included only one paper on manipulation and visceral disease, and it was on the effects of manipulation and COPD (115). In this study of 44 COPD patients, 23 were treated with manipulation and standard medical therapy and 21 with standard treatment only (controls). The experimental group showed tendencies (not significant) toward greater improvement in lung function than the control group; however, subjective improvement, including the ability to walk up stairs and perform physical work was significantly higher in the manipulated group than in the control group.

These results are similar to others in the study of manipulation and COPD. That is, physical improvements in lung capacities are rarely seen in advanced cases of respiratory disease; however, subjective improvement is extremely common. This is why Allen and Kelso made a plea for more research into respiratory disease and manipulative therapy (103). They noted responses similar to Miller's (115), in that "with few exceptions, the patients' subjective response to manipulative treatment was an improved sense of well being and relief from congestion, dyspnea, and the milder forms of air hunger" (103). These comments were based on studying patients over long periods of time (up to 10 years).

The manipulative approach to chronic lung disease has been described in the literature both generally (90, 94–97) and in a specific case (116).

Stiles has taken a fairly philosophical perspective—mentioning the importance of subluxations in causing neural facilitation and its resultant pathophysiology (96). Frymann goes further by describing the nature of musculoskeletal involvement in COPD (97). Regularly applied manipulative care yields gratifying results in chronic lung disease, she states.

Also mentioned is the importance of another result of manipulative therapy, which I have not described in this chapter—the sense of optimism and well-being that is derived from a "hands-on therapy" during chronic disease: "Patient persistance with (manipulative) treatment will result in progressive amelioration, improved thoracic mobility, increased endurance of physical activity, reduced fatigue, and improved well being. Above all, the despair and despondency will give way slowly to a happier, more optimistic attitude, in which life has value once more" (97).

Finally, although structural lung damage from chronic disease (i.e., reduced volume) does not readily change after manipulative therapy, the therapy does have beneficial effects, both subjectively and objectively, (115, 116). The chiropractic model predicts a reduced progression of lung damage during chiropractic care (because of both physical assistance to respiration via increased thoracic compliance and neurological assistance to respiration by removing sources of facilitation and trophic disturbances). This phenomenon has been described (117) when the progression of COPD was studied (vis-à-vis pulmonary functions) during a course of manipulative therapy. As the author concludes, "the trend of values for RV, ERV and FEV [residual volume, expiratory reserve volume, and forced expiratory volume], for this subject during six years of treatment suggests that osteopathic health care may serve an important role in the management of patients with COPD by decreasing the rate at which respiratory function is lost."

Acute Upper Respiratory Disease

Manipulative therapy is important in treating acute respiratory disease (URI) since these infections rank among the highest causes of lost man-hours from work. The manipulative approach is similar to that described above, however, lymphatic drainage techniques are often stressed. Harakal (108) describes eight methods of treatment:

1. Cervical soft-tissue manipulation (patient supine);
2. Lymphatic drainage techniques;
3. Pressure therapy over the paranasal sinuses;
4. Establishment of normal upper rib function (for proper inspiration);
5. Cervical manipulation;
6. Thoracic manipulation;
7. Examination of T12-L2 when cough is present;
8. Establishment of normal craniosacral function.

He recommends this program and states "with treatment early in the course of the disease process, the length of illness can be shortened, inconvenience reduced, and complications minimized."

Manipulative therapy was even studied for its effects on children when bronchiolitis (102). Treatment was given for 60 to 90 seconds, three times per day, on hospitalized patients. Although the results were inconclusive, the author has recommended further investigation to define the role of manipulation in such cases.

Finally, the work of Purse (118) must be mentioned. Purse (a pediatrician) reported the results of thousands of cases of URI treated with antibiotics alone or with antibiotics and manipulation. As expected, he concluded that the most effective therapy was a combination of antibiotics and manipulation.

CONCLUSION

Given the bulk of evidence supporting a positive role for manipulative therapy and given the safe, gentle, and effective nature of the therapy itself, it is difficult to understand why there is not more manipulative care for patients with visceral disease. Whatever the reasons, they are beyond the scope of this chapter.

Manipulative therapy has been described in relation to its role in treating patients with cardiovascular, respiratory, and gastrointestinal problems. Other areas could just as well have been chosen, such as psychiatric disorders, gynecological disease, thyroid disease, renal disease, and others. The goal in this chapter was to illustrate that there *is* a role for manipulative therapy in treating *patients* with dysfunction, disorders, or disease. The role may be primary or secondary, but in all cases, it is designed to remove sources of interference to normal nerve function, so that the body may either heal itself or be assisted in the process of healing.

Remember that chiropractic care, being Hippocratic in nature, seeks to treat the patient with the disease, not the disease within the patient. In this regard manipulative therapy has no boundaries, save for its contraindications. Chiropractors should utilize this therapy in whatever setting or instance they can. By extending manipulative therapy to patients with visceral disease, the most efficient and appropriate role for manipulation will become better understood, and patients under our care will be better served.

References

1. Patterson M, Steinmetz J: Long-lasting alteration of spinal reflexes: a potential basis for somatic dysfunction. *Manual Med* 2:38–42, 1986.
2. Daiber W: Disorders of the kidneys. In Hoag JM (ed): *Osteopathic Medicine.* New York, McGraw-Hill, 1969, p 632.
3. Solheim RN: *Gastroenterology for Chiropractic Physicians.* Northwestern College of Chiropractic, Minneapolis, 1962.
4. Pansky B, House E: *Functional Approach To Neuroanatomy,* ed 2. New York, McGraw-Hill, 1967.
5. Hulten L: Extrinsic nervous control of colonic motility and blood flow. *Acta Physiol Scand Supp* 335, 1969.
6. Sato A, Sato Y, Shimado F, Torigata Y: Change in gastric motility produced by nociceptive stimulation of the skin in rats. *Brain Res* 87:151–159, 1975.
7. Kametani H, Sato A, Sato Y, Simpson A: Neural mechanisms of reflex facilitation and inhibition of gastric motility

to stimulation of various skin areas of rats. *J Physiol (Lond)* 294:407–418, 1979.

8. Jansson G: Effects of reflexes on somatic afferents on the adrenergic outflow to the stomach in the cat. *Acta Physiol Scand* 77:17–22, 1969.

9. Swenson R: Effect of supramaximal electrical stimulation of suboccipital muscle afferents on blood pressure and gastric motility in rats, unpublished.

10. Wiles M: Observations on the effects of upper cervical manipulation on the electrogastrogram. *JMPT* 3:226–228, 1980.

11. Harakal J, Burns CL: An osteopathic approach to disease of the upper gastrointestinal tract. *Osteopath Ann* 6:51–54, 1978.

12. Lewit K, Rychlikova E: Reflex and vertebrogenic disturbances in peptic ulcer. In Lewit K, Gutmann G (eds): *Rehabilitacia: Proceedings of the IV Congress, Prague*. International Federation of Manual Medicine, 1975.

13. Banner R: Thermography, radiography, and osteopathic palpation in the diagnosis of duodenal ulcerations. *JAOA* 73:899–903, 1974.

14. Kamieth H: Pathogenic importance of the thoracic portion of the vertebral columns. *Arch Orthop u Umfall-Chir* 49:585–606, 1958. Abstracted in *JAMA* Nov 15, p 1586, 1958.

15. Nicholas NS: Correlation of somatic dysfunction with visceral disease. *JAOA* 75:425–428, 1975.

16. Stiles E: Osteopathic approach to peptic ulcer disease. *Osteopath Med* 2:57–62, 1977.

17. Vear H: A clinical review of gastric acidity. *Digest Chiro Econ* 14:24–26, 1972.

18. Rivillis J: Immunosympathectomy and gastric secretion. *Arch Surg* 107:618–621, 1973.

19. Djahangiuri B, Taubin HL, Landsking L: Increased sympathetic activity in the pathogensis of restraint ulcer in rats. *J Pharmacol Exp Ther* 184(1):113–118, 1973.

20. Robuck S: Osteopathic management of gastric and duodenal ulcers. *JAOA* 46:465–468, 1947.

21. Magoun H: Gastroduodenal ulcers from the osteopathic viewpoint. *Yr Bk Acad Osteopath*, pp 117–120, 1962.

22. Strong W: Disorders of the digestive system. In Hoag JM (ed): *Osteopathic Medicine*. New York, McGraw-Hill, 1969.

23. Smeyne AL: The effect of stress on the colon. *Osteopath Ann* 7:24–27, 1979.

24. English W: The somatic components of colon disease. *Osteopath Ann* 4:150–157, 1976.

25. Masterton E: Irritable bowel syndrome: an osteopathic approach. *Osteopath Ann* 12:21–31, 1984.

26. Overton RM: Diagnosis and treatment of functional constipation. *J Nat Chiro Assoc* 10:15–18, 1956.

27. Lewit K: Liver and gallbladder disease. In Lewit K: *Manuelle Therapie*. Prague, JA Barth, 1973, p 432.

28. Cole WV: The osteopathic lesion complex: effects of osteopathic lesion, chemical irritants in the muscle at the level of T6, and chemical irritants in the liver. *JAOA* 49:135–141, 1949.

29. Rogers F: Searching for a distinctly osteopathic approach to heart disease. *Osteopath Ann* 13:288–291, 1985.

30. Gooch AS, Maranhao V, Goldberg H: The straight thoracic spine in cardiac diagnosis. *Am Heart J* 74:595–602, 1967.

31. DeLeon AC, Perloff JK, Twigg H: The straight back syndrome: clinical cardiovascular manifestations. *Circulation* 32:193–203, 1965.

32. Rawlings ME: Straight back syndrome; a new heart disease. *Dis Chest* 39:435–443, 1961.

33. Egli AB: Spine and heart, vertebrogenous cardiac syndromes. *Ann Swiss Chiro Assoc* 4:95–105, 1969.

34. Koch RS: A somatic component to heart disease. *JAOA* 60:735–739, 1961.

35. Tilley RM: The role of palpatory diagnosis and manipulation therapy in heart disease. *Osteopathic Ann* 4:272–277, 1976.

36. Beal M: Palpatory testing for somatic dysfunction in patients with cardiovascular disease. *JAOA* 82:822–831, 1983.

37. Tran TA, Kirby JD: The effects of upper cervical adjustment upon the normal physiology of the heart. *ACA J Chiro* 14:S58–62, 1977.

38. Tran TA, Kirby JD: The effects of upper thoracic adjustment upon the normal physiology of the heart. *ACA J Chiro* 14:S25–28, 1977.

39. Busch BW, Danelius BD, Drost SF: Cardiovascular changes after chiropractic—effects of chiropractic adjustment on selected parameters of the cardiovascular system. *ACA J Chiro* 8:S33–39, 1974.

40. Esler MD, Nestel PJ: Sympathetic responsiveness to head-up tilt in essential hypertension. *Clin Sci* 44:213–216, 1973.

41. Roppel RM, Johnston WL: Electrodermographic study of hypertensives. *JAOA* 77:477–478, 1978.

42. Johnston WL, Hill JL, Sealey JW, Sucher BM: Cervicothoracic palpation in hypertensive patients. Proceedings of the 23rd National Osteopathic Research Conference, Chicago, 1979. *JAOA* 79:300–308, 1980.

43. Johnston WL, Hill JL, Elkiss ML, Marino RV: Identification of stable somatic findings in hypertensive subjects by trained examiners using palpatory examination. *JAOA* 81:830–836, 1982.

44. Frumkin K, Nathan RS, Prout MF, Cohem MC: Nonpharmacologic control of essential hypertension in man: a critical review. *Psychosom Med* 40:294–320, 1978.

45. Baldwin W: Hypertension. In Hoag JM (ed): *Osteopathic Medicine*, New York, McGraw-Hill, 1969, p 519.

46. Goodheart G: Hypertension. *Digest Chiro Econ* 11:20–23, 1968.

47. Hood RP: Blood pressure. *Digest Chiro Econ* 16:36–38, 1974.

48. Welberry AE: Chiropractic management of the hypertensive. *J Natl Chiro Assoc* 33:26–27, 1963.

49. Dulgar G, Hill D, Situcek A, Davis BP: Evidence for a possible anti-hypertensive effect of basic technique apex contact adjusting. *ACA J Chiro* 17:S97–102, 1980.

50. Northup TL: Manipulative management of hypertension. *JAOA* 60:973–978, 1961.

51. Wilson PT: Osteopathic cardiology. *Yearbook of the American Academy of Osteopathy*, 1958.

52. Blood HA. Manipulative management of hypertension. *Yearbook of the American Academy of Osteopathy*, 1964, pp 189–195.

53. Norris T: A study of the effect of manipulation on blood pressure. *Yearbook of the Academy of Osteopathy* 1964 pp 184–8.

54. Miller AD: A review of hypertension and its management by osteopathic manipulative therapy. *Yearbook of the Academy of Osteopathy*, 1966, pp 30–36.

55. Celander E, Kuenig AJ, Celander DR: Effect of osteopathic manipulative therapy on autonomic tone as evidenced by blood pressure changes and activity of the fibrinolytic system. *JAOA* 67:1037–1038, 1968.

56. Fischera AP, Celander DR: Effect of osteopathic manipulative therapy on autonomic tone as evidenced by blood pressure changes and activity on the fibrinolytic system. *JAOA* 68:1036–1038, 1969.

57. Kolman S, Getson P, Levin F, Scolthorpe R: Effects of osteopathic manipulation on several different physiological functions: Part IV, absence of crossover effect. *JAOA* 73:669–678, 1974.

58. Stiles EG: Osteopathic approach to the hypertensive patient. *Osteopath Med* 2:41–45, 1977.

59. Mannino JR: The application of neurologic reflexes to the treatment of hypertension. *JAOA* 79:225–231, 1979.

60. Morgan JP, Dickey JL, Hunt HH, Hudgins PM: A controlled trial of spinal manipulation in the management of hypertension. *JAOA* 85:308–313, 1985.

61. Wiles MR, Diakow P: Chiropractic and visceral disease: a brief survey. *JCCA* 26:65–68, 1982.

62. Crawford J, Hickson G, Wiles MR: The management of hypertensive disease: a review of spinal manipulation and the efficacy of conservative therapeusis. *JMPT* 9:27–31, 1986.

63. Burns L: A review of cardiac pathology in certain laboratory animals. *JAOA* 45:115–116, 1945.

64. Rinzler SH, Travell J: Therapy directed at the somatic component of cardiac pain. *Am Heart J* 35:248–258, 1948.

65. Foreman RD, Ohata CA: Effects of coronary artery occlusion on thoracic spinal neurons receiving viscerosomatic inputs. *Am J Physiol* 238:667–674, 1980.

66. Raab W: The nonvascular metabolic myocardial vulnerability factor in coronary artery disease. *Am Heart J* 66:685–706, 1963.

67. Wilson P: Angina pectoris. *Yearbook of the American Academy of Osteopathy*, 1949, pp 176–177.

68. Kletzel E: Chiropractic care for artherosclerosis. *J Natl Chiro Assoc* 33:31–31, 67–68, 1963.

69. Johnson FE: Some observations in the use of osteopathic therapy in the care of patients with cardiac disease. *JAOA* 71:799–804, 1972.

70. Rychlikova E: Reflex and vertebrogenic disorders in ischemic heart disease, their importance in therapy. *Rehabilitacia* 8:109–114, 1975.

71. Monti RL: Chiropractic management of coronary artery disease. *ACA J Chiro* 18:S15-S18, 1981.

72. Miller WD: Disorders of the coronary circulation. In Hoag JD (ed): *Osteopathic Medicine*, New York, McGraw-Hill, 1969, p 448.

73. Richmond W: Somatic manipulation in coronary heart disease. *JAOA* 41:217, 1942.

74. Greenman PE: Manipulative therapy in relation to total health care. In Korr I (ed): *Neurobiological Mechanisms in Manipulative Therapy*. New York, Plenum, 1977 p 43.

75. Rogers JT, Rogers JC: The role of osteopathic manipulative therapy in the treatment of coronary heart disease. *JAOA* 76:71–81, 1976.

76. Cox JM, Gorbis S, Pick LM, Rogers JC, Rojers FJ: Palpable musculoskeletal findings in coronary artery disease: results of a double-blind study. *JAOA* 82:832–838, 1983.

77. Cox JM, Gideon D, Rogers FJ: Incidence of osteophytic lipping in the thoracic spine in coronary heart disease: results of a pilot study. *JAOA* 82:837–838, 1983.

78. Frymann V: The osteopathic approach to cardiac and pulmonary problems. *JAOA* 77:668–673, 1978.

79. Miller WD: Functional aspects of coronary circulation. *Osteopath Ann* 2:8–11, 1974.

80. Becker AD: Manipulative osteopathy in cardiac therapy. *Yearbook of the American Academy of Osteopathy*, 1965.

81. Robuck SV: Osteopathic manipulative therapy in organic heart disease. *Yearbook of the American Academy of Osteopathy*, 1965.

82. Howell RK, Kappler RE: The influence of osteopathic manipulative therapy on a patient with advanced cardiopulmonary disease. *JAOA* 73:322–327, 1973.

83. Baldwin W: Cardiac arrhythmias. In Hoag J (ed): *Osteopathic Medicine*. New York, McGraw-Hill, 1969, p 477.

84. Thomas PH: Congestive heart failure. In Hoag J (ed): *Osteopathic Medicine*, New York, McGraw-Hill, 1969, p 501.

85. Stary O: The concept of research into vertebrogenic disease in CSSR: *Accta Univ Carolinae (Med)* Supp 21:16–18, 1965.

86. Robbins AS, Tamkin JA: *Manual of Ambulatory Medicine*, Philadelphia, WB Saunders, 1979.

87. Lewit K: *Manipulative Therapy in Rehabilitation of the Locomotor System.* London, Butterworth, 1985.

88. Lewit K: Relation of faulty respiration to posture, with clinical implications. *JAOA* 79:525–529, 1980.

89. Bergsmann O, Eder M: Atembewegung und Vitalfunctionen (Breathing movement and vital functions). *Man Medizin* 22:96–99, 1984.

90. Miller KD: An osteopathic approach to respiratory disease. *Osteopath Med* 2:81–89, 1977.

91. Hviid C: A comparison of the effect of chiropractic treatment on respiratory function in patients with & without respiratory distress symptoms. *Bull Eur Chiro Union* 26:17–34, 1978.

92. Murphy AS: The effect of various pulmonary & thoracic mobilization procedures on arterial oxygen saturation. *JAOA* 67:1073–1074, 1968.

93. Droste PL, Beckman DL: Pulmonary effects of prolonged sympathetic stimulation. *Proc Soc Exp Biol Med* 146:352–353, 1974.

94. Hoag M: Musculoskeletal involvement in chronic lung disease. *JAOA* 71:698–706, 1972.

95. Palatini K: Breathing in relation to pathology. *Bull Eur Chiro Union* 26:30–1, 1978.

96. Stiles EG: Manipulation management of chronic lung disease. *Osteopath Ann* 9:300–304, 1981.

97. Frymann VM: The osteopathic approach to cardiac & pulmonary problems. *JAOA* 77:668–673, 1978.

98. Wilson PT: Internal medicine: an osteopathic approach. *Osteopath Ann* 7:259–273, 1979.

99. Beyeler W: Experiences in the management of asthma. *Ann Swiss Chiro Assoc* 3:111–117, 1965.

100. Jamison J, LeoKovec K, Lepore S, Hannan P: Asthma in a chiropractic clinic: a pilot study. *J Aust Chiro Assoc* 16:137–43, 1986.

101. Silvagni AJ: Development of a study to determine the effect of osteopathic manipulation procedures in the treatment of asthma. *JAOA* 83:130–131, 1983.

102. Belcastro MR, Backes CR, Chila AG: Bronchiolitis: a pilot study of osteopathic manipulative treatment, bronchodilators, and other therapy. *JAOA* 83:672–676, 1984.

103. Allen TW, Kelso AF: Osteopathic research and respiratory disease. *JAOA* 79:360, 1980.

104. Davis D: Respiratory manifestation of dorsal spine radiculitis simulating cardiac asthma. *Ann Int Med* 32:954–959, 1950.

105. Swan B: Cervical manipulation. *Med J Aust* 55:811, 1968.

106. Wilson PT: The osteopathic treatment of asthma. *JAOA* 45:491–492, 1946.

107. Harakal J: Manipulative treatment for acute upper-respiratory diseases. *Osteopath Ann* 9:253–257, 1981.

108. O'Donovan D: The possible significance of scoliosis of the spine in the causation of asthma and allied allergic conditions. *Ann Allergy*, 9:184–219, 1951.

109. Goldman SR: A structural approach to bronchial asthma. *Bull Eur Chiro Union* 21:66–71, 1972.

110. Arbiloff B: Bronchial asthma: a case report. *J Clin Chiro* 2:40–42, 1969.

111. Hopfer F: Asthma bronchiale und Neuraltherapie. *Wien Klin Wochenscher* 86:108–111, 1974.

112. Boohuys A: Effect of posture in experimental asthma in man. *Am J Med* 34:470–476, 1963.

113. Zink JG: The osteopathic holistic approach to homeostasis. *Yearbook of the American Academy of Osteopathy*, 1970, pp 1–5.

114. Facto LL: The osteopathic treatment for lobar pneumonia. *JAOA* 46:385–391, 1947.

115. Goldstein M (ed): *The Research Status of Spinal Manipulative Therapy* NINCDS, Bethesda, 1975.

116. Howell RK, Dappler RE: The influence of osteopathic manipulation therapy on a patient with advanced cardiopulmonary disease. *JAOA* 73:322–327, 1973.

117. Mall R: An evaluation of routine pulmonary function tests as indicators of responsiveness of a patient with COPD to osteopathic health care. *JAOA* 73:327–333, 1973.

118. Purse FM: Manipulative therapy of upper respiratory infections in children. *JAOA* 65:964–971, 1966.

CHAPTER 15

In the Patient's Interest

Chiropractors should, in the public interest, be accepted as partners in the general health care system. No other health professional is as well qualified by his general training to carry out a diagnosis for spinal mechanical dysfunction or to perform spinal manual therapy (1).

Chiropractic management of spine-related disorders plays a significant role in the diagnosis and treatment of spinal mechanical dysfunction. Lewit (2) has noted that the functional pathology of the locomotor system is a "no-man's-land" between neurology, orthopaedics, and rheumatology. This medical no-man's-land has long been claimed by chiropractors whose discipline is the science concerned with the pathogenesis, diagnostics, therapeutics, and prophylaxis of functional disturbances, pathomechanical states, pain syndromes, and neurophysiological effects related to the statics and dynamics of the locomotor system, especially of the spine and pelvis (3).

The primary therapeutic modality of chiropractors has been spinal manipulative therapy (the chiropractic adjustment). Incomplete information and the failure to demonstrate a clear, biologic rationale for the use of manipulation may account for the history of skepticism about the efficacy of spinal manipulation. Lewit (1) discusses two main aspects of manipulation. "First it causes marked reflex effects in many types of pain, a feature that it shares with many other methods of physical therapy such as massage, electrical stimulation and local anaesthesia." The second effect of manipulation for which there is no substitute is the reversal of restricted joint movement. It is this restoration of normal joint movement that has earned chiropractic its unique place in the health care system.

Judicious use of manipulation requires that differentiation be made between articular fixation and restricted motion due to muscle hypertonicity that is secondary to joint hypermobility (4). Response to manipulation of blocked joints is rapid, and in most cases the patient experiences some relief immediately. Maigne (5) states, "What is unreplaceable in the manipulative therapy is the rapidity of results, at times instantaneous, generally requiring two to three sessions, only in exceptional cases more than six."

This, of course, refers to patients with simple joint-locking and no tissue pathology. In most cases when manipulation is the treatment of choice, there is some soft tissue damage that requires time to heal and is generally benefited by adjunctive procedures (see Chapter 14).

In this sense, the chiropractor is responsible for two diagnoses. The first diagnosis determines the biomechanical problem. This diagnosis takes into account the site of joint locking and the direction of restricted motion, both of which must be determined before the manipulative thrust can be appropriately employed. The second diagnosis is necessary to ascertain the extent of pathology. It determines the type of adjunctive therapy that will hasten the healing process and is the best determinant of the patient's prognosis with regards to healing time (6, 7). A number of studies have indicated that the average number of visits for patients with back pain treated by manipulation is between 3 and 20 (Table 15.1).

Jaquet (8) has concluded that if there is still no or very little progress after twelve visits, there are four possibilities (Table 15.2). First, the original diagnosis may not have been correct. It is advisable to evaluate the condition further, which usually requires investigation from a specialist. This may involve additional diagnostic procedures such as electromy-

Table 15.1 Frequency of Spine Manipulation in the Treatment of Low Back Pain[a]

Study	Year	Controlled	Method	Outcome
Maitland	1957	No	Review of patients treated by physiotherapist with manipulation (author's view of own patients)	No neurological deficits, acute pain: 90% relief in 6 treatments; chronic pain with neurological deficits: 50% relief in 11 treatments
Edwards	1969	Yes	Survey of patients in several physiotherapy centers comparing heat massage, and exercise with mobilization and manipulation carried out in 2 hospitals, 2 private practices, over 2 years	Average number of treatments ranged from 4.8 to 6.4 for various back statuses to gain acceptable results
Sherman	1973	No	Chart review by treating chiropractor	65% of patients apparently recovered or substantially improved in 10 treatments
Doran	1975	No	Manipulation Physiotherapy Corset, analgesics	6.0 treatments 7.3 treatments Equivalent improvement
Potter	1977	No	Manipulation with variable other treatments	70% recovered with manipulation, much improved treatment frequency for various low back pain states, 3.3 to 5.5 visits
Evans	1978	Yes	Pain medication available to all patients; one group treatment with manipulation once a week for 3 weeks; control group medication only	Manipulated group decreased pain faster & increased spine flexion compared to control
Rasmussen	1979	Yes	Randomized trial with either manipulation or short-wave diathermy, 3 times per week for 2 weeks	92% of patients treated with manipulation free of symptoms in 14 days with 6 visits
Cox	1984	No	Data collection and analysis on 576 cases in a multicenter study	Average days to maximum improvement 43, average number of visits 19

[a]Adapted from information compiled by SG Fechtel.

ography, CT scanning, myelography, or magnetic resonance imaging. In these cases he recommends immediate additional investigation and a complete reevaluation (8).

A second possibility for delayed recovery is that the initial treatment was inappropriate. For example, a patient with an acute herniated disc and progressive neurological deficits likely needs prompt referral for a surgical consultation for possible decompressive surgery. Or, the doctor may be focusing on a herniated disc when a patient's sciatica is caused by a piriformis syndrome. In this example, therapy directed to the involved muscle rather than the spinal joints brings prompt relief.

A third possibility for failure to progress, suggested by Jaquet (8), is that the relationship between the doctor and the patient is not conducive to rehabilitation. This may be due to a personality conflict or to unreasonable expectations by either party. In these cases, it is best to acknowledge that there is something wrong, and Jaquet (8) suggests that even though the diagnosis appears correct and the treat-

Table 15.2 Conditions Delaying Patient Progress[a]

1. Incorrect diagnosis
2. Incorrect treatment
3. Incompatibility between doctor and patient
4. Secondary gain (patient receives benefit from pain behavior)
5. Coexisting conditions

[a]Modified from Jaquet PE: *An Introduction to Clinical Chiropractic* Grounauer. Geneva, Switzerland, 1974.

ment appropriate, the patient might respond better if treated by someone else.

The fourth possibility for a barrier to progress is that the doctor has not understood the patient's actual motivation. The patient may be employing somatization for an emotional problem, seeking more compensation than is justified (compensation neurosis), or may simply by hypochondriacal. In these cases, prompt referral for psychometric evaluation is in the best interest of all concerned (see Chapter 4).

Another point that must be kept in mind when a patient fails to respond in the anticipated length of time is the possibility that more than one condition may exist. Complex cases requiring multiple diagnoses are often frustrating and difficult, and it must be remembered that patients may have more than one disorder. In such cases, the signs and symptoms may be very confusing and even appear contradictory, but with patience and persistence the multiple causative factors can be determined.

The frequency and duration of treatment must always be based on medical necessity, not on false standards such as arbitrary guidelines established for the benefit of overworked claims examiners attempting to clear cluttered desks or quotas established by practice-management entrepreneurs, which benefit the doctor more than the patient.

RECURRENCE

Recurrence of facet-joint locking is relatively frequent following trauma, especially in cases of facet tropism. Facet tropism in the lumbar spine (where one facet articulation is in the coronal plane while the other is in the sagittal or semisagittal plane) predisposes to rotational fixation in the direction of the more coronal facet (9). The classic facet syndrome, in which the facet joints override in extension, also tends to recur following hyperextension injuries. It should not be assumed, without careful examination, that such patients automatically return with the same problem.

A classic facet syndrome can predispose that patient to a disc herniation as the three-joint complex degenerates, and other underlying pathology can mimic back pain of biomechanical origin. While these patients tend to have recurring episodes of facet-joint locking requiring occasional manipulation, maintenance care consisting of repeated manipulation is not recommended and may cause even more harm by repeatedly stretching already traumatized ligaments, the holding elements of the spinal articulations.

The return of symptoms following a brief period of relief following manipulation suggests a reflex effect from reduction of muscle splinting. Patients with hypermobile segments often report relief for several days initially following manipulation. With repeated manipulation, the period of relief is often reduced to several hours (4). In these cases, therapy, to be curative rather than palliative, should be directed specifically to the muscles not to the joints.

The standard criticism that chiropractors foster a dependency on their services, often results from this brief interval of relief followed by a return of symptoms. The subsequent dependency and short duration of relief has kept many medical practitioners from referring patients for a trial of manipulation and kept patients themselves from seeking the benefit of a therapy that can bring lasting relief for specific conditions.

This is not to say that chiropractors should not treat patients with hypermobile segments. On the contrary, hypermobility at one segment is often secondary to hypomobility in an adjacent segment (10). Specific manipulation directed to the fixed segment allows the hypermobile segment to heal gradually, with permanent relief from the painful muscle spasm (see Chapter 8).

RESEARCH AND THE EFFICACY OF SPINAL MANIPULATION

Most research involving spinal manipulative therapy (11–38) has compared the effectiveness of manipulation in the treatment of back pain to other forms of conservative therapy (Table 15.3). Compared with other forms of conservative treatment, spinal manipulative therapy brings faster relief of pain and improved function (Table 15.4). This suggests that manipulation should be the first line of treatment for acute low back pain (39). The long-term effectiveness of repeated manipulation has not been demonstrated, however, and there is no justification for frequent nonspecific manipulation over a

long time (39). Manipulation has also proven effective in the treatment of chronic low back pain, with daily treatment over a two-week period (40). Not just limited to low back pain, spinal manipulation has proven beneficial in the treatment of a variety of neuromusculoskeletal conditions including whiplash injuries and headaches (see Chapters 7–10).

Not as well established is the treatment of visceral conditions (Chapter 14), which have long been observed to respond to spinal manipulation. Spinal lesions that are the result of viscerosomatic reflexes as well as visceral disorders that are initiated by somatovisceral reflexes are appropriately treated by chiropractic physicians. Chiropractic management is directed at the primary spine-related condition and not the secondary organic condition. With appropriate evaluation and monitoring of the secondary condition, a degree of symptomatic relief can often be afforded.

Chiropractors are not autonomous providers, thus patients with disease processes and secondary organic manifestations should be referred to the appropriate medical specialist for evaluation and treatment. Concurrent care for a spinal condition while the patient receives medical care elsewhere is often advantageous.

Consideration must be given to spinal degenerative conditions that may warrant chronic care, including degenerative joint disease, osteoporosis, and discopathy. Unusual or irreversible spinal conditions, including moderate-to-severe scoliosis, failed back syndrome, compressive fracture, and congenital anomalies may produce an underlying structural problem that permanently alters spinal biomechanics, necessitating ongoing care, with consideration for more intense periods of treatment at times of significant exacerbation or reinjury.

In addition to the reductionistic approach to spinal biomechanical dysfunction, in which manipulation is directed to a specific vertebral motion segment, the chiropractor must understand the spine as an organ of posture (Chapter 11). The chain-link concept, in which each vertebral motion segment acts as a link in the chain of articulations forming the vertebral column, allows the chiropractor to treat postural distortion and compensatory lesions in a rational fashion.

Remember that the biomechanics of the spine is a chain reaction. For example, pain where the sartorius muscle attaches at the medial aspect of the knee and where the quadratus lumborum attaches to the 12th rib can both be caused by flexion fixation of the ipsilateral sacroiliac joint. A comprehensive spinal examination will reveal the blocked motion at the sacroiliac joint, which responds to specific manipulation. Stretching the hypertonic muscles alone does not prevent return of the symptoms and is ineffective without appropriately applied manipulation.

Without an understanding of the interaction of the locomotor system, many biomechanical lesions of

Table 15.3 Review of Clinical Trials of Spinal Manipulation, 1984–1989[a]

	Author	Yr	Area of Complaint[b]	Area Manip[b]	Manipulation/Mobilization	Operator[c]	Length of Treatment	Subjects — Manip	Subjects — Total	Improved	Assessment
1	Godfrey et al.	84	LB	LB	Manip	MD/DC	2–5 times	44	81	30	Subj/Obj
2	Terrett & Vernon	84	None	Thor	Manip	DC	Once	25	50	—	Obj
3	Kirkaldy-Willis & Cassidy	85	LB	LB	Manip	DC	2 wks	283	283	202	S/Obj
4	Sikorski	85	LB	LB	Mobil	PT	Unknown	55	116	55	Subj
5	Arkuszewski-1	86	LB	Full	Both	MD	Up to 5 wks	50	100	50	S/Obj
6	Arkuszewski-2	86	LB	Full	Both	MD	Up to 5 wks	47	88	47	S/Obj
7	Brontfort	86	LB	Unknown	Manip	DC	Various	259	259	192	S/Obj
8	Cibulka et al.	86	Hamst	SI	Manip	PT	Once	10	20	10	Obj
9	Meade et al.	86	LB	Full	Manip	DC	6 wks	23	50	—	Subj
10	Mealy et al.	86	Cerv	Cerv	Mobil	PT	8 wks	31	61	—	S/Obj
11	Thabe	86	UC/SI	UC/SI	Manip	MD	Once	—	—	—	Obj
12	Vernon et al.	86	None	Cerv	Manip	DC	Once	9	27	—	Obj
13	Waagen et al.	86	LB	Full	Manip	DC	2 wks	9	19	9	S/Obj
14	Bernard & Kirkaldy-Willis	87	LB	LB	Manip	DC	2 wks	498	736	444	S/Obj
15	Bruckner et al.	87	Thor	Thor	Manip	MD/PT	Unknown	71	73	66	Subj
16	Hadler et al.	87	LB	LB	Manip	MD	Once	26	56	—	Subj
17	Kuo & Loh	87	LB	LB	Both	MD/PT	Various	517	517	434	S/Obj
18	Mathews et al.	87	LB	LB	Manip	PT	2 wks	123	233	98	S/Obj
19	Ongley et al.	87	LB	SI	Manip	MD	Once	40	81	35	Subj
20	Paterson	87	Spine	Full	Manip	unk	3 or more	1037	1037	952	S/Obj
21	Shambaugh	87	Spine	Full	Manip	DC	Once	20	34	20	Obj
22	Turk & Ratkolb	87	Occ	Cerv	Both	MD	3 wks	100	100	75	Subj
23	Berg et al.	88	LB	SI	Manip	DC	Once	10	72	7	Obj
24	Burry & Gravis	88	LB	Unknown	Manip	MD/DC	Unknown	101	420	67	Subj
25	Christian et al.	88	Spine	Full	Manip	DC	Once	20	40	—	Obj
26	Herzog et al.	88	LB	SI	Manip	DC	4 wks	11	11	7	S/Obj
27	McKnight & DeBoer	88	Cerv	Cerv	Manip	DC	Once	53	75	—	Obj
28	Morley	89	LB/LE	LB/LE	Manip	DC	Various	18	18	16	S/Obj

[a]Compiled by Walker A, 1989. References 11–38.
[b]Abbreviations: Cerv, cevical; Full, full spine; Hamst, hamstring; LB, low back; Occ, occipital; Thor, thoracic; SI, sacroiliac joints; UC, upper cervical.
[c]Abbreviations: MD, medical doctor; DC, chiropractor; PT, physical therapist.

the spine go unrecognized and untreated. Referred pain is much more common than radicular pain. Chiropractors have long treated the referring joints and muscles effectively. Chiropractic inclusion in the health care system has continued as a result of patient satisfaction. Typically, chiropractors spend more time than other physicians explaining the condition and providing patient information about the management of activities of daily living (40).

COST EFFECTIVENESS OF CHIROPRACTIC CARE

While chiropractic care may be intensive at the outset, it can produce immediate therapeutic results. A number of studies (Table 15.5) have demonstrated patients treated by chiropractic lose less time from work than those treated by other disciplines. By recognizing and controlling the influence of those seeking exaggerated disability settlements, this trend can continue.

Encouraging prolonged time loss and additional treatment in order to obtain a large disability settlement is rarely in the patient's interest. It serves only those doctors and attorneys promoting disability, while driving up the already high cost of health care. The self-serving few who seek their "piece of the pie" at the expense of the patient and society must be discouraged by ethical chiropractors. Napolitano (41) has warned the profession never to abuse our privileges by such devices as overutilization, double billing, bait-and-switch advertising techniques, or other practices that make chiropractic appear to be a money-making scheme.

Reassurance that the patient will recover with minimal or no disability is in the patient's interest; fostering the "you haven't got it yet but . . ." syndrome is not. Welsh (42) has noted that "Chiropractors who knowingly and routinely misuse the misaligned spine syndrome to lure patients into costly and needless treatments or intentionally instill false fear in their minds are major contributors to the prejudice that exists toward their profession." Savage (43) has stated, "Greed expressed in overutilization, fee gouging and fraudulent billing is found in a minority of practitioners in all professions but the occasional chiropractic miscreant is a convenient target whose action can unfairly produce profession-wide punitive measures." He notes, "as a smaller profession, chiropractic is the easier mark" and "like Caesar's wife, we must be above suspicion."

Table 15.4 Critical Appraisal of Clinical Trials of Spinal Manipulation, 1984–1989[a]

	Author	Comments
1	Godfrey et al.	Manipulation not "clearly superior" to sham physiotherapy; both control and experimental groups improved.
2	Terrett & Vernon	Significant elevation of pain tolerance (140%) in experimental group.
3	Kirkaldy-Willis & Cassidy	71% of totally disabled patients improved with manipulation; 81% success for referred pain syndromes.
4	Sikorski	Study affirms author's treatment regimen; only patients not helped by any other treatment method received mobilization; none were manipulated.
5	Arkuszewski-1	Experimental group shorter duration & improvement more marked; 60% returned to former jobs vs only 36% of control group; compared standard treatment (drug, physical therapy) to full manual treatment.
6	Arkuszewski-2	Drug-treated group averaged 30% longer hospitalization; cervical blockage found in 95% of low back patients; atlantooccipital blockage in 72% experimental grp, 63% control grp.
7	Brontfort	Chiropractor-treated groups better at work, rest & use of drugs; results compared with previous study by orthodox medical practitioner.
8	Cibulka et al.	Suggested relationship between sacroiliac joint dysfunction and hamstring strength.
9	Meade et al.	Feasibility study of hospital vs chiropractic management; improvement for chiropractic patients greater and more rapid; main trial of 2000 patients now ongoing.
10	Mealy et al.	Experimental group showed greatest improvement at 4 and 8 weeks.
11	Thabe	Manipulation results in immediate pain disappearance and spontaneous EMG activity.
12	Vernon et al.	8.5% increase in plasma β-endorphin at 5 min; no response demonstrated in sham group; mobilization used as sham procedure.
13	Waagen et al.	Manipulation more effective at relieving low back pain than sham.
14	Bernard & Kirkaldy-Willis	Manipulation effective for post joint, SI, Maigne's syndrome, segmental instability; SI and post joint syndromes are most common referred pain syndromes.
15	Bruckner et al.	Benign thoracic pain settled by manipulation; authors state benign thoracic pain is probably disc prolapse; this is the third most common chest pain.
16	Hadler et al.	Manipulation had no effect on patients with low back pain less than 2 weeks; patients with 2–4 weeks LBP had 50% more rapid improvement; mobilization used as sham procedure.
17	Kuo & Loh	Describes Chinese manual treatment protocol.
18	Mathews et al.	SLR-limited patients are best candidates for manipulation; manipulation was most beneficial for recovery speed and more effective than standard approach of drugs, support, advice.
19	Ongley et al.	Injections and manipulation effective for treating chronic LBP; by testing both significant variables (injection and manipulation) it is impossible to determine which is responsible for the result.
20	Paterson	Study shows 75% patients improve in 3 manipulation treatments; author calls for reappraisal of manipulative "facts," (e.g., response of chronic/acute, sudden/insidious, obesity).
21	Shambaugh	Manipulation produces significant reduction in back muscle EMG; muscle activity also more symmetrical across spine following manipulation.
22	Turk & Ratkolb	Manipulation effective for chronic headache; at 6 months: 25% patients reported no h/a, 40% improved but use analgesics, 35% had relief 1 month, then h/a reappeared, now take analgesics.
23	Berg et al.	Manipulation effective for severe LBP in pregnancy where diagnosis is sacroiliac dysfunction.
24	Burry & Gravis	Unintended finding that DC manipulation more effective than MD manipulation; subj patient assessment gave negative rating in 4 of 24 (16%) DC manipulation vs 30 of 77 (38%) MD manipulation.
25	Christian et al.	Excludes β-endorphin as analgesic in manipulative therapy; contradicts findings of Vernon et al.
26	Herzog et al.	Manipulation beneficial in restoring sacroiliac mobility function, some in 6 treatments; some force platform measured gait changes apparent with manipulation.
27	McKnight & DeBoer	High normotensive subjects manifest greatest effect; sham procedure was motion palpation; only subjects with manipulable lesions were in experimental group.
28	Morley	Chronic athletic injuries respond to manipulation.

[a]Compiled by A Walker, 1989. References 11–38.

Overcoming the patient's fear of activity, with a graduated return to recreational and work activities, enhances the quality of life and is invaluable. No amount of monetary compensation can make up for the loss of function fostered by dependency and fear of leading an active life. That is not to say that all patients recover without impairment, but in the interest of the patient, emphasis should be on recovery, not on disability.

Selby (44) has noted that there is no prestige in taking longer to correct the same health problems than your colleague and at much greater expense. Our record of cost effectiveness can be speedily eroded if the few "purveyors of profit" are allowed to increase in number and advance unchecked.

Chiropractic care, along with that provided by other health care professionals, is being increasingly scrutinized for cost effectiveness. Tremendous pres-

Table 15.5 Workmans' Compensation Costs on Chiropractic[a]

State	Average Cost/Case	Average Time Loss	Year	Source
Florida	MD cost 27.4% higher than DC	MD 3x longer 311% more costly	1960	Florida workman's compensation records
California	N/A	DC 15.6 days MD 32.0 days	1970	Wolfe, CR
Iowa	DC $ 68.43 MD $117.61	DC average 5 days less than MD	1978	Velie, E
Wisconsin	DC $115.00 MD $243.00	MD 382.4% more than DC	1978	Duffy, DJ
Oregon	MD care 80.3% higher than DC	MD cost 152.9% higher MD days lost 118% higher	1980	Bergemann, B Cichoke, AJ
Kansas	DC $ 68.40 MD $117.61	DC 5.8 days MD 13.1 days	1982	ACA
Florida	Nonsurgery claimants DC $1003.00 MD $1558.00	DC 48.7% shorter disability period for nonsurgical patients	1988	Wolk, S

[a]Adapted from Industrial Health Care Cost and Chiropractors Wisconsin Chiropractic Association

sure is being applied to health professionals to utilize the least expensive method of therapy, and the cost of chiropractic care will become increasingly important (45). It is up to chiropractors to insure that the cost effectiveness of conservative therapy is promoted, based on rational and scientific standards.

OBJECTIVES FOR THE CLINICAL PRACTICE OF CHIROPRACTIC

The Chiropractic Advisory Committee Department of Labor and Industries in the State of Washington, led by Hansen (46), has adopted six objectives for the clinical practice of chiropractic. Based partly on the work of West (47) and Vear (48), these objectives establish criteria for the standardization of chiropractic care.

The first objective in any clinical practice is to establish a satisfactory relationship with patients and determine the nature of the health problem for which they are seeking treatment (46). When they consult a physician, patients usually feel somewhat frightened, insecure, and dependent (47), and establishing rapport and trust is the responsibility of the physician.

Chiropractors, as primary health care providers, act as a portal of entry to the health care delivery system. When they accept responsibility for the chiropractic care of a patient, they must recognize the professional capabilities and limitations in diagnostic and therapeutic procedures utilized by the chiropractic profession (44).

Secondly, through the initial patient interview and consultation, chiropractic physicians must determine if the patient has a health problem requiring the application of clinical chiropractic diagnostic or therapeutic procedures, or whether referral to another primary health care provider is indicated (47, 48). A thorough case history should be elicited and, if referral is indicated, an appropriate referral report should be provided (46).

Each case history should include a description of the patient's chief complaint, past and present health problems, and any relevant psychosocial factors. Particularly important is documentation of any past history of the same or similar conditions, and any previous disability should be noted. A basis should be established for specific diagnostic procedures including physical, orthopaedic, neurological, chiropractic, laboratory, and radiographic (46, 47).

The third objective is to arrive at a professional diagnosis based on the patient's history, diagnostic tests, and radiographs (when indicated) (46, 48). Differential diagnosis is as much an art as a science. It requires the ability to recognize concomitant conditions and any interrelationships between coexisting problems, with prompt referral when appropriate (46, 48).

Objective four is the determination of the appropriate course of care. General and specific contraindications to chiropractic therapeutic care (Chapter 4) should be identified and treatment modified accordingly. Appropriate care should be provided and recorded, based on a specific treatment plan including the expected length of treatment. Patients should be told in understandable terms about anticipated practices and procedures, including the probability of success and the results to be anticipated if nothing is done. Informed consent for chiropractic therapeutics should be recorded in the patient's case record (48).

The fifth objective for the clinical practice of chiropractic is to monitor the patient to ensure that response to therapy is rapid, to ensure that the patient is progressing as expected, and to ensure appropriate changes in case management as required. Chiropractic management should include alleviation of environmental, causal, and irritating factors where possible. Treatment should be modified to the needs of individual patients (48).

The sixth objective is to discharge the patient at the end point of treatment, when no further improvement in the patient's condition can be expected. This responsibility includes follow-up care of the patient when necessary and an outline of active preventive procedures that the patient can pursue to prevent recurrence. This may include counseling and instructing the patient and family members regarding cause, management, need for supportive or maintenance care, and progression for residuals of the condition.

Adequate records should be kept, documenting the stated objectives. These records should be legible and in a format that allows interpretation by others.

FUTURE OF CHIROPRACTIC CARE

The science of chiropractic has traveled a long, tortuous road from its humble beginnings almost a century ago in middle America. From the simplistic theories of Daniel David Palmer to the present, the chiropractic profession has followed many detours in its quest for the scientific validation of manipulation in the management of spine-related disorders.

With today's students graduating from government-accredited colleges, well-steeped in scientific principles, this validation is becoming increasingly apparent. Much suffering has been ameliorated by chiropractors, and in the patient's interest, chiropractic care must be accepted as a synergistic element in the health care arena. As additional research increases the understanding of biomechanical dysfunctions of the spinal chain, the promotion of health and well-being will be enhanced.

References

1. *Chiropractic in New Zealand Report of the Commission of Inquiry.* Reprinted by Palmer College of Chiropractic, Davenport, Iowa, 1979, p 4.
2. Lewit K: *Manipulative Therapy in Rehabilitation of the Motor System.* Boston, Butterworth, 1985, p 358.
3. European Chiropractic Union
4. Muhlemann D: Hypermobility as a common cause for chronic back pain. Submitted for publication in the *Ann Swiss Chiro Assoc.*
5. Maigne R: *Orthopedic Medicine: A New Approach to Vertebral Manipulation.* 1972, p 156.
6. Vear HJ: A pathological basis for prognosis. *JCCA* 3(1):8–9, 1959.
7. Vear HJ: A pathological basis for prognosis. *Digest of Chiro Econ* Mar/Apr, pp 14–15, 1972.
8. Jaquet PE: *An Introduction to Clinical Chiropractic Grounauer.* Geneva, Switzerland, 1974, pp 30–33.
9. Helfet AJ, Gruebell Lee DM: *Disorders of the Lumbar Spine.* Philadelphia, JB Lippincott, 1978, pp 21, 161.
10. Gatterman M: Indications for spinal manipulation in the treatment of back pain. *ACA J Chiro* 16:51–66, 1982.
11. Godfrey CM, Morgan PP, Schatzker J: A randomized trial of manipulation for low-back pain in a medical setting. *Spine* 9(3):301–304, 1984.
12. Terrett CJ, Vernon BA: Manipulation and pain tolerance: a controlled study of the effect of spinal manipulation on paraspinal cutaneous pain tolerance levels. *Am J Phys Med* 63:217–225, 1984.
13. Kirkaldy-Willis WH, Cassidy JD: Spinal manipulation in the treatment of low-back pain. *Can Fam Physician* 31:535–540, 1985.
14. Sikorski JM: A rationalized approach to physiotherapy for low back pain. *Spine* 10:571–579, 1985.
15. Arkuszewski Z: The efficacy of manual treatment in low back pain: a clinical trial. *Manual Med* 2:68–71, 1986.
16. Arkuszewski Z: Involvement of the cervical spine in back pain. *Manual Med* 2:126–128, 1986.
17. Bronfort G: Chiropractic treatment of low back pain, a prospective survey. *J Manipulative Physiol Ther* 9:99–112, 1986.
18. Cibulka MT, Rose SJ, Delitto A, Sinacore DR: Hamstring muscle strain treated by mobilizing the sacroiliac joint. *Phys Ther* 66:1220–1223, 1986.
19. Meade TW and Working Group: Comparison of chiropractic and hospital outpatient management of low back pain: a feasibility study. *J Epidemiol Comm Health* 40:12–17, 1986.
20. Mealy K, Brennan H, Fenelon GCC: Early mobilization of acute whiplash injuries. *Br Med J* 292:656–657, 1986.
21. Thabe H: Electromyography as a tool to document diagnostic findings and therapeutic results associated with somatic dysfunctions in the upper cervical spinal joints and sacroiliac joints. *Manual Med* 2:53–58, 1986.
22. Vernon HT, Dhami MSI, Howley TP, Annet R: Spinal manipulation and β-endorphin: a controlled study of the effects of a spinal manipulation on plasma β-endorphin levels in normal males. *J Manipulative Physiol Ther* 9:1, 1986.
23. Waagen GN, Haldeman S, Lopez D, DeBoer KF: Short term trial of chiropractic adjustments for the relief of chronic low back pain. *Manual Med* 2:63–67, 1986.
24. Bernard TN, Kirkaldy-Willis WH: Recognizing specific characteristics of nonspecific low back pain. *Clin Orthop* 217:266–280, 1987.
25. Bruckner JE, Allard SA, Moussa NA: Benign thoracic pain. *J Soc Med* 80:286–289, 1987.
26. Hadler NM, Curtis MB, Gillings DB, Stinnett MS: A benefit of spinal manipulation as adjunctive therapy for acute low back pain: a stratified controlled trial. *Spine* 12:703–706, 1987.
27. Kuo P-FP, Loh Z-C: Treatment of lumbar intervertebral disc protrusions by manipulation. *Clin Orthop* 215:47–55, 1987.
28. Mathews JA, Mills SB, Jenkins VM, Grimes SM, Morkel MJ, Mathews W, Scott CM, Sittampalam Y: Back pain and sciatica; controlled trials of manipulation, traction, sclerosant and epidural injections. *Br J Rheumatol* 26:416–423, 1987.
29. Ongley MJ, Klein RG, Dorman TA, Eek BC, Hubert LJ: A new approach to the treatment of chronic low back pain. *Lancet* 7:143–146, 1987.
30. Paterson JK: A survey of musculoskeletal problems in general practice. *Manual Med* 3:40–48, 1987.
31. Shambaugh P: Changes in electrical activity in muscles resulting from chiropractic adjustment: a pilot study. *J Manipulative Physiol Ther* 10:300–304, 1987.
32. Turk Z, Ratkolb O: Mobilization of the cervical spine in chronic headaches. *Manual Med* 3:15–17, 1987.
33. Berg G, Hammer M, Moller-Nielsen J, Linden U, Thorblad J: Low back pain during pregnancy. *Obstet Gynecol* 71:71–75, 1988.
34. Burry HC, Gravis V: Compensated back injury in New Zealand. *NZ Med J* 101:542–544, 1988.
35. Christian GF, Stanton GJ, Sissons D, How HY, Jamison J, Alder B, Fullerton M, Funder JW: Immunoreactive ATH, β-endorphin, and cortisol levels in plasma following spinal manipulative therapy. *Spine* 13:1411–1417, 1988.
36. Herzog W, Nigg BM, Read LJ: Quantifying the effects of spinal manipulation on gait using patients with low back pain. *J Manipulative Physiol Ther* 11:151–157, 1988.
37. McKnight ME, DeBoer KF: Preliminary study of blood pressure changes in normotensive subjects undergoing chiropractic care. *J Manipulative Physiol Ther* 11:261–266, 1988.
38. Morley JJ: Treatment of chronic athletic injuries of the low back and lower extremity utilizing manipulation. *Chiro Sports Med* 3(1):4–8, 1989.
39. Fisk JW: An evaluation of manipulation in the treatment of the acute low back syndrome in general practices. In Berergen & Tobis (eds): *Manipulative Therapy.* Springfield, 1977, p 268.

40. Cassidy DJ, Kirkaldy-Willis WH: Manipulation. In Kirkaldy-Willis (eds): *Managing Low Back Pain*. New York, Churchill Livingstone, 1988, pp 287–296.

41. Napolitano EG: Chiropractors of tomorrow must protect their privileges; dedicate themselves to their profession. *ACA J Chiro* 54–55, 1982.

42. Welsh J: How to use advertising to overcome prejudiced minds. *ICA Int Rev of Chiro* Mar-Apr: 51–53, 1987.

43. Savage LJ: Chiropractic crises . . . or opportunities? *ACA J Chiro* 24:5–8, 1987.

44. Selbey LR: Humanitarians or monetarians. *ACA J Chiro* 18:15, 1981.

45. Grieve A, Cassidy JPM: A question of quality and quantity of chiropractic care. *J CCA* 30:1, 19–23, 1986.

46. Hansen DT: *Chiropractic Standards of Practice and Utilization Guidelines in the Care and Treatment of Injured Workers*. Dept of Labor and Industries, State of Washington, 1988, pp 10–12.

47. West HG: Physical and spinal examination procedures utilized in the practice of chiropractic. In Haldeman S (ed): *Modern Development in the Principles and Practice of Chiropractic*. East Norwalk, CT, Appleton-Century-Crofts, 1979, p 269.

48. Vear HJ: *Chiropractic Standards of Practice and Quality Care*. Aspen Press, Rockville, MD (forthcoming).

Glossary

Abduction Movement away from the midline.

Acceleration Rate of change of linear velocity.

Active movement Movement accomplished without assistance; the patient moves the joint or part unassisted.

Activities of daily living Daily living activities include but are not limited to: self-care, personal hygiene, communication, normal living postures, ambulation, travel, nonspecialized hand activities, sexual function, sleep, social and recreational activities.

Acute
1. Of recent onset (hours or days).
2. Sharp, poignant; having a short and relatively severe course.

Adduction Movement toward the midline.

Adhesion Fibrous band or structure by which parts adhere abnormally.

Adjustment Specific form of direct articular manipulation (see manipulation) utilizing either long or short leverage techniques with specific contacts, characterized by a dynamic thrust of controlled velocity, amplitude, and direction (see Chapter 3).

Agonists Muscles, or portions of muscles, so attached anatomically that when they contract, they develop forces that reinforce each other.

Alignment To put in a straight line; arrangement of position in a straight line.

Anatomical position
1. Erect posture, face forward, arms at sides, palms and hands forward with fingers and thumbs in extension.
2. Position of reference for definitions and descriptions of planes and axes.
3. Zero position for measurement of joint motion.

Anecdotal procedure Includes categories and classifications of procedures, technologies, or equipment that have not received the benefit of the experimental method. Items included in this definition originate and depend upon experience and observation only.

Angiolipsis Pressure on an artery, direct or indirect; e.g., in the intervertebral foramen I.V.F. through pressure generated by a discopathy, in the foramina transversarii through osteogenic reactions.

Ankylosis Stiffness or fixation of a joint.

Anomaly Marked deviation from the normal standard.

Antagonistic muscles Muscles or portions of muscles so attached anatomically that when they contract they develop forces that oppose each other.

Anterolisthesis
1. Forward slipping.
2. Anterior translation of the vertebral body.

Arthritis Inflammation of a joint.

Arthrosis Degenerative joint disease of the diarthrodial (freely movable) joints of the spine or extremities.

Articulation
1. Place of union or junction between two or more bones of the skeleton.
2. Active or passive process of moving a joint through its entire range of motion.

Associated myofascial trigger point Focus of hyperirritability in a muscle or its fascia that develops in response to compensatory overload, shortened range, or referred phenomena caused by trigger point activity in another muscle. Satellite or secondary trigger points are types of associated trigger points.

Asymmetry Lack or absence of symmetry of position or motion. Dissimilarity in corresponding parts or organs on opposite sides of the body which are normally alike (see tropism).

Atrophy Acquired reduction in size of an organ that had previously reached a normal size.

Axis Line around which rotatory movement takes place or along which translation occurs. The 3-dimensional description of motion of an object with 3 axes perpendicular to one another. The right-handed Cartesian orthogonal system has 3 axes designated X, Y and Z.

X-axis—Line passing horizontally from side to side. May also be referred to as the coronal axis or the frontal axis. Movement around the X-axis is said to be in the sagittal plane.

Y-axis—Line perpendicular to the ground. May also be referred to as the vertical axis. Movement around the Y-axis is said to be in the horizontal or transverse plane.

Z-axis—Line passing horizontally front to back. May also be referred to as the sagittal axis. Movement around the Z-axis is said to be in the coronal plane.

Axoplasmic flow Flow of neuroplasm along the axon between synapses and toward and away from end organs.

Barrier
1. Anatomical barrier—Limit of anatomical integrity: the limit of motion imposed by an anatomic structure. Forcing movement beyond this barrier would produce tissue damage.
2. Elastic (physiologic) barrier—Elastic resistance that is felt at the end of passive range of movement; further motion toward an anatomic barrier may be induced passively (joint play).
3. Pathologic barrier—Functional limit within the anatomic range of motion, which abnormally diminishes the normal physiologic range (see fixation).

Biomechanics Application of mechanical laws to living structures. The study and knowledge of biological function from an application of mechanical principles.

Body mechanisms Study of the static and dynamic human body to note the mechanical integration of the parts, and to endeavor to restore and maintain the body as nearly as possible in normal mechanical condition.

Bogginess Tissue texture abnormality characterized principally by a palpable sense of sponginess in the tissue, interpreted as resulting from congestion due to increased fluid content.

Brachial Referring to the upper extremity.

Bucket-handle rib motion Movement of the lower ribs during respiration such that with inhala-tion the lateral aspect of the rib elevates, increasing the transverse diameter of the thorax.

Caliper rib movement Movement of lower ribs during respiration such that the ribs move anteriorly with inhalation.

Caudad Toward the tail or inferiorly.

Causalgia Burning pain that is sometimes present in injuries of the nerve, particularly those sensory nerves supplying the extremities.

Center of gravity Point in the body through which the resultant force of gravity acts.

Center of mass Point in the body or body part at which all mass seems to be concentrated.

Cephalad Toward the head.

Cervical Denoting relation to the neck.

Chiropractic
Chiropractic practice—Discipline of the scientific healing arts concerned with the pathogenesis, diagnostics, therapeutics, and prophylaxis of functional disturbances, pathomechanical states, pain syndromes, and neurophysiological effects related to the statics and dynamics of the locomotor system, especially of the spine and pelvis.
Chiropractic science—Investigation of the relationship between structure (primarily the spine) and function (primarily the nervous system) of the human body that leads to the restoration and preservation of health.

Chronic Long-standing (weeks, months, or years) but *not* necessarily incurable. Symptoms may range from mild to severe.

Circumduction of the trunk Combination of forward flexion, right lateral flexion, extension, and left lateral flexion in succession, which produces a circular movement of the trunk.

Clinical evaluation Collection of data by a physician for the purpose of determining the health status of an individual. The data include information obtained by history; clinical findings obtained from a physical examination; laboratory tests including radiographs, electrocardiograms, blood tests, and other special tests and diagnostic procedures; and measurements of anthropometric attributes and physiologic and psychophysiologic functions.

Compensation Changes in structural relationships to accommodate foundation disturbances and maintain balance.

Concussion Shock, the state of being shaken, a severe shaking or jarring of a part; also the morbid state resulting from such a jarring.

Concomitant Accompanying; accessory; joined with another.

Contact point Area of the adjustive hand that makes contact with the patient in the delivery of the chiropractic adjustment. There are 12 contact points:

1. Pisiform
2. Hypothenar
3. Metacarpal (knife-edge)
4. Digital
5. Distal interphalangeal (DIP)
6. Proximal interphalangeal (PIP)
7. Metacarpophalangeal (MP or index)
8. Web
9. Thumb
10. Thenar
11. Calcaneal
12. Palmar

Contraction Physiological development of tension in muscle.

1. Eccentric (isolytic)—Contraction of a muscle against resistance while forcing the muscle to lengthen.
2. Concentric (isotonic)—Approximation of the muscle origin and insertion without change in its tension.

Contracture

1. State of prolonged shortening of a muscle, which persists in the absence of muscle action potential.
2. Pathologic shortening of a muscle.

Contraindication Any condition, especially any condition of disease, that renders one particular line of treatment improper or undesirable.

Contusion Bruise; an injury in which the skin is not broken.

Coupling Phenomenon of consistent association of one motion (translation or rotation) about an axis with another motion (translation or rotation) about a second axis. One motion cannot be produced without the other.

Creep When deformation of a viscoelastic material over time is subjected to a suddenly applied uniform load.

Crepitus Crackling sound produced by the rubbing together of fragments of fractured bone.

Curvature Pathological bend of the spine in the coronal plane.

Curve Anatomical bend of the spine in the sagittal plane. Primary curves of the spine are the embryological curves that persist in the sacral and thoracic regions. Secondary curves of the spine are developmental and occur in the lumbar and cervical regions as a consequence of the assumption of upright posture.

Deformation Change in length or shape.

Degenerative Deterioration or breaking down of a part or parts of the body.

Degrees of freedom Number of independent coordinates required in a coordinated system to completely specify the position of an object in space. One degree of freedom is rotation around one axis or translation along one axis. The spine is considered to have six degrees of freedom because it has the capability of rotatory movement around 3 axes as well as translatory movement of 3 axes.

Diagnosis Art of distinguishing one disease from another; the determination of the nature of a cause of disease.

Disability Legal disqualification or incapacity; something that restricts limitation.

Discopathy Any pathological changes in a disc.

Dislocation Displacement of one or more bones of a joint or of any organ from the original position.

Displacement State of being removed from normal position; vertebral displacement refers to a disrelationship of the vertebra to its relative structures.

Distortion Any mechanical departure from ideal or normal symmetry in the body framework.

Distraction Movement of two surfaces away from each other.

Dynamics Study of motions of bodies and forces acting to produce the motions.

Dyskinesia Impairment of the power of voluntary movement, resulting in fragmentary or incomplete movements, aberrant motion.

Effleurage Form of massage employing slow, rhythmic stroking executed with minimum force and light pressure.

Elastic deformation Any recoverable deformation.

Elasticity Property of a material or structure to return to its original form following the removal of the deforming load.

Electromyogram Electrical activity of whole muscles recorded by surface electrodes, or that of single motor units recorded by intramuscular needle electrodes.

End-play (end-feel) Discrete, short-range movements of a joint, independent of the action of voluntary muscles, determined by springing each vertebra at the limit of its passive range of motion.

Equilibrium State in which a body is at rest with neither translatory nor rotatory motion (static equilibrium), or in which a body is in constant motion with no acceleration or deceleration (dynamic equilibrium).

Exacerbation Increase in the manifestations of a malady.

Experimental procedures Pertaining to, derived from, or found on experiment (a test or trial); of the nature of an experiment; tentative. This includes categories and classifications of procedures, technologies, or equipment not conforming to widespread use within or amongst individual branches of the health disciplines but nevertheless of such a nature (based on testing and trial criteria) that there is no organized scientific opposition to its use in health care. Although not orthodox, such items are far removed from empiricism or quackery.

Extension Separation of two embryologically ventral surfaces; movement away from the fetal position; the return movement from flexion.

Eukinesia Good movement.

Facet asymmetry Vertebral structure in which the orientation of the facets is not anatomically bilaterally comparable (see tropism).

Facilitation Increase in afferent stimuli so that the synaptic threshold is more easily reached; thus there is an increase in the efficacy of subsequent impulses in that pathway or synapse. The consequence of increased efficacy is that continued stimulation produces hyperactive responses.

Fascia Tissue layers under the skin or between muscles, which form the sheaths of muscles or invest other deep, definitive structures, as nerves and vessels.

Fascitis Inflammation of the fascia.

Fibromyalgia syndrome Form of nonarticular rheumatism with diffuse musculoskeletal aches, pain, and stiffness at many sites, associated with exaggerated tenderness at characteristic anatomic locations known as tender points.

Fibrosis Formation of fibrous tissue.

Fibrositis (see fibromyalgia syndrome)

Fixation
1. Absence of motion of a joint in a position of motion, usually at the extremity of such motion.
2. (Dynamic fault.) State whereby a vertebra or pelvic bone has become temporarily immobilized in a position that it may normally occupy during any phase of physiological spinal movement.
3. Immobilization of a vertebra in a position of movement when the spine is at rest, or in a position of rest when the spine is in movement.

Fixation subluxation Lack of movement of a joint, caused by muscular spasm, a shortened ligament, or an intraarticular blocking.

Flat palpation Examination by finger pressure that proceeds across the muscle fibers at a right angle to their length, while compressing them against a firm underlying structure, such as bone. It is used to detect taut bands and trigger points.

Flexibility Ability of a structure to deform under the application of load.

Flexion Approximation of two embryologically ventral surfaces; movement toward the fetal position.

Force Push or pull produced by action of one body on another.

Fracture Breaking of bone or cartilage.

Friction massage Deep circular massage to irritate or stimulate a muscle or increase its tonus and/or its arterial perfusion, or express swelling by moving the skin over the subcutaneous tissue.

Functional Of or pertaining to a function; affecting the functions but not the structure.

Gait Manner of walking.

Gliding Movement in which the joint surfaces are flat or only slightly curved and one articulating surface slides on the other.

Gonimeter Instrument for measuring angles.

Gravitational line Viewing the patient from the side, an imaginary line in a coronal plane which, in the theoretical ideal posture, starts at the external auditory canal, passes through the lateral head of the humerus at the tip of the shoulder, across the greater trochanter, the lateral condyle of the knee, and slightly anterior to the lateral malleolus. If this were a plane through the body, it would intersect the middle of the third lumbar vertebra and the anterior one-third of the sacrum. It is used to evaluate the AP curve of the spine.

Gravity line Action line of force of gravity.

Health
1. State of optimal physical, mental, and social well-being and not merely the absence of disease or infirmity.
2. Adaptive and optimal attainment of physical, mental, emotional, and spiritual well-being.

Herniation Abnormal protrusion of an organ or other body structure through a defect or natural opening.

Homeostasis
1. Maintenance of static or constant conditions in the internal environment.
2. Level of well-being of an individual maintained by internal physiologic harmony.

Hyper Beyond excessive.

Hypochondrosis Chronic condition in which patients are morbidly concerned with their own health, and believe themselves suffering from grave bodily disease.

Hyperextension Excessive or unnatural movement in the direction of extension.

Hyperkinesia Too much movement; hypermobility.

Hypermobile joint Overflexible link in a series of articulated bodies.

Hypo   Under or deficient.

Hypokinesia   Not enough movement; hypomobility.

Iliosacral motion   Motion of the ilia on a transverse axis of the sacrum, as occurs in walking. Considered to be primarily influenced by the attachments and movements of the pelvis, hips, and lower extremities.

Immobility   Condition of not being movable.

Impairment   Loss of, loss of use of, or derangement of any body part, system, or function. *Permanent impairment* is impairment that has become static or well-stabilized with or without medical/chiropractic treatment, or that is not likely to remit despite medical/chiropractic treatment of the impairing condition.

Impinge   To press or encroach upon; to come into close contact; an obstructing lesion causing pressure on a nerve.

Impulse   Integral force of an adjustment with respect to time.

Inflammation   Reaction of tissues to injury. The essential process, regardless of causative agent, is characterized clinically by local heat, swelling, redness, and pain; pathologically by primary vasoconstriction, followed by vasodilation with slowing of the blood current, and accumulation and deposition of fibrin.

Inertia   Property that makes a body resist a change in motion.

Inhibition   Effect of one neuron upon another, tending to prevent it from initiating impulses.

Innate   Inborn; hereditary.

Innate intelligence   Intrinsic biological ability of a healthy organism to react physiologically to the changing conditions of the external and internal environments.

Innervation   Distribution of nerves to a part.

Instability   Quality or condition of being unstable; not firm, fixed, or constant.
Clinical instability of the spine—Loss of the ability of the spine under physiologic loads to maintain relationships between vertebrae in such a way that there is neither damage nor subsequent irritation to the spinal cord or nerve roots, and in addition, there is no development of incapacitating deformities or pain due to structural changes.

Instrumentation   Use of any tool, appliance, or apparatus; work performed with instruments.

Intensity   Grading as follows:
Minimal—When the symptoms or signs constitute an annoyance but cause no impairment in the performance of a particular activity.

Slight—When the symptoms or signs can be tolerated but cause some impairment in the performance of an activity that precipitates the symptoms or signs.
Moderate—When the symptoms and signs cause marked impairment in performance of an activity that precipitates the symptoms or signs.
Marked—When the symptoms or signs preclude any activity that precipitates the symptoms or signs.

Intersegmental motion   Relative motion taking place between two adjacent vertebral segments or within a vertebral motion segment. Described as the upper vertebra moving on the lower.

Intervertebral disk herniation
1. Protrusion—The annulus is intact but stretched by displaced nuclear material.
2. Extrusion—The annulus is not intact but most of the nuclear material hs not herniated beyond the annulus and the posterior longitudinal ligament is intact.
3. Sequestration—(Prolapse.) The nucleus or a portion thereof (free fragment) has herniated entirely beyond the annulus.

Inversion   A turning inward, inside out, upside down, or other reversal of the normal relation of a part. Often used to describe passive inverted traction.

Ischemic compression   Application of progressively stronger painful pressure on a trigger point for the purpose of eliminating the point's tenderness. This action blanches the compressed tissue, which usually becomes hyperemic (flushed) on release of the pressure.

Isokinetic exercise   Exercise using a constant speed of movement of the body part.

Joint dysfunction   Joint mechanics showing area disturbances of function.

Joint play   Discrete, short-range movements of a joint, independent of the action of voluntary muscles, determined by springing each vertebra in the neutral position.

Jump sign   General pain response of a patient, who winces, may cry out, and withdraws in response to pressure applied on a trigger point.

Kinematics   Division of mechanics that deals with the geometry of the motion of bodies, displacement velocity, and acceleration without taking into account the forces that produce the motion.

Kinesiology
1. Science or study of movement and the active and passive structures involved.
2. Science of movement, its anatomical, physiological, mechanical, psychological, and social aspects.

Kinesthesia Sense by which muscular motion, weight, position, etc. are perceived.

Kinesthetic Pertaining to kinesthesia.

Kinetic chain Combination of several successively arranged joints constituting a complex unit, as links in a chain.
 1. Closed kinetic chain—A system in which motion of one link has determined relations to every other link in the system.
 2. Open kinetic chain—A combination of links in which the terminal joint is free.

Kinetics Body of knowledge that deals with the effects of forces that produce or modify body motion.

Kneading Form of massage employing forceful circular and transverse movement of a large, raised fold of skin and underlying muscle.

Kyphoscoliosis
 1. Abnormal kyphosis plus scoliosis.
 2. Backward and lateral curvature of the spinal column.

Kyphosis Abnormally increased convexity in the curvature of the spine.

Latent myofascial trigger point Focus of hyperirritability in a muscle or its fascia that is clinically quiescent with respect to spontaneous pain; it is painful only when palpated. A latent trigger point may have all the other clinical characteristics of an active trigger point, from which it is to be distinguished.

Lateral flexion
 1. Bending to the side away from the midline.
 2. Term used to denote lateral movements of the head, neck, and trunk in a coronal plane. It is usually combined with rotation.

Lateral listhesis Lateral translatory excursion of the vertebral body.

Lever
 1. A rigid bar moving about a fixed joint.
 2. Distance between joint centers of body segments.

Link Distance between joint centers of body segments.

Listing (dynamic) Designation of the abnormal movement characteristic of one vertebra in relation to subadjacent segments.
 Dynamic listing nomenclature
 1. Flexion restriction
 2. Extension restriction
 3. Lateral flexion restriction (right or left)
 4. Rotational malposition (right or left)

Listing (static) Designation of the spatial orientation of one vertebra in relation to adjacent segments.
 Static listing nomenclature
 1. Flexion malposition

 2. Extension malposition
 3. Lateral flexion maplistion (right or left)
 4. Rotational malposition (right or left)
 5. Anterolisthesis
 6. Retrolisthesis
 7. Lateralisthesis

Lordosis Exaggerated (or pathological) posterior concavity in the anteroposterior curvature of the lumbar and cervical spine.

Lordotic Pertaining to or characterized by lordosis, the anterior spinal curve.

Lumbosacral Pertaining to the lumbar vertebrae and the sacrum; as the lumbosacral plexus, made up of the lower lumbar and upper sacral nerves.

Lumbosacral angle Inclination of the superior surface of the first sacral vertebra to the horizontal. Usually measured from standing lateral x-ray films.

Maintenance Regimen designed to provide for the patient's continued well-being or to maintain the optimum state of health while minimizing recurrence of the clinical status.

Malingering To feign illness or disability, usually to secure benefit from an alleged injury.

Malposition Abnormal or anomalous position.

Manipulation Passive maneuver in which specifically directed manual forces are applied to vertebral and extravertebral articulations of the body, with the object of restoring mobility to restricted areas.
 1. Long-lever manipulation—High-velocity force exerted on a point of the body some distance from the area where it is expected to have its beneficial effect.
 2. Short-lever manipulation—High-velocity thrust directed specifically at an isolated joint.

Manual therapy Therapeutic application of manual force. Spinal manual therapy broadly defined includes all procedures in which the hands are used to mobilize, adjust, manipulate, apply traction, massage, stimulate, or otherwise influence the spine and paraspinal tissues with the aim of influencing the patient's health.

Massage Systematic therapeutic use of friction, stroking, and kneading of the body. Maneuvers performed by hand on the skin of the patient and through the skin of the patient upon the subcutaneous tissue. There may be variation in the intensity of pressure exerted, the surface area treated, and the frequency of application.

Medical necessity Patients' conditions to be treated are recognized ones, and the examinations, tests, and treatments are based on scientific studies and principles that are generally accepted by the profession at large as being necessary and appropriate for proper diagnosis and treatment of patients with the particular conditions presented.

Meric system Treatment of visceral conditions through adjustment of vertebrae at the levels of neuromeric innervation to the organs involved.

Midheel line Vertical line used as reference in standing anteroposterior (AP) x-rays, passing equidistant between the heels.

Midmalleolar line Vertical line passing through the lateral malleolus, used as a point of reference in standing lateral x-rays.

Misalignment Not in proper alignment.

Mobility Capability of movement or of flowing freely.

Mobilization Process of making a fixed part movable. A form of manual therapy applied within the physiological passive range of joint motion, characterized by nonthrust increase in passive joint play.

Moment of force Product of force and distance (moment arm) from any point to the action line of force.

Motion
1. Relative displacement with time of a body in space with respect to other bodies or some reference system.
2. Act or process of changing position. An act of moving the body or its parts.
   Active motion—Movement produced voluntarily by the patient.
   Passive motion—Motion induced by the operator while the patient remains passive or relaxed.
   Physiologic motion—Normal changes in the position of articulating surfaces taking place within a joint or region.

Motor That which causes motion.

Motor unit Functional unit of striated muscle comprised of the motor neuron and all the muscle fibers supplied by the neuron.

Muscle Contractile organ composed of muscle tissue, effecting the movements of organs and parts of the body.

Myalgia Pain in a muscle or muscles:
1. Diffusedly aching muscles due to systemic disease such as virus infection.
2. Spot tenderness of a muscle or muscles as in myofascial trigger points.

Myofascial pain syndrome Pain syndrome characterized by pain in regional muscles accompanied by trigger points that refer pain specifically to each muscle.

Myofascial trigger point Hyperirritable spot, usually within a taut band of skeletal muscle or in the muscle's fascia, that is painful on compression and that can give rise to characteristic referred pain, tenderness, and autonomic phenomena.

Myofascitis Pain, tenderness, other referred phenomena, and the dysfunction attributed to myofascial trigger points.

Myofibrosis Replacement of muscle tissue by fibrous tissue.

Myotatic unit A group of agonist and antagonist muscles that function together as a unit because they share common spinal reflex responses.

Nerve interference Chiropractic term used to refer to the interruption of normal nerve transmission (nerve energy).

Nerve transmission Transmission of information along a nerve axon.
   Impulsed based—Nerve transmission involving the generation and transfer of electrical potentials along a nerve axon.
   Non–impulsed based—The transfer of chemical messengers along a nerve axon, i.e., axoplasmic flow.

Neuralgia Severe paroxysmal pain along the course of a nerve, not associated with demonstrable structural changes in the nerve.

Neuritis Lesion of a nerve or nerves, either degenerative or inflammatory, with pain, hypersensitivity, anesthesis or paresthesia, paralysis, muscular atrophy, and decreased reflexes in the part supplied.

Neurodystrophic Disease process within a nerve, resulting from trauma, circulation disorders, or metabolic diseases, e.g., a neurodystrophic factor (diabetes and pernicious anemia).

Neurogenic Often used to mean originating in nerve tissue; "the cause of the disorder is neurogenic."

Neuropathogenic Disease within a tissue, resulting from abnormal nerve performance, e.g., Barre-Lieou syndrome resulting from neuropathogenic reflexes caused by pathomechanics of the cervical spine.

Neuropathy General term denoting functional disturbances and/or pathologic changes in the peripheral nervous system.

Neurophysiologic effects General term denoting functional or aberrant disturbances of the peripheral or the autonomic nervous system. The term is used to designate nonspecific effects related to: (a) motor and sensory functions of the peripheral nervous system; (b) vasomotor activity, secretomotor activity, and motor activity of smooth muscle from the autonomic nervous system, e.g., neck, shoulder, arm syndrome (the extremity becomes cool with increased sweating); (c) trophic activity of both the peripheral and autonomic nervous system, e.g., muscle atrophy in neck, shoulder, arm syndrome.

Neurothlipsis Direct or indirect pressure on a nerve, e.g., in the IVF through congestion of perineural tissues; in the carpal tunnel through direct ligamentous pressure.

Neurovascular Pertaining to both nervous and vascular structures.

Nutation Motion of the sacrum about a coronal axis, in which the sacral base moves anteriorly and inferiorly and the tip of the coccyx moves posteriorly and superiorly; nodding, as of the head.

Counter nutation—Motion of the sacrum about a coronal axis, in which the sacral base moves posteriorly and superiorly and the tip of the coccyx moves anteriorly and inferiorly; nodding, as of the head.

Objective Pertaining to those relations and conditions of the body perceived by another, as objective signs of disease.

Orthodox procedures All categories and classifications of procedures, technologies, or equipment conforming to widespread use within or amongst individual branches of the health disciplines, with such use based in the scientific method.

Osteopathy System of health care founded by Andrew Taylor Still (1828–1917) and based on the theory that the body is capable of making its own remedies against disease and other toxic conditions when it is in a normal structural relationship and has favorable environmental conditions and adequate nutrition. It utilizes generally accepted physical, pharmacological, and surgical methods of diagnosis and therapy, while placing strong emphasis on the importance of body mechanics and manipulative methods to detect and correct faulty structure and function.

Osteophyte Degenerative exostosis secondary to musculotendinous traction.

Pain Disturbed sensation causing suffering or distress.

Palliative care Care designed to relieve the symptoms of exacerbations but which results in no net improvement in the patient's stationary condition.

Palpable band (taut band or nodule) Group of taut muscle fibers that is associated with a myofascial trigger point and is identifiable by tactile examination of the muscle. Contraction of fibers in this band produces the local twitch response.

Palpation
1. Act of feeling with the hands.
2. Application of variable manual pressure through the surface of the body for the purpose of determining the shape, size, consistency, position, inherent motility, and health of the tissues beneath.

Motion palpation—Palpatory diagnosis of passive and active segmental joint range of motion.

Static palpation—Palpatory diagnosis of somatic structures in a neutral static position.

Palpatory diagnosis Process of palpating the patient to evaluate the neuromusculoskeletal and visceral systems.

Palpatory skills Sensory skills used in performing palpatory diagnosis.

Passive motion Movement that is carried through by the operator without conscious assistance or resistance by the patient.

Passive range of motion Extent of movement (usually tested in a given plane) of an anatomical part at a joint when movement is produced by an outside force without voluntary assistance or resistance by the subject. The subject must relax the muscles crossing the joint.

Pelvic extension (anterior pelvic tilt) Position of the pelvis in which the vertical plane through the anterior-superior iliac spines is anterior to the vertical plane through the symphysis pubis. It is associated with hyperextension of the lumbar spine and flexion at the hip joints. Pelvic extension is a rotatory movement of the pelvic ring around the X or coronal axis, with the axis passing through the femoral heads.

Pelvic flexion (posterior pelvic tilt) Position of the pelvis in which the vertical plane through the anterior-superior iliac spines is posterior to a vertical plane through the symphysis pubis. It is associated with flexion of the lumbar spine and extension of the hip joints. Pelvic flexion is a rotatory movement of the pelvic ring around the coronal axis with the axis passing through the femoral heads.

Pelvic lateral shift Movement in the coronal plane of the pelvis in which one anterior-superior iliac spine moves closer to the midline while the opposite anterior-superior iliac spine has moved further away from the midline. It is associated with adduction and abduction of the hip joints: i.e., in lateral shift of the pelvis to the right, the left anterior-superior iliac spine is closer to the midline, resulting in the right hip in adduction and the left hip in abduction. This motion is coupled with lateral pelvic tilt when the feet are on a level surface. Pelvic lateral shift is a translatory movement along the coronal axis, with the axis passing through the femoral heads.

Pelvic lateral tilt Position of the pelvis in which it is not level in the horizontal plane, i.e., one anterior-superior iliac spine is higher than the other. It is associated with lateral flexion of the lumbar spine and adduction and abduction of the hip joints, i.e., lateral tilt of the pelvis in which the right side is higher than the left, the lumbar spine is laterally flexed toward the right, resulting in a curve convex to the left with the right hip joint in adduction and the left in abduction. Pelvic lateral tilt is a rotatory movement about the Z or sagittal axis.

Pelvic neutral position Anterior-superior iliac spines are in the same horizontal plane and in the same vertical plane as the symphysis pubis.

Pelvis rotation Position of the pelvis in which one anterior-superior iliac spine is anterior to the other. Pelvic rotation is a rotatory movement around the Y or vertical axis.

Percussion Act of firmly tapping the surface of the body with a finger or small hammer to elicit sounds, or vibratory sensations, for diagnostic value.

Petrissage Same as kneading.

Physiologic motion Normal changes in the position of articulating surfaces during the movement of a joint or region.

Pincer palpation Examination of a part by holding it in a pincer grasp between the tips of the digits, to detect taut bands of fibers, to identify tender points in the muscle, and to elicit local twitch responses.

Plane Flat surface determined by the position of three points in space. The three basic planes of reference are derived from the dimensions of space and are at right angles to each other.

A sagittal plane is vertical and extends from front to back, deriving its name from the direction of the sagittal suture of the skull. It may also be called an anterior-osterior plane. The median sagittal plane, midsagittal, divides the body into right and left halves.

A coronal frontal plane is vertical and extends from side to side, deriving its name from the direction of the coronal suture of the skull. It is also called the frontal or lateral plane, and divides the body into an anterior and a posterior portion.

A transverse plane is horizontal and divides the body into an upper cranial and lower caudal portion.

Plastic deformation Nonrecoverable deformation.

Plasticity Property of a material to permanently deform when it is loaded beyond its elastic range.

Plumb line Weighted, true vertical line utilized for fisual comparison with the gravitational line.

Postural balance Condition of optimal distribution of body mass in relation to gravity.

Posture
1. Position of the body.
2. Distribution of body mass in relation to gravity.
3. Attitude of the body.
4. Relative arrangement of the parts of the body. Optimal posture is that state of muscular and skeletal balance that protects the supporting structures of the body against injury or progressive deformity irrespective of the attitude (erect, lying, squatting, stooping) in which these structures are working or resting.

Preventative Treatment procedures considered necessary to prevent the development of clinical status.

Primary myofascial trigger point Hyperirritable spot within a taut skeletal muscle band that was activated by acute or chronic overload (mechanical strain) of the muscle in which it occurs, and was not activated as a result of trigger point activity in another muscle of the body.

Prime mover Muscle primarily responsible for causing a specific joint action.

Pronation In relation to the anatomical position, as applied to the hand, the act of turning the hand palmar surface backward (medial rotation). Applied to the foot, a combination of eversion and abduction movements taking place in the tarsal and metatarsal joints, resulting in lowering of the medial margin of the foot.

Prone Lying with the ventral surface downward.

Propriception Sensing the motion and position of the body.

Propriceptors Sensory nerve terminals that give information concerning movements and position of the body. They occur chiefly in the muscles, tendons, joints, and labyrinths.

Pump-handle rib motion Movement of the upper ribs with respiration such that during inhalation, the anterior aspect of the rib elevates and causes an increase in the anteroposterior diameter of the thorax.

Range of motion Range of translation and rotation of a joint for each of its six degrees of freedom.

Reciprocal innervation Inhibition of antagonistic muscles when the agonist is stimulated.

Rectilinear motion Motion in a straight line.

Referred autonomic phenomena Vasoconstriction (blanching), coldness, sweating, pilomotor response, ptosis, and/or hypersecretion that is caused by activity of a trigger point in a region separate from the trigger point. The phenomena usually appear in the area to which the trigger point refers pain.

Referred trigger point pain Pain that arises in a trigger point but is felt at a distance, often entirely remote from its source of origin. The distribution of referred trigger point pain rarely coincides with the entire distribution of a peripheral nerve or dermatomal segment.

Referred trigger point phenomena Sensory and motor phenomena such as pain, tenderness, increased motor unit activity (spasm), vasoconstriction, vasodilation, and hypersecretion caused by a trigger point, which usually occurs at a distance from the trigger point.

Reflex Result of transforming an ingoing sensory impulse into an outgoing efferent impulse without the act of will.

Reflex therapy Treatment that is aimed at stimulating afferent neuromuscular receptors.

Rehabilitative Procedures necessary for reeducation or functional restoration of a disabled body system or part.

Relaxation Decrease in stress in a deformed structure with time when the deformation is held constant.

Resilience Property of returning to the former shape or size after distortion.

Rib fixation Movement or position of one or several ribs is altered or disrupted. For example, an elevated rib is one held in a position of inhalation such that motion toward inhalation is freer and motion toward exhalation is restricted. A depressed rib is one held in a position of exhalation such that motion toward exhalation is freer and there is a restriction to inhalation.

Ropiness Tissue texture abnormality characterized by a cord-like or string-like feeling.

Rotation Movement about a longitudinal axis.

Sacroiliac fixation (sacroiliac joint locking) Absence of normal motion at the sacroiliac joint, demonstrable by motion palpation in which the axis of rotation has shifted to either the superior or inferior portion of the sacroiliac joint, or (rarely) a situation in which there is total joint locking with no axis of rotation.

Sacroiliac extension fixation (PI)—A state of the sacroiliac joint in which the posterior-superior iliac spine is fixed in a posterior-inferior position, with the innominate bone on that side fixed in extension in relation to the sacrum. The axis of rotation then shifts superiorly and the inferior joint remains mobile.

Sacroiliac flexion fixation (AS)—A state of the sacroiliac joint in which the posterior-superior iliac spine is fixed in an anterior superior position, with the innominate bone on that side fixed in flexion in relation to the sacrum. The axis of rotation then shifts superiorly and the inferior joint remains mobile.

Satellite myofascial trigger point Focus of hyperirritability in a muscle or its fascia that became active because the muscle was located within the zone of reference of another trigger point. To be distinguished from a secondary trigger point.

Scalar quantity Quantity having magnitude only, not direction.

Scan Intermediate screening palpatory examination designed to focus the clinician on regional areas of joint dysfunction.

Scoliosis Pathological or functional lateral curvature of the spine.

Functional scoliosis—Lateral deviation of the spine resulting from poor posture, foundation anomalies, occupational strains, etc., that are still not permanently established.

Structural scoliosis—Permanent lateral deviation of the spine such that the spine cannot return to neutral position.

Screening palpation Digital examination of a muscle to determine the absence or presence of palpable bands and tender trigger points using flat or pincer palpation.

Secondary myofascial trigger point Hyperirritable spot in a muscle or its fascia that became overactive because its muscle was overloaded as a synergist substituting for, or as an antagonist countering the tautness of the muscle that contained the primary trigger point.

Shear Applied force that tends to cause an opposite but parallel sliding motion of the planes of an object.

Sherrington laws Every posterior spinal nerve root supplies a specific region of the skin, although fibers from adjacent spinal segments may invade such a region. When a muscle receives a nerve impulse to contract, its antagonist receives, simultaneously, an impulse to relax.

Short leg Anatomical, pathological, or functional leg deficiency leading to dysfunction.

Side bending See lateral flexion.

Somatic dysfunction Impaired or altered function of related components of the somatic (body framework) system; skeletal, arthrodial, and myofascial structures and related vascular, lymphatic, and neural elements.

Somatization Conversion of mental experiences or states into bodily symptoms.

Somatogenic Produced by activity, reaction, and change originating in the musculoskeletal system.

Spasm Shortening of a muscle due to nonvoluntary motor nerve activity. Spasm cannot be stopped by voluntary relaxation.

Spinography Roentgenometrics of the spine.

Spondylitis Inflammation of the vertebrae.

Spondylarthrosis Arthrosis of the synovial joints of the spine.

Spondylolisthesis Anterior displacement of one vertebra over another (usually L5 over the body of the sacrum or L4 over L5).

Spondylolysis Interruption in the pars interarticularis, may be unilateral or bilateral.

Spondylosis Osseous hypertrophic spur formation at the vertebral endplates due to disc degeneration.

Spondylotherapy Therapeutic application of percussion or concussion over the vertebrae to elicit reflex responses at the levels of neuromeric innervation to the organ being influenced.

Sprain Joint injury in which some of the fibers of a supporting ligament are ruptured, but the continuity of the ligament remains intact.

Spur Projection body as from a bone.

Statics Branch of mechanics that deals with the equilibrium of bodies at rest or in motion with zero acceleration.

Stiffness Measure of resistance offered to external loads by a specimen or structure as it deforms.

Strain
1. Deformation (lengthening or shortening) of any body or member.
2. Overstretching and tearing of musculotendinous tissue.

Stress
1. Internal force between molecules.
2. Sum of the biological reaction to any adverse stimulus—physical, mental and/or emotional, internal or external—that tends to disturb the organism's homeostasis; should these compensating reactions be inadequate or inappropriate, they may lead to disorders.

Stretching Separation of the origin and insertion of a muscle or attachments of fascia or ligaments by applying constant pressure at a right angle to the fiber of the muscle or fascia.

Stringiness Palpable tissue texture abnormality characterized by fine or string-like myofascial structures.

Subluxation
1. Partial or incomplete dislocation.
2. Restriction of motion of a joint in a position exceeding normal physiologic motion, although the anatomic limits have not been exceeded.
3. Aberrant relationship between two adjacent articular structures, which may have functional or pathological sequelae, causing an alternation in the biomechanical and/or neurophysiological reflexes of these articular structures, their proximal structures, and/or body systems that may be directly or indirectly affected by them.

Supination
1. Beginning in anatomical position, applied to the hand, the action of turning the palm forward (anteriorly) or upward, performed by lateral external rotation of the forearm.

2. Applied to the foot, it generally applies to movements (adduction and inversion) resulting in raising the medial margin of the foot, hence the longitudinal arch.

Supine Lying with the ventral side upward.

Symmetry Similarity in corresponding parts or organs on opposite sides of the body.

Syndesmophyte Osseous excrescence or bony outgrowth from a ligament. Usually projecting vertically in the spine.

Tappotement Striking the belly of a muscle with the hypothenar edge of the open hand in rapid succession to increase its tone and arterial perfusion.

Technique Any of a number of physical or mechanical chiropractic procedures used in the treatment of patients.

Tender points Local areas of hypersensitivity found at consistent anatomic sites, which do not refer pain pressure but produce a pain response to light palpation (see fibromyalgia).

Therapeutic Any treatment considered necessary to return the patient to a preclinical status or establish a stationary status.

Thrust Sudden manual application of a controlled directional force upon a suitable part of the patient, the delivery of which effects an adjustment.

Tonus Slight continuous contraction of muscle, which in skeletal muscles aids in the maintenance of posture and in the return of blood to the heart.
Myogenic tonus—Tonic contraction of muscle itself or of its intrinsic nerve cells.

Torque Moment of force (term generally applied to rotation of shafts).

Torsion Motion or state where one end of a part is turned about a longitudinal axis while the opposite end is held fast or turned to the opposite direction.

Traction Force acting on a longitudinal axis to draw structures apart.

Translation Motion of a rigid body in which a straight line in the body always remains parallel to itself.

Trigger point (myofascial trigger point) Small hypersensitive site that, when stimulated, consistently produces a reflex mechanism that gives rise to referred pain or other manifestations. The response is specific, in a constant reference zone, and consistent from person to person.

Trophic Of or pertaining to nutrition, especially in the cellular environment.

Tropism Asymmetry of articular facets.

Vector quantity Quantity having both magnitude and direction.

Vertebral motion segment Two adjacent vertebral bodies and the disc between them, the two posterior joints and the ligamentous structures binding the two vertebrae to one another. Junghann's *bewegunnsegment* translated by Beseman as "motor unit."

Vertebral motor unit See vertebral motion segment.

Viscoelasticity Property of a material to show sensitivity to the rate of loading or deformation. Two basic components are viscosity and elasticity.

Viscosity Property of materials to resist loads that produce shear.

Whiplash Whip-like action of the cervical spine as the result of sudden acceleration or deceleration of the body. The lower end of the cervical chain acts like the handle of a whip, allowing the remainder of the neck and head to be whipped forward and back or from side to side.

INDEX

Note: Page numbers followed by *f* or *t* indicate figures or tables, respectively.